Bringing Evidence into Everyday Practice

Practical Strategies for Healthcare Professionals

Bringing Evidence into Everyday Practice
Practical Strategies for Healthcare Professionals

Winnie Dunn, PhD, OTR, FAOTA
Professor and Chair
Department of Occupational Therapy Education
University of Kansas
Kansas City, Kansas

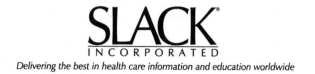

SLACK®
INCORPORATED
Delivering the best in health care information and education worldwide

www.slackbooks.com

ISBN: 978-1-55642-821-0

Instructors: *Bringing Evidence into Everyday Practice: Practical Strategies for Healthcare Professionals, Instructor's Manual,* is also available from SLACK Incorporated. Don't miss this important companion to *Bringing Evidence into Everyday Practice: Practical Strategies for Healthcare Professionals.* To obtain the *Instructor's Manual*, please visit http://www.efacultylounge.com.

The procedures and practices described in this book should be implemented in a manner consistent with the professional standards set for the circumstances that apply in each specific situation. Every effort has been made to confirm the accuracy of the information presented and to correctly relate generally accepted practices. The authors, editor, and publisher cannot accept responsibility for errors or exclusions or for the outcome of the material presented herein. There is no expressed or implied warranty of this book or information imparted by it. Care has been taken to ensure that drug selection and dosages are in accordance with currently accepted/recommended practice. Due to continuing research, changes in government policy and regulations, and various effects of drug reactions and interactions, it is recommended that the reader carefully review all materials and literature provided for each drug, especially those that are new or not frequently used. Any review or mention of specific companies or products is not intended as an endorsement by the author or publisher.

SLACK Incorporated uses a review process to evaluate submitted material. Prior to publication, educators or clinicians provide important feedback on the content that we publish. We welcome feedback on this work.

Published by: SLACK Incorporated
                  6900 Grove Road
                  Thorofare, NJ 08086 USA
                  Telephone: 856-848-1000
                  Fax: 856-853-5991
                  www.slackbooks.com

Contact SLACK Incorporated for more information about other books in this field or about the availability of our books from distributors outside the United States.

Library of Congress Cataloging-in-Publication Data

Dunn, Winnie.
  Bringing evidence into everyday practice : practical strategies for healthcare professionals / Winnie Dunn.
    p. ; cm.
  Includes bibliographical references and index.
  ISBN-13: 978-1-55642-821-0 (alk. paper)
  ISBN-10: 1-55642-821-9 (alk. paper)
 1. Evidence-based medicine. I. Title.
  [DNLM: 1. Evidence-Based Medicine--methods. 2. Meta-Analysis as Topic. 3. Research. 4. Review Literature as Topic. WB 102 D923b 2008]
  R723.7.D86 2008
  610--dc22
                                  2008002325

Printed in the United States of America.

Last digit is print number: 10 9 8 7 6 5 4 3 2 1

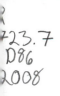
Dedication

I dedicate this workbook to Ellen Pope and Susan Knuth.
They have been my partners in bringing evidence-based practices to Kansas.

Contents

Instructors: *Bringing Evidence into Everyday Practice: Practical Strategies for Healthcare Professionals, Instructor's Manual,* **is** also available from SLACK Incorporated. Don't miss this important companion to *Bringing Evidence into Everyday Practice: Practical Strategies for Healthcare Professionals.* To obtain the *Instructor's Manual,* please visit http://www.efacultylounge.com.

Acknowledgments

This book is a departure from the traditional textbooks on the market, and so it took vision and tenacity from the publishers to move this project into the marketplace. I am grateful to Amy McShane, John Bond, Peter Slack, and Jennifer Cahill for their untiring work to produce this workbook.

It was also a complex task to gather the materials and select what would be the best learning options for students and colleagues. I am grateful to Laura Neely for her steady focus on the details to get permissions, check for consistency, and remind me of the tasks I had yet to complete in a kind, supportive manner. I also acknowledge Michael Ahlers and Candy Conner for their support during this process; I look productive because all of you are back there making sure there are no loose ends.

Material for a workbook requires tryouts to make sure that the activities are understandable and useful to professionals in practice. I acknowledge all the early intervention and school-based providers who have studied evidence-based practices with me; you showed me the way. I also acknowledge all the graduate students who have studied this topic with me; you asked many questions that invited me to understand better and therefore teach better.

About the Author

Winnie Dunn, PhD, OTR, FAOTA, is Professor and Chair of the Department of Occupational Therapy Education at the University of Kansas. She was the Eleanor Clarke Slagle lecturer in 2001, received the Award of Merit from the American Occupational Therapy Association, received the A. Jean Ayres research award and the Chancellor's teaching and research awards, served as a Kemper Teaching Fellow, and is a member of the Academy of Research of the American Occupational Therapy Foundation. She has contributed research and other writings to professional literature across her career. Currently she is involved in a statewide initiative called *KANSAS: From Evidence to Practice*; their purpose is to embed evidence-based practices into all the early intervention and school networks across the state.

Her latest endeavor to translate research into practice involves the publication of a book for the public entitled *Living Sensationally: Understanding Your Senses*. Its focus is to translate her research about sensory processing into everyday language, so that everyone can understand their own, their family's, their coworkers', and their friends' behaviors a little better.

Preface

I just love workbooks! I have loved them all my life. When I was a girl, I would work my way through the puzzle books, and use little scratch pads with notes to myself as I worked. My favorite games were "Who drinks milk and who owns the zebra?" These are the logic games that provide you with a set of statements like "The family in the green house likes to drink milk; they live next to the family that owns a zebra." So you had to create a grid that had every family's house color, pet, drink, car type, and number of members from all these statements. Whew! They were challenging, but boy did I get some brain aerobics from them.

So as I have worked through problems in our profession, this idea of figuring out the puzzle always comes to mind. At first, it was me and an article, trying decipher what the table told me, what the text meant, or figure out what the graph illustrated. As I began to teach, I had to construct methods for introducing this problem solving to others. This workbook is a selection of my puzzles and their solutions; I hope they are as helpful to you as they have been for me and others.

The workbook is in three sections. In the first section, we explore the basic ideas of evidence and research for practice. In the second section, you get a chance to practice with topics that will inform various areas of practice; we use the same general format in each unit, so you can apply that format to other groups of articles that are interesting to you. In the third section, we delve into some advanced ideas about evidence in practice so you have even more tools at your disposal.

Enjoy my professional puzzle book!

Foreword

At the invitation to write this Foreword, I immediately thought to myself that I must say yes. Winnie Dunn is a premiere scientist and teacher, she is a leader in the field of evidence-based practice, and I highly respect her work. My next thoughts were that the field needs a good evidence-based practice training manual, and that I might be able to use this one the next time I teach my course. These thoughts were enough for me to agree to write the Foreword before I read anything but the Table of Contents.

I began my review by flipping through the pages to get a feel for the manual as a student and a teacher. It has the standard structure of a good training manual: short practical chapters, step-by-step strategies for learning how to do evidence-based practice, with strategies tied to concrete examples from the research literature, and many worksheets for students to practice the strategies themselves. It indeed has practical strategies as promised by the title. So I settled into what I thought would be a review of a standard manual that competently addresses the steps of evidence-based practice.

Within a couple of chapters I realized that this is not your typical manual. For over a decade I've been teaching healthcare professionals about evidence-based practice, so I wasn't expecting any experiences of delight or "a-ha" as I read through the manual. Yet my delight and discovery grew with each chapter. To sum up my experience, I found that this manual successfully integrates the art and science of professional reasoning and decision making in healthcare. This accomplishment is very difficult to achieve and is rarely attempted. A more amazing feat in my opinion is that the manual develops scholarship skill at all levels of expertise. It brings both novice and expert to a new depth of understanding about how to think critically and effectively about important problems and issues of healthcare.

What is innovative about this manual is that it confronts the complexities and realities of research evidence and of healthcare practice head on. It tells students how to handle these complexities and realities and gives them the tools to do it. It cultivates confidence that a practitioner can do a good job at evidence-based practice without being an expert in research methods. In contrast to this manual, evidence-based how-to's often teach a simplified and idealized systematic reasoning that doesn't match the complexities and realities of research and practice. These how-to texts generally presume a best-case scenario research literature that has the following attributes:

- The literature contains a set of research studies that have similar research purposes, designs, and measures
- These studies have valid, replicated, consistent findings

- The client samples in the studies are similar to a practitioner's everyday clients
- The assessments and interventions used in the studies are ones can be applied feasibly in a practitioner's setting

Although typical how-to texts coach practitioners to critique and resolve issues around research literature that do not meet best-case standards, the texts are often limited with respect to giving explicit and concrete steps for how to do so. The professional is left to apply best-case scenario techniques to a mixed-case scenario research literature that often has one or more of the following attributes:

- The literature contains studies with different research purposes, designs, or measures, despite having an overlapping relevance for a specific clinical problem or population
- The studies are of mixed quality, with little replication, and often have conflicting findings
- The client samples do not clearly represent the unique needs of a practitioner's everyday clients
- The assessments or interventions in the studies might require modification to be applied feasibly in a practitioner's setting

Given the varieties of human behavior, experience, and research endeavors, especially in fields addressing complex, chronic health conditions, it is likely that the research evidence is mixed rather than best case. By not confronting the complexities of mixed evidence with concrete strategies for handling complexity, the implicit message of many texts is that practitioners cannot adequately perform the tasks of evidence-based practice without advancing their technical training in the interpretation and use of research evidence. In the meantime they must apply the art of practice to use the literature in an intervention setting.

The art of practice is what professionals do in their everyday practice, seemingly intuitively, to make decisions and act quickly in a manner that is expected to bring benefit rather than harm to their clients. Professionals gather bits and pieces of information, not necessarily systematically, into a big picture or a clinical story that guides action. The bits and pieces of information are of variable quality and coherence, and come from a number of sources—clients and their families; team members; their own experience, observations, and training; and the realities of practice contexts. Typically the art of practice is spoken of as if it were distinct from the science of practice.

No one speaks that way in this manual. Rather the teaching is about the integration of the art and science of practice. When art and science are integrated, everyday practice reasoning exemplifies an experienced and informed understanding of the complexity of human living and health. Experience and knowledge are applied artfully and scientifically to the optimization of client benefits within the natural parameters of everyday practice. This manual gives the student concrete strategies at each step in a chain from simple to complex integration of art and science practice, starting with best-case and moving through mixed-case scenario evidence. Although readers are expected to think hard and reflect deeply while making this integration, at no point are they left to flounder without direction.

To accomplish this integration, Winnie Dunn has created a learning path that incorporates evidence-based teaching/learning principles and techniques. For example, she uses a cognitive-behavioral approach that begins with asking students to identify their current thoughts, beliefs, and knowledge about a clinical problem or issue, and then moves on to challenge the students' current position with a lesson that brings in new or counter-evidence. Each lesson steps up the challenge, requiring students to participate in progressively more complex tasks of analysis and integration. Each challenge is accompanied by concrete strategies and pearls of evidence-based wisdom (see the Evidence Detective Tips) to support successful learning outcomes. Students practice the strategies repeatedly across the manual, each time with a novel twist or added challenge. Evidence is continuously compared and contrasted to one's own beliefs, those of other students, and then to other types of evidence. Students practice synthesizing information using both qualitative and quantitative methods and generalizing their understanding of the evidence in broader and broader conceptualizations. For example, one exercise has students combine experimental with descriptive research evidence to form overarching conceptual themes and draw new conclusions from what would appear to be different evidence about assistive devices in rehabilitation practice.

Repetition, practice, and moving back and forth between concrete evidence and abstract conceptualizations creates a skillful set of habits around evidence-based strategies. Habits are useful in evidence-based practice because they are applied quickly, automatically, and effortlessly. They make it possible to use evidence for reasoning and decision making in the busy, time-limited context of everyday practice.

I admire the quality of these methods, which are directed toward developing student knowledge and skill, but the aspects of this manual that I find most delightful and innovative are the exercises that validate the student's lack of knowledge and skill. At the heart of scholarship and wisdom is the recognition of the fact that the more you know the less you can be sure of. Paradoxically, embracing the limits of one's own knowledge allows one to go deeper into the understanding and handling of complexity. My favorite exercises in this manual are the ones that develop skills around paradox and uncertainty, such as practice in writing unanswerable questions, categorizing one's own reactions to data that counter cherished beliefs, and interpreting the findings of statistics that are currently beyond one's full grasp or are unfamiliar.

These and other exercises show students that the recognition of the fallibility of human knowledge is more important than the fallibility itself. This recognition becomes itself the skill, and the fallibility loses its grade F denotation.

I believe that practitioners' recognition of the fallibility of their own and others' knowledge drives optimal client-centered care. From the common ground of fallibility, practitioners and clients participate in the act of discovery and change together. The evidence-based scholar practitioner contributes informed art and science practice to this participation. I'm pleased to conclude that Winnie Dunn's manual is likely to live up to its title's promise to bring evidence into everyday practice. It gives students the practical strategies and scholarship skills they need as healthcare professionals for reasoning with wisdom in a complex world.

Linda Tickle-Degnen, PhD, OTR/L, FAOTA
Professor and Chair
Department of Occupational Therapy
Director, Health Quality of Life Lab
Tufts University
Medford, Massachusetts

Introduction

Professionals are increasingly being asked to base their decisions on evidence. We all agree that this is a good idea; no one wants to spend precious time engaging in strategies that are not likely to be effective. Systematic reviews of the literature provide one excellent resource because scholars summarize a body of literature about a topic for the field. However, there is not a large body of literature to support all the things we encounter in everyday practice.

With Internet access more available, professionals can search for literature on topics of interest to their practice. But just having some articles doesn't ensure evidence-based practice either. Professionals have to know how to mine the gold from these sources to make informed decisions for their everyday practice. With time at a premium, professionals need specific and efficient strategies for using the literature to craft evidence-based plans for their practice.

This book provides the strategies for translating evidence into everyday practices. It provides the initial steps that a single professional, an interdisciplinary team, or a study group can use to build some solid decision-making patterns that will support their practices. This is not a book for scholarly review of the literature; scholars have resources for this task and are increasingly providing us with excellent material we can use on topics with a wealth of information available.

There are textbooks that discuss more formal ways to review the literature (e.g., Law and MacDermid's *Evidence-Based Rehabilitation: A Guide to Practice* [2nd ed., 2008]). There are other texts that will guide you through the research design and statistics used to support research; we will discuss these issues as they arise within an article of interest (e.g., Portney and Watkins' *Foundations of Clinical Research: Applications to Practice* [2000] and Kielhofner's *Research in Occupational Therapy: Methods of Inquiry for Enhancing Practice* [2006]). Use one of these texts or your own design and statistics text to learn more about a study's features.

Instead, this book will help professionals entering practice or in practice to take the first steps toward including evidence in their everyday decisions. We will examine how to access meta-analyses or systematic reviews, but we will also examine how to evaluate the two to three articles a team finds that address the dilemma they are facing that week in their service system. As professionals gain more confidence about how to access and use the literature on a small scale, the concept of evidence-based practice will feel more attainable for everyone.

Resource Book on Evidence-Based Practice for This Book

Law, M., & MacDermid, J. (2008). Evidence-based rehabilitation: A guide to practice *(2nd ed.). Thorofare,
NJ: SLACK Incorporated.*

This book is an excellent reference to help you
understand the concepts of evidence-based practice. The authors provide many good examples of
how professionals formally analyze the literature
to determine what best practices ought to be.

Other Recommended Resources That Address Research Design and Statistics

Portney, L., & Watkins, M. (2000). Foundations of
clinical research: Applications to practice. *Upper
Saddle River, NJ: Prentice Hall Health.*

This book is an excellent reference to help you
understand research designs, methods, statistical
procedures, and results in research articles. As
you read articles, use this text to understand the
methods and results that the authors describe.

Kielhofner, G. (Ed.). (2006). Research in occupational
therapy: Methods of inquiry for enhancing practice. *Philadelphia: F. A. Davis.*

This book is also an excellent reference to
support your learning about research designs and
statistical procedures. This text can serve as a reference when you don't understand something in
an article you are reading.

Overview of This Book

The book is divided into three sections. Section I will introduce the reader to basic evidence-
based practice concepts. Section II provides opportunities for practicing how to gather information
and summarize it for use in practice. Section III
addresses additional issues in evidence-based
practice.

Section I: Learning the Basics

Section I contains basic information about
evidence-based practice principles and methods.

Unit 1
Introduction to the Concepts of Evidence-Based Practice

During this unit, you will explore the general
concepts of evidence-based practice and research.
You will review articles that discuss the core concepts and issues of evidence-based practice, read
about research as a resource for professional practice, have a discussion with your study partners
about what you learned, find a newer article that
adds to your discussion, and share it with your
study partners.

Searching Databases

There is a wealth of information available to
professionals, but one needs to know how to gain
access to this relevant material. In this unit, you
will explore professional databases and learn how
to access relevant information effectively and efficiently.

Determining the Quality of the Evidence

Some studies provide stronger evidence than
other studies because of how they were designed.
You will learn some of the classification systems
that enable you to know the level of a study's contribution to your knowledge for evidence-based
practice.

Unit 2
Handling Anomalous Data

Another really important issue to address
when working to create an evidence-based practice is how you personally react to ideas that come
your way. It is human nature to be attracted to information that agrees with your beliefs and to be
skeptical about information that challenges your
beliefs. We will learn a framework for understanding reactions to new ideas in practice during
this unit.

Unit 3
Basic Characteristics of Research Articles

It is hard to be evidence-based professionals without some understanding of how research
articles are constructed. Professionals can expect
to obtain certain information from different parts
of the research article; these expectations serve as
guideposts for evidence-based practice. You can
compare the population you serve to the study
group; you can decide whether the measures
in the study document behaviors that matter to
you; you can determine whether the intervention
itself might be manageable for your practice. In
this unit, you will explore the parts of a research
article so you can be a better evidence-based professional.

Practice With an Entire Article

We will walk through an article together, studying the details of its structure, creating hypotheses along with the authors, and practicing writing interpretations in your own words.

SECTION II: PRACTICE DERIVING MEANING FROM THE EVIDENCE

It takes practice to learn how to uncover the evidence. In this section you will practice analyzing research articles. You will learn many strategies that you can use in your professional practice. We will cover the following topics in our evidence-based reviews (Units 4 through 9):

- Evidence about the use of assistive devices with older adults and people with disabilities
- Evidence about the use of compensatory strategies with community-dwelling adults who have schizophrenia
- Evidence about caregiving across the life span
- Evidence about the use of sensory processing knowledge in the natural contexts for children
- Evidence about the use of constraint-induced therapy with persons who have had a stroke
- Evidence about diet and exercise for adults

There are many other topics we could cover; this gives you a range of topics to get you started. The first edition of *Evidence-Based Rehabilitation: A Guide to Practice* (Law, 2002) contains examples of reviews of the literature (Chapter 8 contains a review of cognitive behavior interventions and Chapter 14 contains a review of where to provide services for people who have had a stroke). These may be helpful examples as you study.

SECTION III: EXPANDING YOUR KNOWLEDGE AND SKILLS FOR EVIDENCE-BASED PRACTICE

There are additional resources available to support evidence-based practice. Scholars conduct formal reviews of the literature so you can have summaries and recommendations from others. Emerging ideas in professional practice don't have evidence, so you need to have other strategies for evaluating these ideas. Finally, profes-sionals need to collect their own data within their practices to verify the effectiveness of any evidence. We will review these topics in Section III.

Unit 10
Summary and Meta-Analysis Articles

Scholars review sets of articles and provide a summary of the findings in both summary and meta-analysis articles. This is a great resource for professionals who have very little time to conduct exhaustive reviews. You will learn how to read and take advantage of these resources.

Unit 11
Examining Emerging and Controversial Practices

What do professionals do with new ideas? How do we determine whether a new idea is worthy of our attention as evidence-based professionals? This unit will introduce you to some strategies for analyzing new or controversial ideas so you can incorporate promising interventions and set aside other ideas from your practice.

Unit 12
Developing Evidence for Your Own Practice

No matter how much evidence is available, professionals still don't know whether an intervention will work in **their** practices. Collecting data within professional practice provides validity that the intervention is effective with that person in that situation. We can also try out an intervention not typically used in a population by collecting data to determine the appropriateness of the generalization.

HOW TO USE THIS BOOK

This book will take you step by step to learn how to incorporate evidence into your everyday practice. Please read the bulleted list on page xxiii to learn about the different components used throughout this book to help you with the this process.

SUMMARY

Many texts provide academic knowledge about evidence-based practice; this book will give you the tools to implement sound ideas in your professional life.

How to Use This Book

The goal of this book is to help the reader learn how to incorporate evidence into his or her everyday decisions. The book contains several different elements to help achieve this goal.

- Each unit contains activities that assist the reader step by step toward incorporating evidence into everyday decisions.
- Throughout the book, the reader is asked to read certain journal articles that will be used as the basis for the unit activities and worksheets. To help the reader, most of these journal articles have been reprinted in the Appendix of this book, which begins on page 173. The text provides the bibliographic information of each article and what article number it is in the Appendix.
- There are a few articles necessary for completing the activities that are not reprinted in this book. The reader must obtain and review these articles on his or her own.
- Each unit contains worksheets to aid in the reader's practice and learning. The worksheets are mentioned in the text and are located at the end of each respective unit.
- Sidebars include important material to assist in learning, performing the activities, and completing the worksheets. The sidebars are referenced in the text.
- Evidence Detective Tips are included throughout the book, giving the reader additional helpful hints regarding research studies and practice.
- A Bibliography for the entire book begins on page 169.

Section I

Learning the Basics

BACKGROUND KNOWLEDGE FOR EVIDENCE-BASED PRACTICE

In the first section of this manual, you will explore the basic concepts of evidence-based practice, examine your own patterns of accepting or rejecting evidence that challenges your current beliefs, and learn how to look at the Methods and Results sections of professional articles.

Unit 1

Introduction to Evidence-Based Practice

During this unit, we will be exploring the general concepts of evidence-based practice. You will review articles and participate in discussions with classmates or colleagues about the concepts of evidence-based practice. You will also find a newer article that informs this discussion, and share the abstract with your classmates/colleagues (your study partners).

When you complete the work for this unit, you will have the following skills and competencies:

- Identify what you already know about basic research concepts
- Identify new concepts you need to know about research
- Become familiar with evidence-based practice language
- Recognize interdisciplinary issues in evidence-based practice
- Articulate the importance of evidence-based practice
- Identify initial strategies for implementing evidence-based practice in your practice
- Understand how to select key words for searching in library databases
- Identify advanced search strategies to obtain critical information
- Sort through possible citations to identify relevant ones
- Become familiar with the levels of evidence

IDENTIFY WHAT YOU ALREADY KNOW AND IDENTIFY NEW CONCEPTS ENCOUNTERED

Research studies that demonstrate the effectiveness or limitations of particular strategies provide the material for evidence-based practice. Professionals need to have a basic understanding about research concepts so they can decide whether or not the research they are reading is worthy of consideration. You will notice that you are familiar with some of the material as your read about research concepts, while other concepts will be new to you.

Activity 1-1

Read a chapter about research from your own research design textbook (or your can read Chapter 1 in Portney and Watkins [2000] or Chapters 3 and 4 in Kielhofner [2006]). Complete Worksheets 1A and 1B to summarize what is familiar and new to you. There is an example at the beginning of each worksheet.

Activity 1-2

Meet with study partners and discuss what each of you learned about research concepts. If you have examples of these concepts being used in a study you have read, bring them to share with your study partners.

FAMILIARIZE YOURSELF WITH EVIDENCE-BASED PRACTICE LANGUAGE

Knowledge about research concepts is necessary but insufficient for evidence-based practice. Professionals must also know the language and structure for employing evidence-based practices. We must understand what people mean when they say "evidence-based practice" so we can meet the expectations within our work. Law and MacDermid (2008) provide an excellent summary about evidence-based practice to guide your thinking.

Activity 1-3

Read Chapters 1 through 3 in Law and MacDermid (2008). These chapters provide a good background for understanding evidence-based practice. Think about how these ideas might relate to your areas of practice interest; brainstorm ideas about applications in practice with your study partners. Complete Worksheet 1C to summarize your thoughts.

We can obtain information about evidence-based practice from journal articles as well as textbooks. Sometimes articles are helpful because they focus on one aspect of evidence-based practice, enabling the reader to tailor work on an aspect of interest to the reader's practice.

Activity 1-4

Obtain and read the five articles listed below. They discuss the five steps in implementing evidence-based practice (using Worksheet 1D).

Tickle-Degnen, L. (1999). Evidence-based practice forum. Organizing, evaluating and using evidence. American Journal of Occupational Therapy, 53(6), 537-539.

Tickle-Degnen, L. (2000a). Evidence-based practice forum. Communicating with clients, family members, and colleagues about research evidence. American Journal of Occupational Therapy, 54(3), 341-343.

Tickle-Degnen, L. (2000b). Evidence-based practice forum. Gathering current research evidence to enhance clinical reasoning. American Journal of Occupational Therapy, 54(1), 102-105.

Tickle-Degnen, L. (2000c). Evidence-based practice forum. Monitoring and documenting evidence during assessment and intervention. American Journal of Occupational Therapy, 54(4), 434-436.

Tickle-Degnen, L. (2000e). Evidence-based practice forum. What is the best evidence to use in practice? American Journal of Occupational Therapy, 54(2), 218-221.

Activity 1-5

Obtain and read one additional article on evidence-based practice that is applicable to your interests. Be prepared to use what you have learned in the discussion you will have in Activity 1-7.

Ilott, I. (2003). Evidence-based practice forum. Challenging the rhetoric and reality: Only an individual and systemic approach will work for evidence-based occupational therapy. American Journal of Occupational Therapy, 57(3), 351-354.

Lee, C. J., & Miller, L. T. (2003). Evidence-based practice forum. The process of evidence-based clinical decision making in occupational therapy. American Journal of Occupational Therapy, 57(4), 473-477.

Ottenbacher, K. J., Tickle-Degnen, L., et al. (2002). From the desk of the editor. Therapists awake! The challenge of evidence-based occupational therapy. American Journal of Occupational Therapy, 56(3), 247-249.

Rappolt, S. (2003). Evidence-based practice forum. The role of professional expertise in evidence-based occupational therapy. American Journal of Occupational Therapy, 57(5), 589-593.

Tickle-Degnen, L. (2000d). Evidence-based practice forum. Teaching evidence-based practice. American Journal of Occupational Therapy, 54(5), 559-560.

Tickle-Degnen, L. (2003). Evidence-based practice forum. Where is the individual in statistics? American Journal of Occupational Therapy, 57(1), 112-115.

Tickle-Degnen, L., & Bedell, G. (2003). Evidence-based practice forum. Heterarchy and hierarchy: A criti-

cal appraisal of the levels of evidence as a tool for clinical decision making. American Journal of Occupational Therapy, 57(2), 234-237.

EVIDENCE-BASED PRACTICE IS AN INTERDISCIPLINARY ISSUE

No matter what professional background one has, the call for evidence-based practice is strong. Some disciplines have been working on these issues for a long time, while other disciplines are just starting to consider how to incorporate evidence in their practices. Since we all work on interdisciplinary teams, it is important to know how other disciplines are dealing with similar issues.

Activity 1-6

Locate an article about evidence-based practice from another discipline. Read the article and consider similarities and differences from your own discipline. Consider whether this other discipline has ideas that might be useful to your thinking as your plan to implement evidence-based practices.

For this activity, you can use "evidence-based practice" as one of your search phrases. Add to it the name of another discipline (e.g., "nursing"). The search engine will select only articles with both these concepts in them. You could also add "children" and you would get only articles about children, nursing, and evidence-based practice. Some search engines let you select where to search; you might want to limit the search to the title, abstract, and key words, rather than the whole article, so you narrow your list to only those articles that use the search words in these sections of the article.

Activity 1-7

Meet with study partners.
- Discuss what additional information you gained from reading the articles (Activities 1-4 and 1-5).
- Did the articles give your more ideas about how to implement evidence-based practice in your areas of interest?
- Discuss ideas you obtained from reading an interdisciplinary article (Activity 1-6).

- How could this discipline's perspective contribute to your thinking?

SEARCHING PROFESSIONAL DATABASES TO FIND ARTICLES

Professionals need to know how to conduct searches using various search engines and databases. Most professional libraries have learning modules prepared by the librarians to coach you about conducting a search; you can also access these experts to help you in person. If you are inexperienced at using search strategies, you can also take a class at a library, use the Help section of your search engine (e.g., MEDLINE, CINAHL), or try out some strategies on Google Scholar (it has a section on tips for searching).

Chapter 5 of the Law and MacDermid (2008) text also explains how to search in the literature.

Activity 1-8

Practice Searching in Professional Databases

Select a professional database that is relevant to your area of interest. Put in one key word and see how many references you get. Add one or two more words to your list and see how these key words narrow your list. Then go back to your original word and enter two different key words. Compare the two lists. Sometimes narrowing with certain key words makes your list more precise; narrowing can also divert your list away from your specific interest areas.

If you know an author who is an expert in an area, you can also search by that person's name along with key words.

DETERMINING THE QUALITY OF EVIDENCE

In addition to understanding how to look at the parts of a research article, professionals are responsible for considering the quality of the studies because quality helps you to know how much influence the findings need to have in your practice.

Chapter 6 in Law and MacDermid (2008) provides a summary of various methods that researchers use to determine the level of evidence that a particular study contributes to knowledge. They introduce three different classification systems for evidence.

Activity 1-9

Comparing and Contrasting Levels of Evidence

Using the three classification systems introduced in Chapter 6 of Law and MacDermid (2008), complete a comparison of the similarities and differences among the three systems. Discuss the advantages and disadvantages with your study partners. Use Worksheet 1E to analyze the systems next to each other in preparation for your discussion. One part is completed for you; you will see that Greenhalgh (1997) provides a very general statement and the others have much more detail. What are the advantages and disadvantages of these approaches?

Discuss which classification system is most useful for your work. As we encounter articles in this manual, and in your practice, consider the levels of evidence each article represents to your knowledge.

SUMMARY

This unit introduced you to concepts that form the basis for evidence-based practice. Mastering these concepts and skills enables you to understand the evidence you will encounter in your practice.

All references for this unit can be found in the Bibliography, beginning on page 169.

Worksheet 1A
Familiar Research Concepts

List three research concepts that were already familiar to you. Then make notes about where you have encountered these concepts before.

Familiar Research Concept	Where I Have Encountered This Concept Before
Research uses objectivity to avoid bias	*High school science class experiments*
1.	
2.	
3.	

Worksheet 1B
New Research Concepts

List three research concepts that are new to you. Look up some additional information about these concepts and make notes that will help you remember these concepts in the future.

New Research Concept	What I Have Learned About This Concept
Basic research is concerned with generating ideas regardless of their application to practical problems	*The concepts generated from basic research can be helpful in guiding ideas for applied research studies*
1.	
2.	
3.	

Worksheet 1C
Evidence-Based Practice Concepts

List four ideas about evidence-based practice from the units. Jot down an example from practice that illustrates that concept being implemented.

Evidence-Based Practice Idea	Example of This Idea Being Implemented
Evidence-based practice is a combination of clinical expertise and evidence from the literature	*A team of rehab therapists would discuss what to do about a patient who has had a stroke; they discuss their experiences with other patients and an article on constraint-induced therapy*
1.	
2.	
3.	
4.	

Worksheet 1D
Steps in Implementing Evidence-Based Practice

List five steps for implementing evidence-based practice based on the evidence-based practice forum articles you read (see Activity 1-4). Then list one or two tips to remember about each step. An example is provided.

Evidence-Based Practice Steps	Tips to Remember About This Step
(Step 1) Create a clinical question	*Include:* *a. The occupational performance issue* *b. The assessment strategies* *c. The interventions you are wondering about (Tickle-Degnen, 1999)*
1.	a. b.
2.	a. b.
3.	a. b.
4.	a. b.
5.	a. b.

Worksheet 1E
Comparison of Classification Systems

Greenhalgh (1997)	Breast Cancer (1998)	National Health Svc (2004)
Systematic reviews and meta-analyses	*Level 1: Evidence is based on RCTs (or meta-analyses of such trials) of adequate size*	*1++ High quality meta-analyses, systematic reviews of RCTs or RCTs wth very low risk of bias*

Unit 2

Characterizing Responses to Evidence

When professionals encounter evidence that may affect their practices, they must decide what they are going to do with that information. Sometimes research isn't relevant to a particular situation. Research projects may be done poorly and therefore have to be set aside. Research may support a professional's current practices; these studies are easy to embrace. Research may also be relevant to one's practice, but findings may challenge what the professional currently believes to be true. As evidence-based practitioners, professionals need to understand how to handle these various scenarios.

It is human nature to be attracted to information that agrees with our beliefs and to be skeptical about information that challenges our beliefs. However, as professionals, we have a responsibility to remain open to new possibilities. Across one's career it is easy to see that ideas progress; what is considered acceptable practice changes as we understand more. But individually and as a team, it can be easy to get stuck in protocols or routines that were originally based on best avail-able knowledge but become outdated as new information becomes available. We have to acknowledge that this sometimes happens, and we have to push ourselves to consider alternatives every day of our professional careers.

Sometimes it is appropriate and necessary to reject or ignore data; evidence-based practice does not mean professionals accept every new piece of information that comes along. Using evidence in practice does mean that professionals critically analyze their reactions to make sure that new information is given proper consideration.

When you complete the work for this unit, you will have the following skills and competencies:

- Understand the different ways people respond to new or challenging data
- Recognize different ways people will react and what their reactions mean
- Formulate a strategy for analyzing your own responses to new or challenging data in your practice

Sidebar 2-1
Executive Summary of Chinn and Brewer (1993)

Anomalous Data

This article presents a detailed analysis of the ways in which scientists and science students respond to [anomalous] data. We postulate that there are seven distinct forms of response…one…to accept the data… the other six responses involve discounting the data in various ways… (p. 1)

Anomalous data: Evidence that contradicts a person's current theories about how something happens/works.

Seven Possible Responses to Anomalous Data

1.   IGNORE the anomalous data. People ignore data when the data are contradictory to their view about how things work. They don't even bother to "explain" why the data are contrary when they are ignoring them.

Look for examples in which the professional demonstrates lack of interest in the topic, perhaps not seeing the relevance of a particular area of writing for the professional's practice areas.

2.   REJECT the anomalous data. People also reject data when they are contradictory to their current views. The unique feature of rejection is that the person will explain why data should be rejected.

*Look for examples in which the professional provides a justification for rejecting particular information. A therapist might reject findings from an article because measures were weak, there weren't enough subjects, or that it was the **only** study in the area of interest.*

3.   EXCLUDE the anomalous data. People exclude data by deciding that the data reveal information that is relevant for some other discipline or area of expertise, but not their own.

Look for explanations about why particular information doesn't apply to the current practices and beliefs. A therapist might exclude data about spasticity because the study is about children and the therapist serves adults.

4.   Hold the anomalous data in ABEYANCE. People hold the data in abeyance by delaying their willingness to deal with the data. They continue to hold their current beliefs, and acknowledge that someday the ideas in the data will be articulated so that they will change current beliefs.

Look for explanations that focus on current beliefs and how they are not developed enough to account for the new finding. A therapist might hold data showing that traditional neurodevelopmental treatment (NDT) doesn't work in abeyance by saying that there aren't good enough measures yet.

5.   REINTERPRET the anomalous data. People reinterpret the data by formulating an explanation about the data that are consistent with their current beliefs even though the researchers have articulated a different explanation for the findings.

Look for explanations that show two different explanations for the same findings. An occupational therapist thinks that the findings show the power of sensory processing; the behaviorist thinks that the findings show the power of contingencies.

6.   Make PERIPHERAL CHANGES in the theory. People make peripheral changes to their current beliefs by making a minor change to their current beliefs, but retaining the core of their current ideas.

Look for explanations that compartmentalize the findings into one small part. The therapist says that recovery models might be OK for some mental health disorders, but not the ones that she works with.

7.   Accept the data and CHANGE the theory. People accept data by changing a core belief based on data (as we might do as we begin to implement evidence-based practice).

Look for explanations that show a shift in a belief within the practice. The therapist decides that the team needs to stop doing range of motion exercises because studies have shown they don't contribute to the functional outcomes she desires.

WAYS TO HANDLE ANOMALOUS DATA

There is an older article from the education literature that provides some structure for considering alternatives for handling new or unfamiliar data. In 1993, Chinn and Brewer wrote an article about how children learn science; their ideas extend well beyond this initial goal and provide a wonderful framework for considering our reactions to new and potentially challenging information. They discuss "anomalous data" as "evidence that contradicts a person's current theories about how something happens/works."

Chinn and Brewer (1993) propose that people respond in seven possible ways when presented with anomalous data (Sidebar 2-1). Let's review the seven different ways people respond. Think of times you have responded in each of these seven ways.

Activity 2-1

Read the Chinn and Brewer (1993, pp. 1-14) excerpt located in the Appendix (Article 1).

Chinn, C. A., & Brewer, W. F. (1993). *The role of anomalous data in knowledge acquisition: A theoretical framework and implications for science instruction.* Review of Educational Research, 63(1), 1-49.

Take note of the seven ways that people respond to new or challenging information. Think of a situation in practice that would illustrate each of the seven patterns. Complete Worksheet 2A to record your thoughts.

Activity 2-2

Meet with your study partners and be prepared to discuss Terrance's case (Sidebar 2-2)

Sidebar 2-2
Case Study: Terrance

Terrance has been working in a rehabilitation setting for 10 years. He is proud of his work; he focuses on retraining activities of daily living in the early part of rehabilitation and works on functional supports for the individual and his or her family as part of transition planning.

Terrance is part of a study group. Last week they read an article about forced use (also called constraint-induced therapy), a procedure that restrains unaffected limbs, thereby "forcing" use of the affected limb (as with strokes). The study group had a lively discussion. Now Terrance is faced with having to consider whether he needs to change his rehabilitation practices.

based on what you learned from the Chinn and Brewer (1993) article. Write a scenario for each of Chinn and Brewer's responses that would illustrate Terrance's response to this new information (Worksheet 2B).

SUMMARY

Understanding reactions to new information is a critical part of evidence-based practice. Sometimes reactions to reject or hold data in abeyance are appropriate, and other times these reactions represent fear or reluctance to think a new way. Considering all possibilities enables professionals to understand themselves, their colleagues, and the people they serve a little better. Critical analyses of one's reactions to new data ensure that the best possible professional practices are being implemented.

All references for this unit can be found in the Bibliography, beginning on page 169.

Worksheet 2A
Identifying Practice Examples That Illustrate Chinn and Brewer's (1993) Strategies

Think of an example from practice that would illustrate a professional using each of Chinn and Brewer's (1993) ways of responding to anomalous data.

Chinn and Brewer (1993) Responses	Examples From Practice
IGNORE the data (don't even bother to "explain" data away)	
REJECT the data (articulate an explanation for why data should be rejected)	
EXCLUDE the data from the domain of current beliefs (the data are outside the domain of current beliefs)	
Hold the data in ABEYANCE (I promise to deal with it later...assume that someday current beliefs will be articulated so that it can explain these data)	
REINTERPRET the data while retaining current beliefs (accept the data as something that should be explained by current beliefs...opposing forces accept data but interpret the data differently based on their own beliefs)	
Reinterpret the data and make PERIPHERAL CHANGES to current belief (make a relatively minor change to current belief...accepts the data but is unwilling to give up current belief and accept new beliefs)	
Accept the data and CHANGE current beliefs, possibly in favor of a particular new belief (change one or more of the core aspects of current beliefs—when faced with information that is contradictory to current beliefs, accepts alternate beliefs)	

Worksheet 2B
Explaining Terrance's Possible Responses to the Anomalous Data About Forced Use

Response	Terrance's Possible Responses
IGNORE	*Since Terrance is part of a study group, and they are reading articles of interest to his practice, this is not an option for his responses.*
REJECT	
EXCLUDE	
HOLD IN ABEYANCE	
REINTERPRET	
PERIPHERAL CHANGES	
CHANGE	

Unit 3

Understanding and Using the Basic Parts of Research Articles

In this unit, you will explore some of the basic parts of research articles. When you understand the parts of a research article, you will know where to look for information you need to apply evidence in your practice.

When researchers set out to report their findings, there are some conventions everyone follows to report the findings. Each professional journal has a stylized way of presenting the information, but the same basic information is available no matter what style journals select. Portney and Watkins (2000) provide a summary of the parts of research articles in Chapter 31, "Evaluating Research Reports"; use this reference as a guide to your learning.

When you complete the work of this unit, you will have the following skills and competencies:

- Identify the key sections of a research article
- Summarize what you will find in each section of a research article
- Recognize the strengths and weaknesses of operational definitions in an article

- Derive meaning from the Results section of an article
- Read and interpret tables and figures in articles
- Link research questions, methods, results, and discussion

Keep your research design and statistics reference books handy; when you are reviewing an article, look up the design and statistical analyses the authors are using. These texts typically do a great job of explaining what these procedures mean and how to interpret them for your practice. By doing this every time you review an article, you will build your repertoire of background knowledge.

Activity 3-1

Read Chapter 4 in the Law and MacDermid (2008) text to provide you with some background about research articles. Focus on the sections that discuss how to measure outcomes, including the discussion about statistical outcomes. Jot notes about key points that will help you when you read articles.

19

Activity 3-2

Read the chapter in your research design text that provides an overview of the parts of research articles and guidance about what to ask yourself as you read articles (e.g., Chapter 31 in Portney and Watkins [2000] or Sections 2, 5, and 6 in Kielhofner [2006]).

BASIC SECTIONS OF RESEARCH ARTICLES

Traditionally there are five parts to a research article. The *Title* and *Abstract* provide the reader with an overview of the work that will be reported. You can decide whether you are interested in the article by looking at this summary. Because the Title and Abstract are brief, the reader cannot determine the strength of the study or its applicability to certain practice situations from just this part of an article.

The *Introduction* provides background about the subject matter and builds a case for this study. The reader can get familiarized with relevant literature and understand what gaps there may be, which create the need for the study to be reported. Toward the end of the Introduction, the authors provide the research questions, hypotheses, or problem statement that frames the current study's work.

The *Methods* section provides the reader with the blueprint for the study. All the essential elements about who, what, where, when, and how must be reported here. There should also be enough detail that the reader can imagine all parts of the study and another researcher could conduct a similar study.

Because the Methods section provides details about the study structure, there are several sections. The *Participants* section describes who the authors will study. The *Design* section explains how the study is organized. The *Instrumentation* section describes what measures are used in the study. The *Procedures* section explains the sequence of events to complete the study. The *Data Analysis* section describes how the data were analyzed to determine the outcomes.

The *Results* section provides the reader with the findings of the study. The reader should expect only facts in this section of a research article. Interpretive material is reserved for the Discussion section. The reader should expect to see tables and figures summarizing findings. The authors must report on each hypothesis or research question in the Results section.

The *Discussion* section is the place for the authors to reflect on the findings of the study and provide the reader with their insights about the meaning of the study findings. Many times, authors will link their findings to literature, pointing out both similarities and differences with the current study.

Activity 3-3

Read the following article, which is located in the Appendix (Article 2):

Mann, W. C., Belchior, P., Tomita, M. R., & Kemp, B. J. (2005). Barriers to the use of traditional telephones by older adults with chronic health conditions. Occupational Therapy Journal of Research: Occupation, Participation and Health, 25(4), 160-166.

Complete the Worksheet 3A as you review the Mann et al. (2005) article. Observe how your ideas change as you move from the Abstract to the Introduction.

- As you read the Methods section, take note of the new considerations that occur to you.
- Do your reactions change when you encounter the Results?
- Do the authors change your perspective with their insights in the Discussion?

PRACTICE EXAMINING PARTICIPANT CRITERIA (METHODS SECTION)

Now that you have some initial practice, let's look at some of the parts of research articles by themselves. For example, by looking at the details of the Methods sections, we learn whether the articles relate to specific populations or can be generalized. We also learn whether the researchers designed the studies properly. This activity will increase your discrimination ability when engaging in evidence-based practice.

One of the important details is the participant population; this section of the Methods enables you to decide if a study is applicable to your practice. Specifically, researchers provide details about who they will include and exclude in their study. Read the inclusion and exclusion criteria in Worksheet 3B and then consider how you would implement these criteria to select participants.

Activity 3-4

Learning About Inclusion and Exclusion Criteria

You can see from this list of criteria in column 1 of Worksheet 3B that it is not perfectly clear who would be included or excluded from the participant pool. For example, what criteria would be used to decide whether someone is "ambulant"? Use Worksheet 3B to identify what questions you have about these criteria, and then write an improved version of the criteria. For example, what would you observe or what test score would you use to decide whether someone was "ambulant"? The criteria need to be precise enough that when presented with a potential participant, everyone would agree about including or excluding the person. When you can count on understanding who is a participant, you can count on understanding the meaning and application of the findings to appropriate situations. When it is unclear who participated in the study, the applications of the findings also come into question.

PRACTICE REVIEWING METHODS AND RESULTS

Sometimes it is helpful to have models when learning a new skill. You are going to practice analyzing Methods and Results sections using an already-prepared summary so you can compare your analysis to an expert who conducted the same analysis.

The first edition of *Evidence-Based Rehabilitation: A Guide to Practice* (Law, 2002) provides two chapters that include a critical review of articles (Chapter 8 reviews cognitive behavior interventions for people with chronic pain and Chapter 14 reviews interventions for people with strokes). These may be helpful examples as you study.

The authors provide brief summaries of the articles they found in a literature search. We will be examining summary articles that grow from critical reviews such as these in a later unit. For now, you will read a few of the articles and create a summary of them, and then compare your work

to the summaries provided within the Law (2002) text.

Activity 3-5

Summarizing Articles for Reviews

Review two articles from either Chapter 8 or 14 of the Law (2002) text. Mark the material from the Methods and Results sections and then transfer brief comments about this material to Worksheet 3C. After you complete Worksheet 3C, compare your summary to those provided in Chapter 8 or 14. Did you include all relevant information? Did you provide too much detail? Having brief notes makes it easier to summarize across articles.

Baranek (2002) wrote a summary article (Article 3 in the Appendix) in which she reviewed intervention studies for children who have autism.

Baranek, G. T. (2002). *Efficacy of sensory and motor interventions for children with autism.* Journal of Autism and Developmental Disorders, 32*(5)*, 397-422.

We will revisit the article in a later chapter when we discuss summary articles as an excellent source of information for evidence-based practice. For now, we will use one portion of this review to provide a model for summarizing the Methods and Results of articles.

The skill of summarizing the Methods and Results of a research article in a succinct table can be a great way to work in a study group with your colleagues because you can cover more material when everyone can see the overview quickly and don't have to page through the article as you go.

Activity 3-6

Summarizing Methods and Results

Review the four articles (Articles 4 through 7 in the Appendix) listed on Worksheet 3D.

Kern, L., Koegel, R. L., & Dunlap, G. (1984). *The influence of vigorous versus mild exercise on autistic stereotyped behaviors.* Journal of Autism and Developmental Disorders, 14, 57-67.

Kern, L., Koegel, R. L., Dyer, K., Blew, P. A., & Fenton, L. R. (1982). *The effects of physical exercise on self-stimulation and appropriate responding in autistic children.* Journal of Autism and Developmental Disorders, 12, 399-419.

Levinson, L. J., & Reid, G. (1993). *The effects of exercise intensity on the stereotypic behaviors of individuals with autism.* Adapted Physical Activity Quarterly, 10(3), 255-268.

Watters, R. G., & Watters, W. E. (1980). *Decreasing self-stimulatory behavior with physical exercise in a group of autistic boys.* Journal of Autism and Developmental Disorders, 10, 379-387.

These are the articles that Baranek (2002) included in her review of physical exercise interventions for children who have autism. Mark the parts of the article that coincide with the headings on Worksheet 3D, then complete Worksheet 3D on the four articles. Complete the worksheet **before** you look at what Baranek placed into the table. In class with study partners and your teacher, compare what you wrote with what Baranek wrote. What did you forget? Did you provide too many details?

Now that you have practiced two different ways to summarize the Methods and Results of a research article, you likely have a preference for one of these methods. There are other methods as well. Appendix A in Law and MacDermid (2008) provides a Critical Review Form for Quantitative Studies (Appendix B provides guidelines for use) and Appendix C provides a Critical Review Form for Qualitative Studies (Appendix D provides guidelines for use). Professionals will find different formats useful for summarizing a study.

PRACTICING SUMMARIZING FINDINGS FROM A STUDY

When you read a research article, you must understand the findings and the meaning of the findings for practice situations. When you are in a practice situation, colleagues, families, and other care providers expect that you are familiar with the current literature. They want to know what the articles mean for their situation. Therefore you need to understand how to translate the findings into regular words that you can share with others. One way to begin is to think about what you would say to a particular person (e.g., "I just read an article about what we are discussing, and their findings suggest we consider _____ in our interventions").

DEVELOPING TAKE HOME MESSAGES

Professionals want clear, easy-to-understand guidelines about what to do to improve their practices based on the most recent evidence. We will call these summaries "Take Home Messages" to remind ourselves to use understandable language. You will need to consider Take Home Messages for your colleagues (within your discipline and from other disciplines), family members, other care providers, and those receiving your care. When considering what you are going to write, think about these questions:

- What would you say to colleagues about how they might need to change their practices to gain the optimal benefit?
- What would you say to your team regarding the articles' findings based on the articles you have read?
- How would you extrapolate information from these articles to develop hypotheses for other populations than the ones that were studied?

Activity 3-7
Creating Take Home Messages From Research Articles

Read the following article, located in the Appendix (Article 8), which examines the effectiveness of two interventions.

Fetters, L., & Kluzik, J. (1996). *The effects of neurodevelopmental treatment versus practice on the reaching of children with spastic cerebral palsy.* Physical Therapy, 76(4), 346-358.

Review Sidebar 3-1 which summarizes the parts of the Fetters and Kluzik (1996) article. Compare this summary to your understanding of the article from your reading.

Now complete Worksheet 3E to design Take Home Messages using this article as your source of information. Pretend that this is the only article about reaching for children with spastic cerebral palsy.

Activity 3-8
Sharing With Study Partners

Share your Take Home Messages with your study partners and see how each of yours compared. Do you agree with each other about the findings? Did you say something that no one else said?

Sidebar 3-1
Summary of Fetters and Kluzik (1996)

Article Example
Fetters, L., & Kluzik, J. (1996). The effects of neurodevelopmental treatment versus practice on the reaching of children with spastic cerebral palsy. *Physical Therapy. 76*(4), 346-358. (**Note:** Please read the study in its entirety; this is a brief summary.)

Research Question
Does 5 days of NDT and/or practice improve the reaching characteristics of children with spastic cerebral palsy?

Participants
Eight children (two female, six male) age 10 to 15 years, who have spastic quadriplegic cerebral palsy
Inclusion: Understand and carry out spoken directions for reaching task
                Sufficient visual skill to localize object with both eyes
                Sufficient passive range of motion to be able to reach target
                Used computers in classroom or for schoolwork

Instrument
WATSMART: Waterloo Spatial Motion Analysis and Recording Technique
Has validity and reliability; was recalibrated for each session; uses infrared signals to record the movements of interest

Procedure
Children played interactive video game before and after each treatment session
They had at least 10 trials of reaching from a "resting" pad on the table to a switch on the computer positioned within the extended range of motion reach for each child

Treatment Conditions
Daily sessions of physical therapy, 35 minutes each session, 5 days in each condition (counterbalanced)
No treatment week prior to study and in between two conditions
Condition A: NDT by certified NDT physical therapist—goals to improve trunk and shoulder girdle control
                during reaching, improved smoothness and efficiency of movement, and improved ability
                to initiate movement
Condition B: Practice—repeated reaching to play computer games
Week 1:   Rest
Week 2:   Treatment (NDT or practice) 5 days, 35 minutes/day, measure outcomes each day
Week 3:   Rest
Week 4:   Treatment (NDT or practice) 5 days, 35 minutes/day, measure outcomes each day

Outcome Measures
1. Movement unit: number of movement units per reach
2. Movement time: interval between tabletop and computer touches
3. Path: length of path of reaching movement between tabletop and computer touch
4. Reaction time: time between therapist's signal to "go" and tabletop liftoff

Analysis
ANOVA for repeated measures/paired *t* tests

Continued on Next Page

Sidebar 3-1 (Continued)
Summary of Fetters and Kluzik (1996)

Results

? Time in Treatment	Movement Unit	Movement Time	Path/Displacement	Reaction Time
After Week 2	Yes	Yes	No	No
After Week 4	Yes	Yes	Yes	No
? Improvements	Movement Unit	Movement Time	Path/Displacement	Reaction Time
NDT	No	No	No	No
Practice*	No	Yes	No	No

(*Practice differences bigger even though not significant.)

Adapted from Fetters, L., & Kluzik, J. (1996). The effects of neurodevelopmental treatment versus practice on the reaching of children with spastic cerebral palsy. *Physical Therapy, 76*(4), 346-358.

Revise your Take Home Messages based on feedback.

Activity 3-9

Recognizing the Strengths and Limitations of Research Articles

All research articles make a contribution and have limitations. Perhaps a group of articles is only about one age group and diagnosis; then we are not sure whether we can apply their findings to other age groups and other diagnoses. There will always be practice questions that can and cannot be answered by the available research. Sometimes researchers conduct studies about what can be answered; that does not mean that studies reflect the only important topics for practice. Perhaps there are no measures to find out the answer to an important practice question. It might be that a population is so heterogeneous that it is hard to detect changes or to discover who would or would not profit from an intervention. In practice, there will always be answerable and unanswerable questions. Advances in measurement, technology, and knowledge make more questions answerable.

Considering the Fetters and Kluzik (1996) article, complete Worksheet 3F about the "answerable" and "unanswerable" questions for practice.

Meet with your study partners and compare your lists. Discuss the items that were unique on people's lists and add ideas to your original list.

SUMMARY

Now that you have a beginning understanding of the parts of articles and what they provide, you are ready to look at topical articles to derive meaning from a group of studies.

PRACTICE WITH AN ENTIRE ARTICLE

Now that you have practiced with parts of articles, let's take one article and look at several parts at one time. The following article is located in the Appendix (Article 9).

Rogers, S. J., Hepburn, S., & Wehner, E. (2003). *Parent reports of sensory symptoms in toddlers with autism and those with other developmental disorders.* Journal of Autism and Developmental Disorders, 33(6), 631-642.

Rogers, Hepburn, and Wehner (2003) looked at sensory symptoms in various developmental disorders; this is a good article for novices to evidence-based practice because the article is clearly written, contains several types of statistical analyses, includes graphing, and has some thought-provoking ideas to pose for the future. Additionally, it is an interdisciplinary article, so it provides a look at a topic that is of interest to many professionals working with children who have developmental disorders. The article is not an intervention study, so we can focus on the structure of the article itself, rather than on a possible intervention.

Activity 3-10

Summarizing the Article

Complete Worksheet 3G to summarize the key points of the Rogers et al. (2003) article.

You can get most of the information for the worksheet from the Abstract, but you will also need to search through the Methods section to get some of the needed details from the study.

EXAMINING THE INTRODUCTION

During the Introduction, the reader expects to get an overview of the work in the area of interest which builds a case for the study. Since there is limited space, authors have to be selective about how they build their case.

Activity 3-11

Identifying Themes

You can begin to look at the Introduction by looking for the overall themes. The Rogers et al. (2003) study has nine paragraphs leading to the statement of purpose of this study. Read each paragraph and write the theme of that paragraph; sometimes this helps you to see the key points of the authors' argument (Worksheet 3H).

Activity 3-12

Discussing the Introduction With Study Partners

Now meet with your study partners and discuss the themes you see in the Introduction. What argument are Rogers et al. (2003) trying to make? Did they convince you that the study would be an important contribution?

FRAMEWORK FOR THE STUDY

Rogers et al. (2003) state four aims for their study:

1. To examine parental reports of sensory symptoms in young children with several different developmental disabilities
2. To examine relationships of sensory symptoms with intellectual ability, age, and severity
3. To examine external validity by comparing consistency of parental reports and observer reports of sensory symptoms across several different instruments
4. To evaluate the relative contribution of sensory symptoms to the acquisition of adaptive behavior in young children

As the reader, you will want to watch for design and results that meet these aims.

ANALYZING THE METHODS

Participants

The authors tell you how they found children to participate in their study in the first part of this section. Then they tell you the inclusion criteria for participants.

Activity 3-13

Summarizing Inclusion Criteria

Summarize the Rogers et al. (2003) participant criteria in Worksheet 3I.

Measures

The authors list the measures used in the study and summarize the validity and reliability of the measures to familiarize the reader with their assessments.

Activity 3-14

Finding More Information About Measures

Look up further information on one of the assessments to find out more about the measure. Be sure to include information about the measure's validity and reliability. Law, Baum, and Dunn (2005) provide a summary of many measures used in applied science research and may be a good reference for practice settings.

Procedures

The Rogers et al. (2003) study's procedures were primarily about the strategies they used to collect the data since there is not an intervention.

Results

The authors provide a combination of text, tables, and figures to report their results. This is a great strategy because it accommodates all types of readers (i.e., those that understand the text explanation, those that enjoy examining the numbers they reported, and those that prefer graphs to show relationships).

Understanding the Relationship Among Graphs, Tables, and Text

In the Rogers et al. (2003) study, Figure 1 is an illustration of the numbers reported in Table II. Across the bottom of the figure is a list of the subtests of the Short Sensory Profile; these subtests are listed at the top of Table II (the first line is the total score which is not graphed). You will also notice that the "movement" subtest was omitted from the table; this appears to be an editing error. With the means graphed, the numeric comparisons among the groups are illustrated for you. For example, on "taste," the children with autism are separated from the other groups. The "auditory filtering" subtest has a pattern of autism and Fragile X syndrome clustering together, with the other two groups separated from them. The "visual/auditory processing" subtest shows that all the groups cluster together.

You can see these same patterns in the numbers on Table II in Rogers et al. (2003). Additionally, this table contains the significance levels from the statistical comparisons. You will see that all the comparisons yielded some significant differences between groups **except** for the visual/auditory processing subtest ($p=.211$). So the statistical findings are illustrated on Figure 1 as well.

Activity 3-15

Find the Text to Match the Tables and Figures

Find the text in Rogers et al. (2003) that explains Table II and Figure 1, and match up the text with the results on the specific subtests. Meet with your study partners and discuss how the tables and figures enhance the reporting of results.

Decoding the Text Results

Let's use the third full paragraph on page 245 ("It was possible...") of the Rogers et al. (2003)

article to examine the details of statistical results. In this paragraph, the authors are reporting about a specific analysis they did to understand their findings a little further. You will note that they only report what they did and their findings; it is not appropriate to add interpretations to the Results section. This gives the reader the chance to study the results and make some preliminary conclusions and hypotheses before reading what the authors are thinking (their ideas will be in the Discussion section to follow).

In the first sentence, they state their hypothesis: they want to know whether the increased presence of repetitive and restrictive behaviors might be associated with the higher scores on the Sensory Profile. They selected some of the items from the ADI-R that reflect repetitive and restrictive behaviors, and used these items to compare across the groups. They want to know whether repetitive behaviors and sensory symptoms present in the same pattern; if they do, then one might hypothesize that sensory symptoms and repetitive behaviors are related in some way (we will see what the authors have to say about this in the Discussion).

They report "There was a significant difference by group ($F[3,98]=24.21$, $p<.001$)." They are telling the reader that there were differences between the groups that met statistical standards. The brackets tell the reader exactly what the calculations yielded; the F test is the result you get from the Analysis of Variance, and the p level tells how much difference occurred. (In this case, there would be an error 1 time in 1,000 times—that is pretty good!)

The significance finding only goes so far; we don't know where the differences are without further testing. Rogers et al. (2003) report on "post hoc" tests here; this means that they are checking for differences between all the groups to find out where the differences exist. They are telling us that the children with autism were significantly different from all the other groups, suggesting that they have a higher rate of repetitive and restrictive behaviors (as tested by items 70 to 85 on the ADI-R).

Since the reader won't find out what Rogers et al. (2003) think of this finding until the Discussion, the reader can reflect on what this finding might mean. This pattern of autism being different from all athe other groups is a different pattern than the one reported for the sensory symptoms, so they cannot be completely interrelated. (Aren't you excited to know what the authors think too?)

Activity 3-16

Study Other Results Text

Meet with study partners to examine other paragraphs in the Results section of Rogers et al. (2003). Discuss what the authors are telling the readers. Hypothesize what the results might mean so you can compare to the authors' ideas in the Discussion.

Activity 3-17

Answering Research Questions

Rogers et al. (2003) set out four aims for the study. Meet with your study partners to identify which paragraphs, tables, and graphs address each of the four aims. Discuss whether you felt that the authors addressed each of the aims and what the answer to their hypotheses would be.

DISCUSSION

During the Discussion section, the reader expects the authors to examine their findings and derive meaning from them. In their 2003 article, Rogers et al. provide a clear map for the reader about the progression of their Discussion. They use key phrases to alert the reader (e.g., "The first question to be examined...", "However, we also found....", "The second main question...", "The next important finding..."). These marker phrases help the reader to frame the Discussion.

Many times sections of the Discussion will coincide with particular results. We examined the Results paragraph about repetitive behaviors, so let's look at the Discussion about this finding. Rogers et al. (2003) restate the finding in the first sentence, and then go on to tell the reader what they think this means. They say that the repetitive behaviors are what distinguishes children with autism, since they are significantly different on this measure and are not the only group with significant differences in sensory symptoms. The "lore" in practice suggests that repetitive behaviors reflect sensory responses. If that relationship

were true, then the children with Fragile X syndrome would also have had an elevated repetitive behavior score, since they also had elevated sensory symptoms. Now that was worth waiting for, wasn't it?

Activity 3-18

Link Discussion With Results

Find other sections of the Rogers et al. (2003) Discussion that you can link to sections of the Results. Discuss with your study partners to make sure you understand the authors' conclusions and hypotheses. Do you have alternate interpretations of the data? What other explanations could be posed? Are the authors revealing any biases in their Discussion?

Activity 3-19

Handling Anomalous Data

The findings from the Rogers et al. (2003) article may challenge some of your current beliefs. Refer to your Executive Summary (see Sidebar 2-1) of the Chinn and Brewer (1993) article to decide where your reactions to the article findings are occurring (Worksheet 3J). Bring these issues up with your study partners.

DEVELOPING TAKE HOME MESSAGES

The final step in the analysis process for evidence-based practice is to summarize the findings for those who need to use the ideas to improve their practices.

Activity 3-20

Worksheet for Documenting Take Home Messages

Select two constituent groups as the focus of your attention and create some Take Home Messages for them. Pretend that the article you read was the **definitive** article on the topic. Use Worksheets 3K and 3L to summarize your work.

When considering what you are going to write, think about these questions:

- What would you say to colleagues about how they might need to change their practices to gain the optimal benefit?
- What would you say to your team regarding the article's findings based on articles you have read?
- How would you extrapolate information from the article to develop hypotheses for other populations than the ones that were studied?

SUMMARY

Sometimes taking the time to go through one article helps develop skills for deriving meaning for evidence-based practice. In this unit, you learned about the parts of research articles and what to expect from each part. Using this information, professionals can take advantage of what the literature has available to make their practices evidence based.

All references for this unit can be found in the Bibliography, beginning on page 169.

Worksheet 3A

Reviewing the Parts of a Research Article

Parts of the Research Article	Your Reactions to the Material
Mann, W. C., Belchior, P., Tomita, M. R., & Kemp, B. J. (2005). Barriers to the use of traditional telephones by older adults with chronic health conditions. *Occupational Therapy Journal of Research: Occupation, Participation and Health, 25*(4), 160-166.	
Title/Abstract What do you think this article is about from reading the Title and Abstract only?	
Introduction Does the literature seem relevant to the topic? What convinces you that this study needs to be done to fill a gap in the literature? How have your ideas changed about what this study is about?	
Methods Could another researcher conduct this study from the information provided? What are you wondering about after reading the Methods? Now what do you think this study is about?	
Results How would you tell someone else what the findings are? What practices might you change because of these findings?	
Discussion What do the authors add to the story in this section? What surprises you about the authors' insights and conclusions?	

Worksheet 3B
Analyzing and Improving the Precision of Participant Criteria

Inclusion Criteria*	What Questions Do You Have About the Criteria? How Do You Think the Authors Would Verify That Someone Had Met the Inclusion Criteria?	How Would You Make the Criteria More Precise and Observable/Verifiable?
Ages 23 to 50 years		
Preverbal or single word language		
Ambulant		
Sighted		
Apparent tactile defensiveness and/or...		
...Aversive response to movement		

*Headings from Soper, G., & Thorley, C. (1996). Effectiveness of an occupational therapy programme based on sensory integration theory for adults with severe learning disabilities. *British Journal of Occupational Therapy, 59*(10), 475-482.

Worksheet 3C
Summarizing Intervention Studies

Reference:

Purpose of the study:

Design of the study and sample used:

Outcomes and interventions used in the study:

Results:

Conclusions and implications:

Worksheet based on Law, M., & MacDermid, J. (2008). *Evidence-based rehabilitation: A guide to practice* (2nd ed.). Thorofare, NJ: SLACK Incorporated.

Worksheet 3D

Summarize Intervention Studies From Baranek (2002)

Citation	Number of Participants	Characteristics of Participants	Design Elements	Intervention Specifications	Outcomes Measured	Findings
Kern et al. (1982)						
Kern et al. (1984)						
Levinson & Reid (1993)						
Watters & Watters (1980)						

© 2008 SLACK Incorporated. From Dunn, W. *Bringing Evidence into Everyday Practice: Practical Strategies for Healthcare Professionals.* Thorofare, NJ: SLACK Incorporated.

Worksheet 3E
Creating Brief Take Home Messages

Fetters, L., & Kluzik, J. (1996). The effects of neurodevelopmental treatment versus practice on the reaching of children with spastic cerebral palsy. *Physical Therapy, 76*(4), 346-358.

Write a three- to five-sentence summary of the findings of the article.

Write a one- to two-sentence statement for a colleague searching for an effective reaching intervention strategy.

Write a one- to two-sentence statement for a teacher who wants to try one of these strategies in his or her classroom.

Write a one- to two-sentence statement for a parent who heard about one of these strategies and wants you to implement the strategy with his or her child.

Worksheet 3F
Identifying Answerable and Unanswerable Questions

Identify two answerable and two unanswerable questions from the Fetters and Kluzik (1996) article. Discuss your ideas with your study partners. One example is provided.

Answerable Question	What in the Article Enables You to Answer This Question?
Does movement time improve with NDT or practice as interventions?	*They measured the time from the tabletop to the computer in each condition.*

Unanswerable Question	What Else Would We Need to Be Able to Answer This Question?
Does NDT improve computer use?	*The researchers would have to measure the accuracy/efficiency of the computer use.*

Worksheet 3G

Summarizing Characteristics

Summarize the article Rogers, S., Hepburn, S., & Wehner, E. (2003). Parent reports of sensory symptoms in toddlers with autism and those with other developmental disabilities. *Journal of Autism and Developmental Disorders*, 33(6), 631-642.

Citation	Participants	Setting	Measures	Design	Intervention	Findings	Notes
Rogers et al. (2003)							

Citation: Put the reference here.
Participants: List the important characteristics of participants.
Setting: Describe the location of the study.
Measures: List the outcome measures used in the study.
Design: Describe what type of comparisons or relationships are being tested/studied.
Intervention: List the most important aspects of the procedures being tested.
Findings: List the most important outcomes.
Notes: If you have insights or questions, jot them down.

Worksheet 3H
Summarizing Themes in the Introduction

Write a phrase summarizing the theme of each paragraph in the Introduction of the Rogers et al. (2003) article.

1.

2.

3.

4.

5.

6.

7.

8.

9.

Worksheet 3I
Summarizing the Inclusion Criteria

Summarize the Rogers et al. (2003) inclusion criteria in your own words.

Criteria for autism:

Criteria for Fragile X syndrome:

Criteria for developmental delay:

Criteria for typical development:

Worksheet 3J
Reactions to New Data

Think about your reactions to the article. Based on Chinn and Brewer's (1993) ways of responding to anomalous data, what would you say your reaction illustrates?

Chinn and Brewer (1993) Responses	Example Reaction to the Findings
IGNORE the data (don't even bother to "explain" data away)	
REJECT the data (articulate an explanation for why data should be rejected)	
EXCLUDE the data from the domain of current beliefs (the data are outside the domain of current beliefs)	
Hold the data in ABEYANCE (I promise to deal with it later...assume that someday current beliefs will be articulated so that it can explain these data)	
REINTERPRET the data while retaining current beliefs (accept the data as something that should be explained by current beliefs...opposing forces accept data but interpret the data differently based on their own beliefs)	
Reinterpret the data and make PERIPHERAL CHANGES to current belief (make a relatively minor change to current belief...accepts the data but is unwilling to give up current belief and accept new beliefs)	
Accept the data and CHANGE current beliefs, possibly in favor of a particular new belief (change one or more of the core aspects of current beliefs—when faced with information that is contradictory to current beliefs, accepts alternate beliefs)	

Worksheet 3K
Take Home Messages for Group 1

Pretend that the article you just read is the definitive article about the topic. Develop Take Home Messages showing what you would say to a particular constituent group regarding the topic based on the article you have read.

Take Home Messages About:

Name:

These messages are for:

_____ colleagues in my discipline   _____ care providers

_____ colleagues in other disciplines   _____ family members

_____ adults receiving care   _____ children receiving care

Take Home Message	Rationale for This Message From the Literature

Worksheet 3L
Take Home Messages for Group 2

Pretend that the article you just read is the definitive article about the topic. Develop Take Home Messages showing what you would say to a particular constituent group regarding the topic based on the article you have read.

Take Home Messages About:

Name:

These messages are for:

_____ colleagues in my discipline   _____ care providers

_____ colleagues in other disciplines   _____ family members

_____ adults receiving care   _____ children receiving care

Take Home Message	Rationale for This Message From the Literature

Section II

Practice Using Evidence to Design Best Practices

It is all well and good to learn research and evidence concepts, but this doesn't automatically enable professionals to use these concepts to affect their everyday practices. If you want to be an evidence-based practitioner, you have to practice how to harness ideas from the literature. With the tools from Section I, we can begin looking at groups of articles about similar topics and make decisions about what their findings tell us about our professional practices.

In this section, you will examine several selections of articles on particular topics and then develop Take Home Messages from the articles. You will consider what you would say to various audiences about the topics, including colleagues on your team, family members, and other people or agencies you serve. In each chapter, you will explore several topics that are applicable to a wide range of practice situations. Then you will have some opportunities to apply the same strategies to some articles that will inform your areas of practice.

FORMAT FOR WORK IN SECTION II

Throughout Section II, you will follow the same format for your work. You will read a few articles about a similar topic, complete a summary worksheet on those articles, identify similarities and differences among the articles, and get feedback from study partners. You will also examine research designs, statistical procedures, reporting of results, and interpreting discussions in the articles as well. You will have a nice collection of Take Home Messages for your practice when you complete the work of Section II. You will also have an established pattern of systematic analysis you can use for future articles that become available, making your work more efficient.

When you complete the work in Section II, you will have the following skills and competencies:
- Ability to systematically summarize the Methods and Results of research articles
- Ability to compare and contrast findings across articles on similar topics

- Ability to derive meaning from Methods, Designs, Results, and Discussions in research articles
- Ability to discuss insights with colleagues to refine understanding about research findings
- Ability to construct Take Home Messages for communities of interest

Unit 4

Examining Evidence Related to Assistive Devices

During this unit, you will explore some evidence about the impact of assistive devices on a person's ability to participate in his or her everyday life. This topic is applicable to a wide range of populations and settings, and so can be informative to many types of practice. Using adaptations to support everyday life provides people with direct access to the activities they want and need to do each day; understanding evidence about what, how, and when to apply assistive devices can improve our effectiveness at supporting people within their lives.

We make recommendations about how to adapt objects and activities every day and assume that these are good ideas and effective practices. Perhaps we need to wonder which adaptations are most helpful, or which are most cumbersome even though they work when someone actually uses them. Perhaps some adaptations simply don't work in the sense that they take too much time, or the adaptations remove the part of the activity that was satisfying for the person.

So let's delve into this literature and find out what the researchers and their participants have

to say about the use of adaptive devices to support people's lives.

When you complete the work in this unit, you will have the following skills and competencies:

- Understand how assistive device literature may contribute to your effectiveness at supporting people to participate in their everyday lives
- Recognize themes in diverse literature that suggest enduring themes related to assistive devices
- Articulate how to find other articles that would contribute to your knowledge about this topic
- Design an optimal plan for your area of practice based on what you have read
- Construct Take Home Messages for various constituents so they understand quickly what the literature says about the topic

You will be reviewing articles, creating summaries for comparison and contrast, gaining insights from your study partners, and creating Take Home Messages for constituent groups.

Activity 4-1

Read the articles listed below, which are located in the Appendix (Articles 2, 10 through 13). These articles will provide background for your work in this unit and will shed some light on the use of assistive devices. For this unit, focus on the ways that assistive devices contribute to participation and satisfaction in everyday life.

Chiu, C. W. Y., & Man, D. W. K. (2004). *The effect of training older adults with stroke to use home-based assistive devices.* Occupational Therapy Journal of Research: Occupation, Participation and Health, 24(3), 113-120.

Lund, M. L., & Nygård, L. (2003). *Incorporating or resisting assistive devices: Different approaches to achieving a desired occupational self-image.* Occupational Therapy Journal of Research: Occupation, Participation and Health, 23(2), 67-75.

Mann, W. C., Belchior, P., Tomita, M. R., & Kemp, B. J. (2005). *Barriers to the use of traditional telephones by older adults with chronic health conditions.* Occupational Therapy Journal of Research: Occupation, Participation and Health, 25(4), 160-166.

Mann, W. C., Llanes, C., Justiss, M. D., & Tomita, M. (2004). *Frail older adults' self-report of their most important assistive device.* Occupational Therapy Journal of Research: Occupation, Participation and Health, 24(1), 4-12.

Stark, S. (2004). *Removing environmental barriers in the homes of older adults with disabilities improves occupational performance.* Occupational Therapy Journal of Research: Occupation, Participation and Health, 24(1), 32-40.

Activity 4-2

Summarizing the Methods and Results of Research Articles

Create a summary (Worksheet 4A) for the articles listed in Activity 4-1.

Summary articles use tables to show readers the most important aspects of studies. Locate a summary article in an area of your interest and see its tables are organized. Make an organizational table that suits your learning and information needs.

LOOKING FOR PATTERNS AND THEMES

First look for similarities and differences in the structures of the studies.

- Did they study the same populations?

- Did they use similar settings?
- Were the designs similar?
- How did the measures compare to each other?

The answer to these questions can help you understand differences in findings. For example, if one study says that assistive devices are effective and another study says no one uses them, you will need to examine these other factors to see what might have contributed to the differences. One study might have examined younger people who really like technological devices, while another study might have examined older people who were limited in their experience with devices. You can then hypothesize that devices are only effective with a certain group or when outcomes address only certain aspects of everyday life activities.

Now, think about the topic.

- What happened to your thinking from before and after reading the articles?
- How did your ideas change?
- Have you observed that professionals have incorporated these findings into their practices?
- Are you going to do anything differently now that your have read these studies?

Now consider what questions are answerable or unanswerable from these studies.

Activity 4-3

Recognizing the Strengths and Limitations of Research Articles

All research articles make a contribution and have limitations. Perhaps a group of articles is only about one age group and diagnosis; then we are not sure whether we can apply their findings to other age groups and other diagnoses. There will always be practice questions that can and cannot be answered by the available research. Sometimes researchers conduct studies about what can be answered; that does not mean that studies reflect the only important topics for practice. Perhaps there are no measures to find out the answer to an important practice question. It might be that a population is so heterogeneous that it is hard to detect changes or to discover who would or would not profit from an intervention. In practice, there will always be answerable and unanswerable questions. Advances in measurement, technology, and knowledge make more questions answerable.

Considering this group of articles, complete Worksheet 4B about the "answerable" and "unanswerable" questions for practice.

Activity 4-4

Discuss your ideas and queries related to the questions in Worksheet 4B with your study partners.

Activity 4-5

Handling Anomalous Data

The findings from these articles (Chiu & Man, 2004; Lund & Nygård, 2003; Mann et al., 2004, 2005; Stark, 2004) may challenge some of your current beliefs. Refer to your Executive Summary (see Sidebar 2-1) of the Chinn and Brewer (1993) article to decide where your reactions to the article findings are occurring. Bring these issues up with your study partners. Complete Worksheet 4C with the assistive device findings on your mind. Be prepared to discuss the ideas you have with your study partners. Also consider what you might say to someone with each of the responses if you were in a conversation.

Activity 4-6

Expanding the Evidence

Obtain another article (i.e., in the past 6 years) that adds information to your understanding about this topic. Add this citation, etc., to your summary (Worksheet 4A). Make copies of your article for your study partners.

Activity 4-7

Group Discussion

Meet with your study partners and discuss your findings and reactions to the articles listed in Activity 4-1. Add your unique information to the discussion from the article you are contributing on the topic. Refine your notes based on your discussion.

These studies (Chiu & Man, 2004; Lund & Nygård, 2003; Mann et al., 2004, 2005; Stark, 2004) were a combination of experimental and descriptive designs, so we have a mix of information to deal with. The studies also included people with many types of disabilities, which enable us to generalize the information across a wider group. In your practice, you might use the Chiu and Man (2004) findings to hypothesize that training in hospital and in home follow-up is needed for all devices, not just for bathing. You could use the same framework and try their strategies with eating devices or mobility devices to see if the intervention is applicable to more than bathing. You could also add the information about telephone use to see whether adding a training program about additional features of the phone would increase use of these features after people return home. These are examples of how to integrate the findings from these studies together and use them in new ways in service to your particular practice issues. Be prepared to discuss other options with your study partners.

EXTENDING KNOWLEDGE ABOUT METHODS AND RESULTS

In each unit of Section II, each set of articles reflects an overall topic. Additionally, each article illustrates some unique features of studies and ways to report the methods and findings. By examining some aspects of each study, you will accumulate knowledge about designs and statistics while learning more about the evidence. This process will build your capacity as an evidence-based professional because when you encounter other articles with similar features, you will know how to use the information in your decision making.

UNDERSTANDING HOW TO COMBINE EXPERIMENTAL AND DESCRIPTIVE DATA

You will notice that the five articles about assistive devices listed in Activity 4-1 have a combination of experimental and descriptive studies. In this situation, you might be able to hypothesize about intervention options more directly by using the intervention studies as your basis for thinking. You can then use the descriptive study findings to expand your ideas about what conditions might increase the possibility of assistive devices being used and satisfying for the people you serve. Perhaps a team will be able to identify criteria for recommending a device to an individual and criteria for **not** recommending a device.

Evidence Detective Tip

You can extend what you know from experimental studies by looking at the characteristics of descriptive studies on the same topic.

Activity 4-8

Combining Experimental and Descriptive Data

The studies in this unit address issues related to assistive devices. Two of the studies are experimental (Chiu & Man, 2004; Stark, 2004). Let's look at the insights we have gained from these two intervention studies, and then consider how to expand our knowledge about assistive devices using the other three descriptive studies you read (Lund & Nygård, 2003; Mann et al., 2004, 2005).

In the first column of Worksheet 4D, identify a finding from one of the intervention studies. Now review the three descriptive studies' findings to identify something from these studies that could expand your ideas from the experimental studies. You will use these ideas in your discussion group with your study partners. One example is completed on Worksheet 4D to provide a model for your work.

In this example, we are expanding the idea of training and follow-up using the additional information from the descriptive studies. When trying these ideas, a therapist would collect data to see if this new application of the knowledge is also effective.

Now complete a few more rows with your ideas and be prepared to discuss them with your study partners. There are several ways to organize the themes from these studies; there is not one way that is correct.

Activity 4-9

Discussion of Organizing Themes

When you meet with your study partners, share your different ways of organizing the themes and discuss how you identified these themes.

Think about how you would reorganize your thinking about recommending assistive devices. How will you individualize your choices about assistive devices? Will your choices be different depending on how training is set up?

Activity 4-10

Developing Take Home Messages

The final step in the analysis process for evidence-based practice is to summarize the findings for those who need to use the ideas to improve their practices. Professionals want clear, easy-to-understand guidelines about what to do. We will call these summaries "Take Home Messages" to remind ourselves to use understandable language. You will need to consider Take Home Messages for your colleagues (within your discipline and from other disciplines), family members, other care providers, and those receiving your care.

Select two constituent groups as the focus of your attention and create some Take Home Messages for them. Pretend that the articles you read (Chiu & Man, 2004; Lund & Nygård, 2003; Mann et al., 2004, 2005; Stark, 2004) were the **definitive** articles on the topic. Use Worksheets 4E and 4F to summarize your work.

When considering what you are going to write, think about these questions:

- What would you say to colleagues about how they might need to change their practices to gain the optimal benefit?
- What would you say to your team regarding the articles' findings based on the articles you have read?
- How would you extrapolate information from these articles to develop hypotheses for populations other than the ones that were studied?

SUMMARY

In this unit, you reviewed literature related to use of assistive devices. This information enables professionals to make informed choices about how to select, train, and recommend assistive devices.

All references for this unit can be found in the Bibliography, beginning on page 169.

Worksheet 4A

Summarizing Characteristics of Research Articles

Citation	Participants	Setting	Measures	Design	Intervention	Findings	Notes
Study 1: Chiu & Man (2004)							
Study 2: Lund & Nygård (2003)							
Study 3: Mann et al. (2004)							
Study 4: Mann et al. (2005)							
Study 5: Stark (2004)							
Study 6:							

Citation: Put the reference here.
Participants: List the important characteristics of participants.
Setting: Describe the location of the study.
Measures: List the outcome measures used in the study.
Design: Describe what type of comparisons or relationships are being tested/studied.
Intervention: List the most important aspects of the procedures being tested.
Findings: List the most important outcomes.
Notes: If you have insights or questions, jot them down.

Worksheet 4B
Writing Answerable and Unanswerable Questions

Write one question you can and one question you cannot answer from the studies in this unit. Discuss these with your study partners.

Answerable Question	What in the Article Enables You to Answer This Question?
What kind of training will improve adaptive device use for older adults?	*Training in hospital and at home had better outcomes (Chiu & Man, 2004)*

Unanswerable Question	What Else Would We Need to Be Able to Answer This Question?
What kind of training will improve adaptive device use for children?	*Studies on children using adaptive devices*

Worksheet 4C
Reactions to New Data

Think about your reactions to the articles. Based on Chinn and Brewer's (1993) ways of responding to anomalous data, what would you say your reaction illustrates?

Chinn and Brewer (1993) Responses	Example Reaction to the Findings
IGNORE the data (don't even bother to "explain" data away)	
REJECT the data (articulate an explanation for why data should be rejected)	
EXCLUDE the data from the domain of current beliefs (the data are outside the domain of current beliefs)	
Hold the data in ABEYANCE (I promise to deal with it later...assume that someday current beliefs will be articulated so that it can explain these data)	
REINTERPRET the data while retaining current beliefs (accept the data as something that should be explained by current beliefs...opposing forces accept data but interpret the data differently based on their own beliefs)	
Reinterpret the data and make PERIPHERAL CHANGES to current belief (make a relatively minor change to current belief...accepts the data but is unwilling to give up current belief and accept new beliefs)	
Accept the data and CHANGE current beliefs, possibly in favor of a particular new belief (change one or more of the core aspects of current beliefs—when faced with information that is contradictory to current beliefs, accepts alternate beliefs)	

Worksheet 4D

Examining Ways to Expand Knowledge About Assistive Devices

Findings From Intervention Studies About Assistive Devices From Chiu and Man (2004) and Stark (2004)	Expansion of Findings Using Lund and Nygård (2003)	Expansion of Findings Using Mann et al. (2004)	Expansion of Findings Using Mann et al. (2005)
Participants who got specialized training within the hospital and after returning home are more proficient and satisfied with their bath devices (Chiu & Man, 2004)	*Identify whether the person is a "pragmatic," "ambivalent," or "resistant" user and organize training around these issues*	*When possible from data in this study, share with person that many people use the particular device*	*Do a specialized training program about the special features of the telephone, and follow up with some phone calls after he or she is home so that he or she can use the features*

Worksheet 4E
Take Home Messages for Group 1

Pretend that the articles you just read are the definitive articles about the topic. Develop Take Home Messages showing what you would say to a particular constituent group regarding the topic based on the articles you have read.

Take Home Messages About:

Name:

These messages are for:

_____ colleagues in my discipline   _____ care providers

_____ colleagues in other disciplines   _____ family members

_____ adults receiving care   _____ children receiving care

Take Home Message	Rationale for This Message From the Literature

Worksheet 4F
Take Home Messages for Group 2

Pretend that the articles you just read are the definitive articles about the topic. Develop Take Home Messages showing what you would say to a particular constituent group regarding the topic based on the articles you have read.

Take Home Messages About:

Name:

These messages are for:

_____ colleagues in my discipline　　　　_____ care providers

_____ colleagues in other disciplines　　　_____ family members

_____ adults receiving care　　　　　　　_____ children receiving care

Take Home Message	Rationale for This Message From the Literature

Unit 5

Examining Evidence Related to Use of Compensatory Strategies to Enhance Participation

During this unit, you will explore some evidence about the use of compensatory strategies to support participation. Many times, professionals focus their attention on changing the person's skills and abilities so he or she can participate more effectively. Another option in intervention is to adjust environments and activities so that they are more "friendly" to the person; this enables successful participation as well.

We have two articles in this unit that inform our decisions about changing specific situations to support people's participation. Both articles studied application of compensatory strategies with people who have schizophrenia, but we could also study this topic with other populations and other age groups.

When you complete the work of this unit, you will have the following skills and competencies:

- Understand how this literature may contribute to effectiveness
- Articulate how to find other articles that would contribute to your knowledge about this topic

- Design an optimal plan for your area of practice based on what you have read
- Construct Take Home Messages for various constituents so they understand quickly what the literature says about the topic

You will be reviewing articles, creating summaries for comparison and contrast, gaining insights from your study partners, and creating Take Home Messages for constituent groups.

Activity 5-1

Reading the Literature

Read the following articles, which are included in the Appendix (Articles 14 and 15). These articles shed some light on use of compensatory strategies to support participation. For this exercise, focus on how they provided the supports and what measures they used to determine effectiveness.

Velligan, D. I., Bow-Thomas, C. C., Huntzinger, C., Ritch, J., Ledbetter, N., Prihoda, T. J., & Miller, A. L. (2000). Randomized controlled trial of the use of compensatory strategies to enhance adaptive functioning in outpatients with schizophrenia. American Journal of Psychiatry, 157(8), 1317-1323.

Velligan, D. I., Mueller, J., Wang, M., Dicocco, M., Diamond, P. M., Maples, N. J., & Davis, B. (2006). Use of environmental supports among patients with schizophrenia. Psychiatric Services, 57(2), 219-224.

Activity 5-2

Summarizing the Methods and Results of Research Articles

Create a summary (Worksheet 5A) for the articles listed in Activity 5-1.

Summary articles use tables to show readers the most important aspects of studies. Locate a summary article in an area of your interest and see how its tables are organized. Make an organizational table that suits your learning and information needs.

LOOKING FOR PATTERNS AND THEMES

First look for similarities and differences in the structures of the studies.

- Did they study the same populations?
- Did they use similar settings?
- Were the designs similar?
- How did the measures compare to each other?

The answer to these questions can help you understand differences in findings. For example, one study examined three conditions (Velligan et al., 2000) and the more recent study used two conditions (Velligan et al., 2006); you will need to consider why this change occurred. Did the earlier study inform this decision? In these studies, there are some similar and some unique measures; how do the measures lead to similar or different results?

Now, think about the topic.

- What happened to your thinking from before and after reading the articles?
- How did your ideas change?
- Have you observed that professionals have incorporated these findings into their practices?
- Are you going to do anything differently

now that your have read these studies?

These questions enable you to examine how the findings affected yours and others' thinking about practice. A great study that professionals are skeptical about will not have an impact on the practices; as professionals we need to understand the reasons why people may or may not adopt a strategy that has been shown effective through a research study.

Now consider what questions are answerable or unanswerable from these studies.

Activity 5-3

Recognizing the Strengths and Limitations of Research Articles

All research articles make a contribution and have limitations. Perhaps a group of articles is only about one age group and diagnosis; then we are not sure whether we can apply their findings to other age groups and other diagnoses. There will always be practice questions that can and cannot be answered by the available research. Sometimes researchers conduct studies about what can be answered; that does not mean that studies reflect the only important topics for practice. Perhaps there are no measures to find out the answer to an important practice question. It might be that a population is so heterogeneous that it is hard to detect changes or to discover who would or would not profit from an intervention. In practice, there will always be answerable and unanswerable questions. Advances in measurement, technology, and knowledge make more questions answerable.

Considering this group of articles, complete Worksheet 5B about the "answerable" and "unanswerable" questions for practice.

Activity 5-4

Handling Anomalous Data

The findings from these articles (Velligan et al., 2000, 2006) may challenge some of your current beliefs. Refer to your Executive Summary (see Sidebar 2-1) of the Chinn and Brewer (1993) article to decide where your reactions to the article findings are occurring (Worksheet 5C). Bring these issues up with your study partners.

Activity 5-5

Expanding the Evidence

Obtain another article (i.e., in the past 6 years) that adds information to your understanding about this topic. Add this citation, etc., to Worksheet 5A. Make copies of your article for your study partners.

Activity 5-6

Group Discussion

Meet with your study partners and discuss your findings and reactions to the articles listed in Activity 5-1. Add your unique information to the discussion from the article you are contributing on the topic. Refine your notes based on your discussion.

Here are some questions to get you started:

- Why do you think that the more recent study (Velligan et al., 2006) only used two conditions?
- How did two or three conditions affect the findings?
- Why do you think that the group receiving unrelated adaptations in the Velligan et al. (2000) study had such a high relapse rate compared to the others?
- How could you apply these findings to other populations?

Linking Evidence From Different Worlds

Sometimes you can find helpful information about a problem in practice in a place you wouldn't expect. For example, in this unit you are working on studies that show that creating specifically tailored cognitive adaptations increase a person's ability to participate. Both of these studies (Velligan et al., 2000, 2006) examine this concept in persons with schizophrenia. In Unit 4, you examined studies that tested the impact of assistive devices; some participants had physical impairments, others were older adults who needed some adaptations. If you are in a practice that serves people with severe mental illness, you may not think to look at the older adult or physical disability literature, and yet, there may be some helpful information in all these places for several areas of practice.

> ### Evidence Detective Tip
> You can combine findings from different topics and populations to gain a broader view.

Activity 5-7

Practice Linking Evidence Across Populations

Working with your study partners, identify themes from the two articles in this unit (Velligan et al., 2000, 2006) and the five articles from Unit 4 (Chiu & Man, 2004; Lund & Nygård, 2003; Mann et al., 2004, 2005; Stark, 2004). What are some common themes across all seven studies? What is a finding from one group that could inform (and hopefully improve!) the interventions for another group? For example, are there some findings from the cognitive adaptations studies that could improve an assistive device intervention for older adults? Complete Worksheet 5D on your own, and then meet with your study partners to discuss what each of you thought about. Take notes to refine your own thinking. Worksheet 5D has been started for you.

Activity 5-8

Developing Take Home Messages

The final step in the analysis process for evidence-based practice is to summarize the findings for those who need to use the ideas to improve their practices. Professionals want clear, easy-to-understand guidelines about what to do. We will call these summaries "Take Home Messages" to remind ourselves to use understandable language. You will need to consider Take Home Messages for your colleagues (within your discipline and from other disciplines), family members, other care providers, and those receiving your care.

Select two constituent groups as the focus of your attention and create some Take Home Messages for them. Pretend that the articles you read (Velligan et al., 2000, 2006) were the **definitive** articles on the topic. Use Worksheets 5E and 5F to summarize your work.

When considering what you are going to write, think about these questions:

- What would you say to colleagues about how they might need to change their practices to gain the optimal benefit?
- What would you say to your team regarding the articles' findings based on the articles you have read?
- How would you extrapolate information from these articles to develop hypotheses for populations other than the ones that were studied?

Summary

During this unit, you learned about the use of compensatory strategies to support participation. This evidence revealed the impact that changing environments and activities can have on participation. You also practiced integrating articles from this unit with the assistive device articles in Unit 4 to gain a broader evidence-based perspective.

All references for this unit can be found in the Bibliography, beginning on page 169.

Worksheet 5A

Summarizing Characteristics of Research

Citation	Participants	Setting	Measures	Design	Intervention	Findings	Notes
Study 1: Velligan et al. (2000)							
Study 2: Velligan et al. (2006)							
Study 3:							

Citation: Put the reference here.
Participants: List the important characteristics of participants.
Setting: Describe the location of the study.
Measures: List the outcome measures used in the study.
Design: Describe what type of comparisons or relationships are being tested/studied.
Intervention: List the most important aspects of the procedures being tested.
Findings: List the most important outcomes.
Notes: If you have insights or questions, jot them down.

Worksheet 5B
Writing Answerable and Unanswerable Questions

Write one question you can and one question you cannot answer from the studies in this unit. Discuss these with your study partners.

Answerable Question	What in the Article Enables You to Answer This Question?

Unanswerable Question	What Else Would We Need to Be Able to Answer This Question?

Worksheet 5C
Reactions to New Data

Think about your reactions to the articles. Based on Chinn and Brewer's (1993) ways of responding to anomalous data, what would you say your reaction illustrates?

Chinn and Brewer (1993) Responses	Example Reaction to the Findings
IGNORE the data (don't even bother to "explain" data away)	
REJECT the data (articulate an explanation for why data should be rejected)	
EXCLUDE the data from the domain of current beliefs (the data are outside the domain of current beliefs)	
Hold the data in ABEYANCE (I promise to deal with it later...assume that someday current beliefs will be articulated so that it can explain these data)	
REINTERPRET the data while retaining current beliefs (accept the data as something that should be explained by current beliefs...opposing forces accept data but interpret the data differently based on their own beliefs)	
Reinterpret the data and make PERIPHERAL CHANGES to current belief (make a relatively minor change to current belief...accepts the data but is unwilling to give up current belief and accept new beliefs)	
Accept the data and CHANGE current beliefs, possibly in favor of a particular new belief (change one or more of the core aspects of current beliefs—when faced with information that is contradictory to current beliefs, accepts alternate beliefs)	

Worksheet 5D
Looking at Themes Across Studies

Part 1: Looking for Common Concepts Across Studies

Concept That Occurs Across Studies	Where That Concept Comes From
Specifically focused training with adaptations leads to better utilization	*Cognitive adaptation training on specific needs yielded more improvements (Velligan et al., 2000)* *Group with home-based training in devices after discharge had better outcomes (Chiu & Man, 2004)* *Removing environmental barriers significantly improved performance (Stark, 2004)*

Worksheet 5D (Continued)
Looking at Themes Across Studies

Part 2: Looking for Ways to Extend Knowledge
From One Area of Practice to Another

Concept From Study...	That Can Be Joined With Another Study Finding	...That Would Improve Intervention to Another Group
Specific training in adaptations and devices improves function and use (Velligan et al., 2000, 2006)	Older adults use the telephone socially, but don't know about additional features that could be helpful (Mann et al., 2005)	So, we could do specific training in the additional features of the phone that would improve communication and safety, and perhaps more older adults would access these options successfully

Worksheet 5E
Take Home Messages for Group 1

Pretend that the articles you just read are the definitive articles about the topic. Develop Take Home Messages showing what you would say to a particular constituent group regarding the topic based on the articles you have read.

Take Home Messages About:

Name:

These messages are for:

_____ colleagues in my discipline

_____ colleagues in other disciplines

_____ adults receiving care

_____ care providers

_____ family members

_____ children receiving care

Take Home Message	Rationale for This Message From the Literature

Worksheet 5F
Take Home Messages for Group 2

Pretend that the articles you just read are the definitive articles about the topic. Develop Take Home Messages showing what you would say to a particular constituent group regarding the topic based on the articles you have read.

Take Home Messages About:

Name:

These messages are for:

_____ colleagues in my discipline   _____ care providers

_____ colleagues in other disciplines   _____ family members

_____ adults receiving care   _____ children receiving care

Take Home Message	Rationale for This Message From the Literature

Unit 6

Examining Evidence Related to Caregiving

During this unit, you will explore some evidence about how caregiving affects people. This topic is interesting because we can study it across age groups and diagnoses. Many situations require someone to be a caregiver; for example, adults care for their own children, their partners, and their parents. In your practice you are likely to encounter people who are providing everyday care for someone you are serving in your professional role. Even though many systems require us to focus on a specific person who has an injury, disease, or disability, in order to provide best practice care, we must also understand how to support and guide the friends and family who are or will be responsible for the target person in their everyday lives.

So, what does the literature tell us about the experience of caregiving? With these insights, what will we need to change about our approach to those providing care as a means for supporting the person we are serving?

I hope you are also curious about what you will find. Perhaps you are wondering whether people caring for adults have the same issues as people caring for children. Perhaps you want to know about caregiving that spans a short or long period of time. Jot down your ideas before you read; this will enable you to reflect on the literature in a more specific way.

When you complete the work in this unit, you will have the following skills and competencies:

- Understand how caregiver literature may contribute to your effectiveness for serving the person and their friends and family
- Recognize themes in diverse literature that suggest enduring themes related to caregiving
- Articulate how to find other articles that would contribute to your knowledge about this topic
- Design an optimal plan for your area of practice based on what you have read
- Construct Take Home Messages for various constituents so they understand quickly what the literature says about caregiving

You will be reviewing articles, creating summaries for comparison and contrast, gaining insights from your study partners, and creating Take Home Messages for constituent groups.

Activity 6-1

Reading the Literature

Read the articles listed below, which are located in the Appendix (Articles 16 through 18). These articles shed some light on the experience of caregiving. For this unit, focus on the issues of barriers and solutions that caregivers report about their experiences.

Larson, E. (2006). *Caregiving and autism: How does children's propensity for routinization influence participation in family activities?* Occupational Therapy Journal of Research: Occupation, Participation and Health, 26(2), 69-79.

McGuire, B. K., Crowe, T. K., Law, M., & VanLeit, B. (2004). *Mothers of children with disabilities: Occupational concerns and solutions.* Occupational Therapy Journal of Research: Occupation, Participation and Health, 24(2), 54-63.

Vikström, S., Borell, L., Stigsdotter-Neely, A., & Josephsson, S. (2005). *Caregivers' self-initiated support toward their partners with dementia when performing an everyday occupation together at home.* Occupational Therapy Journal of Research: Occupation, Participation and Health, 25(34), 149-159.

Activity 6-2

Summarizing the Methods and Results of Research Articles

Create a summary (Worksheet 6A) for the articles listed in Activity 6-1.

Summary articles use tables to show readers the most important aspects of studies. Locate a summary article in an area of your interest and see how its tables are organized. Make an organizational table that suits your learning and information needs.

LOOKING FOR PATTERNS AND THEMES

First look for similarities and differences in the structures of the studies.
- Did they study the same populations?
- Did they use similar settings?

- Were the designs similar?
- How did the measures compare to each other?

The answer to these questions can help you understand differences in findings. For example, if one study says an intervention worked and another study says it did not, you will need to examine these other factors to see what might have contributed to the differences. One study might have examined caregiving of children and another about caregiving of adults. You can then hypothesize that the intervention is only effective with a certain group or when outcomes are measured in a certain way.

Now, think about the topic.
- What happened to your thinking from before and after reading the articles?
- How did your ideas change?
- Have you observed that professionals have incorporated these findings into their practices?
- Are you going to do anything differently now that your have read these studies?

Now consider what questions are answerable or unanswerable from these studies.

Activity 6-3

Recognizing the Strengths and Limitations of Research Articles

All research articles make a contribution and have limitations. Perhaps a group of articles is only about one age group and diagnosis; then we are not sure whether we can apply their findings to other age groups and other diagnoses. There will always be practice questions that can and cannot be answered by the available research. Sometimes researchers conduct studies about what can be answered; that does not mean that studies reflect the only important topics for practice. Perhaps there are no measures to find out the answer to an important practice question. It might be that a population is so heterogeneous that it is hard to detect changes or to discover who would or would not profit from an intervention. In practice, there will always be answerable and unanswerable questions. Advances in measurement, technology, and knowledge make more questions answerable.

Considering this group of articles (Larson, 2006; McGuire et al., 2004; Vikström et al., 2005), complete Worksheet 6B about the "answerable" and "unanswerable" questions for practice.

Activity 6-4

Handling Anomalous Data

The findings from these articles (Larson, 2006; McGuire et al., 2004; Vikström et al., 2005) may challenge some of your current beliefs. Refer to your Executive Summary (see Sidebar 2-1) of the Chinn and Brewer (1993) article to decide where your reactions to the article findings are occurring (Worksheet 6C). Bring these issues up with your study partners.

Activity 6-5

Expanding the Evidence

Obtain another article (i.e., in the past 6 years) that adds information to your understanding about this topic. Add this citation, etc., to your summary worksheet (Worksheet 6A). Make copies of your article for your study partners.

Activity 6-6

Group Discussion

Meet with your study partners and discuss your findings and reactions to the articles listed in Activity 6-1. Add your unique information to the discussion from the article you are contributing on the topic. Refine your notes based on your discussion.

These studies were descriptive in nature and so they illuminated our understanding about the experience of caregiving. One of the studies was about caring for adults and the others were about caring for children; your additional studies likely covered the life span as well. The three original studies also covered many disabilities, and yet we could identify common themes within the caregiving experience. Discuss your thoughts and insights with your study partners.

EXTENDING KNOWLEDGE ABOUT METHODS AND RESULTS

In each unit of Section II, each set of articles reflects an overall topic. Additionally, each article illustrates some unique features of studies and ways to report the methods and findings. By examining some aspects of each study, you will accumulate knowledge about designs and statistics while learning more about the evidence. This process will build your capacity as an evidence-based professional because when you encounter other articles with similar features, you will know how to use the information in your decision making.

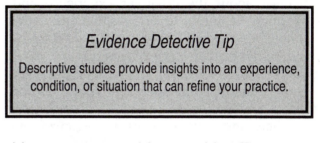

Evidence Detective Tip

Descriptive studies provide insights into an experience, condition, or situation that can refine your practice.

UNDERSTANDING HOW TO USE EVIDENCE FROM DESCRIPTIVE STUDIES

You will notice that the three articles on caregiving (Larson, 2006; McGuire et al., 2004; Vikström et al., 2005) are not intervention studies; they are all descriptive studies. Although they don't explicitly tell us about an intervention, they provide us with insights that guide our thinking about how to approach caregivers and what might be on caregivers' minds. From articles like these, we might work with our colleagues to develop a list of questions to ask the caregivers. We might also keep articles like these in a file to share with caregivers so they can learn what is universal about their experiences.

Each of these studies reported themes they derived from their interviews and discussions. Let's take a little time to look at the themes in more detail. We will use a similar process to the ones the authors used when looking at their interview data.

Activity 6-7

Identifying the Themes

Make a list of the themes reported from each study (Larson, 2006; McGuire et al., 2004;

Vikström et al., 2005) using Worksheets 6D and 6E. When you see something reported in more than one study, write down the concept or idea in the first column of the worksheet. Jot down what each author had to say about that concept. Go back to the first column and write a short rationale for clustering these themes together. Keep doing this until you don't see any more concepts that they share. Then look at unique concepts from each article: do you think these unique features are related to the way the researchers conducted their study, are they about the population, or something else?

This process helps you to see what may be universal about the caregiver experience and what might be unique to certain situations. In the example provided on Worksheet 6D, you'll see all three studies contain some discussion about caregivers feeling a lack of support for their caregiver role. Quotations from caregivers could also be added for validation.

There are several ways to organize the themes from these studies; there is not one way that is correct. When you meet with your study partners, share your different ways of organizing the themes and discuss how you identified these themes.

Activity 6-8

Addressing the Themes

Think about how you might address some of the common themes in your practice. For example, since we saw a theme of "lack of support," what might you put into place ahead of time to ensure that caregivers don't encounter this feeling? Be prepared to discuss your strategies with your study partners.

Activity 6-9

Developing Take Home Messages

The final step in the analysis process for evidence-based practice is to summarize the findings for those who need to use the ideas to improve their practices. Professionals want clear, easy-to-understand guidelines about what to do. We will call these summaries "Take Home Messages" to remind ourselves to use understandable language. You will need to consider Take Home Messages for your colleagues (within your discipline and from other disciplines), family members, other care providers, and those receiving your care.

Select two constituent groups as the focus of your attention and create some Take Home Messages for them. Pretend that the articles you read (Larson, 2006; McGuire et al., 2004; Vikström et al., 2005) were the **definitive** articles on the topic. Use Worksheets 6F and 6G to summarize your work.

When considering what you are going to write, think about these questions:

- What would you say to colleagues about how they might need to change their practices to gain the optimal benefit?
- What would you say to your team regarding the articles' findings based on the articles you have read?
- How would you extrapolate information from these articles to develop hypotheses for other populations than the ones that were studied?

SUMMARY

In this unit, you learned about the experience of caregiving. The articles were descriptive in nature, and so provided a picture of caregiving from various points of view. These perspectives are useful to professionals in practice because they remind us about all the people we serve.

All references for this unit can be found in the Bibliography, beginning on page 169.

Worksheet 6A

Summarizing Characteristics of Research

Citation	Participants	Setting	Measures	Design	Intervention	Findings	Notes
Study 1: Larson (2006)							
Study 2: McGuire et al. (2004)							
Study 3: Vikström et al. (2005)							
Study 4:							

Citation: Put the reference here.
Participants: List the important characteristics of participants.
Setting: Describe the location of the study.
Measures: List the outcome measures used in the study.
Design: Describe what type of comparisons or relationships are being tested/studied.
Intervention: List the most important aspects of the procedures being tested.
Findings: List the most important outcomes.
Notes: If you have insights or questions, jot them down.

Worksheet 6B
Writing Answerable and Unanswerable Questions

Write one question you can and one question you cannot answer from the studies in this unit. Discuss these with your study partners.

Answerable Question	What in the Article Enables You to Answer This Question?
Unanswerable Question	What Else Would We Need to Be Able to Answer This Question?

Worksheet 6C
Reactions to New Data

Think about your reactions to the articles. Based on Chinn and Brewer's (1993) ways of responding to anomalous data, what would you say your reaction illustrates?

Chinn and Brewer (1993) Responses	Example Reaction to the Findings
IGNORE the data (don't even bother to "explain" data away)	
REJECT the data (articulate an explanation for why data should be rejected)	
EXCLUDE the data from the domain of current beliefs (the data are outside the domain of current beliefs)	
Hold the data in ABEYANCE (I promise to deal with it later...assume that someday current beliefs will be articulated so that it can explain these data)	
REINTERPRET the data while retaining current beliefs (accept the data as something that should be explained by current beliefs...opposing forces accept data but interpret the data differently based on their own beliefs)	
Reinterpret the data and make PERIPHERAL CHANGES to current belief (make a relatively minor change to current belief...accepts the data but is unwilling to give up current belief and accept new beliefs)	
Accept the data and CHANGE current beliefs, possibly in favor of a particular new belief (change one or more of the core aspects of current beliefs—when faced with information that is contradictory to current beliefs, accepts alternate beliefs)	

Worksheet 6D
Finding Similarities in Conceptual Themes

Concept/Theme and Rationale for Decision	Study 1: Larson (2006)	Study 2: McGuire et al. (2004)	Study 3: Vikström et al. (2005)
Need for support (they all felt alone or abandoned somehow)	*Inappropriate, inadequate, no support*	*Inadequate support*	*Lack of understanding from others*

Worksheet 6E
Examining the Unique Themes in Caregiving

In the boxes, enter the unique concepts to one study and your hypothesis about why this happened.

Study	Unique Concept Presented in the Study	Why Was This Concept Presented Only in This Study?
Study 1: Larson (2006)		
Study 2: McGuire et al. (2004)		
Study 3: Vikström et al. (2005)		

Worksheet 6F
Take Home Messages for Group 1

Pretend that the articles you just read are the definitive articles about the topic. Develop Take Home Messages showing what you would say to a particular constituent group regarding the topic based on the articles you have read.

Take Home Messages About:

Name:

These messages are for:

_____ colleagues in my discipline   _____ care providers

_____ colleagues in other disciplines   _____ family members

_____ adults receiving care   _____ children receiving care

Take Home Message	Rationale for This Message From the Literature

Worksheet 6G
Take Home Messages for Group 2

Pretend that the articles you just read are the definitive articles about the topic. Develop Take Home Messages showing what you would say to a particular constituent group regarding the topic based on the articles you have read.

Take Home Messages About:

Name:

These messages are for:

_____ colleagues in my discipline   _____ care providers

_____ colleagues in other disciplines   _____ family members

_____ adults receiving care   _____ children receiving care

Take Home Message	Rationale for This Message From the Literature

Unit 7

Examining Evidence Related to Applying Sensory Processing Knowledge in Context

During this unit, you will explore some evidence about how to apply sensory processing knowledge within children's natural contexts. You will see when you review the summary article by Baranek (2002) (see Unit 10) that the data suggest that generalization occurs when knowledge is applied within children's daily life. This unit will give you a good start on how one might accomplish this goal.

When you complete the work of this unit, you will have the following skills and competencies:

- Understand how this literature may contribute to evidence-based practice
- Articulate how to find other articles that would contribute to your knowledge about this topic
- Design an optimal plan for your area of practice based on what you have read
- Construct Take Home Messages for various constituents so they understand quickly what the literature says about the topic

You will be reviewing articles, creating summaries for comparison and contrast, gaining insights from your study partners, and creating Take Home Messages for constituent groups.

Activity 7-1

Reading the Literature

Please obtain and read the articles listed below. These articles shed some light on applying sensory processing knowledge within everyday contexts.

Edelson, S., Edelson, M., Kerr, D., & Grandin, T. (1999). *Behavioral and physiological effects of deep pressure on children with autism: A pilot study evaluating the efficacy of Grandin's hug machine.* American Journal of Occupational Therapy, 53, *145-152.*

Fertel-Daly, D., Bedell, G., & Hinojosa, J. (2001). *Effects of a weighted vest on attention to task and self-stimulatory behaviors in preschoolers with pervasive developmental disorders.* American Journal of Occupational Therapy, 55, *629-640.*

Schilling, D., Washington, K., Billingsley, F., & Deitz, J. (2003). *Classroom seating for children with attention deficit hyperactivity disorder: Therapy balls versus chairs.* American Journal of Occupational Therapy, 57, 534-541.

VandenBerg, N. (2001). *The use of a weighted vest to increase on-task behavior in children with attention difficulties.* American Journal of Occupational Therapy, 55(6), 621-628.

Activity 7-2

Summarizing the Methods and Results of Research Articles

Create a summary (Worksheet 7A) for the articles listed in Activity 7-1.

Summary articles use tables to show readers the most important aspects of studies. Locate a summary article in an area of your interest and see how its tables are organized. Make an organizational table that suits your learning and information needs.

Looking for Patterns and Themes

First look for similarities and differences in the structures of the studies.

- Did they study the same populations?
- Did they use similar settings?
- Were the designs similar?
- How did the measures compare to each other?

The answer to these questions can help you understand differences in findings. For example, if one study examined preschoolers and another study examined school-aged children, you will need to consider whether the interventions are helpful across these age groups. In these studies, there are different amounts of weight applied to the vests; if there are differences in the findings, we might hypothesize about the influence of the weight of the vests on the outcomes reported.

Now, think about the topic.

- What happened to your thinking from before and after reading the articles?
- How did your ideas change?
- Have you observed that professionals have incorporated these findings into their practices?
- Are you going to do anything differently now that you have read these studies?

These questions enable you to examine how the findings affected yours and others' thinking about practice. A great study that professionals are skeptical about will not have an impact on practice; as professionals we need to understand the reasons why people may or may not adopt a strategy that has been shown effective through a research study.

Now consider what questions are answerable or unanswerable from these studies.

Activity 7-3

Recognizing the Strengths and Limitations of Research Articles

All research articles make a contribution and have limitations. Perhaps a group of articles is only about one age group and diagnosis; then we are not sure whether we can apply their findings to other age groups and other diagnoses. There will always be practice questions that can and cannot be answered by the available research. Sometimes researchers conduct studies about what can be answered; that does not mean that studies reflect the only important topics for practice. Perhaps there are no measures to find out the answer to an important practice question. It might be that a population is so heterogeneous that it is hard to detect changes or to discover who would or would not profit from an intervention. In practice, there will always be answerable and unanswerable questions. Advances in measurement, technology, and knowledge make more questions answerable.

Considering the group of articles listed in Activity 7-1, complete Worksheet 7B about the "answerable" and "unanswerable" questions for practice.

Activity 7-4

Handling Anomalous Data

The findings from these articles (Edelson et al., 1999; Fertel-Daly et al., 2001; Schilling et al., 2003; VandenBerg, 2001) may challenge some of your current beliefs. Refer to your Executive Summary (see Sidebar 2-1) of the Chinn and Brewer (1993) article to decide where your reactions to the article findings are occurring (Worksheet 7C). Bring these issues up with your study partners.

Activity 7-5

Expanding the Evidence

Obtain another article (i.e., in the past 6 years) that adds information to your understanding about this topic. Add this citation, etc., to your summary worksheet (Worksheet 7A). Make copies of your article for your study partners.

Activity 7-6

Group Discussion

Meet with your study partners and discuss your findings and reactions to the articles listed in Activity 7-1. Add your unique information to the discussion from the article you are contributing on the topic. Refine your notes based on your discussion.

EXTENDING KNOWLEDGE ABOUT THE RESEARCH ARTICLES

In each unit of Section II, each set of articles reflects an overall topic. Additionally, each article illustrates some unique features of studies and ways to report the methods and findings. By examining some aspects of each study, you will accumulate knowledge about designs and statistics while learning more about the evidence. This process will build your capacity as an evidence-based professional because when you encounter other articles with similar features, you will know how to use the information in your decision making.

COMPARING THE CHARACTERISTICS OF AN INTERVENTION

Two of the studies in this unit are testing the impact of using a weighted vest on children's participation (Fertel-Daly et al., 2001; VandenBerg, 2001). Although they both use the weighted vest as their intervention, they use different criteria to apply this intervention. This occurs frequently across studies that on first consideration seem to be about the same intervention. Let's analyze the similarities and differences between these interventions.

Activity 7-7

Comparing Intervention Characteristics

Complete Worksheet 7D by reviewing the descriptions in the studies (Fertel-Daly et al., 2001; VandenBerg, 2001). One idea is provided to get you started.

Evidence Detective Tip

When you compare the characteristics of an intervention across studies, you learn what parameters of that intervention might matter for your practice.

EXAMINING THE KEY POINTS IN THE INTRODUCTION

These studies (Edelson et al., 1999; Fertel-Daly et al., 2001; Schilling et al., 2003; VandenBerg, 2001) are testing the effectiveness of applying touch pressure and proprioception input within children's daily routines to improve their participation. The purpose of the Introduction is to build a case for the study; therefore, there should be some common themes among these studies in building a case for their research projects.

Activity 7-8

Comparing References and Concepts

Meet with your study partners to complete Worksheets 7E and 7F. Discuss what one group of authors might have included to strengthen their arguments and build their case. We have provided you with an example in each worksheet to get you started.

Evidence Detective Tip

You can search for related articles using a reference the articles have in common.

LEARNING HOW TO INTEGRATE FINDINGS ACROSS STUDIES

These studies (Edelson et al., 1999; Fertel-Daly et al., 2001; Schilling et al., 2003; Vanden-Berg, 2001) investigated different ways to provide touch pressure and proprioception within children's daily routines. The researchers wanted to find out whether they could apply knowledge about how the sensory systems work to support performance. This is what ties these articles together. One might not consider weighted vests, ball chairs, and a hug machine as a homogeneous group of interventions, but when you understand the researchers' underlying beliefs and hypotheses, they have a lot in common with each other. Activity 7-8 illustrates the common themes of touch pressure and proprioception; the fact that the authors used different interventions becomes less important when you understand the themes.

The studies also used small numbers of participants, so one could say the evidence isn't very large. The advantage of this group of studies is that they are accumulating similar findings across children of different ages and diagnoses. The studies suggest that professionals who understand the underlying concepts of touch pressure and proprioception can identify ways to provide these inputs during the course of the day in a way that supports children to participate more successfully.

Activity 7-9

Group Discussion

Thinking across these studies (Edelson et al., 1999; Fertel-Daly et al., 2001; Schilling et al., 2003; VandenBerg, 2001), identify some other everyday interventions you could use that would support a person's participation with touch pressure and proprioception. How could you collect data in persons' everyday lives to document whether or not your idea was working?

Activity 7-10

Developing Take Home Messages

The final step in the analysis process for evidence-based practice is to summarize the findings for those who need to use the ideas to improve their practices. Professionals want clear, easy-to-understand guidelines about what to do. We will call these summaries "Take Home Messages" to remind ourselves to use understandable language. You will need to consider Take Home Messages for your colleagues (within your discipline and from other disciplines), family members, other care providers, and those receiving your care.

Select two constituent groups as the focus of your attention and create some Take Home Messages for them. Pretend that the articles you read (Edelson et al., 1999; Fertel-Daly et al., 2001; Schilling et al., 2003; VandenBerg, 2001) were the **definitive** articles on the topic. Use Worksheets 7G and 7H to summarize your work.

When considering what you are going to write, think about these questions:

- What would you say to colleagues about how they might need to change their practices to gain the optimal benefit?
- What would you say to your team regarding the articles' findings based on the articles you have read?
- How would you extrapolate information from these articles to develop hypotheses for populations other than the ones that were studied?

SUMMARY

In this unit, you studied research that illustrated how to apply theoretically sound principles in everyday practice. Although each study was small, by grounding their ideas and decisions in theory, the authors illustrated how to look across studies to see patterns of effective practice.

All references for this unit can be found in the Bibliography, beginning on page 169.

Worksheet 7A

Summarizing Characteristics of Research

Citation	Participants	Setting	Measures	Design	Intervention	Findings	Notes
Study 1: Edelson et al. (1999)							
Study 2: Fertel-Daly et al. (2001)							
Study 3: Schilling et al. (2003)							
Study 4: VandenBerg (2001)							
Study 5:							

Citation: Put the reference here.
Participants: List the important characteristics of participants.
Setting: Describe the location of the study.
Measures: List the outcome measures used in the study.
Design: Describe what type of comparisons or relationships are being tested/studied.
Intervention: List the most important aspects of the procedures being tested.
Findings: List the most important outcomes.
Notes: If you have insights or questions, jot them down.

Worksheet 7B
Writing Answerable and Unanswerable Questions

Write one question you can and one question you cannot answer from the studies in this unit. Discuss these with your study partners.

Answerable Question	What in the Article Enables You to Answer This Question?
Unanswerable Question	**What Else Would We Need to Be Able to Answer This Question?**

Worksheet 7C
Reactions to New Data

Think about your reactions to the articles. Based on Chinn and Brewer's (1993) ways of responding to anomalous data, what would you say your reaction illustrates?

Chinn and Brewer (1993) Responses	Example Reaction to the Findings
IGNORE the data (don't even bother to "explain" data away)	
REJECT the data (articulate an explanation for why data should be rejected)	
EXCLUDE the data from the domain of current beliefs (the data are outside the domain of current beliefs)	
Hold the data in ABEYANCE (I promise to deal with it later...assume that someday current beliefs will be articulated so that it can explain these data)	
REINTERPRET the data while retaining current beliefs (accept the data as something that should be explained by current beliefs...opposing forces accept data but interpret the data differently based on their own beliefs)	
Reinterpret the data and make PERIPHERAL CHANGES to current belief (make a relatively minor change to current belief...accepts the data but is unwilling to give up current belief and accept new beliefs)	
Accept the data and CHANGE current beliefs, possibly in favor of a particular new belief (change one or more of the core aspects of current beliefs—when faced with information that is contradictory to current beliefs, accepts alternate beliefs)	

Worksheet 7D
Comparing Characteristics of Interventions

Characteristic of Weighted Vest Intervention	Fertel-Daly et al. (2001)	VandenBerg (2001)
Weight of vest	1 pound of weight	5% of body weight

Comparing the Reference Lists of Articles

Bibliography/ References in Common	Edelson et al. (1999)	Fertel-Daly et al. (2001)	Schilling et al. (2003)	VandenBerg (2001)
McClure et al. (1991)	**X**	**X**		**X**

Worksheet 7F
Comparing Introduction Concepts in Articles

Concepts Reflected in Introductions	Edelson et al. (1999)	Fertel-Daly et al. (2001)	Schilling et al. (2003)	VandenBerg (2001)
Deep pressure has a calming effect	Deep pressure can reduce anxiety	Deep pressure has a calming effect		Deep pressure provides a calming effect

Worksheet 7G
Take Home Messages for Group 1

Pretend that the articles you just read are the definitive articles about the topic. Develop Take Home Messages showing what you would say to a particular constituent group regarding the topic based on the articles you have read.

Take Home Messages About:

Name:

These messages are for:

_____ colleagues in my discipline

_____ colleagues in other disciplines

_____ adults receiving care

_____ care providers

_____ family members

_____ children receiving care

Take Home Message	Rationale for This Message From the Literature

Worksheet 7H
Take Home Messages for Group 2

Pretend that the articles you just read are the definitive articles about the topic. Develop Take Home Messages showing what you would say to a particular constituent group regarding the topic based on the articles you have read.

Take Home Messages About:

Name:

These messages are for:

_____ colleagues in my discipline   _____ care providers

_____ colleagues in other disciplines   _____ family members

_____ adults receiving care   _____ children receiving care

Take Home Message	Rationale for This Message From the Literature

Unit 8

Examining Evidence Related to Constraint-Induced Therapy Interventions

During this unit, you will explore some evidence about constraint-induced therapy interventions. There is a growing body of evidence about constraint-induced therapy, so it is important for professionals providing service in rehabilitation to know what these researchers are finding and recommending for practice.

The articles you will review in this unit have some other features that will expand your understanding about how to read research papers; we will practice analyzing these features to give you some experience with the internal structure of research articles.

When you complete the work in this unit, you will have the following skills and competencies:

- Understand how this literature may contribute to our knowledge about effective interventions
- Articulate how to find other articles that would contribute to your knowledge about the subject
- Identify the parameters that seem to make the intervention effective and/or

ineffective based on the evidence you have read
- Design an optimal plan for your area of practice based on what you have read
- Construct Take Home Messages for various constituents so they understand quickly what the literature says about the subject

You will be reviewing articles, creating summaries for comparison and contrast, gaining insights from your study partners, and creating Take Home Messages for constituent groups.

Activity 8-1

Reading the Literature

Read the following articles. The Flinn et al. (2005) and Karman et al. (2003) articles are located in the Appendix (Articles 19 and 20). You will have to obtain the Bonifer et al. (2005) article on your own.

Bonifer, N., Anderson, K., & Arciniegas, D. (2005). *Constraint-induced movement therapy after stroke: Efficacy for patients with minimal upper-extremity motor ability.* Archives of Physical Medicine and Rehabilitation, 86, 1867-1873.

Flinn, N. A., Schamburg, S., Fetrow, J. M., & Flanigan, J. (2005). *The effect of constraint-induced movement treatment on occupational performance and satisfaction in stroke survivors.* Occupational Therapy Journal of Research: Occupation, Participation and Health, 25(3), 119-127.

Karman, N., Maryles, J., Baker, R. W., Simpser, E., & Berger-Gross, P. (2003). *Constraint-induced movement therapy for hemiplegic children with acquired brain injuries.* Journal of Head Trauma Rehabilitation, 18(3), 259-267.

These articles shed some light on the effectiveness of constraint-induced therapy. For this exercise, you will focus on methods used, meaning of the results, and the format of the papers from different journals.

The articles are from interdisciplinary literature and provide insights for professionals in several disciplines. Don't get bogged down in technical details, rather, look at the overall procedures and outcomes. When reading interdisciplinary literature in refereed journals, there must be some level of confidence that the blind review process led to presentation of reasonable procedures to test the hypotheses.

Activity 8-2

Summarizing the Methods and Results of Research Articles

Create a summary (Worksheet 8A) for the articles listed in Activity 8-1.

Summary articles use tables to show readers the most important aspects of studies. Locate a summary article in an area of your interest and see how its tables are organized. Make an organizational table that suits your learning and information needs.

LOOKING FOR PATTERNS AND THEMES

First look for similarities and differences in the structure of the studies (your worksheet will help you because you can look across studies quickly).

- Did they study the same populations?
- Did they use similar settings?
- Were the designs similar?
- How did the measures compare to each other?

The answers to these questions can help you understand differences in findings. For example, these studies (Bonifer et al., 2005; Flinn et al., 2005; Karman et al., 2003) used different amounts of time for restraining movements. What does this mean as you think about evidence-based use of constraint-induced movement? One of the studies involved children; how does this enable generalization? What do the studies have in common? You can use the patterns you see to begin formulating hypotheses for your practice.

Now, think about the topic.

- What happened to your thinking from before and after reading the articles?
- How did your ideas change?
- Have you observed that professionals have incorporated these findings into their practices?
- Are you going to do anything differently now that your have read these studies?

Be prepared to discuss your ideas and queries with your study partners.

Now consider what questions are answerable or unanswerable from these studies.

Activity 8-3

Recognizing the Strengths and Limitations of Research Articles

All research articles make a contribution and have limitations. Perhaps a group of articles is only about one age group and diagnosis; then we are not sure whether we can apply their findings to other age groups and other diagnoses. There will always be practice questions that can and cannot be answered by the available research. Sometimes researchers conduct studies about what can be answered; that does not mean that studies reflect the only important topics for practice. Perhaps there are no measures to find out the answer to an important practice question. It might be that a population is so heterogeneous that it is hard to detect changes or to discover who would or would not benefit from an intervention. In practice, there will always be answerable and unanswerable questions. Advances in measurement, technology, and knowledge make more questions answerable.

Considering this group of articles (Bonifer et al., 2005; Flinn et al., 2005; Karman et al., 2003), complete Worksheet 8B about the "answerable" and "unanswerable" questions for practice.

Activity 8-4

Handling Anomalous Data

The findings from the articles listed in Activity 8-1 may challenge some of your current beliefs. Refer to your Executive Summary (see Sidebar 2-1) of the Chinn and Brewer (1993) article to decide where your reactions to the article findings are occurring (Worksheet 8C). Bring these issues up with your study partners.

Be prepared to discuss the ideas you have with your study partners. Consider what you might say to someone with each of the responses if you were in a conversation.

Activity 8-5

Expanding the Evidence

Obtain another recent article (i.e., in the past 6 years) that adds information to your understanding about this topic. Add this citation, etc., to your summary worksheet (Worksheet 8A). Make copies of your article for your study partners.

Activity 8-6

Group Discussion

Meet with your study partners and discuss your findings and reactions to the articles (Bonifer et al., 2005; Flinn et al., 2005; Karman et al., 2003). Add your unique information to the discussion from the article you are contributing on the topic. Refine your notes based on your discussion.

EXTENDING KNOWLEDGE ABOUT METHODS AND RESULTS

In each unit of Section II, each set of articles reflects an overall topic. Additionally, each article illustrates some unique features of studies and ways to report the methods and findings. By examining some aspects of each study, you will accumulate knowledge about designs and statistics while learning more about the evidence. This process will build your capacity as an evidence-based professional because when you encounter other articles with similar features, you will know how to use the information in your decision making.

The constraint-induced therapy articles you have read in this unit provide an opportunity to learn about other characteristics of articles. In the Methods section, Bonifer et al. (2005) have no subheadings; the other two studies (Flinn et al., 2005; Karman et al., 2003) both use subheadings to alert the reader to the components (e.g., Participants, Measures). This difference is likely related to the format and traditions of these journals. Although subheadings are user friendly for readers, they take up precious space. How does this difference affect you as a consumer of the studies?

UNDERSTANDING DATA IN TABLES AND FIGURES

The Bonifer et al. (2005) article contains tables and figures that help illustrate their findings for the reader. These authors provide information about their findings in three ways. First they provide a summary of the means and standard deviations for their measures at each time point in Table 2. This is a common type of table for a study like this. Second, they report in the text which comparisons are significant. Third, they take some of the information from Table 2 and graph it for you in the figures. Let's use Figure 1 in Bonifer et al. as an example. This figure shows visually the comparisons of the means and standard deviations of the FM totals (see second line on Table 2). Pre-treatment mean is 84. The standard deviation is 10.75. This is what they graphed in the first box and whisker plot. The dot in the center of the first box is at 84; the "whiskers" extend 10.75 in each direction. The next box and whisker corresponds to the post-treatment scores, and the third one illustrates the 1-month follow-up scores (follow across line 2 of Table 2).

If you now refer to the Bonifer et al. text (2005, pp. 1869-1870), you will see that they report a significant difference between pre-treatment and post-treatment. The graph illustrates the magnitude of this change (i.e., comparing the first and second box and whisker plots on Figure 1). They also report no additional changes between post-treatment and follow-up (i.e., comparing the second and third box and whisker plots on Figure 1); this finding indicates that participants maintained the improvement, which is a good finding and you can see the similarity on the graph. Many authors only report the numbers and significance without the graph. Now that you see this example, you can always make a graph like this for yourself using data from any article (using the mean and standard deviation) if a figure would help you see the comparison better.

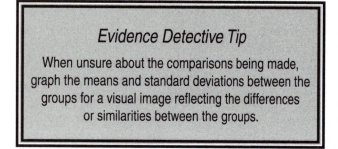

Evidence Detective Tip

When unsure about the comparisons being made, graph the means and standard deviations between the groups for a visual image reflecting the differences or similarities between the groups.

Activity 8-7

Practice With Your Study Partners

Work with your study partners to examine Figures 2 and 3 in Bonifer et al. (2005). Which lines of data from Table 2 are illustrated in these figures? What paragraphs in the text give you the significance data for these comparisons? Why are there only two box and whisker plots on Figure 2?

Now let's look at the Karman et al. (2003) figures. These authors selected a different way to illustrate their data. They stacked their post-test levels on top of the pretest amounts for each child. They are showing you each individual participant, rather than showing you a summary of all the participants, as the box and whisker plots showed in the previous study. You have to look in the text (Results section and Figure 1) to see which children's changes meet the significance criteria. Note that subjects 1 and 2 (see Figure 1) had more use to start with; perhaps the intervention was more helpful for those with lower baseline movement.

The Flinn et al. (2005) article also used graphs to illustrate their findings. Instead of stacking

their pre/post data, they made three bars for each participant (see Figures 1 and 2).

Activity 8-8

Practice With Your Study Partners

Discuss which graphing strategy you like the most/least. Which article provided the clearest link between the numeric data and the illustrations? What was unclear? What suggestions would you make to improve one or all of these articles?

UNDERSTANDING UNFAMILIAR MEASURES

The Karman et al. (2003) study used a measure that may not be familiar to readers. The authors give readers references for learning more about the measure, and then they provide an informative summary so readers can evaluate their findings. They provide six examples of the tasks (e.g., folding paper, opening a box), and then provide tables showing the rating scales. This strategy enables readers to imagine what happened in the study, and then decide whether the measure would be applicable to a practice population (Could the children I serve do these tasks? What would they look like when doing them?).

LEARNING MORE ABOUT INTERVENTIONS

Each of these studies (Bonifer et al., 2005; Flinn et al., 2005; Karman et al., 2003) examined the effectiveness of constraint-induced therapy. However, they did not use exactly the same procedures for their interventions.

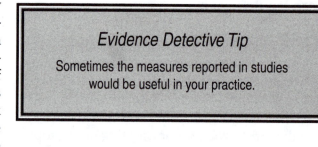

Evidence Detective Tip

Sometimes the measures reported in studies would be useful in your practice.

Activity 8-9

Comparing Features of Interventions

Meet with your study partners to compare and contrast the features of the intervention program for the three studies (Bonifer et al., 2005;

Flinn et al., 2005; Karman et al., 2003). One aspect has been added to Worksheet 8D to get you started; complete Worksheet 8D to plan for your meeting. After your complete your discussion of the similarities and differences, write a summary statement that includes the best intervention features for an effective intervention program based on these studies.

Activity 8-10

Knowing What the Public Might Know

The topic of constraint-induced therapy has gotten a lot of public attention, so you will be able to find newspaper and magazine articles that report on the research for the public. Find an article that journalistically reports on the findings of a research article and share it with your study partners. Consider the following issues in your discussion.

- Sometimes public press articles do not use "person-first" language. Does your article use negative connotations that would be unacceptable in professional literature (e.g., saying "stroke victims" has two negative features—first saying stroke as the initial word, which defines the person as a disability rather than as a person, and second, saying victim, which presumes that the experience of having a stroke is automatically negative)?

- What are the differences between what actual professional authors say about their findings and what journalists say about the findings?

- In what ways might the public be served by this journalist report?

- In what ways might the public be misled by this journalist report?

- How do science and evidence advance with public articles such as this one?

Activity 8-11

Developing Take Home Messages

The final step in the analysis process for evidence-based practice is to summarize the findings for those who need to use the ideas to improve their practices. Professionals want clear, easy-to-understand guidelines about what to do. We will call these summaries "Take Home Messages" to remind ourselves to use understandable language. You will need to consider Take Home Messages for your colleagues (within your discipline and from other disciplines), family members, other care providers, and those receiving your care.

Select two constituent groups as the focus of your attention and create some Take Home Messages for them. Pretend that the articles you read (Bonifer et al., 2005; Flinn et al., 2005; Karman et al., 2003) were the **definitive** articles on the topic. Use Worksheets 8E and 8F to summarize your work.

When considering what you are going to write, think about these questions:

- What would you say to colleagues about how they might need to change their practices to gain the optimal benefit?

- What would you say to your team regarding the articles' findings based on the articles you have read?

- How would you extrapolate information from these articles to develop hypotheses for populations other than the ones that were studied?

Summary

In this unit, you learned about constraint-induced therapy. Although all the studies addressed this topic, they each had individualized ways of applying the concept to their interventions. These distinctions are important to detect in evidence-based practice; professionals have to make decisions about how much, how long, etc. every day.

All references for this unit can be found in the Bibliography, beginning on page 169.

Worksheet 8A

Summarizing Characteristics of Research

Citation	Participants	Setting	Measures	Design	Intervention	Findings	Notes
Study 1: Bonifer et al. (2005)							
Study 2: Flinn et al. (2005)							
Study 3: Karman et al. (2003)							
Study 4:							

Citation: Put the reference here.
Participants: List the important characteristics of participants.
Setting: Describe the location of the study.
Measures: List the outcome measures used in the study.
Design: Describe what type of comparisons or relationships are being tested/studied.
Intervention: List the most important aspects of the procedures being tested.
Findings: List the most important outcomes.
Notes: If you have insights or questions, jot them down.

Worksheet 8B
Writing Answerable and Unanswerable Questions

Write one question you can and one question you cannot answer from the studies in this unit. Discuss these with your study partners.

Answerable Question	What in the Article Enables You to Answer This Question?

Unanswerable Question	What Else Would We Need to Be Able to Answer This Question?

Worksheet 8C
Reactions to New Data

Think about your reactions to the articles. Based on Chinn and Brewer's (1993) ways of responding to anomalous data, what would you say your reaction illustrates?

Chinn and Brewer (1993) Responses	Example Reaction to the Findings
IGNORE the data (don't even bother to "explain" data away)	
REJECT the data (articulate an explanation for why data should be rejected)	
EXCLUDE the data from the domain of current beliefs (the data are outside the domain of current beliefs)	
Hold the data in ABEYANCE (I promise to deal with it later...assume that someday current beliefs will be articulated so that it can explain these data)	
REINTERPRET the data while retaining current beliefs (accept the data as something that should be explained by current beliefs...opposing forces accept data but interpret the data differently based on their own beliefs)	
Reinterpret the data and make PERIPHERAL CHANGES to current belief (make a relatively minor change to current belief...accepts the data but is unwilling to give up current belief and accept new beliefs)	
Accept the data and CHANGE current beliefs, possibly in favor of a particular new belief (change one or more of the core aspects of current beliefs—when faced with information that is contradictory to current beliefs, accepts alternate beliefs)	

Worksheet 8D
Comparing the Intervention Programs

Feature	Bonifer et al. (2005)	Flinn et al. (2005)	Karman et al. (2003)
Length of time spent with restraint	*90% of waking hours*	*3.5 hours per day*	*All waking hours*
Length of intervention period			

Summary Statement About Constraint-Induced Therapy Procedures:

Worksheet 8E
Take Home Messages for Group 1

Pretend that the articles you just read are the definitive articles about the topic. Develop Take Home Messages showing what you would say to a particular constituent group regarding the topic based on the articles you have read.

Take Home Messages About:

Name:

These messages are for:

_____ colleagues in my discipline   _____ care providers

_____ colleagues in other disciplines   _____ family members

_____ adults receiving care   _____ children receiving care

Take Home Message	**Rationale for This Message From the Literature**

Worksheet 8F
Worksheet 8F
Take Home Messages for Group 2

Pretend that the articles you just read are the definitive articles about the topic. Develop Take Home Messages showing what you would say to a particular constituent group regarding the topic based on the articles you have read.

Take Home Messages About:

Name:

These messages are for:

_____ colleagues in my discipline　　　　_____ care providers

_____ colleagues in other disciplines　　　_____ family members

_____ adults receiving care　　　　　　　_____ children receiving care

Take Home Message	Rationale for This Message From the Literature

Unit 9

Examining Evidence Related to Diet and Exercise

During this unit, you will explore some evidence about diet and exercise. Although it might seem that this topic is specific to physical therapists and dieticians, it is a relevant interdisciplinary topic. A dietician may be the expert about the components of food and the characteristics of a healthy diet, but other team members need to understand the overall topic so they can support healthy choices when issues arise. For example, an occupational therapist working on meal preparation is a more effective service provider when guiding recipe selection, etc. to incorporate the general principles of that person's dietary needs.

It is also interesting to read literature from team members' disciplines because each of us understands something differently from the studies based on our backgrounds. Someone who is focused on joint protection might see some alternative ways to get exercise accomplished that are more "friendly" to the joints than the study describes.

Diet and exercise are also important topics for professionals themselves. When we understand this body of knowledge, we can maintain our own health, making us more available for the service we provide in our practices. The therapeutic process includes empathy, and when professionals are seeking to understand topics for themselves, the process of discovery and improvement can be shared between service provider and recipient.

When you complete the work in this unit, you will have the following skills and competencies:

- Understand how this literature may contribute to the effectiveness of your practice
- Articulate how to find other articles that would contribute to your knowledge about this topic
- Design an optimal plan for your area of practice based on what you have read
- Construct Take Home Messages for various constituents so they understand quickly what the literature says about this topic

You will be reviewing article excerpts, creating summaries for comparison and contrast, gaining insights from your study partners, and creating Take Home Messages for constituent groups.

Activity 9-1

Reading the Literature

We are providing you with the Abstracts (Sidebars 9-1 and 9-2) of two articles that shed some light on diet and exercise. Obtain the full articles if this topic is of particular interest to you.

Aldana, S. G., Greenlaw, R. L., Diehl, H. A., Salberg, A., Merrill, R. M., Ohmine, S., & Thomas, C. (2005). *Effects of an intensive diet and physical activity modification program on the health risks of adults.* Journal of the American Dietetic Association, 105(3), 371-381.

Riebe, D., Blissmer, B., Greene, G., Caldwell, M., Ruggiero, L., Stillwell, K. M., & Nigg, C. R. (2004). *Long-term maintenance of exercise and healthy eating behaviors in overweight adults.* Preventive Medicine, 40, 769-778.

Since these articles are from interdisciplinary sources, it is not necessary to understand the intimate details of the studies (e.g., the details about the cholesterol levels, etc.). We will focus on the structure of the Methods and Results in this unit.

Activity 9-2

Summarizing the Methods and Results of Research Articles

Create a summary (Worksheet 9A) using the Aldana et al. (2005) and Riebe et al. (2004) Abstracts (see Sidebars 9-1 and 9-2). You will not have as much detail without the full article, but you will be able to see comparisons and contrasts between the Abstracts.

Sidebar 9-1
Aldana et al. (2005) Abstract

Background. This study assessed the clinical impact of lifestyle change education on chronic disease risk factors within a community. **Design.** Randomized clinical trial. **Setting/participants.** Participants included 337 volunteers age 43 to 81 years from the Rockford, IL, metropolitan area. **Intervention.** The intervention group attended a 40-hour educational course delivered over a 4-week period. Participants learned the importance of making healthful lifestyle choices and how to make improvements in nutrition and physical activity. **Main outcome measures.** Changes in health knowledge, nutrition, and physical activity behavior, and several chronic disease risk factors were assessed at baseline and 6 weeks. **Results.** Beneficial mean changes in scores tended to be significant for the intervention group but not for the control group. Variables with improved scores included health knowledge, percent body fat, total steps per week, and most nutrition variables. Clinical improvements were seen in resting heart rate, total cholesterol, low-density lipoprotein cholesterol, and systolic and diastolic blood pressure. The control group experienced comparatively small but significant improvements in health knowledge, systolic and diastolic blood pressure, glucose, and in some nutrition variables. For almost all variables, the intervention group showed significantly greater improvements. **Conclusions.** This lifestyle modification program is an efficacious nutrition and physical activity intervention in the short term and has the potential to dramatically reduce the risks associated with common chronic diseases in the long term.

Sidebar 9-2
Riebe et al. (2004) Abstract

Background. Most people experience weight regain following the termination of a weight management program. The failure to maintain changes in diet and exercise patterns is a major factor. This study presents 24-month outcomes of a healthy-lifestyle weight management program designed to promote long-term changes in diet and exercise behaviors. **Methods.** Overweight and obese adults ($n = 144$; BMI = 32.5 ± 3.8) completed a 6-month clinic-based weight management program and were followed for an additional 18 months. Assessments completed at baseline, 6, 12, and 24 months included weight, body composition, dietary recalls, self-reported physical activity, and mediator variables based on Transtheoretical Model of Health Behavior Change. **Results.** At 24 months, subjects maintained decreases in weight, % body fat, caloric intake, % kcal saturated fat, and increases in weekly exercise minutes ($P < 0.05$). Individuals who maintained regular exercise at 24 months had higher confidence scores and higher use of experiential and behavioral processes. Individuals who maintained a healthy diet at 24 months had lower temptation scores and higher use of experiential and behavioral processes. **Conclusions.** A healthy-lifestyle weight management program is successful at promoting long-term changes in exercise and dietary behaviors. Individuals who actively engage in the maintenance process are more likely to succeed.

Summary articles use tables to show readers the most important aspects of studies. Locate a summary article in an area of your interest and see how its tables are organized. Make an organizational table that suits your learning and information needs.

LOOKING FOR PATTERNS AND THEMES

First look for similarities and differences in the structures of the studies.

- Did they study the same populations?
- Did they use similar settings?
- Were the designs similar?
- How did the measures compare to each other?

The answers to these questions can help you understand differences in findings. For example, if one study says an intervention worked and another study says it did not, you will need to examine these other factors to see what might have contributed to the differences. In these studies, one intervention lasted for 6 months, while the other intervention lasted for 4 weeks; if there are differences in the findings, we might hypothesize about the influence of these time periods on the outcomes reported.

Now, think about the topic.

- What happened to your thinking from before and after reading the abstracts?
- How did your ideas change?
- Have you observed that professionals have incorporated these findings into their practices?
- Are you going to do anything differently now that your have read these excerpts?

These questions enable you to examine how the findings affected yours and others' thinking about practice. A great study that professionals are skeptical about will not have an impact on the practices; as professionals we need to understand the reasons why people may or may not adopt a strategy that has been shown effective through a research study.

Now consider what questions are answerable or unanswerable from these studies.

Activity 9-3

Recognizing the Strengths and Limitations of Research Articles

All research articles make a contribution and have limitations. Perhaps a group of articles is only about one age group and diagnosis; then we are not sure whether we can apply their findings to other age groups and other diagnoses. There will always be practice questions that can and cannot be answered by the available research. Sometimes researchers conduct studies about what can be answered; that does not mean that studies reflect the only important topics for practice. Perhaps there are no measures to find out the answer to an important practice question. It might be that a population is so heterogeneous that it is hard to detect changes or to discover who would or would not benefit from an intervention. In practice, there will always be answerable and unanswerable questions. Advances in measurement, technology, and knowledge make more questions answerable.

Considering the two Abstracts (Aldana et al., 2005; Riebe et al., 2004), complete Worksheet 9B about the "answerable" and "unanswerable" questions for practice.

Activity 9-4

Handling Anomalous Data

The findings from these excerpts (Aldana et al., 2005; Riebe et al., 2004) may challenge some of your current beliefs. Refer to your Executive Summary (see Sidebar 2-1) of the Chinn and Brewer (1993) article to decide where your reactions to the Abstract findings are occurring (Worksheet 9C). Bring these issues up with your study partners.

Activity 9-5

Expanding the Evidence

Obtain another article (i.e., in the past 6 years) that adds information to your understanding about this topic. Add this citation, etc., to your summary worksheet (Worksheet 9A). Make copies of your article for your study partners.

Activity 9-6

Group Discussion

Meet with your study partners and discuss your findings and reactions to the excerpts (Aldana et al., 2005; Riebe et al., 2004). Add your unique information to the discussion from the article you are contributing on the topic. Refine your notes based on your discussion.

EXTENDING KNOWLEDGE ABOUT METHODS AND RESULTS

In each unit of Section II, each set of articles reflects an overall topic. Additionally, each article illustrates some unique features of studies and ways to report the methods and findings. By examining some aspects of each study, you will accumulate knowledge about designs and statistics while learning more about the evidence. This process will build your capacity as an evidence-based professional because when you encounter other articles with similar features, you will know how to use the information in your decision making.

The diet and exercise studies (Aldana et al., 2005; Riebe et al., 2004) in this unit provide an opportunity to learn about other characteristics of articles. These two studies used different time frames and measured some of the same aspects of diet and exercise in different ways. Some professionals might be more familiar with one of the programs or measures, making that study's findings more inviting to their practice. Professionals might also be in programs that already have a diet and exercise program of a certain length; if their program is longer, the study with a shorter intervention might not be as appealing.

UNDERSTANDING HOW PARTICIPANTS ENTER AND COMPLETE A STUDY

The Aldana et al. (2005) study provides a really helpful figure outlining how people entered the study (see Sidebar 9-3). Many authors tell readers this information in the text, but it can be confusing to figure out what happened. They show who started, who was excluded, and who got into each group.

Activity 9-7

Practice With Your Study Partners

Review the Aldana et al. (2005) figure (see Sidebar 9-3) and discuss whether you think any of the losses of participants might have affected the results of the study (e.g., is it likely that people who were unwilling to commit would have changed the results?).

DIGESTING DATA IN TABLES AND FIGURES

The tables in both of these studies (Aldana et al., 2005; Riebe et al., 2004) are very detailed and provide the reader with a comprehensive view of their findings. This can be overwhelming to readers who are either novices to the topic or those who are unfamiliar with the statistical procedures. We will examine portions of the tables here so you can become more familiar with how to read and make use of their data for these and other studies.

We looked at data in the constraint-induced therapy articles and how graphs of the data could increase understanding about the comparisons. In these diet and exercise articles, the authors use only tables and make notations on the tables indicating what comparisons are significantly different. The Aldana et al. (2005) article contains nearly five full pages of tables with 7 to 10 columns each; the Riebe et al. (2004) article contains seven tables that span about three pages of the article. Whew! This is a lot of information to digest.

The Aldana et al. (2005) article uses a "change score" format for reporting their findings. This means that they report how each group performed initially, and then how much change they made after the program. Other studies (e.g., Riebe et al. [2004]) report actual means and standard deviations; the amount of change isn't immediately apparent.

We are providing you an excerpt from an Aldana et al. (2005) table (Sidebar 9-4) so we can examine this a little further. You will notice that they provide the mean and standard deviation for the baseline and then provide the mean change and standard deviation for the 6-week follow-up (we think the standard deviation is related to the change scores, but are not completely sure from the article). In the last column, the *T* statistic and *p* values indicate that the intervention and control groups are

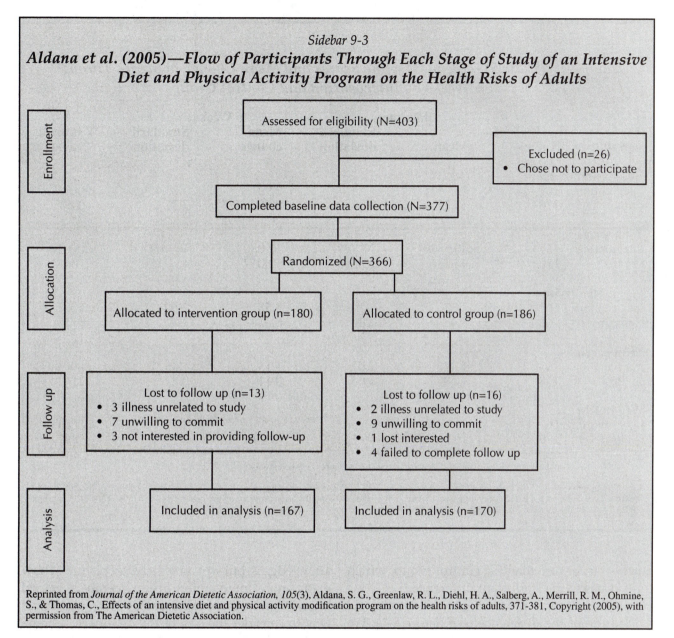

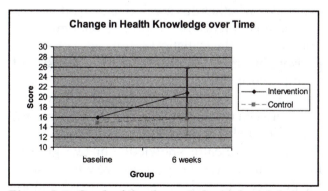

Figure 9-1. *Graph of the change in health knowledge over time (data taken from Aldana et al. [2005]).*

statistically significantly different; <.0001 means that this difference would in error less than 1 in 10,000 times. For most people, this would be convincing.

With a difference of this magnitude you might expect that the two groups are radically different. Let's graph the data and see what <.0001 looks like in this case. Using the data from Health Knowledge (row 1), Figure 9-1 is a graph of that comparison. The first points on the graph are the baseline mean scores. For the second points on the graph, we added the baseline mean plus mean change to get our center point. You can see that the intervention group slopes upward at a

Sidebar 9-4
Aldana et al. (2005)—Mean Baseline Scores and Mean Change in Scores Through 6 Weeks by Intervention and Control Groups

| | | Baseline | | 6 Weeks | | |
Variable	No.	Mean	Standard deviation	Mean change	Standard deviation	T statistic P value[a]
Health knowledge[***]						
Intervention	167	15.95	3.54	7.92	5.01	<.0001
Control	170	14.84	3.26	0.85	3.21	.0087
Total steps[***]						
Intervention	167	40,583	22,777	12,080	16,909	<.0001
Control	170	44,136	23,545	2,057	15,936	.1044
Vegetable servings[***]						
Intervention	163	3.37	2.14	1.58	2.60	<.0001
Control	168	3.42	2.20	0.03	1.80	.8735
Fruit servings[***]						
Intervention	163	1.47	1.07	1.15	1.46	<.0001
Control	168	1.58	1.05	0.11	0.87	.2162
Weight (lb)[***]						
Intervention	167	205.44	53.56	-7.55	4.72	<.0001
Control	170	192.31	56.23	-0.29	8.51	.5817

[***] $P<.0001$, based on the T statistic assessing difference in mean change scores between groups.

Reprinted from *Journal of the American Dietetic Association, 105*(3), Aldana, S. G., Greenlaw, R. L., Diehl, H. A., Salberg, A., Merrill, R. M., Ohmine, S., & Thomas, C., Effects of an intensive diet and physical activity modification program on the health risks of adults, 371-381, Copyright (2005), with permission from The American Dietetic Association.

much sharper rate than the control group, which contributes to the significant difference.

We took one more step to illustrate the magnitude of the difference (see Figure 9-1). We graphed +1 SD and -1 SD from the 6-week means (see 6 Weeks Standard Deviation score in Sidebar 9-4) in a whisker plot format so we could see how much the two groups overlapped. You will see that the mean score for the control group is about at the point of the -1 SD score of the intervention group. If you think about the bell curve, only about 16% of the population falls below -1 SD. So in this graph, about 16% of the intervention group performed lower than the mean score (the 50% mark) of the control group. Clearly, their education program created a change for those who received it.

However, we don't know whether gaining 4.92 points of additional Health Knowledge is useful since we don't know exactly what that knowledge is, but we can see a better picture of how many more intervention group members gained knowledge in the 6 weeks. This is an additional way to consider the size of the difference; when a study is about your interest area, you will have a better idea whether this much change matters.

So an evidence-based professional must not only consider the statistical significance of a comparison, but must also consider the effect size of the difference. The effect size can be calculated several ways and tells us the magnitude of the difference between two conditions (Portney & Watkins, 2000). Figure 9-1 illustrates the magnitude of the differences in health knowledge of two groups. In a later unit on meta-analyses, we will consider the average effect size across a group of studies. Tickle-Degnen (2001), which is located in the Appendix (Article 21) and discussed in Unit 10, also provides a helpful discussion about application of effect size to evidence-based practice.

Sidebar 9-5
Riebe et al. (2004)—Exercise Behavior Outcomes From Baseline to 2 Years for All Subjects (n = 91)

	Baseline	6 Months	12 Months	24 Months
Days of exercise per week				
Overall	2.38 (2.3)[a]	4.30 (1.8)[b]	3.57 (2.0)[c]	3.63 (2.1)[c]
Minutes of exercise per day				
Overall	25.6 (26.2)[a]	41.9 (17.5)[b]	40.2 (25.8)[b]	38.4 (25.2)[b]
Minutes of exercise per week				
Overall	101.7 (118.3)[a]	188.8 (107.2)[b]	169.7 (128.6)[b]	164.1 (140.0)[b]

Note: values with different superscripts for the same variable are significantly different using a Bonferroni correction ($p < 0.05$).

Reprinted from *Preventive Medicine, 40*, Riebe, D., Blissmer, B., Greene, G., Caldwell, M., Ruggiero, L., Stillwell, K. M., & Nigg, C. R., Long-term maintenance of exercise and healthy eating behaviors in overweight adults, 769-778, Copyright (2005), with permission from Elsevier.

Evidence Detective Tip

Sometimes comparisons can be statistically significant and yet reflect changes that are small when considering the person's everyday life behavior. Look at the actual amount of change in a behavior, and ask yourself whether that amount of change would be noticeable in your practice and whether it is likely to contribute to improved satisfaction or participation. (This is what "effect size" calculations will tell you when they are reported in studies.)

Activity 9-8

Practice With Your Study Partners

Work with your study partners to create graphs for the other variables (Total Steps, Vegetable Servings, Fruit Servings, and Weight) from the Aldana et al. (2004) table excerpt (see Sidebar 9-4). Discuss whether you think that the statistically significant changes matter in actual practice. How might the intervention group behave differently, participate differently, feel more satisfied with these differences in steps, etc.? If these amounts of knowledge, steps, servings, and weight seem inadequate, what amounts of these factors would be adequate for your practice decisions?

Now let's look at the Riebe et al. (2004) article tables. These authors used a different strategy to report their findings even though they are also using tables. They report the actual mean and standard deviation scores for the four points

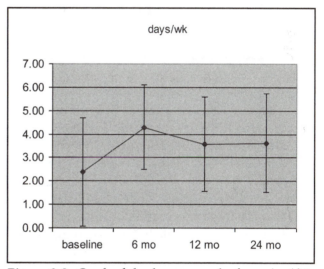

Figure 9-2. Graph of the days per week of exercise (data taken from Riebe et al. [2004]).

in time they measured performance. Sidebar 9-5 contains an excerpt of a Riebe et al. table.

We used the numbers from the first row of the Riebe et al. (2004) table (see Sidebar 9-5) to create Figure 9-2.

Let's look at the first row of table data in Sidebar 9-5. You will see superscript letters a, b, and c. These authors are indicating significant differences from one point to the next using these superscript letters. In the first row (Days of Exercise Per Week), the 6-month point is significantly different from baseline (as indicated by the b) and the 12-month point is significantly different from baseline and the 6-month point (as indicated by the c). The 24-month point is also different from baseline and 6 months, but is not different from the 12-month point (as indicated by another c, matching the 12-month point).

As if that isn't interesting enough, it is also important to note that the significant difference between baseline and 6 months is because of an increase in the number of days of exercise, while the significant difference between 6 months and 12 months is because of a decrease in the number of days of exercise. Significance testing does not tell you the direction of the change. You have to look at the data to know. Even though there was a decline, it is still significantly higher than baseline, and the improvement was stable until 24 months.

Evidence Detective Tip

We only know whether a significant difference is better or worse by looking at the means to see the direction of the change.

Graphing the data can be helpful in this example as well. We graphed the first row of data for you (see Figure 9-2), showing the mean and standard deviation of the four points in time on the graph. You can see the sharp increase, followed by a decline, and then stabilization. You can also see a lot of variation in how many days people walked per week. In the baseline, +1 SD is just under 5 days per week, and -1 SD is practically no walking at all. If you look at the -1 SD point for each time period, the study showed that even these lower performers were walking about 1.5 days per week. Would this be enough of a change to convince you that their strategies were helpful? Would these amounts of changes be enough to make someone feel satisfied and healthier? These questions require professional judgment beyond the statistical significance.

Activity 9-9

Practice With Your Study Partners

Discuss how your feel about the changes in days per week as indicated above. Then graph the other two variables provided (Minutes of Exercise Per Day, Minutes of Exercise Per Week) and discuss whether you think the differences matter

to professionals and adults in exercise programs. Discuss the use of the superscript letters on these comparisons; what do they indicate about the data, and how does that show up on your graphs?

UNDERSTANDING THE TECHNICAL WORDING IN RESULTS

Another challenge for professionals looking for evidence is making sense of the technical reporting of results in the text of articles. Although we cannot be experts at all statistics, it is helpful to know how to acquire a basic understanding of the way researchers report their findings. Knowing this, when you peruse the Results sections of an article, you can make your own decisions about whether the study is applicable to your practice. You can decide whether you agree or disagree with the authors' interpretations (in the Discussion section). Researchers are expected to report only the facts in the Results sections; researchers have more latitude in the Discussion section, where they are explaining what they think the data mean.

Activity 9-10

Practice With Your Study Partners

We have excerpted a paragraph from the Results section of Riebe et al. (2004) (Sidebar 9-6). Meet with your study partners and discuss this information (use Portney and Watkins [2000] or another research design and statistics text for reference). Write in your own words what each part of this paragraph means. Use Worksheet 9D to guide your discussion and documentation.

Activity 9-11

Developing Take Home Messages

The final step in the analysis process for evidence-based practice is to summarize the findings for those who need to use the ideas to improve their practices. Professionals want clear, easy-to-understand guidelines about what to do. We will call these summaries "Take Home Messages" to remind ourselves to use understandable language. You will need to consider Take Home Messages for your colleagues (within your discipline and

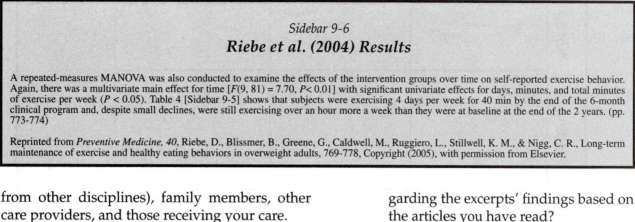

Sidebar 9-6
Riebe et al. (2004) Results

A repeated-measures MANOVA was also conducted to examine the effects of the intervention groups over time on self-reported exercise behavior. Again, there was a multivariate main effect for time [$F(9, 81) = 7.70$, $P < 0.01$] with significant univariate effects for days, minutes, and total minutes of exercise per week ($P < 0.05$). Table 4 [Sidebar 9-5] shows that subjects were exercising 4 days per week for 40 min by the end of the 6-month clinical program and, despite small declines, were still exercising over an hour more a week than they were at baseline at the end of the 2 years. (pp. 773-774)

from other disciplines), family members, other care providers, and those receiving your care.

Select two constituent groups as the focus of your attention and create some Take Home Messages for them. Pretend that the excerpts you read (Aldana et al., 2005; Riebe et al., 2004) were from the **definitive** articles on the topic. Use Worksheets 9E and 9F to summarize your work.

When considering what you are going to write, think about these questions:

- What would you say to colleagues about how they might need to change their practices to gain the optimal benefit?
- What would you say to your team regarding the excerpts' findings based on the articles you have read?
- How would you extrapolate information from these excerpts to develop hypotheses for other populations than the ones that were studied?

SUMMARY

In this unit, you examined research related to diet and exercise. You compared the various strategies used in the interventions and the outcomes associated with those strategies. The ideas in these studies are likely to be applicable across many populations including you.

All references for this unit can be found in the Bibliography, beginning on page 169.

Worksheet 9A

Summarizing Characteristics of Research

Citation	Participants	Setting	Measures	Design	Intervention	Findings	Notes
Study 1: Aldana et al. (2005)							
Study 2: Riebe et al. (2004)							
Study 3:							

Citation: Put the reference here.
Participants: List the important characteristics of participants.
Setting: Describe the location of the study.
Measures: List the outcome measures used in the study.
Design: Describe what type of comparisons or relationships are being tested/studied.
Intervention: List the most important aspects of the procedures being tested.
Findings: List the most important outcomes.
Notes: If you have insights or questions, jot them down.

Worksheet 9B
Writing Answerable and Unanswerable Questions

Write one question you can and one question you cannot answer from the studies in this unit. Discuss these with your study partners.

Answerable Question	What in the Article Enables You to Answer This Question?

Unanswerable Question	What Else Would We Need to Be Able to Answer This Question?

Worksheet 9C
Reactions to New Data

Think about your reactions to the excerpts. Based on Chinn and Brewer's (1993) ways of responding to anomalous data, what would you say your reaction illustrates?

Chinn and Brewer (1993) Responses	Example Reaction to the Findings
IGNORE the data (don't even bother to "explain" data away)	
REJECT the data (articulate an explanation for why data should be rejected)	
EXCLUDE the data from the domain of current beliefs (the data are outside the domain of current beliefs)	
Hold the data in ABEYANCE (I promise to deal with it later...assume that someday current beliefs will be articulated so that it can explain these data)	
REINTERPRET the data while retaining current beliefs (accept the data as something that should be explained by current beliefs...opposing forces accept data but interpret the data differently based on their own beliefs)	
Reinterpret the data and make PERIPHERAL CHANGES to current belief (make a relatively minor change to current belief...accepts the data but is unwilling to give up current belief and accept new beliefs)	
Accept the data and CHANGE current beliefs, possibly in favor of a particular new belief (change one or more of the core aspects of current beliefs—when faced with information that is contradictory to current beliefs, accepts alternate beliefs)	

Worksheet 9D
Worksheet 9D
Analysis of the Results Section of an Article

The Exact Words From the Article Describing the Results*	Explanation of Results From Riebe et al. (2004)
"A repeated-measures MANOVA was also conducted to examine the effects of the intervention groups over time on self-reported exercise behavior."	
"Again, there was a multivariate main effect for time [$F[(9.81)=7.70$, $P<0.01$]"	
"with significant univariate effects for days, minutes, and total minutes of exercise per week ($P<0.05$)."	
"Table 4 [Sidebar 9-5] shows that subjects were exercising 4 days per week for 40 minutes by the end of the 6-month clinical program and, despite small declines, were still exercising over an hour more a week than they were at baseline at the end of the 2 years."	

*Exact Words reprinted from *Preventive Medicine, 40*, Riebe, D., Blissmer, B., Greene, G., Caldwell, M., Ruggiero, L., Stillwell, K. M., & Nigg, C. R., Long-term maintenance of exercise and healthy eating behaviors in overweight adults, 769-778, Copyright (2005), with permission from Elsevier.
Reprinted in Dunn, W. (2008). *Bringing Evidence into Everyday Practice:
Practical Strategies for Healthcare Professionals*. Thorofare, NJ: SLACK Incorporated.

Worksheet 9E
Take Home Messages for Group 1

Pretend that the excerpts you just read are from the definitive articles about the topic. Develop Take Home Messages showing what you would say to a particular constituent group regarding the topic based on the excerpts you have read.

Take Home Messages About:

Name:

These messages are for:

_____ colleagues in my discipline	_____ care providers
_____ colleagues in other disciplines	_____ family members
_____ adults receiving care	_____ children receiving care

Take Home Message	Rationale for This Message From the Literature

Take Home Messages for Group 2

Pretend that the excerpts you just read are from the definitive articles about the topic. Develop Take Home Messages showing what you would say to a particular constituent group regarding the topic based on the excerpts you have read.

Take Home Messages About:

Name:

These messages are for:

_____ colleagues in my discipline   _____ care providers

_____ colleagues in other disciplines   _____ family members

_____ adults receiving care   _____ children receiving care

Take Home Message	Rationale for This Message From the Literature

Section III

Expanding Your Knowledge and Skills for Evidence-Based Practice

In the third section, we will examine some additional sources available to support evidence-based practices. Some scholars have gathered the literature on a particular topic and provide a summary of that work along with their insights about the body of work. Baranek (2002) provides a summary of studies that examine aspects of intervention with children who have autism. We looked at a portion of this summary review in Unit 3. The first edition of *Evidence-Based Rehabilitation: A Guide to Practice* (Law, 2002) contains two examples of summaries as well (Chapter 8 and Chapter 14). There are also research-to-practice websites that provide summaries of the literature. Other scholars conduct a more systematic analysis of studies on a particular topic; these works are called meta-analyses (Chapter 7 in the Law text discusses the characteristics, advantages, and disadvantages of meta-analyses). The authors follow particular conventions to include studies and conduct statistical analyses of the strength of findings to come to an overall conclusion. We will examine examples of summary and meta-analyses in Section III.

Another aspect of evidence-based practice concerns the ability to discern whether an emerging practice meets acceptable standards. In Section III, we will study how to critique an emerging practice to determine its viability for use in practice.

A final additional source of evidence is the data professionals collect in everyday practice. Even when research literature indicates that a practice is effective, professionals still have the responsibility to find out the impact of this practice on the individual/family/system being served. We will discuss some methods for collecting data in everyday practice in Section III. Appendices J and K in the Law (2002) text also provide examples of client outcomes and key indicators of progress for practice.

Unit 10

Understanding Summary and Meta-Analysis Articles

During this unit, you will explore evidence that can be obtained from articles that have summarized a body of literature for us.

In addition to individual studies, you can get good information for your evidence-based practice from summary articles that review all the literature available on a specific topic. A special type of summary information article is called *meta-analysis*, which analyzes the findings of a whole set of studies using specialized statistical procedures.

Summary articles are helpful because you can get a lot of research findings from one source. The author has synthesized findings for you, and so you can get a bigger picture more efficiently. You can find summary articles in typical professional library sources and on some specialized websites on the Internet.

When you complete the work of this unit, you will have the following skills and competencies:

- Be familiar with the format of summary articles and what they tell us about an area of practice

- Understand the special characteristics of meta-analyses as summary articles
- Know how to access websites that provide summary material to guide evidence-based practice
- Construct best practice tips for colleagues from a summary article to guide practice decisions
- Construct Take Home Messages for various constituents so they understand quickly what the literature says about the topic

You will be reviewing articles, analyzing the process of article selection, gaining insights from your study partners, and creating Take Home Messages for constituent groups.

The Law (2002) text has some chapters to help you with this material. Chapter 7 explains systematically reviewing the evidence, including how meta-analyses work. Chapter 8 provides an example of a critical review of cognitive behavioral interventions for people with chronic pain. Chapter 14 provides a summary review on where

to provide services for people who have had a stroke. Look for a summary explanation in your research design text (e.g., Portney and Watkins [2000] or Kielhofner [2006]).

We will examine one meta-analysis article and one summary article in this unit.

INTRODUCTION TO USE OF META-ANALYSIS

Although research and evidence-based practice texts explain what a meta-analysis is, and how to construct and understand the analysis, professionals also need to understand how to **use** the valuable summary information to guide their practice decisions. Tickle-Degnen (2001), which is located in the Appendix (Article 21), provides a very helpful discussion for professionals.

Tickle-Degnen, L. (2001). From the general to the specific: Using meta-analytic reports in clinical decision making. Evaluation and the Health Professions, 24(3), 308-326.

She explains that professionals must consider whether the information in the meta-analysis actually applies to the person(s) in their practice. First, professionals must determine whether the characteristics of the research participants match the characteristics of the persons being served; if they don't match, we must consider whether the outcomes would generalize to our particular client. Second, professionals must determine which research participants responded to which aspects of the interventions; we are more at risk if we apply an intervention that was effective overall, but not with the type of person actually being served. Tickle-Degnen (2001) applies findings of a study about exercise post-stroke to a particular individual, Mrs. Jones. We will use a more recent meta-analysis on this topic here; use the Tickle-Degnen article to guide your work on the meta-analysis.

Let's apply the information from the text and article readings to a portion of a meta-analysis so we can practice.

ANALYSIS OF A META-ANALYSIS

Let's study the components of a meta-analysis. You will find excerpts from the following study here within this unit (Sidebars 10-1 through 10-4). Please obtain the full study so you can review the full work with your study partners.

Kwakkel, G., van Peppen, R., Wagenaar, R. C., Dauphinee, S. W., Richards, C., Ashburn, A., Miller, K., Lincoln, N., Partridge, C., Wellwood, I., & Langhorne, P. (2004). Effects of augmented exercise therapy time after stroke: A meta-analysis. Stroke, 35(11), 2529-2536.

Sidebar 10-1
Kwakkel et al. (2004) Abstract

Background and Purpose—To present a systematic review of studies that addresses the effects of intensity of augmented exercise therapy time (AETT) on activities of daily living (ADL), walking, and dexterity in patients with stroke. **Summary of Review**—A database of articles published from 1966 to November 2003 was compiled from MEDLINE, CINAHL, Cochrane Central Register of Controlled Trials, PEDro, DARE, and PiCarta using combinations of the following key words: stroke, cerebrovascular disorders, physical therapy, physiotherapy, occupational therapy, exercise therapy, rehabilitation, intensity, dose–response relationship, effectiveness, and randomized controlled trial. References presented in relevant publications were examined as well as abstracts in proceedings. Studies that satisfied the following selection criteria were included: (1) patients had a diagnosis of stroke; (2) effects of intensity of exercise training were investigated; and (3) design of the study was a randomized controlled trial (RCT). For each outcome measure, the estimated effect size (ES) and the summary effect size (SES) expressed in standard deviation units (SDU) were calculated for ADL, walking speed, and dexterity using fixed and random effect models. Correlation coefficients were calculated between observed individual effect sizes on ADL of each study, additional time spent on exercise training, and methodological quality. Cumulative meta-analyses (random effects model) adjusted for the difference in treatment intensity in each study was used for the trials evaluating the effects of AETT provided. Twenty of the 31 candidate studies, involving 2686 stroke patients, were included in the synthesis. The methodological quality ranged from 2 to 10 out of the maximum score of 14 points. The meta-analysis resulted in a small but statistically significant SES with regard to ADL measured at the end of the intervention phase. Further analysis showed a significant homogeneous SES for 17 studies that investigated effects of increased exercise intensity within the first 6 months after stroke. No significant SES was observed for the 3 studies conducted in the chronic phase. Cumulative meta-analysis strongly suggests that at least a 16-hour difference in treatment time between experimental and control groups provided in the first 6 months after stroke is needed to obtain significant differences in ADL. A significant SES supporting a higher intensity was also observed for instrumental ADL and walking speed, whereas no significant SES was found for dexterity. **Conclusion**—The results of the present research synthesis support the hypothesis that augmented exercise therapy has a small but favorable effect on ADL, particularly if therapy input is augmented at least 16 hours within the first 6 months after stroke. This meta-analysis also suggests that clinically relevant treatment effects may be achieved on instrumental ADL and gait speed.

Reprinted with permission from Kwakkel, G., van Peppen, R., Wagenaar, R. C., Dauphinee, S. W., Richards, C., Ashburn, A., Miller, K., Lincoln, N., Partridge, C., Wellwood, I., & Langhorne, P. (2004). Effects of augmented exercise therapy time after stroke: A meta-analysis. *Stroke, 35*(11), 2529-2536.

Dissecting the Abstract

As you have been learning, the Abstract provides an overview of the work. Following the format prescribed by this journal, Kwakkel et al. (2004) provide the readers with three subheadings:

1. Background and Purpose
2. Summary of Review
3. Conclusion

Background and Purpose

Kwakkel et al. (2004) succinctly tell what their goal was for the study. Some authors write a statement of purpose, while other authors use a question format to tell readers what they are studying.

Activity 10-1

Dissecting the Abstract

Dissect the Kwakkel et al. (2004) Abstract (see Sidebar 10-1) into your own words (complete Worksheets 10A through 10C). Since these authors made statements, change it to a question (Worksheet 10A) and put it into your own words.

This Abstract is packed with information. The Summary of Review gives the reader all the critical information about how Kwakkel et al. (2004) picked articles they would analyze, the statistical procedures they used, the outcomes that were measured, and the outcomes of their analysis. From this part of the Abstract readers learn about the study and can get a sense about whether this meta-analysis would be applicable to their practices (Worksheet 10B).

The authors summarize the parameters of their findings at the end of the Summary of Review. These are the findings that you can use to guide your practice based on the evidence (Worksheet 10C).

Kwakkel et al. (2004) identified 14 criteria they would use to rate the methodology of the studies; each study got one point for each criteria being met. For example, they looked for reliability and validity of the measurements used in each study. They also rated whether the observers were blind to group assignment. Of the 20 studies they used, methodology scores ranged from 2/14 to 11/14; this represents a very wide range of quality in studies. Fourteen of 20 studies reported a positive effect in their outcome measurement. This variability in study quality is common when searching for evidence on a particular topic. One of the advantages of meta-analyses and summary articles is that by looking across a group of studies, professionals can establish a stronger overall basis for making decisions. We reduce vulnerability that occurs when professional decisions rest on one weaker study design and its outcomes.

Applying Tickle-Degnen (2001) strategies for applying to practice, we would first want to look at the participant characteristics in the included studies and locate those studies that had research participants that are more like our own patients/clients. Then we would look at the reported outcomes and the study quality data to decide whether the meta-analysis contained studies that would be useful to our practice situation. If only weak studies are applicable, then it may not be appropriate to apply the results of the meta-analysis to our practice.

Other meta-analyses use a format similar to the ones you have used in this text for summarizing the characteristics of studies (i.e., they make a table and list the characteristics of the methods and results). This second format provides the reader with more details about each study, but frequently leaves the reader with the responsibility of determining quality of study components. Sometimes this quality decision is more challenging for professionals who are less familiar with research design and statistics.

Studying the Results

Now let's look at a portion of the results of the Kwakkel et al. (2004) study.

Identifying Eligible Studies for the Meta-Analysis

One of the most challenging aspects of meta-analyses is the selection of the studies to be included. In this study, Kwakkel et al. (2004) set some initial criteria and then began looking for articles in professional databases. In this study, the authors considered 7,483 citations before selecting the 20 that they analyzed. They used a systematic process for making decisions about which studies to include.

Sidebar 10-2
Kwakkel et al. (2004) Results

The search strategy resulted in a list of 7483 citations. After selection based on title and abstract, 507 full articles were obtained. Thirty-two studies were identified as being relevant. Five studies used a pretest–posttest assessment design;[20–24] 3 studies included a control condition but no randomization;[25–27] and 25 studies were RCTs.[4–11,28–44] Despite being an RCT, the article by Peacock et al[29] was also excluded because of lack of information about treatment contrast and missing point measures and estimates of variability. Four studies referred to the same patients, who had been reported in 3 RCTs, which had already been included in this meta-analysis.[35,38,39,40] One study also included patients with traumatic brain injury;[41] only the patients with stroke were included in the present analysis.

Table 1 [Sidebar 10-3] shows the main characteristics of the 20 eligible studies included in the meta-analysis. Fourteen of these reported statistically significant effects for functional outcomes in favor of the group with augmented therapy time. In 6 studies, additional exercise therapy did not result in a significant difference in efficacy. In total, 2686 patients with stroke were involved. The start of therapy ranged from within the first week after stroke[9,31,42] to >1 year after stroke onset.[11,33,36] Seventeen of the 20 studies investigated the effects of intensity within the first 6 months after stroke, whereas in 3 studies the research protocol was initiated >6 months after stroke.[11,33,36]

On average, the experimental group received twice as much physical therapy (44.5 minutes; SD, 30.8) and occupational therapy (13.9 minutes; SD, 23.6) daily as the control group (21.1 minute; SD, 18.0 and 7.0 minutes; SD, 16.8, respectively; Table 1). The additional time that exercise therapy was provided to the experimental group ranged from 132 minutes[11] to 6816 minutes,[30] with a weighted average of 959 minutes or ≈16 hours of additional therapy time per patient.

Reprinted with permission from Kwakkel, G., van Peppen, R., Wagenaar, R. C., Dauphinee, S. W., Richards, C., Ashburn, A., Miller, K., Lincoln, N., Partridge, C., Wellwood, I., & Langhorne, P. (2004). Effects of augmented exercise therapy time after stroke: A meta-analysis. *Stroke, 35*(11), 2529-2536.

Activity 10-2

Making a Flow Chart

Using the information in the excerpted Kwakkel et al. (2004) Results section (see Sidebars 10-2 and 10-3), make a flow chart illustrating the process these authors used to go from 7,483 studies to 20 studies for their meta-analysis. This process will help you understand how to make systematic decisions for yourself when selecting studies to review in your practice.

When I constructed my version of the flow chart (Figure 10-1), I wrote down a series of questions the authors asked themselves at each decision point and then what the answers were to the questions. When I completed my flow chart for the Kwakkel et al. (2004), study, there was one part that was unclear, leading to an apparent discrepancy in the numbers. Did you find it also, or was the writing clear enough to you? Check with your study partners about their ideas. It is critically important for writers to be very clear with descriptions of their methods. This does not mean the authors did anything wrong in the study; it does mean that readers don't have exact details about what happened.

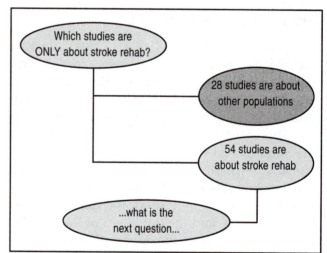

Figure 10-1. Example of a flow chart.

Activity 10-3

Practicing Making Flow Charts for Yourself

With this little bit of practice, what are some questions and criteria you might include in a sorting process for your practice? Create a draft of the decision process you might use for a question in a practice area of interest to you (Worksheet 10D).

Sidebar 10-3

Kwakkel et al. (2004)—Study Characteristics of Trials on Intensity of Stroke Rehabilitation

Reference	No. (E/C)	Stroke Type	Start of Rehab* (E/C)	Type of Intervention (E/C)	Mean Age* y (E/C)	Duration of Rehab* (E/C)	Daily (min) (PT)† (E/C)	Daily (min) OT† (E/C)	Contrast (min) (E/C)
Stern, 1970	62 (31/31)	TEI	29/33 d	PNF vs conventional	64/64	63/56 d	100/60	---	2100
Smith, 1981	133 (46/43/44)	?	31/41/37 d	Intensive conventional care vs self-care	63/66/65	3 mo	E1: 73/14 E2: 36/14	E1: 41/14 E2: 25/14	E1: 6816 E2: 3324
Sivenius, 1985	95 (50/45)	TEI (89%), ICH (11%)	<1<1 wk	Intensive vs normal	72/70	46/37 d	40/24	0.06/0.06	657
Sunderland, 1992	132 (65/67)	SAH and brain stem excluded	9/9 d*	Enhanced vs conventional	66/69*	18/10 wk*	45/28‖	---	1185
Wade, 1992	94 (49/45)	All types	4.4/5.0 y	Treatment vs no treatment¶	72/72	3 mo	8/0	---	496
Richards, 1993‡	27 (18/9)	Middle band strokes	8.5/13 d	Intensive vs conventional	69/70	5 wk	53/22	---	1933
Werner, 1996	40 (28/12)	MCA strokes	2.9/3.3 y	Treatment vs no treatment	59/66	12 wk	48/0	48/0	4608
Logan, 1997	111 (53/58)	All types (first stroke)	39/45 d	Enhanced vs usual service	71/74	<3 mo	---	22/37	167
Feys, 1998	100 (50/50)	TEI or ICH (SAH excluded)	21/24 d	Enhanced vs sensori-motor stimulation	66/63	6 wk	48/18	---	900
Kwakkel, 1999	101 (33/31/37)	MCA (first ever stroke)	7/7 d	Intensive vs immobilization	67/65	20 wk	70/44	69/44	PT: 2620 OT: 2460
Lincoln, 1999	282 (94/93/95)	All types	12/12 d*	Intensive vs routine	73/73*	5 wk	QPT: 65/42 APT: 59/42	----	QPT: 575 APT: 430
Walker, 1999	185 (94/91)	All types	<1/<1 mo	Treatment (OT) vs no treatment	74/75	5 mo	---	3/0	302
Partridge, 2000	114 (54/60)	All types	?/?	Intensive vs standard	77§	6 wk	60/30	---	900
Gilberston, 2000	138 (67/71)	SAH excluded	31/23 d	Domiciliary program vs routine service	71/71	6 wk	---	13/0	380
Parker, 2001	466 (153/156/157)	All types	<6/<6 mo	Leisure/ADL treatment vs no treatment	72/72	6 mo	---	ADL: 4/0 Leisure: 4/0	442 502
Green, 2002	170 (85/85)	All types	>1/>1 y	Routine treatment vs no treatment	72/74	13 wk	2/0	---	132
Slade, 2002	87 (47/40)	All types	47/45 d	Intensive (OT + PT) vs normal therapy	52/54	≈12 wk	30/19‖	---	614
Rodgers, 2003	123 (62/61)	All types	<10/<10 d	Enhanced upper limb therapy time vs interdisciplinary treatment programme	74/75	6 wk	Mean: 52 vs 38		420
Fang, 2003	156 (78/78)	All types	<7 d	Early intensive PT vs routine therapy without early PT	65/62	4 wk	45	---	900
GAPS, 2004	70 (35/35)	All types	22/25 d	Augmented vs standard PT to improve mobility	68/67	≈10 wk	40/25	---	720
Total	2686 (1515/1171)						≈48.6/ ≈23.3 min	≈22.9/ ≈10.9 min	Weighted mean: 956

ADL indicates activities of daily living; APT, assistant physiotherapist; d, day; wk, week; y, year; ?, unknown; E/C, experimental vs control group; ICH, intracerebral hemorrhage; MCA, middle cerebral artery; min, minutes; mo, month; N, number of patients in each group; OT, occupational therapist; PNF, proprioceptive neuromuscular facilitation; PT, physical therapist; QPT, qualified physiotherapist; SAH, subdural arachnoid hemorrhage; TEI, thromboembolic infarctions; SD, standard deviation.

*Only median figures given.

†Only period of different rehabilitation intensities recorded; average of calculated minutes for every working day during intervention.

‡Findings of the experimental (N=10) and early conventional (N=8) are combined and compared with the control group (N=9).

§Average age of experimental and control group together.

¶Randomized crossover design (only first phase of the trial is considered).

‖OT incorporated.

Reprinted with permission from Kwakkel, G., van Peppen, R., Wagenaar, R. C., Dauphinee, S. W., Richards, C., Ashburn, A., Miller, K., Lincoln, N., Partridge, C., Wellwood, I., & Langhorne, P. (2004). Effects of augmented exercise therapy time after stroke: A meta-analysis. *Stroke, 35*(11), 2529-2536.

Sidebar 10-4
Kwakkel et al. (2004) Discussion

The benefits of augmented therapy time were mainly related to studies that focused the extra time on the lower limb or general ADL and not to the 5 RCTs that provided additional therapy time to the upper limb. It is important to note, however, that an ADL outcome, such as the Barthel Index, is more sensitive to lower limb improvement than to that in the upper limb.[9] Moreover, improvements in mobility are more easily obtained than improvements in dexterity...

...The present meta-analysis has several limitations. First, we defined intensity and treatment contrast on the basis of differences in time that therapy was provided to the experimental and control groups. This is, of course, a crude estimate of the actual effort and energy that is spent in performing exercises.[2,3] Other aspects, such as patients' motivation, attention paid by the therapist, and time spent on home exercises, may have confounded the reported outcomes. Second, although all included studies investigated the effects of additional exercise therapy, the content of therapy differed between studies with regard to goals set and the type of reference treatment (or condition) applied. Finally, we may have missed relevant studies not published in scientific journals or published in languages other than English, German, or Dutch.

Reprinted with permission from Kwakkel, G., van Peppen, R., Wagenaar, R. C., Dauphinee, S. W., Richards, C., Ashburn, A., Miller, K., Lincoln, N., Partridge, C., Wellwood, I., & Langhorne, P.. (2004). Effects of augmented exercise therapy time after stroke: A meta-analysis. *Stroke, 35*(11), 2529-2536.

Meet with your study partners and discuss each of your draft plans. Refine the plans based on feedback. Do you notice any patterns as you look at several decision plans for your flow charts? Are there parts that are always present, and other parts that are unique to a particular topic? Share your final versions of your decision plans and flow charts with your study partners so you each have several examples to take with you.

DISCUSSION OF THE DISCUSSION

As you have learned, the Discussion section of an article expands the ideas from the study by providing interpretation and hypotheses about why the findings turned out the way they did. Read the Kwakkel et al. (2004) Discussion (see Sidebar 10-4) to learn what the authors think about the details of their activities of daily living findings.

Activity 10-4

Alternate Interpretations of Data

Kwakkel et al. (2004) looked at the details of the studies and have several insights to offer the readers. List the things they suggest might have contributed to the findings on Worksheet 10E.

Activity 10-5

Limitations of the Study

The Kwakkel et al. (2004) Discussion (see Sidebar 10-4) describes the limitations of the

study. List them on Worksheet 10F.

So as you can see, even though meta-analyses are compiling data across other studies, they have many of the same elements that we have been examining in other single studies.

WHAT DOES THIS STUDY MEAN FOR YOUR PRACTICE?

Activity 10-6

Applying Findings to Practice

The findings from the Kwakkel et al. (2004) meta-analysis are interesting. Meet with your study partners and discuss the usefulness of the findings for different areas of practice within rehabilitation.

- Discuss what would be useful for acute care teams.
- Discuss what would be useful for rehabilitation units.
- Discuss what would be useful for a home health practice.

Activity 10-7

Applying Findings to a Specific Practice Situation

The general findings of a meta-analysis are not always applicable to a specific person in your practice. Let's practice applying findings to a specific situation.

Read Sarah's case (Sidebar 10-5). Pretend that you and your study partners are the home health team serving Sarah. Considering the findings of the Kwakkel et al. (2004) article, what will your plans be for Sarah's home health rehabilitation program? Complete Worksheet 10G with your team.

Sidebar 10-5
Case Study: Sarah

Sarah is a 73-year-old woman receiving home health services after her rehabilitation from a stroke. She is still working on getting up out of bed, getting dressed, and showering. However, she loves to garden, wants to grocery shop on her own, and wants to cook. The home health therapy team needs to decide what they will recommend for Sarah's course of care.

When we look at the articles in the Kwakkel et al. (2004) meta-analysis, we see that some articles contain research participants who are like Sarah. None of the studies look at the particular long-term outcomes Sarah is after, but the team therapists decide that they will look at the findings and discuss what to do.

When looking at the articles that apply to Sarah, the team sees that some of them are not very strong studies according to the article's methodology analysis, and the weaker studies have questionable effect sizes as well (i.e., the magnitude of the difference between intervention and control groups is small). The stronger studies have younger people than Sarah in them, so the team doesn't know from these data whether the additional exercise recommended will apply to Sarah.

ANALYSIS OF A SUMMARY ARTICLE

Summary or review papers examine a set of articles about a particular topic, just as meta-analyses do. The difference is that summary articles do not have the same requirements for searching and analyzing the findings (i.e., there are more restrictions in a meta-analysis). We will now be looking at parts of the Baranek (2002) study, which is Article 3 in the Appendix.

Baranek, G. T. (2002). *Efficacy of sensory and motor interventions for children with autism.* Journal of Autism and Developmental Disorders, 32(5), 397-422.

DISSECTING THE ABSTRACT

As you have been learning, the Abstract provides an overview of the work. Following the format prescribed by this particular journal, Baranek then provides the reader with a summary paragraph (see Purpose, Search Procedure, and Scope).

Activity 10-8

Finding the Purpose

Baranek (2002) states that she wishes to address a controversy in the literature. Describe her purpose for this summary article in your own words (Worksheet 10H). Use a question format.

EXAMINING THE PURPOSE AND PROCEDURES OF THE REVIEW

This review article has a number of topics to consider, so Baranek (2002) succinctly describes the purpose and procedures at the very beginning of the article. You will notice that much of the information in this initial section is contained in the Abstract of the Kwakkel et al. (2004) meta-analysis; this difference is a function of the journals' styles.

Activity 10-9

Finding the Purpose

Baranek (2002) states three purposes for the study (see Purpose, Search Procedures, and Scope) that reflect the process the readers will need to go through to integrate the findings into their practice. List them on Worksheet 10I in your own words.

Activity 10-10

Comparing Strategies

Under Purpose, Search Procedures, and Scope, you will notice that Baranek (2002) used a similar beginning strategy for locating articles to include. Key words were identified and used to locate articles that might be informative. There are some unique aspects of the process when comparing to the Kwakkel et al. (2004) meta-analysis. Compare and contrast the search strategies (Worksheet 10J).

So you can see that the review article has more latitude to include studies that are related to the topic of review based on the expert judgment of the author. This would not typically occur when conducting a meta-analysis.

Baranek (2002) divided articles into seven categories:

1. Classical SI therapy (three articles)
2. SI-based approach (three articles)
3. Sensory stimulation (five articles)
4. Patterning (two articles)
5. Auditory integration training (nine articles)
6. Prism lenses (three articles)
7. Exercise therapy (four articles)

Activity 10-11

Creating a Summary

Baranek (2002) created a table similar to the ones you have been creating in other units to summarize the methods and results of these articles. Review the rows for the Kern et al. (2002, 2004), Levinson and Reid (1993), and Watters and Watters (1980) articles in Baranek's Table 1. Complete Worksheet 10K and be ready to discuss your ideas with your study partners.

Now that you have become familiar with aspects of these studies, let's look at what Baranek had to say about these studies. She expresses caution in making overarching conclusions from a small sample size, but she acknowledges the consistency of findings across these investigations of the same intervention.

CREATING TAKE HOME MESSAGES FROM SUMMARY ARTICLES

Many times summary articles provide conclusive statements and recommendations for use of the knowledge reported in the study. The Baranek (2002) study provides recommendations for practice based on the findings of the review. Baranek provides the reader with nine recommendations; if this is your area of practice, be

sure to study the findings and recommendations carefully. To summarize her recommendations for education:

1. Best practice must include ways to adjust for children with autism's individual sensory processing patterns.
2. Interdisciplinary teams are needed to design specialized interventions.
3. Specialized interventions are not a substitute for solid educational curricula and must be integrated.
4. Modifications occur within the context of education and are feasible ways to incorporate sensory and motor needs within education.
5. Evidence is limited; sensory and motor services need to be provided with documentation of individual progress, and termination of intervention when progress is not occurring.
6. Outcomes from the interventions reported are short lived; safety needs to be considered, along with appropriate documentation; interventions need to be provided within the context of child's environment.
7. Not all children benefit equally from interventions.
8. Addressing underlying skills may not generalize to functional gains.
9. More studies are needed that include systematic control.

Read the details of these recommendations to make sure you agree about these brief summary statements.

Activity 10-12

Considering the Recommendations for Your Practice

Some of these recommendations may be easy to consider while others may be more difficult to address. Refer to your Executive Summary (see Sidebar 2-1) of the Chinn and Brewer (1993) article to decide where your reactions to the study findings are occurring (Worksheet 10L). Bring these issues up with your study partners.

Activity 10-13

What Does This Study Mean for Your Practice?

The findings from the Baranek (2002) review article are interesting. Meet with your study partners and discuss the usefulness of the findings for different constituent groups.

- Discuss what would be useful for preschool and elementary teachers.
- Discuss what would be useful for parents.
- Discuss what would be useful for other therapists.

ADDITIONAL RESOURCES

Here are some other articles that might be in your areas of interest. Select one of these articles and conduct an analysis like the ones we have just practiced. Share with your study partners so you all have more information.

Ahmad, S., Mu, K., & Scott, S. (2001). Meta-analysis of functional outcome in Parkinson patients treated with unilateral pallidotomy. Neuroscience Letters, 312, *153-156.*

Bond, G. (2004). Supported employment: Evidence for an evidence-based practice. Psychiatric Rehabilitation Journal, 27(4), 345-359.

Cole, J. (1996). Intervention strategies for infants with prenatal drug exposure. Infants and Young Children, 8(3), 35-39.

Hanft, B., & Pilkington Ovland, K. (2000). Therapy in natural environments: The means or end goal for early intervention? Infants and Young Children, 12(4), 1-13.

McWilliam, R. A. (1995). Integration of therapy and consultative special education: A continuum in early intervention. Infants and Young Children, 7(4), 29-38.

Prizant, B. M., & Wetherby, A. M. (1998). Understanding the continuum of discrete-trial traditional behavioral to social-pragmatic developmental approaches in communication enhancement for young children with autism/PDD. Seminars in Speech and Language, 19(4), 329-353, 424.

Schneck, C. (2001). The efficacy of a sensorimotor treatment approach by occupational therapists. In R. Huebner (Ed.), Autism: A sensorimotor approach to management. *Gaithersberg, MD: Aspen.*

Sullivan, M., & Lewis, M. (2000). Assistive technology for the very young: Creating responsive environments. Infants and Young Children, 12(4), 34-52.

WEBSITES

There are also websites that provide summary material for practice. Two excellent websites for information about serving children are CanChild (www.canchild.ca/) and Bottomlines (www.researchtopractice.info/productBridges.php).

You can also get information from the Cochran Collaboration and from professional societies which have evidence material for their constituents and the public (e.g., AOTA Evidence Briefs and OT Seeker from the American Occupational Therapy Association).

Activity 10-14

Using Legitimate Websites

Visit one of the websites listed above and scan the topics available from this website. Obtain a review to share with your study partners.

Go to one other website that provides summaries of research for professionals and consumers. Be sure that you find legitimate websites that would meet professional standards.

Activity 10-15

Group Discussion

Meet with your study partners and discuss the summary articles you have found. How are these types of articles helpful to your practice? Are you surprised by the findings and recommendations these authors report? What future studies are possible now that this work has been summarized?

Activity 10-16

Developing Take Home Messages

The final step in the analysis process for evidence-based practice is to summarize the findings for those who need to use the ideas to improve their practices. Professionals want clear, easy-to-understand guidelines about what to do. We will call these summaries "Take Home Messages" to remind ourselves to use understandable language. You will need to consider Take Home Messages for your colleagues (within your discipline and from other disciplines), family members, other care providers, and those receiving your care.

Select two constituent groups as the focus of your attention and create some Take Home Messages for them. Pretend that the articles you read were the **definitive** articles on the topic. Use Worksheets 10M and 10N to summarize your work.

When considering what you are going to write, think about these questions:

- What would you say to colleagues about how they might need to change their practices to gain the optimal benefit?
- What would you say to your team regarding the articles' findings based on

the articles you have read?

- How would you extrapolate information from these articles to develop hypotheses for populations other than the ones that were studied?

Summary

Scholars who prepare summary and meta-analysis articles provide a great service to professionals in practice. These materials integrate findings across a large group of studies, enabling those in practice to obtain a wealth of information in one source.

All references for this unit can be found in the Bibliography, beginning on page 169.

Worksheet 10A
Research Questions

Question being addressed in the Kwakkel et al. (2004) study in my own words:

Worksheet 10B
Inclusion Criteria

List the inclusion criteria for the Kwakkel et al. (2004) meta-analysis.

1.

2.

3.

Worksheet 10C
Considering the Findings

List the aspects of the findings that you would need to consider in your practices based on this study (Kwakkel et al., 2004).

1.

2.

3.

4.

Worksheet 10D
Creating a Flow Chart

Flow chart for _____

Worksheet 10E
Alternate Interpretations

List the additional factors that might have contributed to the findings of Kwakkel et al. (2004).

1.

2.

3.

Worksheet 10F
Limitations of the Study

List the limitations of the Kwakkel et al. (2004) study.

1.

2.

3.

4.

Worksheet 10G
Applying Evidence to a Specific Situation

Discuss with your study partners what you will plan for Sarah's home health rehabilitation program based on her particular situation and the findings of Kwakkel et al.'s (2004) meta-analysis. Provide a rationale for your decisions. Write a script of what you will say to Sarah (another form of Take Home Messages).

Decision	Rationale	What You Will Say to Sarah (Refer to Tickle-Degnen [2001])

Worksheet 10H
What Is Being Addressed in the Study

Controversy and purpose being addressed in the Baranek (2002) study in my own words:

Worksheet 10I
Stating the Purpose

List the purposes of the Baranek (2002) study.

1.

2.

3.

Worksheet 10J
Comparing Strategies

Same Strategies	Unique Strategies to Baranek (2002)

Worksheet 10K
Summary of Exercise Articles From Baranek (2002)

Questions	Your Summary Statement
How many children do these studies represent?	
What is the age range of the children?	
What designs were used to test the intervention?*	
What are some common themes in the interventions?	
What are some common aspects of the outcome measurements?	
What overall findings can you report from these studies?	

*Use your research design text to understand the different study methods if needed.

Worksheet 10L
Reactions to New Data

Think about your reactions to the articles. Based on Chinn and Brewer's (1993) ways of responding to anomalous data, what would you say your reaction illustrates?

Chinn and Brewer (1993) Responses	Example Reaction to the Findings
IGNORE the data (don't even bother to "explain" data away)	
REJECT the data (articulate an explanation for why data should be rejected)	
EXCLUDE the data from the domain of current beliefs (the data are outside the domain of current beliefs)	
Hold the data in ABEYANCE (I promise to deal with it later...assume that someday current beliefs will be articulated so that it can explain these data)	
REINTERPRET the data while retaining current beliefs (accept the data as something that should be explained by current beliefs...opposing forces accept data but interpret the data differently based on their own beliefs)	
Reinterpret the data and make PERIPHERAL CHANGES to current belief (make a relatively minor change to current belief...accepts the data but is unwilling to give up current belief and accept new beliefs)	
Accept the data and CHANGE current beliefs, possibly in favor of a particular new belief (change one or more of the core aspects of current beliefs—when faced with information that is contradictory to current beliefs, accepts alternate beliefs)	

Worksheet 10M
Take Home Messages for Group 1

Pretend that the articles you just read are the definitive articles about the topic. Develop Take Home Messages showing what you would say to a particular constituent group regarding the topic based on the articles you have read.

Take Home Messages About:

Name:

These messages are for:

_____ colleagues in my discipline	_____ care providers
_____ colleagues in other disciplines	_____ family members
_____ adults receiving care	_____ children receiving care

Take Home Message	Rationale for This Message From the Literature

Worksheet 10N
Take Home Messages for Group 2

Pretend that the articles you just read are the definitive articles about the topic. Develop Take Home Messages showing what you would say to a particular constituent group regarding the topic based on the articles you have read.

Take Home Messages About:

Name:

These messages are for:

_____ colleagues in my discipline   _____ care providers

_____ colleagues in other disciplines   _____ family members

_____ adults receiving care   _____ children receiving care

Take Home Message	Rationale for This Message From the Literature

Unit 11

Examining Evidence Related to Emerging and Controversial Practices

Another issue you will encounter in evidence-based practice is how to handle emerging and controversial practices. In this unit, you will explore this issue and learn how to obtain information and then evaluate whether a particular practice is worthy of attention as an evidence-based practice.

There are two primary reasons why professionals need to understand how to examine emerging and controversial practices. First, younger disciplines (e.g., those that are less than 100 years old!) have not had the time to develop substantial and longitudinal evidence about their practices; data are only available about some of the profession's practices. Second, disciplines are always evolving, so new ideas are always emerging and they need to be tested. There will never be a time when we know all there is to know and have the final evidence on the effectiveness of practices.

When you complete the work in this unit, you will have the following skills and competencies:

- Learn the factors that might make a practice controversial

- Analyze an emerging practice area to determine whether it is controversial
- Construct a summary for colleagues to inform them about an emerging or controversial practice
- Prepare materials for families and clients to inform them about an emerging or controversial practice

You will be reviewing articles and website materials, creating summaries for comparison and contrast, gaining insights from your study partners, and creating summaries for constituent groups.

Activity 11-1

Reading the Literature

Read the articles listed here, which are located in the Appendix (Articles 22 and 23). They provide background for your work in this unit and shed some light on how to decide about the viability of a practice.

McWilliam, R. A. (1999). *Controversial practices: The need for a reacculturation of early intervention fields.* Topics in Early Childhood Special Education, *19(3), 177-188.*

Nickel, R. E. (1996). *Controversial therapies for young children with developmental disabilities.* Infants and Young Children, *8(4), 29-40.*

Professionals know that they need to provide evidence-based practice, and you have been learning some strategies in this book. However, when new ideas emerge, it is hard to know what to do with them. Has there been enough time to test the ideas? Are the new ideas based on sound foundational knowledge? How would others judge the ideas? In this unit, we will explore some ways to organize your thinking about emerging and sometimes controversial practices.

There are always new ideas forming and being tested in every profession; this is a necessary part of the evolution of a discipline and a body of knowledge. New ideas are enticing and exciting and challenge the status quo. But just because something is new doesn't mean that the ideas are preferable to current trends. When professionals have some systematic ways of considering the feasibility of new ideas for providing directions for evidence-based practice, then professionals are not subject to bias because "new" is interesting and "better."

The two readings in this unit are from interdisciplinary childhood journals. The authors provide a structure for considering whether a set of ideas will meet professional standards. These are not the only ways to analyze emerging practices; if you have others you know about, add them to your resources.

Summarizing the Key Points of These Articles

Since these (McWilliam, 1999; Nickel, 1996) are not research articles, they do not contain the typical sections we have come to expect in an article. Instead, these authors provide a set of guidelines about how to analyze an emerging practice to decide if it is controversial.

Activity 11-2
Creating a Summary Worksheet

Create a summary (Worksheet 11A) for yourself that contains brief definitions of the key points

from the articles listed in Activity 11-1. This will serve as a tip sheet when you are analyzing a controversial or emerging practice of your own.

Activity 11-3
Handling Anomalous Data

You will encounter many lively debates over emerging and controversial practices during your career. Those that are passionately in favor (or against) an emerging practice will have many things to say about their point of view. Challenging one's beliefs will be a regular part of your professional life. Some of the controversial practices cited in the McWilliam (1999) and Nickel (1996) articles may be practices you have seen implemented. Perhaps there is an emerging practice you are drawn to and want to try. Take time to think about all points of view before making any specific decision about what you believe and how you will practice.

Select one of the controversial practices summarized in the McWilliam (1999) or Nickel (1996) articles. Refer to your Executive Summary (see Sidebar 2-1) of the Chinn and Brewer (1993) article to decide where a colleague's reactions might fall related to handling anomalous data (Worksheet 11B). Bring these issues up with your study partners.

Activity 11-4
Analyzing an Emerging or Controversial Practice

Now that you have some ideas about what to look for as a controversial practice, let's practice applying these ideas to a specific situation.

Internet Search

First, conduct an Internet search (e.g., Google) on your topic. Print the hits you get from each search. You may need to discuss what key words to use with your study partners and/or your instructor. Select three to five sites to review and take notes on what you find, with particular attention to information that will help you conduct your "controversial therapies" analysis. Write a three- to five-sentence summary of your findings.

Professional Literature Search

Next, conduct a professional literature search (e.g., CINAHL, ERIC, PsycINFO, PubMed, Ovid) using the same key words, key authors, or other distinct terms used in the practice you are examining. Remember, these resources have been independently reviewed by non-interested parties. Print the hits you get from these searches as well. Review the material and write a three- to five-sentence summary of what you find.

Summarizing the Findings From These Searches

Now compile a summary of your findings. After you collect and review the materials, complete an analysis using McWilliam (1999) and Nickel (1996) criteria. Then, construct an overall summary statement about the emerging or controversial practice.

WORKING THROUGH AN EXAMPLE TOGETHER

Let's go through the steps using a particular practice. There is a practice being implemented in some schools called Bal-A-Vis-X.

Internet Search

An Internet search of this topic yields a number of hits; one of them is an "official website."

The website informs the reader that Bill Hubert is the creator of this approach. The site also provides explanations of the practices and tells who will benefit from this intervention.

Professional Literature Search

When using key words from the Internet site (e.g., "Bal-A-Vis-X," "Bill Hubert," "balance," "coordination"), there are zero results from the name of the intervention and from the creator (we searched on ERIC, CINAHL, and PsycINFO). This suggests that the author has not published the findings of any studies in refereed journals (i.e., professional journals have independent reviewers to examine studies and decide whether they are acceptable). There were studies about coordination and balance, but none included this particular procedure. Some studies reported about movement programs, so theoretically these studies could provide support for the Bal-A-Vis-X program. However, we would have to conclude that this program does not have professional evidence to support it.

Summarizing the Findings From These Searches

Sidebar 11-1 is a summary of the searches based on the McWilliam (1999) and Nickel (1996) articles.

Sidebar 11-1

Analyzing Intervention Practices to Determine Whether They Are Controversial

Using the McWilliam (1999) and Nickel (1996) articles as a guide, analyze one emerging practice to determine whether it is controversial.

Attach the results and your summary of a Google search, which will provide you with a public assessment of what is available about the practice. Remember that material on public access does not always meet the standards expected by professionals as acceptable evidence.

Attach the results and your summary of a professional search (using professional resources that have been independently reviewed [e.g., journals]) of what is available about the practice.

Group members:

1.   5.
2.   6.
3.   7.
4.   8.

Topic:
Bal-A-Vis-X

Continued on Next Page

Sidebar 11-1 (Continued)

Analyzing Intervention Practices to Determine Whether They Are Controversial

Summary from Google search:
There are a number of websites that come up when searching this topic. The "official website" contains information about who will benefit, what needs to happen, and contains testimonials from families, therapists, children, and teachers.

Summary from professional search:
There were no hits when searching "Bal-A-Vis-X" and "Bill Hubert." Studies related to movement are available, but none of them tested this program.

Analysis based on McWilliam (1999) criteria:

McWilliam Criteria	*Information from the website*
Cure Claims	*The only ones that don't profit are those who refused to follow instructions (per website)*
Practitioner Specialization	*Three levels of training plus three additional special versions of the program for special needs/individualization*
Questionable Research	*We couldn't find information on the professional website listing journal articles* *The website provides testimonials from teachers, students, and therapists*
Intensity	*There are specific exercise routines, equipment, and training* *There are required amounts of training for providers*
Legal Action	*There was no indication of legal action*

Analysis based on Nickel (1996) criteria:

Nickel Criteria	
Oversimplified Theories	*States that activities are built on "Educational Kinesiology"*
Effective for Many	*Learning disabled, behaviorally disordered, ADD/ADHD, gifted, regular, students who have trouble with pronunciation, auditory perception, verbal instructions, discussion, ocular motility, binocularity, visual form perception, eye-hand coordination (from website)*
Dramatic Results	*There are a range of reports from schools, teachers, therapists, and students in the testimonial section of the website*
Case Reports vs. Studies	*Case reports available, but no studies found*
Treatment Objectives	*Full body coordination, attention, cooperation, self-challenge, peer teaching* *Also outcomes related to populations listed above*
Side Effects	*No side effects were reported*

Conclusions regarding this intervention practice:
There is an enthusiastic following for this program. There is no research to help determine the effectiveness, so we cannot use it in evidence-based professional practice. This may be a good recreational option.

Activity 11-5

Complete an Analysis of a Controversial Practice

Select an emerging or controversial practice with your professor's assistance (you may select one of the topics covered in the articles, a "hot topic" in your area of the country, or a topic you have encountered in your readings or field experiences). Meet with your study partners to complete Worksheet 11C using the McWilliam (1999) and Nickel (1996) criteria and the materials you have gathered.

Activity 11-6

Looking for Patterns and Themes

Think about the similarities and differences in the two methods of searching and the two methods for analyzing the practice. McWilliam (1999) and Nickel (1996) have some overlapping criteria and some distinct criteria; discuss these with your study partners.

- What did each author draw out of the material with his particular point of view?
- What do you know because of using both articles that you would have missed with only one article as a reference?
- What are the differences between the Internet search results and the professional search results?
- Did the material support or complement each other, or were the two search methods in conflict?

Seeing the differences in these two search methods is important because many families and individuals you serve will use the Internet to find out about their situation. Your job as a professional is to help families and individuals evaluate that information in light of evidence-based practice standards. Without your help, the people you serve do not know how to evaluate the information on the Internet; it all looks informative and impressive to an untrained eye.

- What are the benefits and risks of this access?
- How can you, as a professional, guide families and individuals so they find legitimate information for their decision making?

Now, think about the topic.

- What happened to your thinking from before and after each of the searches?
- How did your ideas change?
- Have you observed that professionals have incorporated appropriate findings into their practices?
- Are you going to do anything differently now that your have searched and analyzed this emerging or controversial practice?

Activity 11-7

Group Discussion

Meet with your study partners and discuss your findings and reactions to the emerging and controversial practices.

Activity 11-8

Developing Take Home Messages

When you have completed your analysis of an emerging or controversial practice, you will need to create a summary statement about that practice based on the articles you read about the emerging and controversial practice. Professionals, families, and individuals want clear, easy-to-understand guidelines about what to do. We call these summaries "Take Home Messages" to remind ourselves to use understandable language. You will need to consider Take Home Messages for your colleagues (within your discipline and from other disciplines), family members, other care providers, and those receiving your care.

Select two constituent groups as the focus of your attention and create some Take Home Messages for them. Use Worksheets 11D and 11E to summarize your work.

When addressing emerging and controversial practices, ask yourself a few different questions:

- What would you say to colleagues about using this emerging or controversial practice?

- What would you say to your team regarding the emerging or controversial practice?
- What resources from the professional and Internet literature would you want to make your colleagues aware of?
- How would you counsel a family/individual about how to evaluate the emerging or controversial practice for themselves?

SUMMARY

There are always new ideas emerging in professional practice. We need to consider these ideas with an open mind and critical eye. This unit provided you with strategies for considering these emerging trends as part of an ever-evolving professional practice.

All references for this unit can be found in the Bibliography, beginning on page 169.

Worksheet 11A
Summarizing Key Points for Analysis

Criteria from McWilliam (1999)	Definition	Examples/Notes
1.		
2.		
3.		
4.		
5.		

Criteria from Nickel (1996)	Definition	Examples/Notes
1.		
2.		
3.		
4.		
5.		

Other notes:

Worksheet 11B
Reactions to New Data

Think about reactions to one of the controversial practices described in the McWilliam (1999) and Nickel (1996) articles. Based on Chinn and Brewer's (1993) ways of responding to anomalous data, what would professionals with each of these responses actually say?

Controversial practice being analyzed: _____

Chinn and Brewer (1993) Responses	Example Reaction to the Findings
IGNORE the data (don't even bother to "explain" data away)	
REJECT the data (articulate an explanation for why data should be rejected)	
EXCLUDE the data from the domain of current beliefs (the data are outside the domain of current beliefs)	
Hold the data in ABEYANCE (I promise to deal with it later...assume that someday current beliefs will be articulated so that it can explain these data)	
REINTERPRET the data while retaining current beliefs (accept the data as something that should be explained by current beliefs...opposing forces accept data but interpret the data differently based on their own beliefs)	
Reinterpret the data and make PERIPHERAL CHANGES to current belief (make a relatively minor change to current belief...accepts the data but is unwilling to give up current belief and accept new beliefs)	
Accept the data and CHANGE current beliefs, possibly in favor of a particular new belief (change one or more of the core aspects of current beliefs—when faced with information that is contradictory to current beliefs, accepts alternate beliefs)	

Worksheet 11C
Analyzing Intervention Practices to Determine Whether They Are Controversial

Using the McWilliam (1999) and Nickel (1996) articles as a guide, analyze one emerging practice to determine whether it is controversial.

Attach the results and your summary of a Google search, which will provide you with a public assessment of what is available about the practice. Remember that material on public access does not always meet the standards expected by professionals as acceptable evidence.

Attach the results and your summary of a professional search (using professional resources that have been independently reviewed [e.g., journals]) of what is available about the practice.

Group members:

1.

2.

3.

4.

5.

6.

7.

8.

Topic:

Summary from Google search:

Summary from professional search:

Analysis based on McWilliam (1999) criteria:
McWilliam Criteria

Cure Claims

Practitioner Specialization

Questionable Research

Intensity

Legal Action

(Continued)

Worksheet 11C (Continued)
Analyzing Intervention Practices to Determine Whether They Are Controversial

Analysis based on Nickel (1996) criteria:

Nickel Criteria

Oversimplified Theories

Effective for Many

Dramatic Results

Case Reports vs. Studies

Treatment Objectives

Side Effects

Conclusions regarding this intervention practice:

Worksheet 11D
Take Home Messages for Group 1

Pretend that the articles you just read are the definitive articles about the topic. Develop Take Home Messages showing what you would say to a particular constituent group regarding the topic based on the articles you have read.

Take Home Messages About:	
Name:	
These messages are for:	
_____ colleagues in my discipline	_____ care providers
_____ colleagues in other disciplines	_____ family members
_____ adults receiving care	_____ children receiving care

Take Home Message	Rationale for This Message From the Literature

Worksheet 11E
Take Home Messages for Group 2

Pretend that the articles you just read are the definitive articles about the topic. Develop Take Home Messages showing what you would say to a particular constituent group regarding the topic based on the articles you have read.

Take Home Messages About:

Name:

These messages are for:

_____ colleagues in my discipline   _____ care providers

_____ colleagues in other disciplines   _____ family members

_____ adults receiving care   _____ children receiving care

Take Home Message	Rationale for This Message From the Literature

Unit 12

Creating Evidence Within Your Own Practice

Throughout this book, we have been exploring ways to examine the evidence available in the professional literature. All of the skills you have learned will enable you to access the literature so you can provide evidence-based practices to the people you serve in your practice. However, regardless of whether you identify evidence to support a particular practice or not, you have the responsibility to collect data within your practice to evaluate whether a practice is effective **for that particular person/family/setting.** Even proven practices may not be the right intervention for a specific situation. In this unit you will learn some basic strategies for collecting evidence within your practice to guide your decisions about whether the interventions are effective. When you are applying evidence-based practices from the literature, your data collection confirms and verifies the effectiveness of the practice within your situation. When you are extending ideas from the literature to new populations or settings, you are creating evidence about this new application. In any case, collecting data to guide your practice is

another everyday way to provide evidence-based practice.

When professionals share information with each other without data, we can call this "professional folklore." This refers to information that professionals share with each other based on their experiences and ideas without a systematic structure. Professionals passing on folklore might say "It really works when you…." An evidence-based professional says "Studies have shown…" or "We have some evidence that…" We might need to add "This intervention idea hasn't been tested with children this age" or "We don't have evidence for this intervention, so let's try it for 2 weeks, measure progress, and then decide if we are going to continue." As you become more skilled at collecting data in your practice, you can share your systematic findings with colleagues. Because you have collected data, you are not passing along professional folklore, you are sharing evidence. Everyday evidence builds just as research studies build, to illustrate patterns we can rely on for better decision making.

When you complete the work in this unit, you will have the following skills and competencies:

- Understand the importance of everyday evidence in your practice
- Learn specific strategies for collecting evidence within your practice
- Recognize how to decide when interventions are not effective and need to be changed based on your data
- Construct a data collection and monitoring plan that extends evidence from the literature
- Practice reporting data-based information to colleagues and families

BASIC STRUCTURE FOR EVIDENCE-BASED DATA COLLECTION IN YOUR PRACTICE

When professionals take the time to collect data, it is important to make sure that these efforts will yield useful findings. If you collect information that is unreliable, then others may not agree with or believe your conclusions. Take the time to organize your efforts so you have reliable data.

Collect Information, Not Interpretations

There are two levels of information gathering; they each have an important purpose, but must not be confused with each other in evidence-based practice. The first level of information gathering is factual; anyone gathering the same information will obtain the same information. For example, if you are doing a skilled observation in a classroom, a factual observation is the number of times the student leaves his desk. Anyone watching this student would be able to see whether the student left his chair (as long as you set clear operational definitions about "leaving the chair," see Unit 3 about operational definitions).

The second level of information gathering involves making a hypothesis about what the observed behavior means. An occupational therapist using a sensory processing frame of reference might say "The student needs movement input, so he leaves the chair frequently to get this movement." A teacher using a behavioral frame of reference might say "The student is trying to get my attention, so he leaves his chair a lot." A psychologist using a psychosocial frame of reference might say "The student is anxious and is moving around

to manage his anxiety." Professionals won't agree about this level of information gathering unless they are using the same frame of reference. When planning on an interdisciplinary team, members negotiate which hypotheses seem most plausible for the student and begin their planning based on these hypotheses. The team then establishes factual ways to collect data on the desired outcomes (e.g., in this example, the student getting his seatwork completed in a timely manner) so they can measure the accuracy of their hypothesis and the effectiveness of their intervention.

Measure Something That Matters

It is tempting to measure things that are easy to measure, but this does not advance your evidence-based practice. For example, you can count how many times a person looks away from her hands while trying to crochet, but this may not be relevant to the person getting back to a satisfying experience with her hobby of crocheting. Perhaps the woman didn't used to watch her hands while crocheting and looking away gives her the chance to feel other sensory inputs while crocheting. Perhaps looking at her hands reminds her that her arthritis is bad, and this reduces her optimism about getting back to crocheting. If we are working with a woman to reconnect her with her hobby of crocheting, then we have to measure the **crocheting experience** somehow. Getting at the most important factors requires some planning. In this example, you would want to ask the woman what makes crocheting satisfying for her, and then find a way to document what she tells you. If she tells you she likes to stack up the squares for a blanket, you can count the number of squares (and you might have her start with small squares, so she sees progress quickly). If she tells you she just likes to spend some time crocheting every day, then you might record the number of minutes she crochets or the number of times per day she picks up her crocheting, and ask her to rate her satisfaction each day (you would hope to see a relationship between the amount of time and increasing satisfaction to indicate you were making progress).

Measure Participation, Not Interventions

Since professionals spend a lot of time working out creative interventions, it is easy to slip into the pattern of measuring the procedures rather than the outcomes you desire. For example, if you are running a community reintegration program, you could get focused on member attendance and involvement with the training activities. This is good information for your records about the intervention; it will help you know whether those that were more involved had better outcomes, but it does not indicate effectiveness. You have to measure the desired outcomes to know the effectiveness of your intervention. In this example, you might record how long it takes members to get housing or employment and how many secure housing or employment.

Measure During Living, Not During Therapy

When we stay focused on the person's participation, it is clear that in order to know whether our interventions are effective, they must change the person's life. Changing how he or she performs in a clinical situation is a step toward increased competence, but it does not substitute for actual changes in participation during the times when the person really needs to participate. If we train adolescents in social skills in a planned social group, it is a good place to learn and practice (this is part of the intervention). If we want to know whether those adolescents manage better with their peers, we will have to watch them during class, in transitions between classes, in a club, or at a party. In this example, we can also rely on the adolescents to report their satisfaction with socializing because they are in the class, hallways, clubs, and parties. You have read studies that use parent, self, or partner reports of participation in natural contexts. You can also have people videotape in the natural setting, and you can code the behaviors of interest later.

Record What You Are Measuring

Writing down what happens creates a record of your hypotheses and outcomes. When your interventions are working to improve participation, your documentation verifies this. When your interventions are not having the desired effect, documentation helps you remember your clinical reasoning processes, so you can reformulate your hypotheses and plans. Find simple ways to document:

- Use bullet-point lists to characterize the behaviors of interest

- Make graphs showing the data points and progress
- Design simple illustrations or take pictures of desired behaviors
- Add notations to your graphs and lists so you don't have to go back to a full report or record each time you need to review your documentation

Simple recording plans become a great communication tool for you; everyone involved (including persons, families, and other professionals) gets the picture about what is going on very quickly.

DATA COLLECTION METHODS

Many authors have written about ways to document the effectiveness of your interventions. Let's examine a few examples, and then you can practice.

Copy Measurement Strategies in Journal Articles

The first resources you have are all the intervention studies you have read or will read. When a study tests an intervention that is applicable to your practice, examine the measurement strategies used. Are there any that you can use in your practice to document participation outcomes? Did the authors make an interesting table or graph?

Activity 12-1
Let's Practice

Select a journal article whose findings are applicable to an area of practice that is interesting to you. Make a worksheet showing how you could use their measurement strategies within a practice situation.

FIND OUT EXACTLY WHAT THE OUTCOME NEEDS TO BE

A big barrier to documenting the effectiveness of practices is having unclear ideas about what the desired outcome is. Families and individuals might say "We want her to walk"; does this mean getting around with a cane, using a walker, or only walking independently of other supports? When professionals don't get specific, they can be at crossed purposes to the people being served.

So, how do we get specific? We ask the right questions, and listen to the answers. Here are some questions that can get you started:

- What will it look like when your mom can walk again?
- How will we know that your son has more friends?
- What would a perfect morning routine be for your family?
- What would a successful job be for you?

You will be surprised about the answers. As professionals we are predisposed to thinking about problems a certain way. Although this is mostly helpful, sometimes this characteristic can cause us to jump to incorrect conclusions. The family may think independence upon returning home means mom can indicate what she wants for dinner, while the occupational therapist may think independence means mom has to make dinner. Intervention plans would not look the same in these two scenarios.

Activity 12-2

Let's Practice

Meet with a study partner and interview each other in this way. Start with a general statement ("I want to be more fit"). Jot notes about what you think this means, and then ask the other person what it means to him or her (e.g., What would "being more fit" look like for you?). Compare your answers.

USE A REFERENCE PERSON TO GET IDEAS

Sometimes you will struggle to identify an appropriate level of a behavior for your outcome goal. In these cases, you can observe an average person in the same setting to get an idea about what would be an appropriate amount of the behavior. Let's say the family says they want dad to socialize more. Dad is in a nursing home; how much social interaction is appropriate during certain times of the day at the nursing home? You can go into the dining room or game room and record what other men do. What does their interaction look like (e.g., are they talking, watching, moving, smiling?)? What is the frequency of these behaviors? Knowing this baseline information in

concert with Dad and the family's ideas about interacting will help you craft a great measurement of his progress.

DEVELOP A PROGRESS MONITORING PLAN

Linder and Clark (2000) provide an excellent summary of the progress monitoring method (Table 12-1). They provide a six-point structure for designing a theoretically sound way to collect evidence for your practice. With a simple worksheet, you have cues about what to think about next, and soon you are finished writing your plan.

Let's look at an example. Stella is having a hard time with independent work in the classroom. Table 12-2 shows what her team documented for Stella.

Stella's team discussed their test results, observations, interviews with teachers, and an ecological assessment and hypothesized that Stella needed more intense sensory input to help her focus and complete her seatwork. They reviewed the literature and found some evidence for using weighted vests and flexible seating to improve work product (see Unit 7) to support their decisions.

This team didn't want to take any chances on having success! They added three interventions together to try to increase her participation; we might call this an "intervention package." They won't know if only one selection might have worked; they will only know if the intervention package works. You will also notice that the teacher did not care about accuracy of work in this plan. She just wanted Stella to keep working; she felt that accuracy and getting the work to be just the right level for Stella could come later. The teacher said "We can't know whether Stella has skills because she doesn't work long enough to show us what she can do." The teacher agreed to record the length of time Stella worked during independent work time and felt confident that she would make swift progress.

GRAPHING STELLA'S PROGRESS

Figure 12-1 is a simple graph to chart Stella's progress. We made a 5 (number of weeks) x 10 (number of minutes) graph to make it easy to record her time working. We drew a line from 0 to the endpoint (5 and 10) to show how much progress she needed to make each week. Then the

Table 12-1
Summary of the Parts of the Progress Monitoring Plan

Outline of Tasks for Progress Monitoring	Summary of Components
Behavior	Describe what the person is doing currently, with emphasis on what participation is challenging
Goal	Describe the participation goal
Hypothesis for observed behavior	This is an If...Then statement In the If part, tell what your hypothesis is and link it to a theoretically sound idea In the Then part, tell your general intervention idea based on the theoretically sound hypothesis
Intervention plan	Describe specifically what your intervention will look like so other people could implement it
Measurement strategy	Describe how you will measure and who will measure the behavior
Decision-making plan	State the criteria for success on the goal

Table 12-2
Sample Progress Monitoring Plan for Stella

Outline of Tasks for Progress Monitoring	Stella's Plan
Behavior	*Stella is constantly repositioning herself and fidgeting in her chair, making it difficult to complete her seatwork*
Goal	*Stella will continue working independently for 10 minutes*
Hypothesis for observed behavior	*If Stella's distractibility is due to her need to obtain additional sensory input,* *Then interventions that increase this input during independent work will make it possible for Stella to complete seatwork*
Intervention plan	*Provide Stella with a weighted vest, flexible cushion, and heavy lap pillow during seatwork*
Measurement strategy	*Teacher will record number of minutes Stella continues working independently*
Decision-making plan	*Within 5 weeks, Stella will work for 10 minutes in a row*

teacher could just color in the boxes indicating the average number of minutes each week.

We want Stella to work at least as many minutes as the diagonal line indicates for each week. She meets this standard during weeks 1 and 2. During week 3 she makes no more progress, but continues at the same level. The team intervenes immediately to adjust the plan so Stella will make more progress.

Activity 12-3

Let's Practice

As you can see from Figure 12-1, Stella made progress the first 2 weeks of the program, then she stalled in the third week. Because the team was collecting data, they knew right away that the intervention was only partially effective. Meet with your study partners and decide what to do next so that Stella continues to make progress during her independent work.

You might want to make a new hypothesis. What are some additional reasons why Stella could be inattentive (e.g., the work is too hard for her)? This hypothesis will guide the planning process.

Activity 12-4

Let's Practice Some More!

Saul is a 16-month-old boy who is happy and playful with his family. He is the only boy, with two sisters and grandparents close by. His parents are concerned that he is still not moving around by himself to play. When the team completed their assessments, they had several hypotheses about why Saul wasn't moving:

- Saul is weak when compared to age peers.
- Saul has poor biomechanical alignment and instability.
- Saul has low registration (he misses sensory cues).
- Saul has sensation avoiding (he gets overwhelmed easily with sensory input).
- The family caters to Saul, so he doesn't have to move to play.

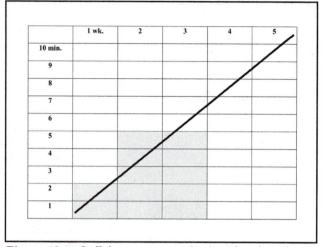

Figure 12-1. *Stella's progress monitoring plan data sheet. Reprinted from* Sensory Profile Supplement. *Copyright © 2006 by NCS Pearson Inc. Reproduced with permission. All rights reserved.*

Saul's family is very involved with their children. The team decided to make more than one progress monitoring plan, so they could discuss the options with the family and make the decision about where to begin with them.

Meet with your study partners and write three progress monitoring plans for Saul's family (Worksheets 12A through 12C). Table 12-3 shows the one they wrote related to lack of strength, so pick three other hypotheses for your work.

DESIGN A CHART OR GRAPH TO RECORD BEHAVIOR

The progress monitoring plans typically invite the team to make a graph of the behavior. You can make charts for just about anything. Visual prompts about progress are helpful because they serve as a reminder about the goal and show what progress we are making.

Activity 12-5

Let's Practice

Chart your own progress on something. Make a chart showing which food groups you have had in your diet each day. Graph the times you remember where your keys are. How does graphing and charting change your behavior?

When you go into a practice situation, create a way to graph the progress of a person you are

Table 12-3
Sample Progress Monitoring Plan for Saul

Outline of Tasks for Progress Monitoring	Saul's Plan
Behavior	*Saul doesn't move; he sits in one place to play*
Goal	*Saul will move to play with toys*
Hypothesis for observed behavior	*If Saul's immobility is due to lack of strength, Then improving his strength will enable him to move to play*
Intervention plan	*Provide progressively more resistance to Saul's play schemas including use of gravity*
Measurement strategy	*Saul will reach for and obtain toys from surfaces above his head (later we will have the family move toys to other positions that require both reaching and shifting body position)*
Decision-making plan	*Within a month, Saul will obtain a toy from a surface above shoulder level within 10 seconds of a cue*

serving. Share the graph with the individual and see how that changes the behavior.

DEVELOP A SPECIFIC SCALE FOR OUTCOME ATTAINMENT

Some research programs use a method called goal attainment scaling. When using this method in research, there are very specific criteria about how to establish the scale. The precision is related to making sure that each step along the scale represents exactly the same amount of change as every other step along the scale.

We can take this idea and adapt it for the purpose of documenting progress. First you identify the current behavior; this behavior becomes the -1 point on the scale. Then you ask "How would the behavior look if it got worse?"; this behavior becomes -2 on the scale. Next, you ask "What will the behavior look like when we have reached our goal?"; this becomes the neutral (or 0) point on the scale. Next, find out what a dream behavioral outcome would be: "What would the behavior look like if we exceeded our expectations?"; this becomes the +1 point on the scale. If you like, you can go to utopia and ask one more question: "If this person had perfect behavior, what would it

look like?"; this is the +2 point on the scale. Now you have a ready-made way to document progress on behaviors that might be too complicated to characterize other ways.

Let's look at an example. Kim has trouble with the bus. She is disruptive with her classmates when they are going to the bus at the end of the school day. Figure 12-2 is an example of what the teacher, parent, bus driver, and principal came up with for their outcome scale.

The team laughed about the utopia possibility and thought it was silly to write it down. But an interesting thing happened: by talking about the specific behaviors (they had a list of what "without incident" meant and a list of "positive bus behaviors") among themselves, and with Kim, she started to remind everyone when she did one of the behaviors (e.g., "I said something nice to the driver today"). So consider the long view when you do this yourself.

The principal and bus driver made the judgments each day, and the teacher made a chart with Kim showing her progress. They did it on a computer program so they could email it to Kim's parents as well, providing an additional way to reinforce desirable behaviors.

| -2
Worse | -1
Current | 0
Goal | +1
Exceeds Goal | +2
Utopia! |
|---|---|---|---|---|
| *Kim has to be pulled out of the bus line and have her parents pick her up* | *Kim pushes and bumps people while going to the bus* | *Kim gets to the bus without incident* | *Kim gets to the bus and seated without incident* | *Kim gets positive reports about the bus ride after getting on the bus without incident* |

Figure 12-2. *Goal attainment example.*

This outcome attainment plan does not tell us what interventions the team used to change Kim's behavior; it focuses attention on measuring the participation and that is what will indicate how effective the interventions were.

Activity 12-6

Let's Practice

Think of something you want to improve about yourself or your life. Write an outcome attainment scale for this area of your life. Post it in a prominent place, so you remember what you want to accomplish. Use graph paper to graph your progress.

RECORD OUTCOMES IN CONTEXT

An ecological assessment is an evaluation of the contexts in which behaviors occur. As professionals, we want to look for situations that are easier and harder for the persons we are serving, so we can tailor our recommendations according-

ly. We think about what might be contributing to or interfering with participation in each setting of interest.

When designing data collection to document the effectiveness of our interventions, contexts matter as well. Here is an example of an ecological assessment for a young woman who wants to make more friends. Assessments indicated that she is sensitive to noise in her environment. The therapist wants to identify settings that were more or less likely to support making new friends.

Figure 12-3 is a shortened version of an ecological assessment. The therapist and woman decide that lunch and after work have the biggest potential for developing friends, and that the woman has some control over these situations. The intervention is the therapist making recommendations to the woman about how to manage her auditory sensitivity to maximize the possibility of being able to interact successfully. The measurement of outcomes in this example will be related to the woman's satisfaction with developing friends (e.g., number of times per week she goes

	Riding the Bus to Work	**Working at Her Office**	**Going to Lunch**	**Socializing After Work**
Auditory Sensitivity	*Lots of people talking, moving around, bus noises as people enter and exit*	*Has own office with a door*

Plays soft music in the background | *Variable depending on where she eats*

Invitation to join big groups may trigger sensitivity | *Venues vary and therefore have varying levels of sound* |

Figure 12-3. *Partial ecological assessment.*

out to lunch with others; number of people she visits with after work).

RECORD PERFORMANCE AND SATISFACTION WITH PERFORMANCE

The Canadian Occupational Performance Measure (COPM) evaluates a person's level of performance and the person's satisfaction with current performance. There are data on the COPM itself, documenting its ability to record changes in participation. Combining performance with satisfaction is a way to acknowledge that people can be satisfied with average performance in some as-pects of their lives. The COPM is a great tool for documenting the effectiveness of an intervention in daily life.

SUMMARY

In this unit, you learned some basic ways to collect data within your practice so you can document the actual progress being made. Collecting data is a way to verify the effectiveness of your evidence-based practice decisions and extends the literature into the lives of the people you are serving.

All references for this unit can be found in the Bibliography, beginning on page 169.

Worksheet 12A
Progress Monitoring Plan 1

Outline of Tasks for Progress Monitoring	Plan for: Participation Focus:
Behavior	
Goal	
Hypothesis for observed behavior	
Intervention plan	
Measurement strategy	
Decision-making plan	

Worksheet 12B
Progress Monitoring Plan 2

Outline of Tasks for Progress Monitoring	Plan for: Participation Focus:
Behavior	
Goal	
Hypothesis for observed behavior	
Intervention plan	
Measurement strategy	
Decision-making plan	

Worksheet 12C
Progress Monitoring Plan 3

Outline of Tasks for Progress Monitoring	Plan for: Participation Focus:
Behavior	
Goal	
Hypothesis for observed behavior	
Intervention plan	
Measurement strategy	
Decision-making plan	

Bibliography

Ahmad, S., Mu, K., & Scott, S. (2001). Meta-analysis of functional outcome in Parkinson patients treated with unilateral pallidotomy. *Neruoscience Letters, 312,* 153-156.

Aldana, S. G., Greenlaw, R. L., Diehl, H. A., Salberg, A., Merrill, R. M., Ohmine, S., & Thomas, C. (2005). Effects of an intensive diet and physical activity modification program on the health risks of adults. *Journal of the American Dietetic Association, 105*(3), 371-381.

Baranek, G. T. (2002). Efficacy of sensory and motor interventions for children with autism. *Journal of Autism and Developmental Disorders, 32*(5), 397-422.

Bond, G. (2004). Supported employment: Evidence for an evidence-based practice. *Psychiatric Rehabilitation Journal, 27*(4), 345-359.

Bonifer, N., Anderson, K., & Arciniegas, D. (2005). Constraint-induced movement therapy after stroke: Efficacy for patients with minimal upper-extremity motor ability. *Archives of Physical Medicine and Rehabilitation, 86,* 1867-1873.

Chinn, C. A., & Brewer, W. F. (1993). The role of anomalous data in knowledge acquisition: A theoretical framework and implications for science instruction. *Review of Educational Research, 63*(1), 1-49.

Chiu, C. W. Y., & Man, D. W. K. (2004). The effect of training older adults with stroke to use home-based assistive devices. *Occupational Therapy Journal of Research: Occupation, Participation and Health, 24*(3), 113-120.

Cole, J. (1996). Intervention strategies for infants with prenatal drug exposure. *Infants and Young Children, 8*(3), 35-39.

Dunn, W. *Sensory profile supplement.* (2006). San Antonio, TX: Harcourt.

Edelson, S., Edelson, M., Kerr, D., & Grandin, T. (1999). Behavioral and physiological effects of deep pressure on children with autism: A pilot study evaluating the efficacy of Grandin's hug machine. *American Journal of Occupational Therapy, 53,* 145-152.

Fertel-Daly, D., Bedell, G., & Hinojosa, J. (2001). Effects of a weighted vest on attention to task and self-stimulatory behaviors in preschoolers with pervasive developmental disorders. *American Journal of Occupational Therapy, 55,* 629-640.

Fetters, L., & Kluzik, J. (1996). The effects of neuro-developmental treatment versus practice on the reaching of children with spastic cerebral palsy. *Physical Therapy, 76*(4), 346-358.

Flinn, N. A., Schamburg, S., Fetrow, J. M., & Flanigan,

J. (2005). The effect of constraint-induced movement treatment on occupational performance and satisfaction in stroke survivors. *Occupational Therapy Journal of Research: Occupation, Participation and Health, 25*(3), 119-127.

Greenhalgh, T. (1997). Assessing the methodological quality of published papers. *British Medical Journal, 315*, 305-308.

Hanft, B., & Pilkington Ovland, K. (2000). Therapy in natural environments: The means or end goal for early intervention? *Infants and Young Children, 12*(4), 1-13.

Ilott, I. (2003). Evidence-based practice forum. Challenging the rhetoric and reality: Only an individual and systemic approach will work for evidence-based occupational therapy. *American Journal of Occupational Therapy, 57*(3), 351-354.

Karman, N., Maryles, J., Baker, R. W., Simpser, E., & Berger-Gross, P. (2003). Constraint-induced movement therapy for hemiplegic children with acquired brain injuries. *Journal of Head Trauma Rehabilitation, 18*(3), 259-267.

Kern, L., Koegel, R. L., & Dunlap, G. (1984). The influence of vigorous versus mild exercise on autistic stereotyped behaviors. *Journal of Autism and Developmental Disorders, 14*, 57-67.

Kern, L., Koegel, R. L., Dyer, K., Blew, P. A., & Fenton, L. R. (1982). The effects of physical exercise on self-stimulation and appropriate responding in autistic children. *Journal of Autism and Developmental Disorders, 12*, 399-419.

Kielhofner, G. (Ed.). (2006). *Research in occupational therapy: Methods of inquiry for enhancing practice.* Philadelphia: F. A. Davis.

Kwakkel, G., van Peppen, R., Wagenaar, R. C., Dauphinee, S. W., Richards, C., Ashburn, A., Miller, K., Lincoln, N., Partridge, C., Wellwood, I., & Langhorne, P. (2004). Effects of augmented exercise therapy time after stroke: A meta-analysis. *Stroke, 35*(11), 2529-2536.

Larson, E. (2006). Caregiving and autism: How does children's propensity for routinization influence participation in family activities? *Occupational Therapy Journal of Research: Occupation, Participation and Health, 26*(2), 69-79.

Law, M. (2002). *Evidence-based rehabilitation: A guide to practice.* Thorofare, NJ: SLACK Incorporated.

Law, M., Baum, C., & Dunn, W. (2005). *Measuring occupational performance: Supporting best practice in occupational therapy.* (2nd ed.). Thorofare, NJ: SLACK Incorporated.

Law, M., & MacDermid, J. (2008). *Evidence-based rehabilitation: A guide to practice* (2nd ed.). Thorofare, NJ: SLACK Incorporated.

Lee, C. J., & Miller, L. T. (2003). Evidence-based practice forum. The process of evidence-based clinical decision making in occupational therapy.

American Journal of Occupational Therapy, 57(4), 473-477.

Levinson, L. J., & Reid, G. (1993). The effects of exercise intensity on the stereotypic behaviors of individuals with autism. *Adapted Physical Activity Quarterly, 10*(3), 255-268.

Linder, J., & Clark, G. (2000). Best practices in documentation. In W. Dunn (Ed.), *Best practice occupational therapy in community service with children and families.* Thorofare, NJ: SLACK Incorporated.

Lund, M. L., & Nygård, L. (2003). Incorporating or resisting assistive devices: Different approaches to achieving a desired occupational self-image. *Occupational Therapy Journal of Research: Occupation, Participation and Health, 23*(2), 67-75.

Mann, W. C., Belchior, P., Tomita, M. R., & Kemp, B. J. (2005). Barriers to the use of traditional telephones by older adults with chronic health conditions. *Occupational Therapy Journal of Research: Occupation, Participation and Health, 25*(4), 160-166.

Mann, W. C., Llanes, C., Justiss, M. D., & Tomita, M. (2004). Frail older adults' self-report of their most important assistive device. *Occupational Therapy Journal of Research: Occupation, Participation and Health, 24*(1), 4-12.

McGuire, B. K., Crowe, T. K., Law, M., & VanLeit, B. (2004). Mothers of children with disabilities: Occupational concerns and solutions. *Occupational Therapy Journal of Research: Occupation, Participation and Health, 24*(2), 54-63.

McWilliam, R. A. (1995). Integration of therapy and consultative special education: A continuum in early intervention. *Infants and Young Children, 7*(4), 29-38.

McWilliam, R. A. (1999). Controversial practices: The need for a reacculturation of early intervention fields. *Topics in Early Childhood Special Education, 19*(3), 177-188.

National Health Service (NHS) in the United Kingdom. (2004). *Section 6: Forming guideline recommendations.* Retrieved October 22, 2007 from http://www.sign.ac.uk/guidelines/fulltext/50/section6.html.

Nickel, R. E. (1996). Controversial therapies for young children with developmental disabilities. *Infants and Young Children, 8*(4), 29-40.

Ottenbacher, K. J., Tickle-Degnen, L., et. al. (2002). From the desk of the editor. Therapists awake! The challenge of evidence-based occupational therapy. *American Journal of Occupational Therapy, 56*(3), 247-249.

Portney, L., & Watkins, M. (2000). *Foundations of clinical research: Applications to practice.* Upper Saddle River, NJ: Prentice Hall Health.

Prizant, B. M., & Wetherby, A. M. (1998). Understanding the continuum of discrete-trial traditional behavioral to social-pragmatic developmental approaches in communication enhancement for young children with autism/PDD. *Seminars in Speech and Language, 19*(4), 329-353, 424.

Rappolt, S. (2003). Evidence-based practice forum. The role of professional expertise in evidence-based occupational therapy. *American Journal of Occupational Therapy, 57*(5), 589-593.

Riebe, D., Blissmer, B., Greene, G., Caldwell, M., Ruggiero, L., Stillwell, K. M., & Nigg, C. R. (2004). Long-term maintenance of exercise and healthy eating behaviors in overweight adults. *Preventive Medicine, 40*, 769-778.

Rogers, S. J., Hepburn, S., & Wehner, E. (2003). Parent reports of sensory symptoms in toddlers with autism and those with other developmental disorders. *Journal of Autism and Developmental Disorders, 33*(6), 631-642.

Schilling, D., Washington, K., Billingsley, F., & Deitz, J. (2003). Classroom seating for children with attention deficit hyperactivity disorder: Therapy balls versus chairs. *American Journal of Occupational Therapy, 57*, 534-541.

Schneck, C. (2001). The efficacy of a sensorimotor treatment approach by occupational therapists. In R. Huebner (Ed.), *Autism: A sensorimotor approach to management.* Gaithersberg, MD: Aspen.

Soper, G., & Thorley, C. (1996). Effectiveness of an occupational therapy programme based on sensory integration theory for adults with severe learning disabilities. *British Journal of Occupational Therapy, 59*(10), 475-482.

Stark, S. (2004). Removing environmental barriers in the homes of older adults with disabilities improves occupational performance. *Occupational Therapy Journal of Research: Occupation, Participation and Health, 24*(1), 32-40.

Steering Committee on Clinical Practice Guidelines for the Care and Treatment of Breast Cancer. (1998). *Clinical practice guidelines for the care and treatment of breast cancer.* Retrieved October 22, 2007, from http://www.cmaj.ca/cgi/content/full/158/3/DC1.

Sullivan, M., & Lewis, M. (2000). Assistive technology for the very young: Creating responsive environments. *Infants and Young Children, 12*(4), 34-52.

Tickle-Degnen, L. (1999). Evidence-based practice forum. Organizing, evaluating and using evidence. *American Journal of Occupational Therapy, 53*(6), 537-539.

Tickle-Degnen, L. (2000a). Evidence-based practice forum. Communicating with clients, family members, and colleagues about research evidence. *American Journal of Occupational Therapy, 54*(3), 341-343.

Tickle-Degnen, L. (2000b). Evidence-based practice forum. Gathering current research evidence to enhance clinical reasoning. *American Journal of Occupational Therapy, 54*(1), 102-105.

Tickle-Degnen, L. (2000c). Evidence-based practice forum. Monitoring and documenting evidence during assessment and intervention. *American Journal of Occupational Therapy, 54*(4), 434-436.

Tickle-Degnen, L. (2000d). Evidence-based practice forum. Teaching evidence-based practice. *American Journal of Occupational Therapy, 54*(5), 559-560.

Tickle-Degnen, L. (2000e). Evidence-based practice forum. What is the best evidence to use in practice? *American Journal of Occupational Therapy, 54*(2), 218-221.

Tickle-Degnen, L. (2001). From the general to the specific: Using meta-analytic reports in clinical decision making. *Evaluation and the Health Professions, 24*(3), 308-326.

Tickle-Degnen, L. (2003). Evidence-based practice forum. Where is the individual in statistics? *American Journal of Occupational Therapy, 57*(1), 112-115.

Tickle-Degnen, L., & Bedell, G. (2003). Evidence-based practice forum. Heterarchy and hierarchy: A critical appraisal of the levels of evidence as a tool for clinical decision making. *American Journal of Occupational Therapy, 57*(2), 234-237.

VandenBerg, N. (2001). The use of a weighted vest to increase on-task behavior in children with attention difficulties. *American Journal of Occupational Therapy, 55*(6), 621-628.

Velligan, D. I., Bow-Thomas, C. C., Huntzinger, C., Ritch, J., Ledbetter, N., Prihoda, T. J., & Miller, A. L. (2000). Randomized controlled trial of the use of compensatory strategies to enhance adaptive functioning in outpatients with schizophrenia. *American Journal of Psychiatry, 157*(8), 1317-1323.

Velligan, D. I., Mueller, J., Wang, M., Dicocco, M., Diamond, P. M., Maples, N. J., & Davis, B. (2006). Use of environmental supports among patients with schizophrenia. *Psychiatric Services, 57*(2), 219-224.

Vikström, S., Borell, L., Stigsdotter-Neely, A., & Josephsson, S. (2005). Caregivers' self-initiated support toward their partners with dementia when performing an everyday occupation together at home. *Occupational Therapy Journal of Research: Occupation, Participation and Health, 25*(34), 149-159.

Watters, R. G., & Watters, W. E. (1980). Decreasing self-stimulatory behavior with physical exercise in a group of autistic boys. *Journal of Autism and Developmental Disorders, 10*, 379-387.

Appendix

Journal Articles for Activities

The Role of Anomalous Data in Knowledge Acquisition: A Theoretical Framework and Implications for Science Instruction

Clark A. Chinn, William F. Brewer

Understanding how science students respond to anomalous data is essential to understanding knowledge acquisition in science classrooms. This article presents a detailed analysis of the ways in which scientists and science students respond to such data. We postulate that there are seven distinct forms of response to anomalous data, only one of which is to accept the data and change theories. The other six responses involve discounting the data in various ways in order to protect the preinstructional theory. We analyze the factors that influence which of these seven forms of response a scientist or student will choose, giving special attention to the factors that make theory change more likely. Finally, we discuss the implications of our framework for science instruction.

Center for the Study of Reading, University of Illinois at Urbana—Champaign. We thank Jack Easley, Paul Thagard, Punyashloke Mishra, and three anonymous reviewers for helpful comments on earlier drafts of this article.

This article addresses an issue that is crucial for understanding how people learn science and how to improve science instruction: How do students respond when they encounter scientific information that contradicts their current theories[1] about the physical world? In other words, how do students respond when their current beliefs about the physical world conflict with the information presented during science instruction?

This issue is crucial for two reasons. The first is that encountering contradictory information is a very common occurrence when one is learning science. Science students' preinstructional beliefs about the natural world conflict sharply with many of the accepted scientific theories taught in school, and this is true across a wide variety of domains within biology, chemistry, and physics (for reviews, see Carey, 1985; Champagne, Klopfer, & Gunstone, 1982; Confrey, 1990; Driver & Easley, 1978; Driver, Guesne, & Tiberghien, 1985; Eylon & Linn, 1988; Osborne & Freyberg, 1985; Perkins & Simmons, 1988; Roth, 1990). Thus, the encounter with contradictory information is at the heart of knowledge acquisition in science.

The second reason why the encounter with contradictory information is crucial for science education is that students typically resist giving up their preinstructional beliefs. Instead of abandoning or modifying their preinstructional beliefs in the face of new, conflicting data and ideas, students often staunchly maintain the old ideas and reject or distort the new ideas. For instance, some children who are told that the earth is round preserve their preinstructional belief that the earth is flat by concluding that the earth is disc shaped (Vosniadou & Brewer, 1992). Similarly, children can spend days or weeks studying photosynthesis and yet persist in their preinstructional belief that plants get their food from the soil (C. Anderson & Smith, 1984). And a number of researchers have found that many young adults go through high school and university physics courses without ever giving up their pre-Newtonian views of motion (e.g., Champagne, Klopfer, & Anderson, 1980; Clement, 1982; McCloskey, Caramazza, & Green, 1980). It is clear that a key to improved science education is to find better ways of convincing students to change their preinstructional theories in response to new, contradictory scientific ideas.

The Role of Anomalous Data

The current literature on science education includes many new instructional approaches that take students' preinstructional theories into account and are designed to convince students to change their theories. Virtually all of these approaches share one key ingredient: the use of anomalous data, that is, presenting students with evidence that contradicts their preinstructional theories. The anomalous data are intended to cause students to become dissatisfied with their current theories, which cannot account for the anomalous data, and to adopt instead the target scientific theory, which successfully explains the data (e.g., Posner, Strike, Hewson, & Gertzog, 1982).

Educational researchers who have advocated using anomalous data to spur students to change their preinstructional theories include Alvermann and Hynd (1989); R. Anderson (1977); Brown and Clement (1992); Champagne, Gunstone, and Klopfer (1985); A. Collins (1977); diSessa (1982); Dreyfus, Jungwirth, and Eliovitch (1990); Finegold and Gorsky (1988); M. Hewson and Hewson (1983); P. Hewson (1981); Inagaki (1981); Johsua and Dupin (1987); Minstrell (1989); Neale, Smith, and Johnson (1990); Nussbaum and Novick (1982); Pines and West (1986); Posner et al. (1982); Roth (1990); Roth, Anderson, and Smith (1987); Rowell and Dawson (1983); Wang and Andre (1991); Watson and Konicek (1990); and White and Frederiksen (1990). The particulars of these approaches vary widely, and the anomalous evidence itself is presented in different ways, sometimes through laboratory work or live demonstrations, sometimes through computers, and sometimes through discussions. Regardless of the details of the method, the presentation of anomalous data is always a key step intended to precipitate theory change.

We agree that presenting students with anomalous data is a promising instructional technique. In the history of science, anomalous data have played an important role in scientific revolutions (Humphreys, 1968; T. Kuhn, 1962), and it is plausible to assume that persuasive data are needed to convince students to abandon well-entrenched preinstructional theories. But the use of anomalous data is no panacea. Science students frequently react to anomalous data by dis-

Article Reprint Information: Chinn, C. A., & Brewer, W. F. (1993). The role of anomalous data in knowledge acquisition: A theoretical framework and implications for science instruction. *Review of Educational Research, 63*(1), 1-49. Copyright (1993) by the American Educational Research Association. Reproduced with permission of the publisher.

counting the data in some way, thus preserving their preinstructional theories. For example, Champagne et al. (1985) report a study in which students who believed that heavy objects fall faster than light objects subsequently watched the teacher attempt to refute their belief by dropping two blocks of different weights from a common height. Although the blocks appeared to strike the ground simultaneously, many students refused to accept the anomalous data. Two middle school students "reasoned that the blocks had, in fact, fallen at different rates, but that the difference in descent times was too small to be observed over the short distance (approximately one meter) used in the original demonstration" (p. 65). Other students declared that the blocks must, in fact, have been of equal weight. Thus, anomalous data do not always lead to belief change. Students often find ways to discredit anomalous data and protect their preinstructional beliefs against the data.

Core Questions

In order to use anomalous data in science instruction, educators must gain a better understanding of how students deal with data that contradict their preinstructional theories. In order to use anomalous data effectively in instruction, it is necessary to know the answers to three questions:

1. What are the different responses a student can make to anomalous data?
2. What are the conditions that lead to different responses to anomalous data? That is, why does a student ignore anomalous data in one instance, reject anomalous data in another instance, and abandon his or her preinstructional theory in a third instance?
3. Drawing on the answers to the first two questions, what can educators do to make theory change more likely in the classroom? How can instruction be designed to make theory change more likely and to make the discrediting of anomalous data less likely?

The purpose of this article is to suggest answers to these three questions. We propose a theoretical framework for understanding how students respond to contradictory data and *why* they respond as they do. Then we use this framework to make recommendations for science instruction.

Although the issue of how scientists and science students respond to anomalous information is critical for science education, no one, to our knowledge, has yet developed a detailed framework for understanding responses to anomalous information. Several researchers, such as P. Hewson (1981) and

R. Schank, Collins, and Hunter (1986), have listed some ways in which people may react to anomalous information, and many relevant insights are scattered throughout Thomas Kuhn's (1962) *The Structure of Scientific Revolutions*. Other relevant observations are dispersed widely in the literatures on the history of science, philosophy of science, science education, cognitive science, cognitive psychology, developmental psychology, and social psychology.

As we have searched the literatures on the history of science and on education and psychology for instances of people responding to anomalous data, we have been struck by the similarities in the descriptions of the responses of scientists, nonscientist adults, and science students. The fundamental ways in which scientists react to anomalous data appear to be identical to the ways in which nonscientist adults and science students react to such data. Thus, our analysis will provide support for the thesis that the scientific reasoning processes of children are similar to those of scientists (Brewer & Samarapungavan, 1991; Carey, 1985).

The rest of this article is composed of three parts, corresponding to the three questions raised above. In the first part, we classify the forms of response to anomalous data. We discuss each postulated form of response and provide evidence for our position with examples from the history of science and from psychology and science education. In the second part, we discuss the factors that influence how people respond to anomalous data, giving particular attention to what causes a person to be convinced by the anomalous data instead of attempting to shield the preexisting theory from change. In the third part, we discuss the implications of our analysis for science instruction.

Forms of Psychological Response to Anomalous Data

In idealized form, we conceptualize the situation in which anomalous data occur as follows: An individual currently holds theory A. The individual then encounters anomalous data, data that cannot be explained by theory A. The data may be anomalous because they clearly conflict with theory A or simply because theory A cannot be used to marshal any explanation for the data. The anomalous data may or may not be accompanied by theory B, which is intended to explain much of the body of data explained by theory A, plus the anomalous data.

What are the possible responses of the individual to the anomalous data? We postulate that there are seven basic responses:

(a) *ignore* the anomalous data, (b) *reject* the data, (c) *exclude* the data from the domain of theory A, (d) hold the data in *abeyance*, (e) *reinterpret* the data while retaining theory A, (f) reinterpret the data and make *peripheral changes* to theory A, and (g) accept the data and *change* theory A, possibly in favor of theory B. We think this is close to an exhaustive set of the possible responses to anomalous data.

In the next sections of the article we will discuss each of these forms of response to anomalous data. After that, we will present a theoretical justification for choosing just these seven forms of response and for concluding that these are an exhaustive set of possible responses.

As we discuss each form of response, we will support our analysis with selected examples from the history of science and experimental evidence from psychology and science education. We have included historical examples for four reasons. First, the history and philosophy of science has been a fruitful source of ideas and evidence for science educators (e.g., Duschl & Gitomer, 1991; Snir, 1991). Second, the examples from the history of science are often particularly clear and compelling. Third, a classification that aims to account for how people respond to anomalous data about the physical world ought to be able to account for both the responses of scientists and the responses of science students. Finally, we want to illustrate the similarities between scientists and science students. When we juxtapose examples from the history of science with examples from psychology and science education, it becomes clear that science students frequently respond in the same essential ways that scientists do.

Ignoring Anomalous Data

The most extreme way to dispose of a piece of anomalous data is simply to ignore it. When an individual ignores data, he or she does not even bother to explain the data away. Theory A remains intact and totally unscathed.

History of science. The popular press frequently publishes "data" that contradict received scientific ideas, but these data are typically ignored by scientists. Thus, physicists ignore reports of new perpetual motion machines. Psychologists ignore claims for the existence of ESP. Astronomers ignore the predictions of astrology. Biologists ignore the reports of sightings of the Loch Ness monster.

However, it is not merely fringe ideas like ESP and astrology that get ignored by scientists. Data that are later accepted by the scientific community may be similarly ignored. An example can be seen in the reception of the meteor impact theory of mass extinctions at the end of the Cretaceous period. In 1980, Luis Alvarez and his colleagues (Alvarez, Alvarez, Asaro, & Michel, 1980) reported that the K-T boundary in Italy (the K-T boundary is the boundary between Cretaceous and Tertiary sediments) contained an anomalously high amount of iridium and argued that the iridium could have come only from a meteor or comet; therefore, the mass extinction of species at the end of the Cretaceous period must have been caused by the impact of a meteor or comet. But at a later conference attended by Alvarez at which paleontologists discussed mass extinctions, there was no mention of the word *iridium*. The paleontologists ignored Alvarez's data (Muller, 1988, p. 72).

Psychology and education. In a study of middle school students reading science texts, Roth and Anderson (1988) provided evidence that students sometimes ignore information in science texts that contradicts their existing schemas. In their study, several students gleaned almost no new information from the texts; instead, they used a few key words in the text to call up a preexisting schema. One such student, Maria,

read a section of one text that used milk as an example of how all foods can ultimately be traced back to green plants, the food producers. Maria announced that "most of this stuff I already knew.... It's just about milk...how we get our milk from cows." In fact, the text did not discuss people at all in this example. Maria never picked up any notion of the main ideas the text was developing—that plants make food. This is typical of her pattern of reading to find familiar ideas, ignoring the rest of the text, and relying on prior knowledge to fill in the details. (Roth & Anderson, 1988, p. 114)

From this description, it is not clear whether Maria simply did not read the new information or whether she read it extremely superficially. But either behavior fits into the category of ignoring new information.

Deanna Kuhn (1989) reported a study that indicated that students may ignore data that contradict their favored causal hypothesis. As an example, one ninth grade girl believed that eating a Mars Bar (a kind of candy bar) is unrelated to whether one catches a cold, whereas eating mustard causes one to catch a cold. Presented with a pattern of noncovariation between the type of candy bar and catching cold, the girl said, "With the Mars Bar you get a cold off and on, because here's one they got colds and over

here they didn't....so it really doesn't matter" (p. 677). But presented with the same pattern of noncovariation for mustard, the girl interpreted the evidence very differently: "Mostly likely all the time you get a cold with the mustard. Like there you did [instance 2] and there you did [instance 7]" (p. 677). The girl appears to have ignored the two instances where mustard was not associated with colds. The girl's prior theory asserted that mustard causes colds, so she ignored the data that contradicted her causal hypothesis.

Rejecting Anomalous Data

Rejecting data is similar to ignoring data in that the individual does not accept the data in either case, nor does he or she make any changes to theory A. The difference is that in ignoring data, the individual does not even attempt to explain the data away; in rejection, the individual can articulate an explanation for why the data should be rejected.

Rejection is very common among scientists. It can vary from a detailed methodological or theoretical critique to a vague "There must be something wrong with the experiment." According to Richard Muller (1988), professor of physics at the University of California at Berkeley:

When presented with a new, startling, and strange result, it is easy to find flaws and come up with reasons to dismiss the finding. Even if the skeptic can't find an outright mistake, he can say, "I'm not convinced." In fact, most scientists (myself included) have found that if you dismiss out of hand all claims of great new discoveries, you will be right 95% of the time. (p. 73)

By this standard, it appears that compared with scientists, science students may be remarkably open to new data!

Individuals who reject data use a wide variety of reasons for the rejection; however, three very common forms of rejection are (a) arguing that there was a fundamental methodological error in the way the data were obtained, (b) arguing that the data were merely due to random variation, and (c) declaring the data to be fraudulent.

Methodological error. Perhaps the most common ground for rejecting data is methodological error. The individual asserts that the procedure by which the data were collected is flawed.

History of science. One of the classic cases of rejection based on methodological error occurred when Galileo published the results of his first observations with the telescope. These observations were inconsis-

tent with the then current Aristotelian world view. It appears that, initially, most astronomers and philosophers rejected the data as due to methodological artifacts introduced by the telescope itself (Drake, 1980, p. 44).

Psychology and education. Science students sometimes reject data presented in science classes on methodological grounds. Johsua and Dupin (1987) report a classroom study in which students were debating different explanatory models of a simple electrical circuit, in which a battery was connected to a light bulb. Most of the students incorrectly believed that electrical current "wears out" as it travels from a battery around the circuit. That is, these students believed that some of the current gets used up in order to light up the bulb, so that the current entering the bulb is greater than the current leaving it. The teacher attempted to refute this incorrect belief by inserting two ammeters into the circuit, one on each side of the light bulb. The ammeters showed that the current on each side of the bulb was the same. But instead of changing their beliefs, many students rejected the data on methodological grounds. They stated, for example, that "the apparatus is bust" and that "the bulb was bad, then the battery; let's change them" (p. 129).

Pickering and Monts (1982) studied undergraduates in a chemistry laboratory who, in the course of carrying out a laboratory experiment, generated data that contradicted their prior beliefs. Although their data were, in fact, correct, 45% of the subjects asserted that the data were in error and explained the data away by attributing them to methodological error. Among the subjects who stated that the data were in error, 53% offered a specific methodological explanation and 47% offered only a vague explanation or merely asserted that there was a methodological error.

Random error. Another form of rejection is to assert that the anomalous finding is just a random occurrence.

History of science. Wegener argued that the close fit between the east coastline of South America and the west coastline of Africa supported his theory of continental drift. However, his opponents argued that the degree of fit was simply chance (Hallam, 1973). Similarly, when Weber claimed to have found evidence for gravity waves, one of his critics stated, "By massaging data again and again, knowing what you want for an answer, you can increase the apparent statistical significance of any bump... I'm pretty sure he could get there out of pure noise" (H. Collins, 1981, p. 40).

Psychology and education. Gorman

(1986,1989) has conducted a series of studies to examine how people respond when they are told that there is a chance that the anomalous data they receive are in error. Using a rule discovery task, Gorman (1986) found that when subjects were told that there was a 20% chance that data that contradicted their hypothesis were in error, subjects often rejected the contradictory data. These subjects apparently assumed that data that contradicted their hypothesis must have been among the 20% of the data that were in error. Gorman (1986) also found that "the possibility of errors seems to make it harder for groups to abandon a rule even when they have clearly disconfirmed it" (p. 94).

Fraud. This is the most extreme form of rejection. The individual dismisses the anomalous data as a joke or as outright fraud.

History of science. When Lord Kelvin first heard about X rays, he apparently believed that the reports were a hoax (Thompson, 1976, p. 1125). Similarly, the chemist Kauffman (1988, p. 264) reports that when he first heard that Bartlett had formed a compound with one of the noble gases, he assumed that the announcement was a joke.

Psychology and education. We know of no experimental studies in psychology in which subjects rejected data as a hoax. The demand characteristics of most studies appear to preclude such a response. But Hesse (1987) provides an example from science education. Hesse hung two balls of steel wool on an equal arm balance. Because the two balls had equal mass, the arm of the balance remained level. Then Hesse placed a Bunsen burner under one of the balls. Most students predicted that the heated ball would weigh less. "After the demonstration students were astonished that the heated side weighed more. Several students in disbelief claimed that I somehow rigged the balance" (p. 199).

Excluding Anomalous Data

Another possible response to contradictory data is to declare the data to be outside the domain of the theory. Suppe (1974) notes:

Theories have as their subject matter a certain range of phenomena and they are developed for the purpose of providing answers to a variety of questions about the phenomena in that range.... The range of questions the theory is intended to answer about the phenomena is quite selective; the theory is not expected to be able to answer all possible

questions which could be asked about the phenomena in its range. (p. 211)

Thomas Kuhn (1962) makes a similar generalization and notes that one response to anomaly is for scientists to treat it as "the concern of another discipline" (p. 37). Thus, one approach to anomalous data is simply to assert that one's theory is not intended to account for those data.

In contrast to the individual who rejects anomalous data, the individual who excludes data from his or her theory does not have to make a judgment about the validity of the data. When anomalous data are excluded from the domain of a theory, they obviously do not lead to any theory change.

History of science. Laudan (1977) discusses the example of Brownian motion, which was a phenomenon in search of an explanation beginning in 1828. For nearly a century, it was not clear to which scientific discipline Brownian motion belonged. It was regarded at various times as a biological problem (the motion being caused by small "animalcules"), as a chemical problem, as a problem of electrical conductivity, and as a problem in heat theory. Laudan concludes, "So long as the problem remained unsolved, any theorist could conveniently choose to ignore it simply by saying that it was not a problem which theories in his field had to address" (1977, pp. 19-20).

Psychology and education. One of the first experiments in psychology to discuss the issue of anomalous data was the work of Karmiloff-Smith and Inhelder (1975; Karmiloff-Smith, 1988). These researchers investigated children attempting to balance blocks on a narrow metal support. Some of the blocks had their weight evenly distributed so that they balanced at their geometric center. Other blocks were uneven, with a mass of lead hidden at one end so that they balanced far off center. By the age of 6 or 7, children had developed a geometric-center hypothesis of balancing; they believed that blocks balance in the middle. But with this hypothesis, they were unable to balance the uneven blocks. When children tried to make the uneven blocks balance in the center, the blocks kept falling off the rail. Instead of changing their geometric-center hypothesis, the children declared that the uneven blocks were impossible to balance, and they did not worry about them further. From our perspective, it appears that the children declared those blocks to be outside the domain of the theory they were developing. In this way, they were able to preserve their theory unaltered.

The commonly observed phenomenon

of compartmentalization among science learners can also be viewed as a form of exclusion. Many researchers (e.g., Osborne & Wittrock, 1983; Pines & West, 1986; Roth & Anderson, 1988) have noted that students compartmentalize the science learned in school, keeping it segregated from their theories about how the real world operates. Compartmentalization amounts to excluding classroom science data from everyday theories about how the physical world works.

Holding Anomalous Data in Abeyance

An individual need not come up with an immediate explanation for anomalous data. Individuals who hold a particular theory can place the anomalous data in abeyance, promising to deal with it later. In common with all of the earlier forms of response, placing the data in abeyance leaves the individual's initial theory unchanged. Yet with abeyance, the individual assumes that theory A will someday be articulated so that it can explain the data.

History of science. Thomas Kuhn (1962) has argued that what we have called abeyance is widespread among scientists when they encounter discrepant data: "Even a discrepancy unaccountably larger than that experienced in other applications of the theory need not draw any very profound response. There are always some discrepancies. Even the most stubborn ones usually respond at last to normal practice" (p. 81). A good example of responding to anomalous data by placing it in abeyance is the treatment of the orbit of Mercury by Newtonian physicists during the late 1800s. It was known for a long period that the details of the orbit were inconsistent with Newtonian mechanics, but no astronomers chose to give up the Newtonian theory. They just assumed that there would eventually be a solution within the Newtonian framework (see T. Kuhn, 1962; Whittaker, 1951).

Psychology and education. Brewer and Chinn (1991, 1992) had undergraduate subjects read a text that offered a nonmathematical explanation of several principles of quantum mechanics. These principles violated certain deeply entrenched beliefs held by most people, such as the belief that physical objects like protons and electrons exist as discrete particles. Then subjects were asked to respond to descriptions of experimental data that supported the quantum mechanics principles but contradicted the subjects' own beliefs. One subject, an undergraduate who had taken five physics courses, held the data in abeyance, confident that physicists would eventually solve the paradoxes of quantum mechanics so that he need not give up his commitment to realism. He wrote, "I do not believe that [quantum mechanics] is true. Though we might not know the answers yet—I do believe that everything exists—whether it is observed or not, and has certain properties either way." In answer to another question, he wrote, "Not sure—I'll tell you in 20 years," indicating his belief that scientists will solve the problem within the realist framework.

Reinterpreting Anomalous Data

An individual can accept anomalous data yet preserve his or her prior theory by reinterpreting the data. The difference between reinterpreting data and rejecting data is that when an individual reinterprets data, that individual accepts the data as something that should be explained by his or her theory. In the case of reinterpretation, supporters of theory A and theory B can agree at some level about the data, but at a theoretical level, they give different interpretations of the data. As with all of the previous forms of response to anomalous data, reinterpretation does not require a change in the existing theory.

History of science. The decade-long history of scientists' reactions to Alvarez's impact theory of Cretaceous extinctions is rife with reinterpretations. According to Raup (1986), an early reaction to the iridium anomaly was to argue that the iridium might have seeped down into the K-T boundary from layers of limestone above the K-T boundary. This explains the anomalously high concentration of iridium without the need to posit an extraterrestrial source. Note that the data were not rejected: The scientists who advanced the limestone explanation accepted as fact that there was an unusually high concentration of iridium in the K-T boundary layer. But the high concentration of iridium was reinterpreted, and Alvarez's interpretation was not accepted.

Psychology and education. Wisniewski and Medin (1991) provided clear evidence that people sometimes reinterpret evidence in order to avoid giving up a favored hypothesis. They presented undergraduates with 10 drawings, one at a time. Five of the drawings were allegedly drawn by city children and the other five by farm children. Upon being shown a drawing, subjects guessed whether it had been done by a city child or by a farm child; subjects also explained the rule or rules they used to make this guess. Then subjects were given feedback about whether their guesses were correct or not, and they were invited to modify

their rules if they wished. After receiving the feedback, subjects seldom abandoned their rules; instead, they sometimes reinterpreted features in the drawings. For example, one subject originally said that

a drawing was done by a city child because it depicted a television character, and city children watch more television. However, when told that the drawing was done by a farm child, the person reinterpreted the character as one created from a farm child's imagination. (Wisniewski & Medin, 1991, p. 265)

Instead of giving up the hypothesis that city children watch more television, the subject chose to reinterpret the evidence.

Piaget (1974/1980, chap. 6) presented children with a balance scale task and asked them to predict what would happen when one weight was put in each pan. Most young children predicted that one pan would go down and the other up, like a seesaw. After watching the experimenter place one weight in each pan and finding that nothing happened, a 6-year-old hesitated and scrutinized the scale closely. Then the child declared that the pans were in the same place because both weights were light. The child did not reject the data; there was no attempt to deny that the pans were level. But the data were reinterpreted to show that it was only because the weights were too light that the seesaw effect did not occur.

Chinn and Brewer (1992b) have obtained some very extreme examples of reinterpretation. For example, after reading about some anomalous data that were designed to be clearly inconsistent with the meteor impact theory of mass extinctions, one student who supported the meteor impact theory wrote, "This further proves the meteor impact theory," and he actually increased his rating of how strongly he believed the theory.

Peripheral Theory Change

Philosophers of science have argued that anomalous data can never logically compel a scientist to abandon a particular hypothesis because the hypothesis is embedded in a network of beliefs, any one of which might be wrong (Duhem, 1914/1954; Quine, 1951). Lakatos (1970) has distinguished between two types of propositions within a theory: *hard core* propositions and *protective belt* propositions. Hard core propositions cannot be altered without scrapping the entire theory, but protective belt propositions can be altered while preserving the key, central hypotheses. Thus, another response to anomalous data is for the individual to make a relatively minor modification in his or her current theory. An

individual who responds in this way clearly accepts the data but is unwilling to give up theory A and accept theory B. This is the first response to anomalous data that we have discussed that involves any change in an individual's initial theory.

A variety of modifications to a theory can fall under the category of peripheral theory change. For example, the individual can add or abandon auxiliary theoretical hypotheses, change beliefs about how experiments in the theoretical domain should be conducted, adjust the definition of a theoretical construct, or alter the domain of the theory. In all of these cases, however, the changes leave the theory's central hypotheses intact.

History of science. The early responses to Galileo's first telescope observations provide a good example of a peripheral theory change. A core assumption of Galileo's opponents was that celestial objects were perfect spheres. After looking through Galileo's telescope, one of Galileo's opponents conceded that he saw mountains on the moon through the telescope. However, he argued that the mountains were embedded in a perfectly transparent crystal sphere (Drake, 1980, p. 48). This peripheral modification of the theory accounted for the anomalous data but allowed the philosopher to retain the core belief that the moon was a perfect sphere.

Psychology and education. There are many psychological and educational studies that provide evidence that nonscientist adults and children frequently respond to anomalous data by making peripheral changes to their theory (e.g., Brewer & Chinn, 1991; Dunbar, 1989; Heller & Finley, 1992; Piaget, 1974/1980; Reiner & Finegold, 1987; Rowell & Dawson, 1983; Schauble, 1990). Here we describe only two representative studies.

Vosniadou and Brewer (1992) have provided evidence for peripheral theory change in children's beliefs about the shape of the earth. They discovered that young children (ages 4-6 years) tend to have a flat earth theory of the shape of the earth. As a result, when young children are told by adults that "the earth is round," they are faced with anomalous information. Some of the children account for this anomalous information by making peripheral changes in their flat earth view. These children interpret the information from the adults to indicate that the earth is a flat disc. Other children adopt a two-earth theory in which there is a flat earth on which people live and a round earth up in space. Both of these belief modifications account for the anomalous information about the earth being round but leave the basic flat earth belief intact.

Lawson and Worsnop (1992) investigated the effects of science instruction on students' beliefs about evolution, and their data suggest that some students who supported creationism made a peripheral change to their creationist theory. More than half of the students in the classes that Lawson and Worsnop studied were creationists. The 3-week instructional unit on evolution included a section on fossil evidence for evolution. Before instruction, only 1% of the students agreed with the statement "Fossils were intentionally put on the earth to confuse humans." After instruction, however, 7% of the students agreed with the same statement. Our interpretation of this change is that some of the creationist students who were confronted with compelling fossil evidence for evolution adjusted their peripheral beliefs in order to protect their core belief in special creation. By adding to their theory the peripheral hypothesis that God placed fossils on earth to confuse humans, these students could explain away the anomalous data about fossils.

Subtyping. A very common form of peripheral change is subtyping. As an example, consider the case of an individual who encounters a zebra without stripes. One of the individual's options is to differentiate the category zebra into two subtypes: zebras with stripes and zebras without stripes (cf. R. Schank et al., 1986).

An example of subtyping from the history of science comes from the work of Wallace, who developed some components of the theory of evolution independently of Darwin. Although Wallace believed that natural selection and evolution accounted for the bodily structure of humans and all other forms of life, he believed, unlike Darwin, that the theory of evolution did not account for the advent of the human intellect. The advent of human intellect could be explained only by invoking the theory of divine intervention (Wallace, 1889). Thus, Wallace differentiated between the human body and the human intellect and developed separate theories to account for the origins of the two subtypes.

In science education, Brown and Clement (1992) found that children subtyped the principles of physics into three different subdomains. They applied one set of principles to the domain of physics in outer space, a second set to the domain of objects falling on earth, and a third set to the domain of objects on the earth.

Table 1
Features of each of the seven responses to anomalous data

| Type of response | Features of the response | | |
	Does the individual accept the data?	Does the individual explain the data?	Does the individual change theories?
Ignoring	No	No	No
Rejecting	No	Yes	No
Excluding	Yes or maybe[a]	No	No
Abeyance	Yes	Not yet[b]	No
Reinterpreting	Yes	Yes	No
Peripheral change	Yes	Yes	Yes, partly[c]
Theory change	Yes	Yes	Yes[d]

[a]The individual may either accept the data as valid or remain agnostic about whether the data are valid. [b]The individual expects that the data will be explainable by the current theory at some future date. [c]Only beliefs in the protective belt are changed. [d]Core beliefs are changed.

Theory Change

The strongest effect that anomalous data can have on an individual is to impel the individual to change to a new theory. By theory change, we mean change in one or more of the theorist's core beliefs. In this form of response to contradictory information, the individual accepts the new data and explains it by changing the core beliefs of theory A or by accepting an alternate theory.

History of science. The history of science suggests that theory change often requires a series of empirical anomalies, which collectively appear to be better explained by an alternate theory (T. Kuhn, 1962; Thagard, 1992). The chemical revolution provides a good example of this type of theory change. After more than a decade of active experimentation, major phlogiston theorists switched one by one to become proponents of Lavoisier's oxygen theory (Musgrave, 1976).

Psychology and education. Most psychological and educational experiments in which some subjects ignore, reject, or reinterpret data or change peripheral beliefs also report that a few subjects do change core beliefs in response to contradictory data. In some studies, major belief change takes more time and shows up only over years as students acquire additional knowledge (e.g., Karmiloff-Smith, 1988; Vosniadou & Brewer, 1992). In other studies, some theory change in response to anomalous data occurs within one or a few experimental sessions or within several classroom lessons (e.g., Alvermann & Hynd, 1989; Brown & Clement, 1989; Burbules & Linn, 1988; Dunbar & Schunn, 1990; Johsua & Dupin, 1987; Levin, Siegler, Druyan, & Gardosh, 1990; Ranney & Thagard, 1988; Rowell & Dawson, 1983; Zietsman & Hewson, 1986). For example, Rowell and Dawson (1983) found that 3 of 12 subjects who held a weight theory of water displacement changed to a volume theory after observing anomalous data that supported the volume theory. Using the same domain, Burbules and Linn (1988) devised an educational intervention using anomalous data that convinced more than 70% of adolescents to shift from a weight theory of displacement to a volume theory of displacement within a single session.

Summary

When confronted with anomalous data, an individual can make one of seven responses to the data. We think that the evidence we have provided suggests that these seven categories provide a descriptively adequate account of actual responses to anomalous data. However, we also think that the seven categories can be derived from a logical analysis of the data evaluation and theory change process.

Responding to anomalous data involves an endeavor to coordinate theory and data (cf. D. Kuhn, 1989; Thagard, 1989, 1992). There are three different decisions an individual must make in order to coordinate new anomalous data with an existing theory. First, the individual must decide whether the data are believable. This is important because if the data are not believable, then there is no further need to attempt to coordinate data and theory. Second, the individual must decide whether (and, if so, how) the data can be explained. A successful coordination of theory and data requires that the individual be able to explain the data. Third, the individual must determine whether (and, if so, how) the theory needs to be changed in order to achieve a successful coordination of theory and data. We do not assert that the individual makes these three decisions in any particular order; the decisions may be made in parallel. But all three decisions must be made, either implicitly or explicitly, when anomalous data are encountered.

Thus, attempts to coordinate theory and data involve three fundamental dimensions: (a) whether the individual accepts the data as valid, (b) whether the individual can provide an explanation for why the data are accepted or not accepted, and (c) whether the individual changes his or her prior theory. As Table 1 shows, the seven forms of response to anomalous data differ systematically across these three dimensions.

Not all possible permutations across the three dimensions are shown in Table 1. We believe that those permutations not shown are psychologically implausible. For example, it is psychologically implausible that individuals would reject data as invalid yet change their prior theory. It is similarly unlikely that individuals would change their prior theory yet fail to explain the data; the only reason to change a theory in response to anomalous data is to explain the data. Therefore, we believe that the seven categories shown in Table 1 exhaust the psychologically plausible forms of response to anomalous data.

Note

[1]We want to clarify our usage of three terms: *knowledge*, *beliefs*, and *theories*. In philosophy, the term *knowledge* has traditionally been taken to be justified true belief. However, we will use the word in a more general way to refer to the total set of beliefs held by an individual. We use the term *belief* to refer to any piece of knowledge within this knowledge base. *Theories* are collections of beliefs that have explanatory force. We use the term *belief* rather than some other term to emphasize the fallibility of the knowledge; scientific beliefs and other beliefs often turn out to be mistaken or only partially correct in light of later discoveries. The term *belief* does not imply that beliefs are based on careful reflection; our notion of belief includes unexamined assumptions, including what diSessa (1988) has called "p-prims."

References

Alvarez, L., Alvarez, W., Asaro, F., & Michel, H. V. (1980). Extraterrestrial cause for the Cretaceous-Tertiary extinction: Experimental results and theoretical interpretation. *Science, 208*, 1095-1108.

Alvermann, D. E., & Hynd, C. R. (1989). Effects of prior knowledge activation modes and text structure on nonscience majors' comprehension of physics. *Journal of Educational Research, 83*, 97-102.

Anderson, C. W., & Smith, E. L. (1984). Children's preconceptions and content-area textbooks. In G. G. Duffy, L. R. Roehler, & J. Mason (Eds.), *Comprehension instruction: Perspectives and suggestions* (pp. 187-201). New York: Longman.

Anderson, R. C. (1977). The notion of schemata and the educational enterprise: General discussion of the conference. In R. C. Anderson, R. J. Spiro, & W. E. Montague (Eds.), *Schooling and the acquisition of knowledge* (pp. 415-431). Hillsdale, NJ: Erlbaum.

Brewer, W. F., & Chinn, C. A. (1991). Entrenched beliefs, inconsistent information, and knowledge change. In L. Birnbaum (Ed.), *The International Conference of the Learning Sciences: Proceedings of the 1991 conference* (pp. 67-73). Charlottesville, VA: Association for the Advancement of Computing in Education.

Brewer, W. F., & Chinn, C. A. (1992). *Learning scientific theories that contradict entrenched beliefs*. Manuscript in preparation.

Brewer, W. F., & Samarapungavan, A. (1991). Children's theories vs. scientific theories: Differences in reasoning or differences in knowledge? In R. R. Hoffman & D. S. Palermo (Eds.), *Cognition and the symbolic processes: Applied and ecological perspectives* (pp. 209-232). Hillsdale, NJ: Erlbaum.

Brown, D. E., & Clement, J. (1992). Classroom teaching experiments in mechanics. In R. Duit, F. Goldberg, & H. Niedderer (Eds.), *Research in physics learning: Theoretical issues and empirical studies* (pp. 380-397). Kiel, Germany: Institut fiir die Padagogik der Naturwissenschaften an der Universitat Kiel.

Burbules, N. C., & Linn, M. C. (1988). Response to contradiction: Scientific reasoning during adolescence. *Journal of Educational Psychology, 80*, 67-75.

Carey, S. (1985). Conceptual change in childhood. Cambridge, MA: MIT Press. Carey, S., Evans, R., Honda, M., Jay, E., & Unger, C. (1989). 'An experiment is when you try it and see if it works': A study of grade 7 students' understanding of the construction of scientific knowledge. *International Journal of Science Education, 11*, 514-529.

Champagne, A. B., Gunstone, R. F., & Klopfer, L. E. (1985). Instructional consequences of students' knowledge about physical phenomena. In L. H. T. West & A. L. Pines (Eds.), *Cognitive structure and conceptual change* (pp. 61-90). Orlando, FL: Academic Press.

Champagne, A. B., Klopfer, L. E., & Anderson, J. H. (1980). Factors influencing the learning of classical mechanics. *American Journal of Physics, 48*, 1074-1079.

Champagne, A. B., Klopfer, L. E., & Gunstone, R. F. (1982). Cognitive research and the design of science instruction. *Educational Psychologist, 17*, 31-53.

Chinn, C. A., & Brewer, W. F. (1992b). *Responding to anomalous scientific data: Effects of entrenchment, background knowledge, and an alternative theory*. Manuscript in preparation.

Clement, J. (1982). Students' preconceptions in introductory mechanics. *American Journal of Physics, 50*, 66-71.

Collins, A. (1977). Processes in acquiring knowledge. In R. C. Anderson, R. J. Spiro, & W. E. Montague (Eds.), *Schooling and the acquisition of knowledge* (pp. 339-363). Hillsdale, NJ: Erlbaum.

Collins, H. M. (1981). Son of seven sexes: The social destruction of a physical phenomenon. *Social Studies of Science, 11*, 33-62.

Confrey, J. (1990). A review of the research on student conceptions in mathematics, science, and programming. In C. B. Cazden (Ed.), *Review of research in education* (Vol. 16, pp. 3-56). Washington, DC: American Educational Research Association.

Cooper, J., & Croyle, R. T. (1984). Attitudes and attitude change. *Annual Review of Psychology, 35*, 395-426.

diSessa, A. A. (1982). Unlearning Aristotelian physics: A study of knowledge-based learning. *Cognitive Science, 6*, 37-75.

diSessa, A. A. (1988). Knowledge in pieces. In G. Forman & P. B. Pufall (Eds.), *Constructivism in the computer age* (pp. 49-70). Hillsdale, NJ: Erlbaum.

Drake, S. (1980). *Galileo*. New York: Hill and Wang.

Dreyfus, A., Jungwirth, E., & Eliovitch, R. (1990). Applying the "cognitive conflict" strategy for conceptual change-Some implications, difficulties, and problems. *Science Education, 74*, 555-569.

Driver, R., & Easley, J. (1978). Pupils and paradigms: A review of literature related to concept development in adolescent science students. *Studies in Science Education, 5*, 61-84.

Driver, R., Guesne, E., & Tiberghien, A. (Eds.). (1985). *Children's ideas in science*. Milton Keynes, England: Open University Press.

Duhem, P. (1954). *The aim and structure of physical theory* (P. P. Wiener, Trans.). Princeton, NJ: Princeton University Press. (Original work published 1914)

Dunbar, K. (1989). Scientific reasoning strategies in a simulated molecular genetics environment. In *Proceedings of the Eleventh Annual Conference of the Cognitive Science Society* (pp. 426-433). Hillsdale, NJ: Erlbaum.

Dunbar, K., & Schunn, C. D. (1990). The temporal nature of scientific discovery: The roles of priming and analogy. In *Proceedings of the Twelfth Annual Conference of the Cognitive Science Society* (pp. 93-100) Hillsdale, NJ: Erlbaum.

Duschl, R. A., & Gitomer, D. H. (1991). Epistemological perspectives on conceptual change: Implications for educational practice. *Journal of Research in Science Teaching, 28*, 839-858.

Eylon, B., & Linn, M. C. (1988). Learning and instruction: An examination of four research perspectives in science education. *Review of Educational Research, 58*, 251-301.

Finegold, M., & Gorsky, P. (1988). Learning about forces: Simulating the outcomes of pupils' misconceptions. *Instructional Science, 17*, 251-261.

Gorman, M. E. (1986). How the possibility of error affects falsification on a task that models scientific problem solving. *British Journal of Psychology, 77*, 85-96.

Hallam, A. (1973). *A revolution in the earth sciences*. Oxford, England: Clarendon Press.

Heller, P. M., & Finley, F. N. (1992). Variable uses of alternative conceptions: A case study in current electricity. *Journal of Research in Science Teaching, 29*, 259-275.

Hesse, J. J., III. (1987). The costs and benefits of using conceptual change teaching methods: A teacher's perspective. In J. D. Novak (Ed.), *Proceedings of the Second International Seminar on Misconceptions and Educational Strategies in Science and Mathematics* (Vol. 2, pp. 194-209). Ithaca, NY: Cornell University.

Hewson, M. G., & Hewson, P. W. (1983). Effect of instruction using students' prior knowledge and conceptual change strategies on science learning. *Journal of Research in Science Teaching, 20,* 731-743.

Hewson, P. W. (1981). A conceptual change approach to learning science. *European Journal of Science Education, 3,* 383-396.

Humphreys, W. C. (1968). *Anomalies and scientific theories.* San Francisco: Freeman, Cooper & Company.

Johsua, S., & Dupin, J. J. (1987). Taking into account student conceptions in instructional strategy: An example in physics. *Cognition and Instruction, 4,* 117-135.

Karmiloff-Smith, A. (1988). The child is a theoretician, not an inductivist. *Mind & Language, 3,* 183-195.

Karmiloff-Smith, A., & Inhelder, B. (1975). "If you want to get ahead, get a theory." *Cognition, 3,* 195-212.

Kauffman, G. G. (1988). The discovery of noble-gas compounds. *Journal of College Science Teaching, 17,* 264-268, 326.

Kuhn, D. (1989). Children and adults as intuitive scientists. *Psychological Review, 96,* 674-689.

Kuhn, T. S. (1962). *The structure of scientific revolutions.* Chicago: University of Chicago Press.

Lakatos, I. (1970). Falsification and the methodology of scientific research programmes. In I. Lakatos & A. Musgrave (Eds.), *Criticism and the growth of knowledge* (pp. 91-196). London: Cambridge University Press.

Laudan, L. (1977). *Progress and its problems: Toward a theory of scientific growth.* Berkeley: University of California Press.

Lawson, A. E., & Worsnop, W. A. (1992). Learning about evolution and rejecting a belief in special creation: Effects of reflective reasoning skill, prior knowledge, prior belief and religious commitment. *Journal of Research in Science Teaching, 29,* 143-166.

Levin, I., Siegler, R. S., Druyan, S., & Gardosh, R. (1990). Everyday and curriculum- based physics concepts: When does short-term training bring change where years of schooling have failed to do so? *British Journal of Developmental Psychology, 8,* 269-279.

McCloskey, M., Caramazza, A., & Green, B. (1980). Curvilinear motion in the absence of external forces: Naive beliefs about the motion of objects. *Science, 210,* 1139-1141.

Minstrell, J. A. (1989). Teaching science for understanding. In L. B. Resnick & L. E. Klopfer (Eds.), *Toward the thinking curriculum: Current cognitive research* (pp. 129-149). Alexandria, VA: Association for Supervision and Curriculum Development.

Muller, R. (1988). *Nemesis.* New York: Weiden-feld & Nicolson.

Musgrave, A. (1976). Why did oxygen supplant phlogiston? Research programmes in the chemical revolution. In C. Howson (Ed.), *Method and appraisal in the physical sciences: The critical background to modern science, 1800-1905* (pp. 181-209). Cambridge, England: Cambridge University Press.

Neale, D. C., Smith, D., & Johnson, V. G. (1990). Implementing conceptual change teaching in primary science. *Elementary School Journal, 91,* 109-131.

Nussbaum, J., & Novick, S. (1982). Alternative frameworks, conceptual conflict and accommodation: Toward a principled teaching strategy. *Instructional Science, 11,* 183-200.

Osborne, R., & Freyberg, P. (Eds.). (1985). *Learning in science: The implications of children's science.* Auckland, New Zealand: Heinemann.

Osborne, R. J., & Wittrock, M. C. (1983). Learning science: A generative process. *Science Education, 67,* 489-508.

Perkins, D. N., & Simmons, R. (1988). Patterns of misunderstanding: An integrative model for science, math, and programming. *Review of Educational Research, 58,* 303-326.

Piaget, J. (1980). *Experiments in contradiction* (D. Coltman, Trans.). Chicago: University of Chicago Press. (Original work published 1974)

Pickering, M., & Monts, D. L. (1982). How students reconcile discordant data: A study of lab report discussions. *Journal of Chemical Education, 59,* 794-796.

Pines, A. L., & West, L. H. T. (1986). Conceptual understanding and science learning: An interpretation of research within a sources-of-knowledge framework. *Science Education, 70,* 583-604.

Posner, G. J., Strike, K. A,, Hewson, P. W., & Gertzog, W. A. (1982). Accommodation of a scientific conception: Toward a theory of conceptual change. *Science Education, 66,* 211-227.

Quine, W. V. O . (1951). Two dogmas of empiricism. *The Philosophical Review, 60,* 20-43.

Ranney, M., & Thagard, P. (1988). Explanatory coherence and belief revision in naive physics. In *Proceedings of the Tenth Annual Conference of the Cognitive Science Society* (pp. 426-432). Hillsdale, NJ: Erlbaum.

Reiner, M., & Finegold, M. (1987). Changing students' explanatory frameworks concerning the nature of light using real time computer analysis of laboratory experiments and computerized explanatory simulations of e.m. radiation. In J. D. Novak (Ed.), *Proceedings of the Second International Seminar on Misconceptions and Educational Strategies in Science and Mathematics* (Vol. 2, pp. 368-377). Ithaca, NY: Cornell University.

Roth, K. J. (1990). Developing meaningful conceptual understanding in science. In B. F. Jones & L. Idol (Eds.), *Dimensions of thinking and cognitive instruction* (pp. 139-175). Hillsdale, NJ: Erlbaum.

Roth, K., & Anderson, C. (1988). Promoting conceptual change learning from science textbooks. In P. Ramsden (Ed.), *Improving learning: New perspectives* (pp. 109-141). London: Kogan Page.

Roth, K. J., Anderson, C. W., & Smith, E. L. (1987). Curriculum materials, teacher talk and student learning: Case studies in fifth grade science teaching. *Journal of Curriculum Studies, 19,* 527-548.

Rowell, J. A, & Dawson, C. J. (1983). Laboratory counterexamples and the growth of understanding in science. *European Journal of Science Education, 5,* 203-215.

Schank, R. C., Collins, G. C., & Hunter, L. E. (1986). Transcending inductive category formation in learning. *Behavioral and Brain Sciences, 9,* 639-686.

Schauble, L. (1990). Belief revision in children: The role of prior knowledge and strategies for generating evidence. *Journal of Experimental Child Psychology, 49,* 31-57.

Snir, J. (1991). Sink or float---What do the experts think?: The historical development of explanations for floatation. *Science Education, 75,* 595-609.

Suppe, F. (1974). The search for philosophic understanding of scientific theories. In F. Suppe (Ed.), *The structure of scientific theories* (pp. 3-241). Urbana: University of Illinois Press.

Thagard, P. (1989). Explanatory coherence. *Behavioral and Brain Sciences, 12,* 435-502.

Thagard, P. (1992). *Conceptual revolutions.* Princeton, NJ: Princeton University Press.

Thompson, S. P. (1976). *The life of Lord Kelvin,* Vol. 2 (2nd ed.). New York: Chelsea.

Vosniadou, S., & Brewer, W. F. (1992). Mental models of the earth: A study of conceptual change in childhood. *Cognitive Psychology, 24,* 535-585.

Wallace, A. R. (1889). *Darwinism: An exposition of the theory of natural selection with some of its applications.* London: Macmillan.

Wang, T., & Andre, T. (1991). Conceptual change text versus traditional text and application questions versus no questions in learning about electricity. *Contemporary Educational Psychology, 16,* 103-116.

Watson, B., & Konicek, R. (1990). Teaching for conceptual change: Confronting children's experience. *Phi Delta Kappan, 71,* 680-685.

White, B. Y., & Frederiksen, J. R. (1990). Causal model progressions as a foundation for intelligent learning environments. *Artificial Intelligence, 42,* 99-157.

Whittaker, E. (1951). *A history of the theories of aether and electricity: Vol. I. The classical theories.* New York: Philosophical Library.

Wisniewski, E. J., & Medin, D. L. (1991). Harpoons and long sticks: The interaction of theory and similarity in rule induction. In D. H. Fisher, M. J. Pazzani, & P. Langley (Eds.), *Concept formation: Knowledge and experience in unsupervised learning* (pp. 237-278). San Mateo, CA: Morgan Kaufmann.

Zietsman, A. I., & Hewson, P. W. (1986). Effect of instruction using microcomputer simulations and conceptual change strategies on science learning. *Journal of Research in Science Teaching, 23,* 27-39.

Barriers to the Use of Traditional Telephones by Older Adults With Chronic Health Conditions

William C. Mann, Patrícia Belchior, Machiko R. Tomita, Bryan J. Kemp

Key words: aging, disability, telephone

Abstract: As people age, they face motor, sensory, and cognitive decline that may compromise their performance of activities of daily living and instrumental activities of daily living. Telephone use is an important instrumental activity of daily living for older adults, but many have difficulty in making and receiving calls. Today, there are many features that can be added to the telephone that can help compensate for impairments, but often these features are not used. To better understand the problems of older adults in using their telephones, we surveyed 609 older adults living in the community who had chronic health conditions. Interviews were conducted face-to-face, by telephone, or by mail. The most common reasons for not using more telephone special features were cost, lack of perceived need, and lack of knowledge of the features.
Occupational therapists who work with older adults must understand the importance of telephones in their lives and offer them information and assistance in finding telephones with features that match their special needs. The findings of this study suggest that a significant number of older adults with chronic health conditions are unaware of low-cost, feature-laden telephones that could make their communications easier or, for some, possible.

William C. Mann, OTR, PhD, is Chair and Professor, Department of Occupational Therapy, University of Florida, Gainesville, Florida. Patrícia Belchior, OT, is Research Assistant, Rehabilitation Science Doctoral Program, University of Florida, Gainesville, Florida. Machiko R. Tomita, PhD, is Clinical Associate Professor, Department of Rehabilitation Science, University of Buffalo, Buffalo, New York. Bryan J. Kemp, PhD, is Professor and Director, Rehabilitation Research and Training Center on Aging with Disabilities, University of California, Irvine, Program in Geriatrics, Irvine, California. Address correspondence to William C. Mann at wmann@phhp.ufl.edu.

As people age, they face declines in motor performance (Light, 1990) and sensory functions such as vision, hearing, taste, and olfaction (Nusbaum, 1999). These changes may compromise performance of activities of daily living and instrumental activities of daily living (IADLs). Among all of the IADLs performed by older adults in the course of a day, the use of the telephone is rated most important (Fricke & Unsworth, 2001). The telephone is used for emergencies, arranging for in-home care, and socializing with family and friends (Cream & Teaford, 1999). The use of a telephone decreases loneliness and increases feelings of connectedness among nursing home residents (Gueldner et al., 2001). Telephone services for older adults can provide health information and monitor their health. Telehealth services can decrease the number of visits to emergency departments and physician offices, which can save health care dollars (MacMaster, Goldenberg, Beynon, & Iwasiw, 1999).

Many older adults experience difficulties in using their telephone. Telephone menu systems are frustrating for all of us, but even more so for older adults. Menu options are often presented too rapidly. The location of the telephone in a house can also impede access. Having a telephone in the kitchen is useful for daily calls, but having a telephone in the bedroom is helpful for emergencies (Cream & Teaford, 1999).

Today, telephones offer many features, some of which compensate for impairments faced by older adults (Mann, 1997). Fine motor impairment can be compensated for by telephones with bigger buttons, redial, and memory features. Ringer amplification control and voice amplification control can compensate for hearing impairment. If the individual is deaf, special telephones called telecommunication devices for the deaf (TDDs) can be used. TDDs "provide a keypad for sending messages and a digital display for reading the message from the sender. It requires either that users on both ends of a call have a TDD or that a relay service be used" (Mann, 1997, p. 326). Visual impairment is another common problem experienced by older adults that can be compensated for with bigger buttons, buttons that light up, and buttons with better contrast. To address mobility impairment, telephones that can be answered across the room, such as a remote speaker telephone, can be used. Another option is a cordless telephone or mobile telephone that the person can always have close by.

Although telephones with special features can be easily found in stores, many older adults who need them do not have them, or are not using them. Furthermore, some older adults have difficulties with certain features. The problems they have with their telephones can be categorized as: need for repair, maintenance, or both; poor device performance; and poor person-to-device fit. Older adults are often unaware of the telephone features that make it easier to use and perform more functions (Mann, Hurren, Charvat, & Tomita, 1996).

This study complements an earlier study on the use of the telephone (Mann et al., 1996) by exploring the needs and barriers of the use of the telephone and its features from the perspective of older adults. The study also provides more information about older adults' awareness and use of telephone features.

Methods

The purpose of this study was to better understand how older adults use their standard telephones, if they are satisfied with them, and what features they would like to add to their telephones. In meeting the University of Florida Rehabilitation Engineering Research Center on Technology and Aging mission to advance the utility and ease-of-use of products for older adults, consumer feedback was sought on communication technologies and assistive technology. Consumer feedback in this study was structured around the following research questions:

1. *Telephone ownership, use, and satisfaction:* How many telephones, by type,

Article Reprint Information: Reprinted with permission from Mann, W. C., Belchior, P., Tomita, M. R., & Kemp, B. J. (2005). Barriers to the use of traditional telephones by older adults with chronic health conditions. *Occupational Therapy Journal of Research: Occupation, Participation and Health, 25*(4), 160-166.

were owned by study participants? How often were they used? Are participants satisfied with their telephones? Are their telephones important to them? For what purpose do they use their telephones?

2. *Problems experienced with telephones:* Do they have enough time to get to the telephone when they receive a call? Do they have problems with wiring across the floor? What prevents them from using more features?

3. *Use of telephones in emergencies:* Have they ever needed their telephones in an emergency and, if so, were they able to use them successfully?

4. *Telephone features:* What features could be added to their telephones that would help them? Which features do they have in their telephones, and which features do they use?

The protocol and consent form for this study was reviewed and approved by the University of Florida Institutional Review Board.

Sample

Six hundred and nine older adults with chronic health conditions that limit activities were surveyed from 2001 to 2002. Among older Americans, 28.8% of those aged 65 to 74 years and 50.6% of those older than 75 years have chronic health conditions that limit activities (Fowles, 2001). All of the participants had at least one telephone in their home and were at least 60 years old with a mean age of 74.4 years. Women represented 68.3% of the sample, 91.5% were white, 47.8% had completed college, 40.4% were married, 48.2% lived alone, and 69.8% owned their own home (Table 1).

The most common chronic conditions reported by participants were fatigue (65.0%), joint problems (58.0%), muscular weakness (57.4%), difficulty with hand tasks (50.6%), bladder and bowel control problems (49.0%), and back problems (44.5%) (Table 2). The activities reported as being most difficult to perform were climbing stairs (77.2%), walking (70.4%), doing housework (60.8%), getting out of a chair (51.1%), shopping (48.6%), driving (46.1%), and bending (44.9%) (Table 3).

Data Collection

Data for this study were collected with a questionnaire that included yes or no, multiple-choice, open-ended, and Likert scale questions and answers. Basic demographic data were requested along with the responses to the questionnaire. Prior to distributing the questionnaire, it was reviewed by professionals and older adults with chronic

Table 1
Demographic Data of the Participants
(n = 609)

Characteristic	No. (%)
Age (y)	
Mean	74.4
Standard deviation	8.4
Gender (n = 602)	
Female	411 (68.3)
Male	191 (31.7)
Race (n = 604)	
White	553 (91.5)
Black	35 (5.8)
Hispanic	4 (0.7)
Asian	3 (0.5)
Other	9 (1.5)
Education level (n = 604)	
College (bachelor's degree or higher)	289 (47.8)
Some college, no degree	102 (16.8)
High school or less	213 (35.3)
Marital status (n = 602)	
Married	243 (40.4)
Not married	359 (59.76)
Living status (n = 598)	
Live alone	288 (48.2)
Live with someone	310 (51.8)
Housing status (n = 589)	
Own	411 (69.8)
Rent	133 (22.6)
Other	45 (7.6)
Type of house (n = 576)	
Single-family detached home	320 (55.6)
Senior apartment	51 (8.8)
Retirement community	48 (8.3)
Townhouse or condominium	38 (6.6)
Walk-up apartment building	29 (5.0)
Elevator apartment building	27 (4.7)
2-unit building	19 (3.3)
Mobile home in mobile park	11 (2.0)
Isolated mobile home	9 (1.6)
Other	24 (4.2)

Table 2
Chronic Conditions Reported by Study Participants
(n = 605)

Condition	No. (%)
Fatigue	393 (65.0)
Joint problems	351 (58.0)
Muscular weakness	347 (57.4)
Difficulty with hand tasks	306 (50.6)
Bladder/bowel control problems	296 (49.0)
Back problems	269 (44.5)
Poor hearing	202 (33.4)
Low vision	194 (32.1)
Paralysis of legs	178 (29.4)
Memory difficulties	177 (29.3)
Paralysis of arms	100 (16.6)
Speech difficulties	81 (13.4)
Learning disability	32 (5.3)
Blind	28 (4.6)
Deaf	20 (3.3)
Other	125 (20.7)

health conditions and revised in response to reviewer feedback.

Appointments were scheduled at times convenient for study participants. Occupational therapists and nurses experienced in research interviewing conducted the interviews, which required approximately 1 hour to complete. Six hundred and nine study participants were surveyed; 53 surveys were conducted face-to-face in the participants' homes, 168 interviews were conducted by telephone or home interview, and 388 were completed using a mailed survey. The telephone and in-home interviews included older adults from Western New York, Southern California, and Northern Florida. The mailed survey included older adults with disabilities throughout the United States. The use of a combination of in-home and telephone interviews and a mailed survey made it possible to include a larger sample.

The Southern California sample (n = 18) were drawn from patients who received services at Ranchos Los Amigos Medical Center in Downey, California. The in-home interviews were completed at a continuous care retirement community in Naples, Florida, and with study participants identified by the Rehabilitation Engineering Research Center on Technology and Aging in Northern Florida and Western New York. The mailed survey included older adults with disabilities from across the United States who had subscribed to an assistive technology information service called Project Link (Mann, 1994).

Table 3
Activities Difficult to Perform
(n = 544)

Activity	No. (%)
Climbing stairs	420 (77.2)
Walking	383 (70.4)
Doing housework	331 (60.8)
Getting out of chair	278 (51.1)
Shopping	264 (48.6)
Driving	251 (46.1)
Bending	244 (44.9)
Preparing meals	194 (35.7)
Writing	180 (33.1)
Getting on and off the toilet	175 (32.2)
Bathing	174 (32.0)
Getting dressed	165 (30.3)
Using a computer	130 (23.9)
Managing bowel/ bladder tasks	103 (18.9)
Reading	101 (18.6)
Using the telephone	89 (16.7)
Grooming	76 (14.0)
Holding eating utensils	71 (13.1)
Other	72 (13.2)

Table 4
Telephone Use

Criteria	No. (%)
Frequency	
Daily	521 (86.1)
3–6 days/week	54 (9.0)
1–2 days/week	18 (3.0)
1 day/week	12 (2.0)
Reason	
Social contacts	591 (98.2)
Medical appointments	544 (90.3)
Refilling prescriptions	489 (81.2)
Business	335 (55.6)
Calling for help/ assistance	295 (49.0)
Connecting to the Internet	262 (43.5)
Shopping	245 (40.7)
Banking	238 (39.5)
Other	50 (8.3)

Analysis

Descriptive statistics were used to report sample characteristics. All analyses were completed using SPSS version 11.0 software (SPSS, Inc., Chicago, IL). Frequencies for categorical variables, means, standard deviations, and ranges for non-categorical variables and cross-tabulation of study participants were reported.

Results

Telephone Ownership, Use, and Satisfaction

Touch-tone telephones had the highest ownership rate (1,294; mean = 2.12), followed by cordless telephones (723; mean = 1.2), rotary telephones (133; mean = 0.21), and TDD telephones (35; mean = 0.10). There were 66 telephones in the category of Other (mean = 0.10). Daily telephone use was reported by 86.1% of the participants (Table 4). Although a previous study (Cream & Teaford, 1999) found that daily telephone calls were usually made from a telephone located in the kitchen, the current study did not explore telephone location in the participants' homes. However, most of the participants had more than one telephone.

The most common reasons for using a telephone were social contact (98.2%), setting up medical appointments (90.3%), refilling prescriptions (81.2%), business (55.6%), and calling for help/assistance (49.0%). More than twice as many study participants used the telephone for social contact than for connecting to the Internet.

Most of the participants were very satisfied with their telephones. The highest rate of satisfaction (64.1%) was with touch-tone telephones (Table 5). More than half of the participants stated that the telephone was a very important device (Table 6). This finding is consistent with Fricke and Unsworth (2001), who reported that the use of the telephone is one of the most important IADLs performed in the course of a day. Touch-tone telephones had the highest proportion of the study participants (90.3%) rating them as important.

Problems Experienced With Telephones

The participants were almost evenly divided when asked whether they had enough time to get to the telephone when they received a call; 272 (45.9%) of the participants responded yes, whereas 320 (54.1%) responded no. Approximately 1 in 10 (65; 10.1%) had problems with long telephone wires across the floor. Cost was cited as the major reason that prevented participants from using more features (53.6%), followed by a lack of perceived need (32.3%), lack of knowledge of the device (27.1%), too

complicated or confusing (14.5%), mobility (10.3%), access (9.2%), and too difficult to learn (9.0%) (Table 7).

Use of Telephones in Emergencies

Participants were asked whether they had ever needed to use their telephone in an emergency; 394 (65.9%) responded yes and 204 (34.1%) responded no. Of those who had used their telephone in an emergency, 358 (91.8%) had used it successfully and 32 (8.2%) were not able to use it successfully.

Telephone Features

Few of the study participants provided responses when asked what features could be added to their telephones that would help them. Of those who did respond, 13.3% would like to be alerted when mail (traditional land mail) arrived, 8.2% would like to be alerted about time and weather and conditions, 5.7% would like to be alerted when someone was at the door, 5.1% would like to have a feature to block telemarketers, and 3.4% would like to have a voice-activated telephone (Table 8). The participants were also asked which telephone features they had and which features they actually used. Participants who had particular features on their telephones did not always use them (Table 9).

Discussion

This study confirms earlier findings about the importance of the standard telephone for older adults (Fricke & Unsworth, 2001; Mann et al., 1996). Overall, they were satisfied with their telephones and considered them to be important devices. Almost all participants used their telephones every day.

Among all of the activities that participants find difficult to perform, using the telephone was rated very low. Only 16.7% of participants reported having problems performing this activity. However, approximately half of the participants reported not being able to get to the telephone in time to answer, which can be explained by their difficulties in climbing stairs, walking, and getting out of a chair. This finding suggests that the location of the telephone in a house is more problematic than the use of the telephone itself. An earlier study reported that the location of the telephone in the house can be a barrier to its use (Cream & Teaford, 1999).

Occupational therapists could play a role in suggesting better placement of existing telephones, such as next to a favorite chair or couch. Rearrangement of furniture and providing additional furniture such as

Table 5
Telephone Satisfaction

Type	Missing	Not at All Satisfied (%)	Not Satisfied (%)	Somewhat Satisfied (%)	Very Satisfied (%)	Total
Touch-tone	22	9 (1.7)	18 (3.4)	164 (30.8)	341 (64.1)	554
Cordless	23	27 (5.8)	28 (6.1)	135 (29.2)	272 (58.9)	485
Rotary	8	5 (5.9)	7 (8.2)	36 (42.3)	37 (43.5)	93
TDD	4	3 (15.8)	—	5 (26.3)	11 (57.9)	23
Other	4	2 (4.2)	7 (14.6)	13 (27.1)	26 (54.2)	52

TDD = telecommunication device for the deaf.

Table 6
Telephone Importance

Type	Missing	Not at All Important (%)	Not Important (%)	Somewhat Important (%)	Very Important (%)	Total
Touch-tone	25	7 (1.3)	16 (3.0)	91 (17.2)	478 (90.3)	554
Cordless	29	9 (2.0)	14 (3.0)	79 (17.3)	354 (77.6)	485
Rotary	9	7 (8.3)	10 (12.0)	17 (20.2)	50 (59.5)	93
TDD	4	4 (21.0)	1 (5.2)	2 (10.5)	10 (52.6)	23
Other	4	3 (6.2)	2 (6.2)	6 (12.5)	37 (77.1)	52

TDD = telecommunication device for the deaf.

a bedside table are other options. Likewise, therapists could recommend the use of a cordless or mobile telephone and additional devices or features such as an answering machine or a remote speaker telephone that can be answered from across the room.

Another concern raised by this study is wires running across the floor that could cause a fall. Use of cordless telephones, better placement or wiring, installation of new jacks, or additional telephones could serve as alternatives to this unsafe practice.

More than half of the participants had used the telephone for emergency purposes and most of them were able to use it successfully. However, the main reason for using the telephone was to make social contacts and to set up medical appointments.

When asked about the features they would like to have on their telephones, few participants provided an answer. Several of those who did respond suggested an "alert" function so they would be alerted when mail arrives and about time and weather conditions.

Common features used by participants included redial, ringer volume control, and an answering machine. More than half of the participants did not use more features because of the cost of getting a telephone with additional features. Some participants lacked the knowledge of the features. Speaker, amplification, and large buttons

Table 7
Factors That Prevent Use of Telephone Special Features
(n = 601)

Factor	No. (%)
Cost	322 (53.6)
Lack of perceived need	194 (32.3)
Lack of knowledge of devices	163 (27.1)
Too complicated or confusing	87 (14.5)
Mobility	62 (10.3)
Access	55 (9.2)
Too difficult to learn	54 (9.0)
Hearing impairment	46 (7.6)
Visual impairment	41 (6.8)
Training not available	31 (5.1)
Lack of user manual	26 (4.3)
Pain	24 (4.0)
Privacy/trust	21 (3.5)
Cognitive impairment	16 (2.7)
Not interested	8 (1.3)
Other	65 (10.8)

are features that can help with sensory declines, but these features are underutilized. Telephones with these features are relatively low-cost; therefore, it may be that

Table 8
Telephone Features That Participants Thought Would Be Helpful

Feature	No. (%)
No opinion	89 (25.2)
Alert when mail has arrived	47 (13.3)
Alert about time and weather	29 (8.2)
Alert when someone is at the door	20 (5.7)
Block telemarketers	18 (5.1)
Voice activated	12 (3.4)
Caller identification	10 (2.8)
Reminder to take medication	8 (2.3)
Button for emergency	4 (1.1)
Other	116 (32.9)

many older adults are not aware that they are affordable (Mann et al., 1996). Occupational therapists could play a role in providing information on sources of assistance for acquiring telephones with special features. Every state has a program to provide telephones for individuals with disabilities below a set income level.

This study strongly suggests a role for occupational therapists relative to traditional

Table 9
Telephone Features That
Participants Have and Use[a]

Feature	Have No. (%)	Use No. (%)
Redial	491 (88.5)	384 (76.5)
Ringer volume control	486 (86.6)	358 (73.1)
Answering machine	441 (76.9)	414 (91.2)
Memory dial	404 (75.1)	263 (60.2)
Lighted keypad	243 (43.7)	198 (68.5)
Speaker	221 (41.7)	153 (55.6)
Amplification	215 (40.0)	151 (52.4)
Big buttons	151 (28.1)	137 (62.0)
Call waiting	141 (25.3)	128 (61.8)
Paging ringer	119 (23.4)	48 (27.7)
Caller identification	114 (21.3)	96 (50.3)
Voice mail	74 (13.4)	62 (40.8)
Visual ring signal	73 (14.6)	55 (36.2)
Headset	60 (11.0)	46 (32.6)
Hearing compatibility	58 (11.4)	34 (26.7)
Photographs/ pictures	7 (1.3)	1 (1.2)
Braille keypad	3 (0.6)	—

[a]Not all participants provided an answer for this question. The percentage was computed after removing respondents with missing values.

telephones. Therapists should be prepared to address issues related to telephone placement and wiring, furniture placement, and provision of information about cost and telephone features that address specific impairments. Therapists can also address issues about background noise, telephone maintenance, nuisance calls, and special services.

As underlying technologies develop, the traditional telephone is being replaced by new devices or integrated into multi-purpose devices. Smart telephones are available that offer Internet connectivity, personal digital assistant functions, and camera functions, as well as traditional voice communication. The Internet offers the opportunity for "visual" social contact by sending e-mails with attached pictures, or using a Web camera. Future research should address the challenges older adults may face when using new communication devices to ensure their successful use.

Acknowledgment

This is a study of the Rehabilitation Engineering Research Center on Technology for Successful Aging, funded by the National Institute on Disability and Rehabilitation Research of the Department of Education under grant number H133E010106. The opinions contained in this article are those of the grantee and do not necessarily reflect those of the Department of Education.

References

Cream, A., & Teaford, M. (1999). Maintaining independence through home modifications: A focus on the telephone. *Physical & Occupational Therapy in Geriatrics, 16*(3/4), 117-134.

Fowles, D. G. (2001). *A profile of older Americans: 2001.* Washington, DC: Administration on Aging, U.S. Department of Health and Human Services. Retrieved August 22, 2005, from http://assets.aarp.org/rgcenter/general/profile_2001.pdf.

Fricke, J., & Unsworth, C. (2001). Time use and importance of instrumental activities of daily living. *Australian Occupational Therapy Journal, 48*, 118-131.

Gueldner, S. H., Smith, C. A., Neal, M., Penrod, J., Ryder, J., Dye, M., et al. (2001). Patterns of telephone use among nursing home residents. *Journal of Gerontological Nursing, 27*, 35-41.

Light, K. E. (1990). Information processing for motor performance in aging adults. *Physical Therapy, 70*, 820-826.

MacMaster, E., Goldenberg, D., Beynon, C., & Iwasiw, C. (1999). Health information telephone service for seniors. *The Canadian Nurse, 95*, 38-41.

Mann, W. (1994). Project LINK: Consumer information for persons with disabilities. *Information Technology and Disabilities E-Journal, 1*(2). Retrieved August 20, 2004, from http://www.rit.edu/~easi/itd/itdv01n2/mann.htm.

Mann, W. (1997). An essential communication device: The telephone. In R. Lubinski & D. J. Higginbotham (Eds.), *Communication technologies for the elderly: Vision, hearing, and speech* (pp. 323-339). San Diego, CA: Singular Publishing Group.

Mann, W., Hurren, D., Charvat, B., & Tomita, M. (1996). The use of phones by elders with disabilities: Problems, interventions, costs. *Assistive Technology, 8*, 23-33.

Nusbaum, N. J. (1999). Aging and sensory senescence. *Southern Medical Journal, 92*, 267-275.

Efficacy of Sensory and Motor Interventions for Children with Autism

Grace T. Baranek[1]

Idiosyncratic responses to sensory stimuli and unusual motor patterns have been reported clinically in young children with autism. The etiology of these behavioral features is the subject of much speculation. Myriad sensory- and motor-based interventions have evolved for use with children with autism to address such issues; however, much controversy exists about the efficacy of such therapies. This review paper summarizes the sensory and motor difficulties often manifested in autism, and evaluates the scientific basis of various sensory and motor interventions used with this population. Implications for education and further research are described.

KEY WORDS: Sensorimotor therapies; evidence-based treatments; sensory integration.

[1]The Clinical Center for the Study of Development and Learning, Room 111 Medical School Wing E—CB #7120 University of North Carolina at Chapel Hill, Chapel Hill, NC 27599-7120; e-mail: gbaranek@med.unc.edu.

Purpose, Search Procedures, and Scope

The purpose of this paper is threefold: (1) briefly summarize the empirical literature with respect to sensory and motor development/abnormalities in children with autism, (2) evaluate the scientific basis of sensory and motor interventions used with children with autism, and (3) describe implications of these findings for education and further research. Subject headings and keywords were searched for terms related to sensory and motor deficits (e.g., arousal, sensory reactivity/processing, habituation, posture, praxis, gross/fine/oral motor development, etc.), and categorical terms specific to sensory and motor interventions (e.g., sensory integration, prism lenses, etc.). Searches were conducted using MEDLINE, CINAHL, & PSYCINFO databases to find empirical studies specific to children with autism spectrum disorders (i.e., autistic disorder, pervasive developmental disorder) available in the English language for the past 30 years with a focus on the past 10 years. Also, manual searches of key references from articles were completed. In a few noted cases, studies of individuals with related disorders (e.g., mental retardation), or slightly older children (over 8 years) were included provided the results had implications for young children with autism.

Literature Review of Sensory and Motor Development

Empirical studies about sensory and motor development in children with autism are limited compared to studies of other aspects of development. Those that exist often suffer from a variety of methodological limitations; however, these studies provide both a foundation of scientific knowledge critical for understanding the early development of children with autism and guidance for intervention planning. Empirical evidence converges to confirm the existence of sensory and motor difficulties for many children with autism at some point in their early development (Adrien et al., 1987; 1992; 1993; Baranek, 1999; Dahlgren & Gilberg, 1989; Hoshino et al., 1982; Ohta, Nagai, Hara, & Sasaki, 1987; Ornitz, Guthrie, & Farley, 1977; Scharre & Creedon, 1992), although much variability is present in specific symptoms or patterns expressed. These types of behaviors appear neither universal nor specific to the disorder of autism; however, qualitative aspects of these patterns have not been well studied, and prospective, longitudinal investigations that systematically document developmental trajectories from infancy through childhood are yet to be accomplished. The majority of evidence stems from parental reports, which themselves are prone to some biases and methodological weaknesses. Empirical data from retrospective video studies (Adrien et al., 1992; Baranek, 1999) and clinical evaluations (Gillberg et al., 1990) are emerging to suggest that patterns of sensory and motor features in autism may differ qualitatively from those in other developmental disorders. Furthermore, unusual sensory-perceptual features appear to be manifest quite early in the development of children with autism (i.e., by 9 to 12 months of age). Though not well understood, sensory processing and motor patterns may be related to core features, development of other aberrant behaviors, and later prognosis; thus these patterns have implications for early diagnosis and intervention.

Unusual sensory responses (e.g., hypo- and hyper-responses; preoccupations with sensory features of objects, perceptual distortions; paradoxical responses to sensory stimuli) have been reported in 42 to 88% of older children with autism in various studies (Kientz & Dunn, 1997; LeCouteur et al., 1989; Ornitz et al., 1977; Volkmar, Cohen, & Paul, 1986), indicating that these are common concerns in this population. Percentages vary depending on how specifically items were sampled. Auditory processing problems are particularly noted, with one study (Greenspan & Weider, 1997) purporting that 100% of subjects demonstrated these difficulties. Visual spatial skills are often more advanced than other areas of development, although individual differences are noted. Sensory processing abilities also appear to be uneven and of a fluctuating nature in autism, such that both hyper- and hypo-responses are evident in the same child. These aberrant sensory reactions are thought to reflect poor sensory integration and/or arousal modulation in the central nervous system, although the underlying nature of these symptoms remains speculative (e.g., neurological structures and systems involving the cerebellum, limbic system, cortical mechanisms, etc). Both patterns of under- and over-arousal have been reported (Hutt, Hutt, Lee, & Ounsted, 1964; James & Barry, 1984; Kinsbourne, 1987; Kootz & Cohen, 1981; Kootz, Marinelli, &

Article Reprint Information: Reprinted from Springer/*Journal of Autism and Developmental Disorders*, 32(5), 2002, 397-422, Efficacy of sensory and motor interventions for children with autism, Baranek, G. T., with kind permission from Springer Science and Business Media.

Cohen, 1982; Rimland, 1964; Zentall & Zentall, 1983). Children with autism tend to show these abnormal sensory responses to both social and nonsocial stimuli and in the absence of known peripheral dysfunction (e.g., hearing acuity, visual defect) *per se*. Thus some researchers have suggested shifting toward the investigation of more complex levels of information processing including attentional control mechanisms and executive functions to help explain some of these unusual sensory features or motor deficits (e.g., Lincoln *et al.*, 1995; Minshew, Goldstein, & Seigel, 1997; Wainwright & Bryson, 1996). Given that many conventional educational environments are sensorily complicated and unpredictable, interventions likely need to consider the individualized sensory processing needs of children demonstrating such difficulties to optimize successful participation in such programs.

With respect to developmental milestones, unevenness between domains is often reported, indicating a relative sparing of general motor skills compared to language or social skills in children with autism (Klin, Volkmar, & Sparrow, 1992; Stone *et al.*, 1999). However, not all children with autism demonstrate prowess in motor skills and considerable variability exists (Amato & Slavin, 1998; DeMyer *et al.*, 1972; Jones & Prior, 1985; Johnson, Siddons, Frith, & Morton, 1992; Ohta *et al.*, 1987; Ornitz *et al.*, 1977; Rapin, 1997; Rinehart, Bradshaw, Brereton, & Tonge, 2001). Many demonstrate atypical features (e.g., low muscle tone, oral-motor problems, repetitive motor movements, dyspraxia) or test in the delayed ranges on standardized motor assessments particularly as the complexity of tasks increases. Whether or not these difficulties are purely motoric is unclear, because other areas also affect test-taking abilities. Furthermore, delayed motor development is not a unique characteristic of children with autism, because it is often associated with the level of mental retardation in general. However, because more than 75% of children with autism have concomitant mental retardation, the presence of motoric concerns, regardless of whether they are primary or secondary to autism, still has substantial implications for individualized educational interventions. Developmental motor delays, although only minimally different during infancy, may become magnified with progressive age (e.g., Ohta *et al.*, 1987). Especially during early foundational years, motor skills provide a means for learning important skills in other domains (e.g., social skills, academics) and thus motor-related difficulties may need to

be addressed in the educational curricula or through related therapy services. At least one study (Perez & Sevilla, 1993) demonstrates a predictive relationship between motor skills in children with autism to functional outcomes in other domains such as vocational and leisure skills 5 years later.

Motor planning deficits are an area of particular interest, given that several studies point out that both younger and older children with autism may demonstrate difficulties with aspects of praxis (Adams, 1998; Jones & Prior, 1985; Rinehart *et al.*, 2001; Rogers *et al.*, 1996; Smith & Bryson, 1998; Stone *et al.*, 1990). These difficulties are certainly exaggerated in tasks that require execution of a social imitation, either motor or object related, but may also be present in nonimitated simple goal-directed motor tasks (e.g., reaching, grasping, and placing) (Hughes & Russell, 1993). Motor planning deficits are sometimes mistaken for general clumsiness; however, Rinehart *et al.* (2001) separated out two components of action and found that highly functioning children with autism spectrum disorders, ages 5 to 19 years, had intact movement *execution* but atypical movement *preparation* during a simple motor reprogramming task compared with typical, IQ-matched controls. Specifically, children with autistic disorder were characterized by a lack of anticipation during movement preparation phases, findings suggestive of difficulties in motivational aspects of behavior or attention for action. Children with Asperger's disorder showed slower preparations for movement at phases in which movement should be optimal—implicating additional dysfunction in the frontal-striatal system, according to the authors.

Although it is possible that the formulation of motor plans is deficient, it is also possible that simple motor planning is intact but that the use of externally guided visual feedback is diminished, affecting the quality of motor performance, postural stability, and the lack of effective sequencing of actions (Masterton & Biederman, 1983; Gepner, Mestre, Masson, & de Schonen, 1995; Smith & Bryson, 1998; Stone *et al.*, 1990; Kohen-Raz, Volkmar, & Cohen, 1992). Thus, perceptually challenging tasks that require smooth integration of visual with vestibular-proprioceptive information, for example, may be particularly difficult to perform and could result in poor quality of motor performance on complex tasks. These findings taken together with evidence that motor imitation skills in young children with autism predict later expressive language skills and play skills (Stone *et al.*, 1997), have signifi-

cant implications for educational interventions and future research.

Efficacy of Sensory and Motor Interventions

Because "interventions for sensory and motor deficits" are not synonymous with "sensory and motor interventions," the following *inclusion* criteria were used to define the parameters for the review: (a) remedial interventions that target specific sensory or motor components *per se*, broader performance outcomes that are thought to be the result of the sensory-motor treatment, or both; (b) compensatory skills training approaches; and/or (c) task/environmental modifications targeted for sensory and motor difficulties. A variety of other interventions exist that may be at least partially aimed at improving sensory and motor skills; however, only those interventions that have a primary basis in sensory processing or motor theories were included. Traditional behavioral interventions and psychopharmacological treatments were *excluded*. Likewise, comprehensive educational models (e.g., Greenspan—DIR Model; TEACCH) were *excluded*, even though these programs frequently include a sensory processing or motor development component. Although a variety of professionals (e.g., occupational therapists, adaptive physical educators, physical therapists, speech pathologists, etc.) may utilize various sensory-motor strategies listed within the context of any given child's individualized educational plan, this paper is not intended to be a critique of the efficacy of those related services. Sensory-motor interventions are not presumed to represent the full scope of therapeutic/educational services offered by specialized professionals. Sensory or motor treatments often are used as an adjunct to a more holistic intervention plan. For example, the occupational therapist provides therapeutic interventions aimed at improving a child's occupational performance (e.g., play, school functional skills, self-care) within the educational context. Remediation of sensory or motor deficits (as well as other components including cognitive or psychosocial functions) may occur if indicated, but only within the larger context of occupational performance problems within the learning environment. Compensatory interventions and environmental adaptations are also utilized and often preferred because of the more immediate effects on meaningful participation.

To judge the validity of each category of interventions, first a description of each intervention approach is provided that includes the underlying assumptions of the intervention, proposed mechanisms thought to be responsible for the therapeutic changes purported, and the service delivery model utilized to provide the intervention. In addition, the scientific evidence (i.e., efficacy research from peer-reviewed sources) of each intervention category is reviewed. Table 1 provides a comparative summary of the empirical studies reviewed for children with autism spectrum disorders.

Sensory Integration Therapy

Description and Assumptions. Sensory integration (SI) therapy, based on the work of Dr. A. Jean Ayres, is intended to focus directly on the neurological processing of sensory information as a foundation for learning of higher-level (motor or academic) skills. Some of the neurological assumptions upon which this model is based (i.e., hierarchically organized nervous system) have received criticism as being outdated; recent theorists are reconceptualizing this theory (Bundy & Murray, 2002). The assumption that sensory experiences have an effect on learning is less controversial, although the mechanisms through which this occurs are somewhat ambiguous and often debated. Disruptions in subcortical (sensory integrative) functions are treated by providing controlled therapeutically designed sensory experiences for a child to respond to with adaptive motor actions. Through somatosensory and vestibular activities actively controlled/sought out by the child, the nervous system is thought to be able to better modulate, organize, and integrate information from the environment, which in turn provides a foundation for further adaptive responses and higher-order learning. Other necessary components of the classical SI model include a child-centered approach, providing a just-right challenge (scaffolding), facilitating progressively more sophisticated adaptive motor responses, and engaging the child in affectively meaningful and developmentally appropriate play interactions. The child's focus is intended to be placed on the occupation of play (intrinsically motivated) and not on cognitive-behavioral strategies or repetitive drills—as is the focus of other sensorimotor and behavioral approaches. Treatment goals may center on improving sensory processing to either (a) develop better sensory modulation as related to attention and behavioral control, or (b) integrate sensory information to form better perceptual schemas and practic abilities as a precursor for academic skills, social interactions, or more independent functioning.

Service Delivery Model and Approach. SI therapy is *classically* provided utilizing a direct one-on-one intervention model in a clinic environment that requires specialized equipment (e.g., suspended swings). Treatment plans are designed individually and carried out by a trained therapist (OT) approximately 1 to 3 times per week, 1-hour sessions. Duration typically entails several months and in some cases years. Consultative services, home/school programs, or task/environmental adaptations are often provided in tandem with the direct intervention. Cost varies depending on the location, frequency, and duration of the treatment, but it is comparable to hourly rates of other therapy services. Equipment is generally low-tech, but can be moderately expensive. The feasibility of doing classical SI in a school setting is low because of the need for specialized equipment and the "pull-out" model that may conflict with inclusionary principles.

Empirical Studies. Three studies investigated interventions that matched the criteria of classical SI therapy. Two utilized prospective AB designs with several subjects and adequate controls to look at SI treatment efficacy (Case-Smith & Bryan, 1999; Linderman & Steward, 1999); one utilized a retrospective design to identify predictors of positive outcomes within a group of children with autism receiving SI (Ayres & Tickle, 1980). Although outcome measures included aspects of proximate (sensory processing/modulation) functions and/or broader outcomes (e.g., play skills, social interactions), none of the studies directly attempted to remediate deficits in praxis.

Case-Smith & Bryan (1999) studied five boys across a 3-week baseline phase and a 10-week intervention that consisted of a combination of classical SI treatment and consultation with teachers. Independent coding of videotaped observations of free play indicated that three of the five boys demonstrated significant improvements in mastery play, and four of five demonstrated less "nonengaged" play. Only 1 subject had significant improvements with adult interactions, and none changed in level of peer interaction. Outcome measures more directly related to intrinsic features of the intervention (e.g., individual mastery play) appeared more improved than measures that were not directly addressed in treatment (e.g., peer interaction). Although it is possible that the positive results could be attributed to factors other than the intervention itself (i.e., maturation, caregiving effects), the authors note that the behaviors did not change systematically across all outcome measures. How-

ever, because sensory processing variables were not directly assessed, it is not known whether the positive outcomes are directly due to improvements in sensory processing mechanisms *per se*, as would be purported by sensory integration theory. It is also possible that the improvements evidenced are a function of other components of the intervention (e.g., play coaching, motivational strategies).

Linderman & Steward (1999) also utilized a single subjects AB design with two 3-year-olds with pervasive developmental disorder (mild autism) to track the functional behavioral changes in the home environment associated with classical SI (clinic-based 1 hour per week for 7 to 11 weeks). Subject 1 (who was noted to have tactile hypersensitivity) demonstrated gains in all intended outcomes (social interactions, approach to new activities, response to holding). Subject 2 (who had both hypo-responsiveness to vestibular and hyper-responsiveness to tactile sensations) made gains in activity level and social interaction, but not in functional communication. This study purports that SI may result in some functional gains that generalize to naturalistic contexts. However, given the limitations inherent in this single subject design, it is also possible that other co-occurring interventions (e.g., education), maturational effects, and parent participation in evaluation procedures may have also contributed to the positive outcomes, thus limiting definitive conclusions about the efficacy of the treatment.

The last study by Ayres and Tickle (1980) utilized a retrospective (within group) design to explore variables that predicted positive or negative outcomes following one year of SI therapy in 10 children (mean age 7.4 years) with autism. They found that subjects who tended to have average to hyper-responsive patterns to the various stimuli (e.g., touch, movement, gravity, and air puff) showed better outcomes than those with a hypo-responsive pattern. Numerous limitations (i.e., small sample size, variability of the outcome measures used, lack of control over maturational effects, retrospective nature of the study) make conclusive statements difficult; however, the study raises the possibility that differences in outcomes may be partially dependent on specific subject attributes including patterns of sensory processing.

Numerous efficacy studies of SI exist with other populations (e.g., children with MR or LD) (e.g., Arendt, Maclean, & Baumeister, 1988; Ayres, 1972; Clark et al., 1978; Hoehn & Baumeister, 1994; Humphries et al., 1990; 1992; 1993; Kanter, Kanter, &

Table 1.
Sensory and Motor Intervention Studies

Study	Treatment category[a]	n	Subjects	Int. val.[b]	Ext. val.[c]	Gen[d]	Design elements	Intervention specifications	Outcomes measured	Findings
Ayres & Tickle (1980)	SI-classical	10	Mild-severe autism; 3–13 yr	III	IV	III	Retrospective case-control of treatment responders versus nonresponders	2x week for one year	Language, awareness of environment, purposeful activities, self-stimulation, social and emotional behavior	Subjects with hyper-responsivity to tactile and vestibular stimuli had better outcomes than hypo-responsive subjects
Case-Smith & Bryan (1999)	SI-classical	5	Autism/MR; 4–5 yr	IV	II	I	Single-subject AB design; 3 wk baseline, 10 wk treatment	30 min treatment sessions plus teacher consultation	Mastery play, engaged behaviors, peer and adult interactions	General improvements in mastery play, engaged behaviors, and adult interactions. No significant changes in peer interactions
Linderman & Steward (1999)	SI-classical	2	Autism; 3–4 yr	IV	IV	I	Single-subject AB design; 2 wk baseline, 7 or 11 wk treatment	1 hr/wk in clinic	Functional behavior measures varied between subjects (e.g., social interactions, communication)	Increase in social interactions, response to movement and affection, and approach to new activities
Larrington (1987)	SI-based	1	Autism/severe MR; 15-yr-old boy	IV	IV	III	Descriptive case study	Varied sensory treatment (vest./prop/oral motor) treatment in school and group home; 2 yr	Variety of behaviors (e.g., SIB, play skills, social interactions)	Positive effects reported in many domains of behavior
Reilly *et al.* (1983)	SI-based	18	Autism 6–11 yr	III	I	III	Counter-balanced alternating treatments design; random assignment to activity order	2 sessions 30 min vestibular treatment versus 2 sessions 30 min fine motor treatment (alternating); provided within a 3 wk	Quantity and quality of vocalizations measured during treatment only. (No pre-post measures).	Fine motor activities elicited more variety of speech and mean length of vocalizations and decreased autistic speech than the vestibular treatment
Stagnitti, Raison, & Ryan (1999)	SI-based (Sensory Diet)	1	Sensory Defensiveness and Possible Autism spectrum; 5-yr-old boy	IV	IV	II	Descriptive case study	Brushing, joint compression 3–5x/day for 2 wk (other techniques were also used); repeated again at 5 mo post treatment	Anecdotal reports of tactile tolerance, affect, activity level, temper tantrums at home, school/community	Improvements in all areas following treatment; benefits faded by 5 months post-treatment; 6- and 9-mo assessments (following 2nd phase of treatment) showed sensory defensiveness cured
Edelson *et al.* (1999)	SS-touch pressure	12	Autism 4–13 yr	I	I	III	RCT with placebo; Pre- and post-treatment measures	Hug Machine (pressure) versus placebo (no pressure) 2x 20-min sessions per week; 6 wk total	Behavioral (tension, anxiety, hyperactivity) and physiological (galvanic skin response)	Decreased tension and anxiety for treatment group. Subjects with initially higher anxiety level had better outcomes

continued

Table 1.
Sensory and Motor Intervention Studies *(Continued)*

Study	Treatment category[a]	n	Subjects	Int. val.[b]	Ext. val.[c]	Gen[d]	Design elements	Intervention specifications	Outcomes measured	Findings
Field *et al.* (1997)	SS-touch therapy	22	Autism; mean age 4.5 yr	I	I	III	RCT with alternative treatment; Pre- and post-treatment measures	Touch therapy versus one-to-one quiet play (read) 2x 15-min sessions per week; 4 wk total	Touch aversions, off-task behaviors, orientation to sounds, stereotypic behavior, teacher report	Both groups showed positive changes; treatment group improved in response to sounds, stereotypic behavior, and social behaviors
McClure & Holtz-Yotz (1990)	SS-touch pressure	1	Autism/MR; 13 yr-old boy in psychiatric unit	IV	IV	III	Descriptive case report	Elastic (pressure) wrappings administered over 4 treatment sessions	Self-stimulatory behaviors, self-abuse, social interactions	Generally positive outcomes in all areas during treatment
Ray *et al.* (1988)	SS-vestibular	1	Autism; 9-yr-old male	IV	IV	II	Descriptive case report; Pre-, mid-, and post-treatment measurement	Self-initiated vestibular stimulation; 5-min sessions 2x week over 4 wk	Time spent vocalizing	Increased vocalizations during treatment; most prominent in first week
Zisserman (1991)	SS-touch pressure	1	Autism; 8-yr-old female	IV	IV	III	Descriptive case report	Pressure garments (vest and gloves) worn in classroom	Self-stimulatory behavior (e.g., hand slapping)	Decrease in self-stimulatory behaviors with gloves, slight (nonsignificant) decrease with vest
Bettison (1996)	AIT (Berard)	80	Autism or Asperger (sound hypersensitivity), ages 3-17 yr	I	I	III	RCT with alternative treatment; Pre- and post-measures at 1, 3, 6, 12 mo	Treatment group had AIT (filtered/modulated music); control group had structured listening treatment (unprocessed music), 2 x 30 min per day, 10 days	Aberrant behavior (ABC), sensory problems, sound sensitivity, IQ, language, audiometric tests.	Similar gains noted in both groups. 75% of subjects improved in 1st month. Much variability and attenuation of improvements over course of 12-mo follow-up. Two subjects had significant adverse effects
Brown (1999)	AIT (Berard)	2	Autism; 3.5 and 5 yr	IV	IV	III	Descriptive case reports	AIT 2 x 30 min per day, 10 days	Descriptions of sensory, motor, and functional behaviors	General improvements noted in a variety of domains (e.g., attention and speech)
Gilberg *et al.* (1997)	AIT (Berard)	9	Autism (all with MR; 3-16 yr	III	III	IV	Pre- and post-design (parents/raters aware of treatment)	AIT 30 min daily, 10 days	Pre and post-tests of autism symptoms on CARS and ABC	No significant differences on CARS and ABC; sensory problems declined slightly
Link (1997)	AIT (Berard)	3	Autism; ages 6, 7, and 15 yr; 2 nonverbal	IV	IV	III	Descriptive case reports (pre- and post-measures)	AIT 30 min daily, 10 days	Descriptions of hearing acuity, sound sensitivity, and behavior at home/ school reported by caregivers	One child improved; one child had mixed results; one child deteriorated following a seizure during AIT and was D/C on day 5

continued

Table 1.
Sensory and Motor Intervention Studies (Continued)

Study	Treatment category[a]	n	Subjects	Int. val.[b]	Ext. val.[c]	Gen[d]	Design elements	Intervention specifications	Outcomes measured	Findings
Mudford *et al.* (2000)	AIT (Berard)	16	Autism (low functioning); ages 5-14 yr (M = 9.4)	II	I	I	Balanced cross-over experimental design (parents blind to treatment conditions)	AIT versus placebo (disengaged headphones), 30 min 2x/day, 10 days; 3-5 mo baseline; treatment and control phases in random order for all subjects	Aberrant behavior (ABC, Nisonger; observational recordings), IQ, adaptive behavior (Vineland), language measure (Reynell)	Several drop-outs due to problems tolerating treatment; placebo slightly more beneficial (less aberrant behavior) than AIT for subjects that completed treatment
Neysmith-Roy (2001)	AIT (Tomatis)	6	Severe Autism; ages 4-11 yr	II	III	IV	Pre- and post-design with independent evaluation (repeated across subjects)	20 (30-min) sessions repeated for 4-8 blocks. Treatment phases followed by 3-8 weeks of no treatment/evaluation phases	CARS scores (from independent ratings of videotaped play observations and teacher/parent interviews)	Pre-treatment, all subjects were "severely autistic" on CARS. After treatment 3 (younger) children had reduced severity of autism; 3 older children had few changes
Rimland & Edelson (1994)	AIT (Berard)	445	Autism; primary or secondary dx; 4-41 yr (M = 10.7)	III	II	III	[Part 1: Compared 3 AIT devices using RCT.] Part 2: Retrospective case control (treatment group compared to no treatment, control group of 9 subject from a previous pilot study). Follow-up from 1 to 9 mo in 191 subjects.	AIT 2x 30 min per day for 10 days; one of three AIT device conditions (EERS, Audiokinetron, or Audio Tone Enhancer).	Audiograms, behavioral reactions to sound, parent reports of sound sensitivity, aberrant behavior, and behavior problems checklists	No significant differences among 3 AIT devices. Slightly improved sound sensitivity & acuity. Decreased audiogram variability associated with improved behavior. Age and degree of sound sensitivity not related to behavioral improvement.
Rimland & Edelson (1995)	AIT	18	Autism; 4-21 yr	I	I	III	RCT w/alt. treatment; Pre-, mid-, and post-treatment measures at 2 wk and at 1, 2, 3 mo post-treatment. (raters and parents blind to conditions)	AIT versus alternative treatment (unprocessed music) 2x 30 min per day for 10 days	Audiograms, parental reports of hypersensitivity to sound and aberrant behavior (stereotypy, hyperactivity, speech, etc)	Treatment group had decreased auditory problem behaviors and aberrant behaviors 3 months post-treatment. No significant changes in sound sensitivity; however, subjects were not necessarily hyper-sensitive pre-treatment

continued

Table 1.

Sensory and Motor Intervention Studies (Continued)

Study	Treatment category[a]	n	Subjects	Int. val.[b]	Ext. val.[c]	Gen[d]	Design elements	Intervention specifications	Outcomes measured	Findings
Zollweg, Palm, & Vance (1997)	AIT	30	Autism/MR; ages 7-24 yr; M = 14 yr, 5 mo (included 1 AUT <8 yr)	I	I	III	RCT w/alt. treatment; pre- and post-treatment at 1 wk, and at 1, 3, 6, and 9 mo post-treatment (double blind)	AIT vs. alt. treatment. (unprocessed music) 2x/ day for 10 days, 30 min/ session	Audiograms, sensitivity and loudness tolerance; aberrant behaviors (ABC)	No significant difference in audiological or behavioral outcomes between the groups; control group showed slightly less aberrant behavior at 6 mo post-treatment
Carmody et al. (2001)	Prisms	24	Autism; Ages 3-18 yr; (Median = 8)	III	II	III	Cross-over design (within subjects) with three conditions. [Independent ratings from video used to validate initial optometric readings.]	Three brief optometric assessment conditions for each subject; no lens (baseline) versus base-up or base-down lenses (randomly ordered treatment) for each subject	A single session assessment period with 60-90 sec trials for each task: Recorded spatial orienting behaviors (i.e., head and body posture, facial expression) while seated watching TV and ball catching performance while standing	Head posture, body posture, facial expression, and ball catching increased with correct (facilitating) prism lenses as compared to incorrect and habitual lenses
Kaplan et al. (1996)	Prisms	14	Autism; ages 5-14 yr; (Mean = 8 yr)	III	II	III	Cross-over design (within subjects) with three conditions. [Independent ratings by two authors made later from video to validate initial optometric ratings.]	Performance described under three assessment conditions: no lens (baseline) versus base-up or base-down lenses (randomly ordered treatment) for each subject	A single session assessment period with 60-90 sec trials for each task. Recorded ratings on visual-spatial orientation behaviors (i.e., head position, body posture, facial expression) during various lab tasks (i.e., watch TV seated and standing on balance board;	Overall posture and performance was better with correct prism lenses for group as a whole
Kaplan et al. (1998)	Prisms	18	Autism/PDD; ages 7-18 yr; (Mean = 11.5 yr) (39% with strabismus)	I	II	III	Double-blind cross-over design with placebo control	Subjects match/randomly assigned; 1/2 received placebo (clear lens); 1/2 got treatment (ambient prism lens) conditions for 3-4 mo; then conditions were reversed	Measured behavior problems (Aberrant Behavior Checklist); visual-spatial orientation and attention pre-, mid-, and post-treatment for both treatment and control conditions.	Improved behavior in treatment condition (short term). No significant differences between tx and control conditions for postural orientation and attention. No significant differences between children with and without strabismus; trend for more behavior problems with placebo lenses.

continued

Table 1.
Sensory and Motor Intervention Studies (Continued)

Study	Treatment category[a]	n	Subjects	Int. val.[b]	Ext. val.[c]	Gen[d]	Design elements	Intervention specifications	Outcomes measured	Findings
Neman et al. (1974)	Patterning	66	Institutionalized subjects with MR; (M = 15 yr)	I	I	III	RCT with alt treatment (physical activities with sensory stimulation and attention) and no-treatment control group	Doman-Delcato method patterning treatment 2 hr/day 5x per week for 2.5 mo, then 7x per wk for 4 mo	Cognitive performance, developmental tests for vocabulary, visual-perceptual, and motor skills	No dramatic changes in individuals; no significant changes in IQ or motor skills. Significant increases for treatment group in two categories most related to treatment skills taught; visual competence and mobility. No treatment control fared worst on most measures
Bridgman et al. (1985)	Patterning	12	Various DD—CP, MR, autism/seizure (M = 8 yr)	III	II	III	Prospective cohort design (nonrandom group assignments); pre, mid-(3 and 6 mo) and post-treatment measurements (at 10 mo)	Doman-Delcato method patterning 8 hr per day; control group received Special Education services; 10 mo	Developmental profile, IQ with Bayley mental scale or Stanford-Binet (measurements not uniformly applied)	Treatment group slightly better in language and socialization at 3 mo but findings were short-lived and no significant differences found at 10 mo.
Kern et al. (1982)	Exercise	7	Autism 4-14 yr	II	II	III	Repeated reversal design (ABAB); 45 reversals; Multiple pre- and post-treatment measures	5-20 min structured individual jogging sessions; variable settings (e.g., clinic and home) and variable duration of treatment 4-17 days	Percent of self-stimulation as well as number of correct responses on academic (matching task) and ball playing (catching task).	Consistent decrease in self-stimulatory behaviors and improvements in academic and play responses following treatment
Kern et al. (1984)	Exercise	3	Autism 7-11 yr	II	II	IV	Counter-balanced, alternating treatments design. Baseline and multiple post-treatment measures	15 min vigorous activity (jogging) followed by 15 min mild activity (ball playing) and return to 1st condition; condition order reversed on second day	Time sampling of stereotyped behaviors	Reduction in self-stimulatory behaviors after vigorous jogging exercise.

continued

Table 1.
Sensory and Motor Intervention Studies (Continued)

Study	Treatment category[a]	n	Subjects	Int. val.[b]	Ext. val.[c]	Gen[d]	Design elements	Intervention specifications	Outcomes measured	Findings
Levinson & Reid (1993)	Exercise	3	Autism (low functioning) 11 yr	II	II	IV	Counterbalanced, alternating treatments design; multiple pre-, during, post-treatment measurements	15 min group walking (mild exercise) for 5 sessions versus 15 min individual jogging (vigorous exercise) x 4 sessions across 9 wk	Heart rates, individualized measures of self-stimulatory behaviors	Reduction in self-stimulatory behaviors after vigorous exercise treatment. Effects wear off after 90 min
Watters & Watters (1980)	Exercise	5	Autism; ages 9-11 yr	II	II	IV	Alternating treatments design with three pre-task conditions in randomized order. Pre- and post-treatment measures	Compared three conditions; 8-10 min jogging versus 15 min TV viewing versus varied academic tasks; given 1 session per day, 1-4 X per week (total weeks varied)	Rates of self-stimulatory behaviors and academic performance during a language training session post treatment	Decrease in self-stimulatory behaviors following exercise condition

KEY:

[a]*Treatment Category Codes*
- SI, Sensory Integration Therapy (classical)
- SI-based, Sensory-Integration Based Approach
- SS, Sensory Stimulation Technique
- Patterning, Sensorimotor Patterning
- AIT, Auditory Integration Training
- Prism, Ambient Prism Lenses (Visual Therapy)
- Exercise, Exercise Therapy

[b]*Internal Validity Classification Criteria:*
- I: Prospective study comparing treatment to alternative or placebo (e.g., RCT) where evaluators are blind to treatment status.
- II: Multiple baseline, ABAB, reversal/withdrawal with measurement of outcome blind to treatment conditions, or prepost design with indep. evaluation.
- III: Prepost or historical designs or multiple baseline, ABAB, reversal/withdrawal (not "blind").
- IV: Other (e.g., single subject [AB or ABA] designs without multiple baselines; case study reports).

[c]*External Validity Classification Criteria:*
- I: Random assignment of well-defined cohorts and adequate sample size for comparisons.
- II: Nonrandom assignment, but well-defined cohorts with inclusion/exclusion criteria and documentation of attrition/failures. In addition, adequate sample size for group designs or replication across three or more single subjects.
- III: Well-defined population of three or more subjects in single-subject designs or sample of adequate size in group designs.
- IV: Other.

[d]*Generalization Classification Criteria:*
- I: Documented changes (i.e., generalization) in at least one natural setting outside of treatment setting.
- II: Generalization to one other setting or maintenance beyond experimental intervention in natural setting in which intervention took place.
- III: Intervention occurred in natural setting or use of outcome measures with documented relationship to functional outcome.
- IV: Not addressed or other.

Clark, 1982; Polatajko *et al.*, 1991; 1992; Wilson *et al.*, 1992). Although these are excluded from this review, it is noteworthy that these studies have sparked much controversy, given the lack of consistent empirical support. Some difficult issues surround the nature of the intervention and whether or not these studies were truly representative of SI therapy versus some other variation of sensorimotor or perceptual-motor treatments. Several meta-analyses (Ottenbacher, 1982; Vargas & Camilli, 1999) are also available; these report that effect sizes vary from low to moderately high depending on the populations studied, recency of the studies, and specific parameters measured. Outcomes in psychoeducational and motor categories are stronger than in other areas, at least for SI studies compared to no treatment conditions; however, effects appeared to be equivocal when compared with alternative treatments.

Other Sensory Integration-Based Approaches

Description and Assumptions. This section groups several types of approaches that are based on the foundations of SI theory, but deviate from classical SI in one or more criteria: (a) somatosensory and vestibular activities are provided but suspended equipment is not used; (b) treatment is more adult-structured or passively applied (i.e., not conducive to child-directed play), and/or (c) treatment is more cognitively focused than found in classical SI. For example, structured perceptual-motor training approaches may fall into this category. Although these were popular 10 to 30 years ago, they are less often used today with children with autism.

One example of a popular modernized version of an SI-based program is the "Sensory Diet" (or sometimes referred to as a sensory summation approach), in which the child is provided with a home or classroom program of sensory-based activities aimed at fulfilling the child's sensory needs. A schedule of frequent and systematically applied somatosensory stimulation (i.e., brushing with a surgical brush and joint compressions) is followed by a prescribed set of activities designed to meet the child's sensory needs are integrated into the child's daily routine. Another example that melds together aspects of sensory integration theory with a cognitive-behavioral approach is the "Alert Program," in which a child (usually with a higher functioning level and verbal abilities) is given additional cognitive strategies to assist with his/her arousal modulation.

Service Delivery Model and Approach. These models often utilize a direct intervention (one-on-one or group). Consultative/collaborative models are common; caregivers under the supervision of a therapist may carry out school programs. Treatments generally require less equipment than classical SI and can often be provided in an inclusive setting. Cost is comparable to SI, depending on the length and duration of intervention.

Empirical Studies. No studies of specific perceptual-motor treatments for autism were found. Two studies (Larrington, 1987; Reilly, Nelson, & Bundy, 1983) using structured sensorimotor interventions based on SI principles were found. Despite documenting numerous positive outcomes, the descriptive case study by Larrington (1987) provides limited internal validity as a result of multiple methodological weaknesses, probable maturation effects, and a focus on an older age-group (teenager) that has limited generalizability to young children. The more rigorous study by Reilly *et al.*, (1983) utilized a counter-balanced alternating treatments design with 18 children diagnosed with autism (ages 6 to 11 years) to measure the comparative effects of two interventions on production of vocalizations. The authors expected that structured vestibular-based activities would facilitate higher amounts of language in their subjects during the intervention than the table-top fine motor activities. Order of the two treatment conditions was randomly assigned, and each subject received two 30-minute sessions of each type. No significant differences were found with respect to function of speech, articulation, total language, or rate of vocalizations during the intervention sessions. In contrast to the hypotheses, significant differences in favor of the fine motor group were found for variety of speech, length of vocalizations, and amount of autistic speech. Limitations of these findings included: (a) the children's vocalizations had been previously reinforced by teachers during fine motor activities in the classroom—which may have proved in favor of the alternative therapy; (b) a short duration of the intervention period may not have been sufficient to provide an adequate sampling of behaviors, and (c) outcome measures outside of the treatment sessions were not provided, thus it is not known if the vocalizations generalized to other contexts.

Although the Sensory Diet interventions are commonly used, only one study of a child suspected of having an autistic spectrum disorder was found (Stagnitti, Raison, & Ryan, 1999). This case report described a 5-year-old boy with severe sensory defensiveness who underwent a treatment program consisting of brushing (i.e., sensory summation) followed by joint compressions an average of 3 to 5 times daily for 2 weeks. The program included integration of appropriate sensory activities interspersed throughout the child's daily activities and routines (i.e., sensory diet) and was carried out by the parents at home under the supervision of a therapist trained in these methods. Following initial improvements, the treatment program was repeated several months later when the child's behaviors seemed to again deteriorate. Post-treatment parental reports suggested improvements in tolerance of tactile stimulation, fewer temper tantrums, an increase in activity level, and better coordination. The authors concluded that the child was cured of his sensory defensiveness, and autistic symptoms appeared to resolve. These anecdotal claims appear unfounded given that no systematic data were collected and that adequate methodological controls were not instituted (e.g., a variety of competing treatments were implemented during the 9-month period).

No empirical studies on the Alert Program were found for children with autism or related populations. It may be that some of these programs have been too recently developed to have been subjected to empirical tests; more likely they are utilized by clinicians who report outcomes via individualized education plans (IEPs) and not through the peer-reviewed research literature.

Sensory Stimulation Techniques

Description and Assumptions. These approaches are varied and usually involve passively providing one type of sensory stimulation through a circumscribed modality (e.g., touch pressure, vestibular stimulation) with a prescribed regimen. Sometimes these techniques are incorporated within the broader sensory-integration–based programs described above; other times they are used in isolation. The assumptions vary with the treatment, but most are based on neurophysiological principles stipulating that a given sensory experience may provide facilitatory or inhibitory influences on the nervous system that result in behavioral changes such as arousal modulation. An example of a commonly used technique is "deep pressure" (i.e., firm touch pressure providing calming input), which can be applied via therapeutic touch (e.g., massage; joint compression), or an apparatus (e.g., Hug Machine, pressure garments, weighted vests). Vestibular stimulation, another example, is often used to modulate arousal, facilitate postural tone, or increase vocalizations. Auditory integration training and visual therapies will be discussed in separate sections.

Service Delivery Model and Approach. The service delivery models vary, depending on the intervention provided. Both direct and consultative approaches are used, although the direct intervention approach is more often described in research. Cost varies depending on the equipment used (e.g., minimal cost of brushes vs. moderate to significant costs of Hug Machine) and staff time allocated.

Empirical Studies. Five studies specific to children with autism were found in this category. Three of the studies utilized case study descriptions (McClure & Holtz-Yotz, 1990; Ray, King, & Grandin, 1988; Zisserman, 1991), and two provided more rigorous and controlled methodologies with randomization of subjects to two alternative treatment conditions (Edelson, Goldberg, Edelson, Kerr, & Grandin, 1999; Field *et al.*, 1997). One study reviewed the effects of vestibular stimulation (Ray *et al.*, 1988), and four studies investigated the effects of somatosensory stimulation on a variety of behaviors. All of these studies report effects of some type of touch pressure/deep pressure.

Although several limitations (e.g., a tendency to use numerous measures with small sample sizes) exist in the majority of these studies, they yield some useful information that may guide educational planning. The two prospective controlled studies provide preliminary evidence that touch pressure may have a calming effect on children with autism (Edelson *et al.*, 1999; Field *et al.*, 1997). Field *et al.* (1997) measured the effects of touch therapy (massage) on attentiveness and responsivity in 22 preschool children with autism. Massage was provided for 15 minutes per day, 2 days per week for 4 weeks (i.e., eight sessions). Results indicated that both groups showed positive changes with respect to all the observational variables (i.e., touch aversion, off-task behavior, orienting to sounds; stereotypies) post-treatment; the touch therapy group demonstrated significantly greater changes in responsiveness to sound and stereotypies and significant improvements on measures of social communication. Although hypothetically links were made to changes in autonomic (vagal) activity, these claims are unsubstantiated, because no physiological measures were taken.

Edelson *et al.*, (1999) investigated the efficacy of the Hug Machine—a touch pressure device designed by Temple Grandin

to decrease arousal and anxiety by self-administration of lateral body pressure—in 12 children with autism that had varying levels of anxiety. The treatment group (Hug Machine twice for 20 minutes per week for 6 weeks) showed a significant reduction on a tension scale and a marginally significant change on anxiety. Physiological measures (galvanic skin responses) were not significantly different between groups overall; however, variability in the experimental group increased over the course of treatment. The authors concluded that children in the treatment group with higher initial levels of arousal/anxiety were more likely to benefit from the intervention. Although the small sample size and marginally significant findings limit the conclusions in this study, there is some convergence of findings with the Ayres and Tickle (1980) study that children with hyper-responsive patterns may benefit more from these types of sensory-based interventions than those who are under-responsive.

Both McClure and Holtz-Yotz (1990) and Zisserman (1991) provide interesting but methodologically weak case reports using variations of touch pressure garments to diminish self-stimulatory behaviors. Neither study provided a functional analysis of the self-stimulatory behaviors prior to the interventions, but both assumed the function of the behaviors was sensation seeking and/or arousal modulation based and hypothesized that providing a sensory substitute would yield calming effects and decreased stereotypy. Zisserman (1991) described clinical improvements using pressure gloves (overall 46% decrease) but not for pressure vest (11.8% decrease). Additionally, no carry-over effects could be demonstrated once the gloves were removed. Similarly, McClure & Holtz-Yotz (1990) using elastic wraps to effect behavioral changes (i.e., social interactions, self-stimulation) reported some positive effects in an institutionalized 13-year-old boy with autism/mental retardation; however, investigator biases, cointerventions (medication, physical agent modalities), and poor reliability/validity for the measures used significantly limited conclusive statements. The final case study by Ray *et al.* (1988) describes the effects of vestibular stimulation on speech sounds in a 9-year-old low-functioning boy with autism and dyspraxia. Self-controlled vestibular stimulation (i.e., spinning in circles 5 minutes for 17 days across a 4-week period). Speech sounds were greater in the treatment (17% time) than the pre- (2% time) or post-intervention (1.3% time) phases. Because no measures of vestibular process-

ing were directly collected, it is unclear whether the increased speech production was directly linked to vestibular processing changes. The child was simultaneously receiving other SI treatments in school, which may have confounded results.

Auditory Integration Training (AIT) and Related Acoustic Interventions

Description and Assumptions. AIT is based on the concept that electronically modulated/filtered music provided through earphones may be helpful in remediating hypersensitivities and overall auditory processing ability that is thought to be problematic in children with autism. Although exact neurological mechanisms underlying AIT and other listening therapies are not known, various hypotheses have been proposed (e.g., improved functioning of the reticular activating system, reorganization of the cerebellar-vestibular system, modification of brain serotonin levels). AIT is said to "massage" the middle ear (hair cells in the cochlea) and enhance auditory perception. Methods and equipment vary depending on the specific philosophical approach (i.e., Tomatis or Berard); the most commonly used approach for children with autism in the United States is the Berard method, developed by the French otolaryngologist during the 1960s–1990s. In the Berard method, a modulating and filtering device (e.g., Ears Education & Retraining System [EERS], Audiokinetron or Audio Tone Enhancer [ATE]) accepts music input from CDs and transforms sounds by (a) randomly modulating high and low frequencies and (b) filtering out selected frequencies in accordance with the child's performance on an audiogram (test of auditory thresholds to a series of frequencies that measures hearing ability). Sound frequencies that are 5 to 10 dB different from their adjacent frequencies (i.e., "peaks") are filtered out for the listening sessions. Volume level for the left ear is sometimes reduced in order to stimulate language development in the left hemisphere. Although improved sound modulation is one goal of treatment, other goals include enhancement of generalized behaviors (attention, arousal, language, social skills, etc.).

The Tomatis method is similar, but integrates a psychodynamic with a psychophysiological perspective. In the passive phase, the individual listens to filtered sounds of the maternal voice, as well as prepared music through a modulating apparatus (i.e., Electronic Ear that attenuates low frequencies and amplifies higher frequencies). The earphones have an attached bone conductor to facilitate sounds through vibration and air conduction methods. Later, in the active phase, the subject is introduced to language and audio vocal exercises that provide feedback of his/her own voice through headphones to reinforce more normal auditory perception and overall quality of life.

Variations of listening programs applied to children with autism include Stephen Porges' Acoustic Intervention. This treatment is based on Porges' (1998) Polyvagal Theory—a phylogenetic theory of autonomic nervous system control that is the substrate for emotional and affective experiences. By providing filtered sounds of the human voice (as opposed to any filtered music), the listening stimulation is designed to alternatively challenge and relax the middle ear muscles to enhance speech perception.

Service Delivery Model and Approach.
The Berard AIT treatments are usually provided individually in a small sound-quiet room for 30 minutes 2 times per day for 10 to 20 days (i.e., minimum of 10 hours) by a professional trained in the techniques. Fees can range from $1000 to $3000 for the 2-week treatment. The equipment itself is highly technical and expensive. The Tomatis method is performed in similar ways but often with repeated blocks of intervention with longer overall durations, sometimes spanning years of treatment. The Porges acoustic intervention uses five sessions at 45 minutes each. Occasionally, such auditory treatments are provided within a school setting if the trainer brings the equipment to the school.

Empirical Studies.
Nine studies were found using various methods of AIT with children with autism. Eight of these studies were utilized the Berard AIT method (Bettison, 1996; Brown, 1999; Gillberg, Johansson, Steffenburg, & Berlin, 1997; Link, 1997; Mudford, et al., 2000; Rimland & Edelson, 1994; 1995; Zollweg, Palm, & Vance, 1997). The Tomatis AIT approach was used in one study (Neysmith-Roy, 2001) for the population of interest. An additional study of the Tomatis AIT method demonstrating no positive benefits for children with significant learning disabilities is also published (Kershner et al., 1990) but is not included in this review. Although Porges' acoustic intervention is currently undergoing some scientific experiments with children with autism, no published studies in peer-reviewed journals were found.

Of the nine AIT studies reviewed in total, three used randomized, controlled methods with either no treatment or an alternate treatment/placebo, (Bettison, 1996; Rimland & Edelson, 1995; Zollweg et al., 1997), two utilized other methodological designs with various levels of control (Neysmith-Roy, 2001; Mudford, et al., 2000), one was a pre-post open trial (Gillberg et al., 1997), two were descriptive case reports (Brown, 1999; Link, 1997), and one compared various types of AIT devices (Rimland & Edelson, 1994). These are summarized below.

Bettison (1996) utilized a randomized controlled trials design with AIT as the treatment condition and an alternative structured listening task for the control condition for 80 children with autism (ages 3 to 17 years) with concomitant sound sensitivities. At 1 month post-treatment, both groups demonstrated significant but equal amounts of improvement for all measures showing nonspecific treatment effects. Significant improvements were maintained for the audiogram scores only; patterns of change across other behavioral measures (behavior checklist; development, sensory checklist, and sound sensitivity questionnaire) was so variable that it is difficult to interpret clinically, even though some of the changes were positive. By 12 months, most of the improvements seen reverted to initial post-treatment levels taken at 1 month. It is not clear what aspect of the interventions was responsible for the outcomes—maturation, practice effects, or other aspects of the treatment may have also influenced the results. Moreover, this study documents negative side effects for two subjects who had documented psychiatric problems.

Rimland & Edelson (1995) present some positive effects with 18 subjects (4 to 21 yrs of age) in a randomized controlled trial using AIT (EERS) versus unfiltered music. Results indicated that the treatment group demonstrated fewer auditory problem behaviors and aberrant behaviors than the control; these improvements were maintained across 3 months. However, neither the pure tone discomfort test nor the hearing sensitivity questionnaire provided evidence of reduction in sound sensitivity post-treatment. Treatment and control groups did not significantly differ in their hearing acuity at any of the six points tested. Positive results were not limited to those with hypersensitive hearing. In a large scale study, these same authors (Rimland & Edelson, 1994) investigated the differential effectiveness of three types of auditory filtering devices for 445 subjects with primary or secondary diagnoses of autism (CA = 4 to 41 years; M = 10.73 years). Because no differences were found across the three devices, data were collapsed across treatment condi-

tions. Results indicated a significant but small improvement in hearing sensitivity, as well as decreased variability in audiograms for some subjects, mostly during the first 3 months. Lower-functioning individuals seemed to make greater gains. However, there was no significant relationship between level of sensitivity pre-AIT and the behavioral outcomes post-treatment.

Zollweg, Palm, & Vance (1997) used a well-controlled, double-blind design with an alternative treatment to study the effects of AIT on 30 low-functioning, multihandicapped, institutionalized residents. Nine of the 30 residents had autism; only 1 of the 9 with autism was a child under the age of 8 years. Participants were assigned randomly to treatment (filtered/modulated music) or control (unfiltered/unmodulated music) groups and provided with twenty 30-minute sessions by trained practitioners who were blind to the treatment conditions. Participants were allowed to engage in other activities (e.g., eating, toy play, magazine browsing) simultaneously with treatment to facilitate cooperation. Subjects were assessed for hearing sensitivity and tolerance for loud sounds pre- and post-treatment (1- 3-, 6-, and 9-month time periods) by a licensed audiologist, also blind to treatment conditions. Results of audiological assessments demonstrated that there was a small magnitude change of 200 Hz on pure tone thresholds between the two groups at only one of seven frequencies tested. This finding was likely spurious given the number of comparisons and was not deemed clinically significant by the authors. No significant group differences were found with respect to loudness discomfort levels at any frequency for any of the follow-up time points; in fact, only one subject demonstrated an increased tolerance between the pre-AIT and the 9 month, post-AIT condition. Behavioral data indicated that both groups were reported to improve over time; slight differences favored the control group at 6 months post-treatment for overall scores on the Aberrant Behavior Checklist (ABC), but groups had similar levels of improvement on this measure at 9-months after treatment. No significant differences between groups were noted for any of the subscales of the ABC at any of the post-treatment time points. Although both groups were reported to improve over time, notable fluctuations across the subscales of aberrant behavior on post-treatment assessment phases were not easily interpretable. These findings are similar to those of Bettison (1996) suggesting that factors other than AIT (e.g., extra attention; caregiver expectations, etc.) could be responsible for reductions in aberrant behaviors.

Mudford *et al.* (2000) used a balanced cross-over design to assess the effects of AIT (twenty 30-minute sessions) with 16 children with autism ages 5 to 14 years. Four were girls; all of the subjects were low-functioning. Parents and AIT practitioners were blind to the treatment conditions that included either AIT (modulated music) without the filtering component, or the placebo control (headphones disengaged, music playing in background of room). Baseline and follow-up assessments were used for each condition, including standardized measures of aberrant behavior, cognitive functioning, adaptive levels, language levels, and observational data. Notably, several children dropped out of the study as a result of inability to tolerate the procedures and/or severe behavioral difficulties. Of the 16 children completing the study, there were no positive findings in favor of the AIT condition, despite a liberal alpha level used in the statistical tests. In fact, small but significant differences on measures of aberrant behavior favored the control condition for this low-functioning group.

Neysmith-Roy (2001) describes outcomes of the Tomatis AIT method with six children with severe autism ranging from 4 to 11 years. Several blocks of "Intensives" (i.e., twenty 30-minute sessions repeated from four to eight times) were each followed by a 3- to 8-week unsystematic evaluation period spanning 6 to 21 months, depending on the individual child's program. Pre- and post-measures of autistic symptoms on the Childhood Autism Rating Scale (CARS) were recorded on videotapes of two separate play conditions and parent/teacher reports during both the intervention and evaluation phases. Videos were randomized and coded by two raters who were blind to the conditions of the study for each subject. Reductions in autistic symptoms overall including an improvement in prelinguistic behaviors were noted in three of the six boys (50%), who also happened to be among the youngest subjects, but no improvements were seen in the other three (older) boys. Audiological/physiological measures were not employed because the boys were unable to cooperate for the testing.

A case report by Brown (1999) on two preschool-age siblings with autism describes improvements in sensory-motor functions, attention, social interest, praxis, eye control, and speech for two children who underwent AIT for two 30-minute sessions for 10 days. Similarly, Link (1997) presented a case report for three children with autism, documenting mixed findings. Sound sensitivity (using unvalidated measures) was noted to be unchanged for two of the three children and inconclusive for the third. Informal behavioral observations were found to be improved for one child (across parent and teacher ratings) and mixed a second child. One child unfortunately suffered a psychomotor seizure during the AIT procedure and was removed from the protocol on day 5. Parent and teacher reports on day 5 indicated deterioration in behaviors possibly related to the seizure. Both studies were weak methodologically such that no systematic data was collected and pre- and post-measures lacked independence, as well as validity and reliability data; thus findings are speculative.

In summary, the nine available studies using various methods of AIT with children with autism demonstrate mixed results. Studies with sample selection biases and unmasked evaluation processes would tend to favor outcomes for the treatment groups; however, this was not always the case. Some studies, using various types of methodologies, reported improvements in either behavior or audiological measures (e.g., Brown, 1999; Link, 1997; Neysmith-Roy, 2001; Rimland, 1994; 1995) at some points in time for some children. However, it is important to note that if changes are seen in behaviors without concomitant changes in hearing sensitivity, an alternative mechanism than that proposed by AIT theory may be responsible for the improvements. Furthermore, significant fluctuations of behavior over time, and inconsistency of performance across measures seen in several studies (e.g., Bettison, 1996; Zollweg et al., 1997) are difficult to interpret. Adverse effects (i.e., seizures, behavioral problems) and drop-out rates require special attention given that these are reported in several AIT studies.

Methodologically stronger studies (Bettison; 1996; Mudford et al., 2000; Zollweg et al., 1997) demonstrated that improvements in behavior often were not significantly different between treatment (AIT) and control (unfiltered/unmodulated music) conditions (Bettison, 1996; Zollweg et al., 1997). In two studies (Mudford et al., 2000; Zollweg et al., 1997) the control group showed a subtle advantage in reduction of aberrant behaviors at at least one point in time. Similar improvements for subjects in both treatment and control conditions suggest that effects are due to factors that are peripheral to the treatment (e.g., extra attention; caregiver expectations; compliance training)

and/or other co-occurring treatments (i.e., behavioral and educational interventions) may be influencing outcomes. Future replication studies need to better control for such effects. Although the hypothesis that music in general (filtered or unfiltered) may have a beneficial effect on behavior is plausible, it is yet to be tested empirically. Gravel (1994) provided a detailed critique of AIT studies, stressing the importance of distinguishing between statistical and clinical significance. She states that small differences between frequencies (i.e., 5 dB) or fluctuations in hearing sensitivity in some children with autism may be attributable to attentional/behavioral difficulties that preclude reliable responses on behavioral audiometry. Furthermore, electrophysiological measures (ABRs) fail to demonstrate differences in hearing sensitivity between children with autism and controls—a finding that may challenge the overall premise of AIT.

Visual Therapies

Description and Assumptions. A variety of visual therapies including but not limited to oculomotor exercises, ambient prism lenses, and colored filters (i.e., Irlen lenses) have been applied to children with autism. These visual or behavioral optometric therapies and are aimed at improving visual processing or visual-spatial perception that may be related to autistic symptomatology (e.g., unusual visual stereotypies, coordination problems, strabismus, attention, etc.). In particular, the ambient (i.e., visual-spatial system) as opposed to the focal (i.e., visual acuity system) is hypothesized to be dysfunctional in children with autism. Thus prism lenses transform the light through an angular displacement of 1 to 5 degrees (base up or base down), producing a shift in the field of vision. These are thought to lead to more stable perception and improved behavior or performance.

Service Delivery Model and Approach. Visual therapies and corrective lenses are prescribed individually through a licensed optometrist. In some cases, programs are carried out by parents or other professionals. Various visual treatments may also be combined, as in the case of ambient lenses and oculomotor exercises. Costs may be moderate and include the optometrist's fees for the initial and follow-up evaluations and cost of prescriptive eyewear.

Empirical Studies. Anecdotal data are plentiful; however, empirical studies regarding the efficacy of visual therapies specific to children with autism are limited. No published studies were found on the use of Irlen lenses or independent use of oculomotor therapies for children with autism. Three studies (all by the same group of researchers) investigating prism lenses were found (Carmody, Kaplan, & Gaydos, 2001; Kaplan, Carmody, & Gaydos, 1996; Kaplan, Edelson, & Seip, 1998).

The study by Kaplan et al. (1998) used the most rigorous methodological design (double-blind crossover). It was an extension of the earlier pilot investigation (Kaplan et al., 1996) and used 18 children with autism (CA = 7 to 18 years; M = 11.53 yrs). Thirty-nine percent had strabismus. All subjects were prescribed prism lenses with modification determined individually for the visual direction (base up or base down) and angular displacement. Five subjects were lost as a result of non-compliance with the eyewear. The remaining 18 were matched and randomly assigned to one of the two conditions (placebo lenses or treatment with prism lenses) for 3 months; then treatment conditions were switched for the second phase (4 months). Pre-, mid-, and post-treatment measures were taken for postural orientation, attention, and visual-spatial performance tasks, as well as ratings of behavioral problems. Results indicated short-term positive effects—behavioral findings were most apparent at the mid-evaluation (1½ or 2 months), with less improvement at follow-up (3 or 4 months). Performance on orientation and visual-spatial tasks was not significantly different between conditions. Given these findings, it is unclear what specific mechanisms were responsible for the behavioral improvements because the visual performance measures were unchanged, at least in the context of the laboratory tasks. Children were not engaged in simultaneous visual training tasks that are usually prescribed in conjunction with prism lenses, which may have limited long-term effects. Treatment effects did not appear related to whether or not the children had a prediagnosed strabismus; however, a slight trend toward more behavioral problems during the clear lens (placebo) condition for the strabismus subgroup was reported.

Unfortunately, the above results were less encouraging than those from the original pilot study (Kaplan et al., 1996) and a more recent study (Carmody et al. 2001), both of which demonstrated significantly better performance on orientation and visual-spatial performance when children with autism were wearing correct ("facilitating") prism lenses. Carmody et al. (2001) assessed responses to prism lenses for a convenience sample of 24 children (2 girls, 22 boys) with autism, ages 3 to 18 years, in Hong Kong. Optometric evaluations revealed that 18 children had normal visual acuity, 3 were far-sighted, and 3 were near-sighted. All children were assessed on measures of spatial orientation/spatial management abilities with two functional tasks (i.e., television viewing and ball catching) during each of three visual assessment conditions: (1) habitual viewing (no lenses), (2) eyeglasses with prisms using base-up condition, or (3) eyeglasses with prisms using base-down conditions. Both prism conditions used a mild displacement of the visual scene (5.6 degrees); however, one condition was judged to be the child's favored or correct condition (facilitating lenses) and one was judged to be an incorrect condition (interfering lenses) based on observational measures during the trials by the initial rater. Assessments were videotaped. The full performance assessments were then reviewed by an independent rater, and results were analyzed statistically to validate whether or not the facilitating condition was superior. Results validated the initial rater's assessment that head position, body posture, facial expressions, and ball catching skills significantly improved in the "facilitating lens" condition as opposed to the habitual or interfering lens conditions.

Differences in the ages of the samples and the relative strength of the methodological designs across the three studies could have contributed to the inconsistent findings. The Kaplan et al. (1996) and the Carmody et al. (2001) studies used considerably weaker designs with relatively short trial periods across the three assessment conditions (i.e., no lenses, incorrect prism lenses or correct prism lenses). Replication studies by independent investigators, using well-controlled designs and longer-term follow-up are needed. Likewise, outcome measures used in naturalistic contexts are needed to demonstrate generalizability of these findings.

Sensorimotor Handling Techniques

Description and Assumptions. Several types of sensorimotor handling techniques (e.g., reflex integration, neurodevelopmental therapies, patterning, etc.) have been applied to children with developmental disabilities. Neurodevelopmental therapy (NDT) is a specific sensorimotor (physiotherapy) treatment that originated with the Bobaths in England in the·1950s–1960s. Its focus is on normalization of muscle tone, integration of primitive reflexes, and facilitation of more normal movement patterns through specific handling techniques.

Sensorimotor patterning is a remedial technique that uses a series of very structured, passively manipulated exercises to the limbs to reprogram the central nervous system. Originally designed by Doman and Delcato in the 1950s–1960s, this treatment is based on an older and simplistic recapitulation theory. Developmental gross motor patterns that may have been "missed" (e.g., creeping or crawling) are patterned passively for neurological reorganization. Although it is not used extensively for children with autism, there has been a recent resurgence of interest, particularly as a last-resort therapy. Although craniosacral (C-S) therapy (Upledger, 1996) is not a sensorimotor treatment *per se*, it's similarities to other handling techniques combined with recent anecdotal data of its increased use with children with autism warranted inclusion in this paper. This osteopathic treatment involves physical manipulation (e.g, repeated treatments using gentle and noninvasive traction and decompressions) to alleviate restrictions in the craniosacral system.

Service Delivery Model and Approach. These interventions are administered individually by persons trained in the procedures through attendance in specialized workshops. Contact with the child must be direct physical contact. Interventions may be short or long term for NDT or C-S. Home programs for patterning therapies are eventually carried out by families and tend to be particularly long in duration (8 hours per day for several months or years). Cost of treatments is dependent on frequency and duration (therapists' fees).

Empirical Studies. No empirical studies specific to autism or related disorders (e.g., mental retardation) were found for NDT. From a clinical perspective, it appears that this treatment is rarely applied in any systematic way for use with children with autism unless other accompanying and significant neuromotor problems are present (e.g., cerebral palsy). No empirical studies were found in peer-reviewed journals for C-S. No empirical studies of sensorimotor patterning were found specific to autism. However, two older empirical studies with children with mental retardation were found (Bridgman, Cushen, Cooper, & Williams, 1985; Neman et al., 1974). Both studies provide similar findings and limitations. In the more rigorous study (Neman et al., 1974), the patterning group out-performed the other groups in visual competence and mobility. On other measures, the patterning group out-performed the passive control but not the alternative intervention group; no measurable differences were found in

IQ, and no case made dramatic improvement on any measure. Results from methodologically weaker study (Bridgman *et al.*, 1985) indicated that the treatment group slightly out-performed the control group on language and socialization, whereas the control group fared better in self-help skills. Given that in both studies improvements were more pronounced in the earlier assessments, it appears that findings may reflect early enthusiasm of participants. High drop-out rates are particularly noted with this treatment method.

Physical Exercise

Description and Assumptions. Although physical exercise is included in many regular education curricula, it is not systematically or consistently utilized with children with autism. Health benefits of various exercise programs have been touted, including changes in physical as well as mental well-being. Researchers have been interested in the application of physical exercise particularly as it effects maladaptive or self-stimulatory behaviors. Assumptions frequently made are that aerobic exercise would diminish stress or modulate self-stimulatory or hyperactive behavior through physiological changes related to release of neurotransmitters such as acetylcholine or beta-endorphins.

Service Delivery Model and Approach. Physical education programs are provided easily via individual or group methods by teachers within an educational curriculum given adequate physical space. Frequency or interventions vary from multiple times per day to not at all. The majority of research studies conducted utilize approximately 15 minutes of treatment time per day. The cost of providing services is usually modest, although larger physical spaces are often necessitated (e.g., running track or gym) in lieu of expensive equipment (e.g., exercise bicycle).

Empirical Studies. Four studies of the efficacy of physical exercise for children with autism were found (Kern, Koegel, & Dunlap, 1984; Kern *et al.*, 1982; Levinson & Reid, 1993; Watters & Watters, 1980). All of these studied effects of antecedent exercises on self-stimulatory/stereotyped behaviors using some variation of single-subject designs with controls (e.g., alternating treatments designs). Two of these studies also measured aspects of academic and play tasks in children with autism (Kern *et al.*, 1982; Watters & Watters, 1980). All studies found some beneficial, albeit short-lived, effects of exercise for decreasing self-stimulatory behaviors and mixed findings for im-

proving other simple cognitive/play tasks. Effects were greater for more intensive aerobic activity (relative to mild exertion). A maximum effect was noted at about 1 to 1½ hours with attenuation over time. Limitations of these studies included relatively small sample sizes, large variability in the independent measures, and the potential confounds of extra attention/social interaction that may have contributed to the beneficial effects of the program. The Watters & Watters (1980) study also concluded that there was no evidence to support that decreases in self-stimulatory behavior would automatically generalize to improved academic performance. Two additional studies on general physical education effectiveness for children with autism were found (Schleien, Heyne, & Berken, 1988; Weber & Thorpe, 1992). Weber & Thorpe (1992) found that for older children (ages 11 to 15) greater learning/retention of gross motor skills occurred in a task variation condition. Schleien *et al.*, (1988) found that physical education activities in an integrated physical education class with typical children did not appear to significantly affect performance of motor or play skills over a short term (9-week intervention). Short treatment length or poor sensitivity of motor measures may have limited the findings. It is also possible that general physical exercise and recreational activities do not necessarily generalize to improving social play without specific play skills being taught within the context of treatment.

Other Categories of Sensory or Motor Interventions

Although searches were attempted for many other specific sensory-motor intervention categories (e.g., developmental motor therapies, motor skills training, compensatory approaches, etc.), no empirical studies on autism were found. Clinical observation suggests that providing developmental motor training (i.e., skills training in hierarchically sequenced developmental stages) and compensatory teaching strategies are commonly utilized approaches in many educational and therapeutic programs for children with various diagnoses; thus it was surprising to find so little. However, it appears that these strategies are being provided as part of a broader therapeutic consultation program or via comprehensive educational models; thus empirical data specific to these components may be obscured in the literature. Future reviews may wish to address these components more specifically.

Summary of Efficacy and Motor Interventions

The theoretical strength of many sensory and motor interventions, particularly sensory integration (SI), rests on empirical findings that children with autism indeed have measurable deficits in various sensory processing and motor functions. Some of the treatments reviewed (e.g., sensorimotor handling) provide a questionable rationale for their use with children with autism and have no empirical evidence to evaluate their efficacy with this population. In particular, sensorimotor patterning is based on an older neurological theory that has been essentially disproven; several other programs based on sensory integration theory also suffer from partially outdated assumptions and are being modernized. Although the sheer volume of studies was low across categories reviewed, it was encouraging that several new studies were conducted in recent years. Findings from these studies were often mixed. Several studies in the area of SI, sensory stimulation, auditory integration training, prism lenses, and physical exercise yielded some positive, albeit modest outcomes; however, methodological constraints (e.g., use of small and convenience samples, weak/uncontrolled designs, observer bias, etc.) limit conclusive statements and generalizability of much of this work. In some areas, such as AIT, a few well-controlled studies have been recently conducted but with little overwhelming support for the treatment.

The biggest limiting factor is that many studies fail to directly link changes in the purported dysfunctional mechanism (e.g., auditory sensitivity, visual distortions, vestibular dysfunction) to the functional changes in behavior. Studies either provide outcome measures of the proximate sensory behaviors (e.g., auditory sensitivity, arousal, tactile defensiveness) or the broader functional behaviors (e.g., social interactions, play skills, academic performance), and rarely do they link both in systematic and measurable ways. A few preliminary studies of AIT and sensory stimulation treatments have attempted this; however, the results are still tenuous and inconsistent across studies, indicating need for replications. Furthermore, it is still unclear what specific processes may be responsible for the gains reported, even in the studies that had reasonable controls and sample sizes. Are treatment effects truly reflective of the intervention, or are there other nontreatment effects (e.g., parent's expectations, maturation, imposed structure, added attention, practice, etc.) that influenced the results? Other aspects of the tasks, not central to the treatment protocol, may also be producing beneficial effects. For example, children in one AIT study (Bettison, 1996) responded favorably under both the treatment and the alternative condition, thus, processed (filtered/modulated) music did not appear to be the critical treatment component. Although music "in general" may prove to be beneficial, an alternative explanation could involve the repeated demands for compliance and structured attention to task that are not specific to auditory processing. Another AIT study (Zollweg et al., 1997) demonstrated that both groups improved but the control group outperformed the treatment group on some measures, further questioning the efficacy of the treatment. Similarly, one of the core principles and strengths of classical sensory integration is that the therapy is child-directed and based in an individualized play context. Thus, purported gains in engagement and functional play skills may be influenced by play coaching techniques employed by an expert therapist as much as they are by improvements in sensory processing per se. Only further research with adequate specificity and controls (e.g., multiple baseline conditions in single-subject designs) can tease apart the effective from the noneffective components of these interventions.

Given that autistic symptoms are manifested differently across development and that heterogeneity exists within the autism spectrum, it is likely that individualized patterns of reactivity may be associated with differential treatment outcomes irrespective of the intervention category reviewed. Although outcomes for individual children have been mixed, it is possible that significant individual differences in subject characteristics may be masking significant group effects. That is, we don't know which children will benefit the most from which treatments and under which specific conditions. Several studies in the areas of SI and sensory stimulation indicated that specific sensory processing subtypes (e.g., hyper- versus hypo-responsive) and other subject variables (e.g., age, developmental levels) may affect prognosis for treatment outcomes. Though small sample sizes and retrospective designs limit generalizability, there appeared to be some converging evidence to suggest that a hyper-responsive pattern (i.e., high anxiety, arousal, or sensitivities) may be more amenable to sensory techniques aimed at arousal modulation and resultant gains in performance. Physiological studies of arousal indicate that younger (or less ma-

ture) children may have a higher tendency to display hypersensitive reactions and reject sensory stimuli that interfere with other aspects of functioning. If so, one implication of these findings may be that perhaps beginning some types of sensory-motor interventions at earlier ages would be more beneficial. Some studies have only been conducted with older children and adults (e.g., exercise treatments), and these results cannot be generalized to preschool populations. We cannot know the answers to these types of questions until more systematic research with increased specificity of subject variables is conducted to help distinguish various levels of response to treatments; however, these findings indicate that when provided, sensory and motor interventions need to be individualized for a given child with autism.

A further concern of this area of intervention is that most of the studies provide limited follow-up after intervention, and so it is not known whether positive effects are sustained in the long-term. A few better-controlled follow-ups have been included in some of the AIT studies; however, in those studies in which positive effects were noted initially, an attenuation of responses occurred over time (over the course of 9 to 12 months). These types of findings were also true for one study on prism lenses and two on exercise treatments. This could indicate that either the treatments were not useful in the long term or, conversely, that more frequent application of treatment is needed to maintain such effects. Repeated treatments were certainly useful with exercise therapies where physiological and behavior changes were sustained for approximately 90 minutes following each treatment. The effects of treatment frequency, duration, and intensity on both short- and long-term outcomes need to be further addressed.

Finally, issues of generalizability and feasibility of sensory and motor interventions need to be addressed more fully. The majority of studies across sensory and motor treatment categories, particularly those conducted less recently, have not attempted to investigate broader issues of generalizability. Two SI studies were conducted in naturalistic contexts and documented some functional gains outside of the treatment context. Others have been unable to prove that the intervention has substantial effects on academic performance, beyond the scope or context of the treatment per se. For example, several exercise studies have demonstrated positive effects on primary reduction of aberrant behaviors, but more limited improvements in secondary effects

on academic skills, play, and recreation. AIT studies demonstrate much variability across studies and lack of replication for broader behavioral effects—in some cases, control treatments produced stronger reductions in aberrant behaviors. Gains in areas of mastery play and engagement as a result of SI (i.e., Case-Smith & Bryan, 1999) are interesting to note; however, it is not surprising that behaviors less directly addressed in the context of therapy (e.g., peer interactions and functional communication) show the least improvement. Without direct practice in generalizing to functional tasks and in naturalistic environments, the effects of therapeutic gains in sensory processing or motor components may be limited. Studies of motor development in typical children have demonstrated that behaviors emerge from the confluence of multiple dynamic systems; thus, task-relevant information and perceptions of affordances in the environment can substantially alter movement patterns (Connolly & Elliott, 1989; Thelen & Ulrich, 1991), and motor skills learned in one context may not automatically generalize to naturalistic functional activities (Case-Smith, 1995). In fact, several studies have found that performance of children with autism on goal-directed motor and imitation tasks appears to be better in meaningful and purposeful contexts than in decontextualized situations (e.g., Hughes & Russell, 1993; Rogers, et al., 1996; Stone, et al., 1997). Thus one would expect that difficulties in applying newly acquired sensory or motor components to functional tasks and/or generalizing motor skills learned out of context would be magnified for children with autism.

The feasibility of carrying out specific sensory and motor interventions varies tremendously and is dependent upon such variables as cost, qualifications of needed professionals, and congruence with the philosophical orientation of the broader educational program. With respect to cost, all treatments require specialized training and varying amounts of staff time; however, some require much more technologically sophisticated and expensive equipment (e.g., AIT, Hug Machine, prism lenses) than do others (e.g., massage, C-S). Some treatments (e.g., exercise therapies, some SI-based approaches, prism lenses) are certainly more easily administered within the context of inclusive educational programs than other treatments (e.g., sensorimotor patterning). Of all the treatments summarized, classical SI provides the strongest child-centered and playful approach; this type of approach is often appealing to even the most unmotivated or disengaged child. In the case of sensory stimulation treatments (e.g., brushing, massage), AIT, patterning, and C-S, the child must be able to tolerate various sensory applications or physical manipulations provided by the therapist and usually in a restricted space. For some children with autism, however, structure and repetition are not necessarily aversive, although passive application of stimulation may be; the effects on stress need to be documented better in future studies. No negative side effects have been reported in most of the literature reviewed, with the exception of AIT, in which two studies documented increased behavior problems and some adverse health effects with some children. In addition, compliance has been an issue in several treatments, such as limited tolerance for eyewear or headphones, causing drop-outs from treatment.

Feasibility solutions, however, must go beyond ease of integration and cost effectiveness, they must also answer questions of best practice within the scope of educational goals. Because most of these interventions are used to augment comprehensive educational programs, it is important to know whether or not these treatments actually facilitate progress or hinder it by taking away valuable instruction time. The effects of specific sensory and motor interventions combined with various types of educational models need to be further investigated in large outcome studies. At least one case study report of three preschool children (Schwartz et al., 1998) indicates that there may be multiple means to achieving promising outcomes in young children with autism. Various combinations of specific intervention strategies (including SI in one case) were integrated into the curriculum and produced positive effects. Although classical SI therapy originated with a clinic based, noninclusive model, newer approaches are attempting to utilize a more naturalistic context with sensory-based activities integrated into the classroom routine. However, it will be important to investigate to what degree specific treatments can be "altered" to fit an inclusive education model while still retaining their essential therapeutic elements and purported benefits. Comparisons of such treatments need to be systematically investigated in future efficacy research.

As Rogers (1998) eloquently summarized in her review of comprehensive educational programs, we must keep in mind that a lack of empirical data does not infer that the treatment is ineffective, but rather that efficacy has not been objectively demonstrated. Funding will be critical to this

increasingly urgent investigation. Relying on nonharmful but potentially ineffective treatments can squander valuable time that could be used in more productive educational or therapeutic ways. Given that at least some positive findings are noted with respect to the sensory and motor interventions reviewed, future research must move from the current level of small-scale, poorly controlled, unsystematic studies of effectiveness, to a level that demands scientific rigor and well-controlled large-scale designs. Only such research can provide answers to important questions of not only what is effective but with whom and under what conditions.

Recommendations for Education

1. Although not all children with autism display sensory processing and motor dysfunction, these types of difficulties are prevalent in the population and are reported to interfere with performance in many broader developmental and functional domains. Therefore, at a minimum, "best practice" guidelines would indicate that educational programs for young children with autism need to incorporate appropriately structured physical and sensory environments that accommodate these unique sensory processing patterns and provide opportunities for developmentally appropriate sensory-motor experiences within the context of functional educational goals.

2. Comprehensive educational programs may benefit from consultation with knowledgeable professionals (e.g., occupational therapists, speech and language therapists, physical therapists, adaptive physical educators, etc.) to provide guidance about potential interventions for children whose sensory processing or motoric difficulties interfere with educational performance, as well as to provide support for families struggling with these issues. It is important to note that related services may provide many meaningful interventions that go well beyond the scope of this paper. Thus sensory and motor interventions are not synonymous with the terms for professionals employing these interventions (e.g, occupational therapy, physical therapy, or speech pathology); these terms should not be interchanged when making decisions for provision of therapeutic services.

3. It is important to note that none of the specific interventions reviewed claim to be a substitute for core educational cur-

ricula. If and when utilized, these should be viewed as supplementary interventions integrated at various levels into the broader individualized educational program.

4. Specific task/environmental modifications for sensory processing or motoric deficits tend to be described within the context of broader educational approaches or in combination with specific interventions more so than they are reported in the empirical literature. For example, adaptations may take the form of changing performance expectations, modifying classroom activities to minimize negative sensory reactions, perceptual distortions or motoric difficulties, teaching compensatory strategies, and/or maximizing the child's strengths to bypass sensory and motor difficulties and facilitate fuller participation. Such adaptations for sensory processing or motor difficulties would be feasible in many educational programs and could be used in tandem with other interventions.

5. Given the limited scientific basis of many of the remedial sensory and motor intervention approaches reviewed in this paper, a conservative approach is recommended for prescribing specific sensory or motor treatments. Best practice would suggest that decisions be made on an individualized clinical basis by expert professionals. If indicated, it behooves the professional to provide treatments in shorter-term increments (e.g., 6 to 12 weeks) and document progress in a systematic manner. Treatments need to be discontinued if effects are not apparent within an expected time frame or if negative reactions are documented. Certainly, regression in skills following discontinuation of services merits special attention.

6. With respect to specific interventions, the following points are made:
   a. Most categories of sensory and motor interventions, including SI, sensory stimulation approaches, AIT, and prism lenses have shown mixed effects for children with autism primarily through uncontrolled, descriptive studies; large-scale experimental studies are often lacking. Furthermore, beneficial effects of sensory and motor treatments on atypical behaviors in some children have been shown to be short-lived in several studies that followed children longitudinally.
   b. There is no available empirical evidence to support the use of sensorimotor

handling therapies for general educational purposes in young children with autism.

c. Potential risks of AIT (adverse side effects in some cases, lack of safeguards for hearing loss) need to be seriously weighed against the potential benefits for each individual case undergoing such an intervention.

d. SI and SI-based approaches appear to be relatively safe and anecdotally have shown some benefits in a few children with autism. However, given the mixed findings across uncontrolled, small sample studies, these treatments need to be individually determined and carefully monitored until better-controlled replication studies are completed with children with autism.

e. Deciding how much to pull a child away from his or her educational program is a difficult decision, and thus providing treatments within the context of an inclusive environment needs to be addressed.

7. Given the variability in developmental profiles of children with autism, it should be expected that not all children benefit equally from sensory or motor interventions. There is not a "one-size-fits-all" treatment for a diagnosis of autism. Thus the indiscriminate use of any sensory- or motor-based intervention is unethical. Comprehensive assessments should be the basis for service decisions, and, if necessary, sensory and motor interventions must be prescribed in an individualized manner consistent with the functional goals for each child.

8. Although, in general, intervention strategies need to be developmentally appropriate, remediation of component-level sensory processing functions or developmental motor skills may not automatically result in functional gains or generalize to relevant contexts. Thus, best practice would suggest that functional activities integrated into daily routines within naturalistic contexts increase retention and generalization of skills.

9. The paucity of available scientific research in this area leaves many questions yet to be answered. However, these preliminary findings may provide direction for future studies. The following are recommended:

a. Cross-sectional and longitudinal studies are needed to document the developmental progressions of unusual sensory processing features and qualitative motor functions and their relationships to broader behavioral and educational

outcomes.

b. Replication studies by independent investigators are needed for all sensory and motor treatment categories that have shown positive effects.

c. Methodologically more rigorous designs (e.g, multiple baseline single-subject designs; randomized controlled trials) with better-defined intervention components (duration/course, stimulus type/intensity/frequency, contextual conditions) and more reliable/valid and systematic outcome measures are recommended to directly test effects of a given treatment.

d. Studies that identify specific behavioral and physiological patterns (individual differences) that differentiate responders from nonresponders to specific treatments are warranted.

e. Studies linking the purported neurological mechanisms with both proximate measures of the phenomenon and functional measures of performance in broader domains (e.g., play skills, social skills, academic performance, independent functioning) are needed.

f. Studies providing information on earlier intervention, preventive benefits of sensory and motor interventions, and/or long-term impact on educational programming and functional outcomes of children in naturalistic contexts should be encouraged.

g. Studies documenting the relative contributions of sensory or motor interventions within comprehensive educational curricula are needed because it is unknown whether educational goals are facilitated or inhibited by these various interventions.

Acknowledgments

I extend my gratitude to Alice Blair, Angela Suratt, and Lorin McGuire for their assistance in preparation of this manuscript. I also thank Ruth Humphry, Linn Wakeford, Cathy Lord, Sally Rogers, and Pauline Filipek for their helpful reviews. An earlier draft of this manuscript was commissioned by the National Academy of Sciences, National Research Council's Committee on Educational Interventions for Children with Autism, and presented at the first committee meeting in December of 1999.

References

Adams, L. (1998). Oral-motor and motor-speech characteristics of children with autism. *Focus on Autism and Other Developmental Disabilities, 13,* 108–112.

Adrien, J. L., Lenoir, P., Martineau, J., Perrot, A., Haneury, L., Larmande, C., & Sauvage, D. (1993). Blind ratings of early symptoms of autism based upon family home movies. *Journal of the American Academy of Child and Adolescent Psychiatry, 33,* 617–626.

Adrien, J. L., Ornitz, E., Barthelemy, C., Sauvage, D., & Lelord, G. (1987). The presence or absence of certain behaviors associated with infantile autism in severely retarded autistic and nonautistic retarded children and very young normal children. *Journal of Autism and Developmental Disorders, 17,* 407–416.

Adrien, J. L., Perrot, A., Sauvage, D., Leddet, I., Larmande, C., Hameury, L., & Barthelemy, C. (1992). Early symptoms in autism from family home movies: Evaluation and comparison between 1st and 2nd year of life using I.B.S.E. Scale. *Acta Paedopsychiatrica: International Journal of Child and Adolescent Psychiatry, 55,* 71–75.

Amato, J., & Slavin, D. (1998). A preliminary investigation of oromotor function in young verbal and nonverbal children with autism. *Infant-Toddler Intervention 8,* 175–184.

Arendt, R. E., Maclean, W. E., & Baumeister, A. A. (1988). Critique of sensory integration therapy and its application in mental retardation. *American Journal of Mental Retardation, 92,* 401–429.

Ayres, J. (1972). Improving academic scores through sensory integration. *Journal of Learning Disabilities, 5,* 338–343.

Ayres, A. J., & Tickle, L. S. (1980). Hyper-responsivity to touch and vestibular stimuli as a predictor of positive response to sensory integration procedures by autistic children. *American Journal of Occupational Therapy, 34,* 375–381.

Baranek, G. T. (1999). Autism during infancy: A retrospective video analysis of sensory-motor and social behaviors at 9–12 months of age. *Journal of Autism and Developmental Disorders, 29,* 213–224.

Baranek, G. T., Foster, L. G., & Berkson, G. (1997). Tactile defensiveness and stereotyped behaviors. *American Journal of Occupational Therapy, 51,* 91–95.

Bettison, S. (1996). The long-term effects of auditory training on children with autism. *Journal of Autism and Developmental Disorders, 26,* 361–374.

Bridgman, G. D., Cushen, W., Cooper, D. M., & Williams, R. J. (1985). The evaluation of sensorimotor patterning and the persistence of belief. *British Journal of Mental Subnormality, 31,* 67–79.

Brown, M. M. (1999). Auditory integration training and autism: Two case studies. *British Journal of Occupational Therapy, 62,* 13–17.

Bundy, A. C., & Murray, E. A. (2002). Sensory Integration: A. Jean Ayre's Theory Revisited. In A. C. Bundy, E. A. Murray & S. Lane (Eds.), *Sensory integration: Theory and practice.* Philadelphia: F.A. Davis.

Carmody, D. P., Kaplan, M., & Gaydos, A. M. (2001). Spatial orientation adjustments in children with autism in Hong Kong. *Child Psychiatry and Human Development, 31,* 233–247.

Case-Smith J. (1995). The relationships among sensorimotor components, fine motor skills, and functional performance in preschool children. *American Journal of Occupational Therapy, 49*, 645–652.

Case-Smith, J., & Bryan, T. (1999). The effects of occupational therapy with sensory integration emphasis on preschool-age children with autism. *American Journal of Occupational Therapy, 53*, 489–497.

Clark, F. A., Miller, L. R., Kucherawy, D. A., & Azen, S. P. (1978). A comparison of operant and sensory integrative methods on developmental parameters in profoundly retarded adults. *American Journal of Occupational Therapy, 32*, 86–92.

Connolly, K., & Elliott, J. (1989). The emergence of a tool-using skill in infancy. *Developmental Psychology, 25*, 894–912.

Dahlgren, S. O., & Gillberg, C. (1989). Symptoms in the first two years of life. *European Archives of Psychiatry and Neurological Science, 238*, 169–174.

DeMyer, M., Barton, S., & Norton, J. A. (1972). A comparison of adaptive, verbal and motor profiles of psychotic and nonpsychotic subnormal children. *Journal of Autism and Childhood Schizophrenia, 2*, 359–377.

Edelson, S. M., Goldberg, M., Edelson, M. G., Kerr, D. C., & Grandin, T. (1999). Behavioral and physiological effects of deep pressure on children with autism: A pilot study evaluating the efficacy of Grandin's Hug Machine. *American Journal of Occupational Therapy, 53*, 145–152.

Field, T., Lasko, P. M., Henteleff, T., Kabat, S., Talpins, S., & Dowling, M. (1997). Brief report: Autistic children's attentiveness and responsivity improve after touch therapy. *Journal of Autism and Developmental Disorders, 27*, 333–339.

Gepner, B., Mestre, D., Masson, G., & de Schonen, S. (1995). Postural effects of motion vision in young autistic children. *Neuroreport, 6*(8), 1211–1124.

Gillberg, C., Ehlers, S., Schaumann, H., Jakobsson, G., Dahlgren, S. O., Lindblom, R., Bagenholm, A., Tjuus, T., & Blidner, E. (1990). Autism under age 3 years: A clinical study of 28 cases referred for autistic symptoms in infancy. *Child Psychology and Psychiatry, 31*, 921–934.

Gillberg, C., Johansson, M., Steffenburg, S., & Berlin, O. (1997). Auditory integration training in children with autism: Brief report of an open pilot study. *Autism, 1*(1), 97–100.

Gravel, J. S. (1994). Auditory integrative training: Placing the burden of proof. *American Journal of Speech and Language Pathology, 3*, 25–29.

Greenspan, S., & Weider, S. (1997). Developmental patterns and outcomes in infants and children with disorders in relating and communicating. A chart review of 200 cases of children with autistic spectrum diagnoses. *Journal of Developmental and Learning Disorders, 1*, 87–141.

Hoehn, T. P., & Baumeister, A. A. (1994). A critique of the application of sensory integration therapy to children with learning disabilities. *Journal of Learning Disabilities, 27*, 338–350.

Hoshino, Y., Kumashiro, H., Yashima, Y., Tachibana, R., Watanabe, M., & Furukawa, H. (1982). Early symptoms of autistic children and its diagnostic significance. *Folia Psychiatrica et Neurologica Japonica, 36*, 367–374.

Hughes, C., & Russell, J. (1993). Autistic children's difficulty with mental disengagement from an object: Its implications for theories of autism. *Developmental Psychology, 29*, 498–510.

Humphries, T. W., Snider, L., & McDougall, B. (1993). Clinical evaluation of the effectiveness of sensory integrative and perceptual motor therapy in improving sensory integrative function in children with learning disabilities. *Occupational Therapy Journal of Research, 13*, 163–182.

Humphries, T. W., Wright, M., McDougall, B., & Vertes, J. (1990). The efficacy of sensory integration therapy for children with learning disability. *Physical and Occupational Therapy in Pediatrics, 10*, 1–17.

Humphries, T. W., Wright, M., Snider, L., & McDougall, B. (1992). A comparison of the effectiveness of sensory integrative therapy and perceptual-motor training in treating children with learning disabilities. *Journal of Developmental and Behavioral Pediatrics, 13*, 31–40.

Hutt, C., Hutt, S. J., Lee, D., & Ounsted, C. (1964). Arousal and childhood autism. *Nature, 204*, 909–919.

James, A. L., & Barry, R. J. (1984). Cardiovascular and electrodermal responses to simple stimuli in autistic, retarded and normal children. *International Journal of Psychophysiology, 1*, 179–193.

Johnson, M. H., Siddons, F., Frith, U., & Morton, J. (1992). Can autism be predicted on the basis of infant screening tests? *Developmental Medicine and Child Neurology, 34*, 316–320.

Jones, V., & Prior, M. (1985). A comparison of adaptive, verbal and motor profiles of psychotic and non-psychotic subnormal children. *Journal of Autism and Childhood Schizophrenia, 2*, 359–377.

Kanter, R. M., Kanter, B., & Clark, D. L. (1982). Vestibular stimulation effect on language development in mentally retarded children. *American Journal of Occupational Therapy, 36*, 46–41.

Kaplan, M., Carmody, D. P., & Gaydos, A. (1996). Postural orientation modifications in autism in response to ambient lenses. *Child Psychiatry and Human Development, 27*, 81–91.

Kaplan, M., Edelson, S. M., & Seip, J. L. (1998). Behavioral changes in autistic individuals as a result of wearing ambient transitional prism lenses. *Child Psychiatry and Human Development, 29*, 65–76.

Kern, L., Koegel, R. L., & Dunlap, G. (1984). The influence of vigorous versus mild exercise on autistic stereotyped behaviors. *Journal of Autism and Developmental Disorders, 14*, 57–67.

Kern, L., Koegel, L. R., Dyer, K., Blew, P. A., & Fenton, L. R. (1982). The effects of physical exercise on self-stimulation and appropriate responding in autistic children. *Journal of Autism and Developmental Disorders, 12*, 399–419.

Kershner, J. R., Cummings, R. L., Clarke, K. A., Hadfield, A. J., & Kershner, B. A. (1990). Two year evaluation of the Tomatis listening training program with learning disabled children. *Learning Disability Quarterly, 13*, 43–53.

Kientz, M. A., & Dunn, W. (1997). A comparison of the performance of children with and without autism on the Sensory Profile. *American Journal of Occupational Therapy, 51*, 530–537.

Kinsbourne, M. (1987). Cerebral-brainstem relations in infantile autism. In E. Schopler & G. B. Mesibov (Eds.), *Neurobiological issues in autism* (pp. 107–125). New York: Plenum Press.

Klin, A., Volkmar, F. R., & Sparrow, S. S. (1992). Autistic social dysfunction: Some limitations of the theory of mind hypothesis. *Journal of Child Psychology and Psychiatry, 33*, 861–876.

Kohen-Raz, R., Volkmar, F. R., & Cohen, D. (1992). Postural control in children with autism. *Journal of Autism and Developmental Disorders, 22*, 419–432.

Kootz, J. P., & Cohen, D. J., (1981). Modulation of sensory intake in autistic children: Cardiovascular and behavioral indices. *Journal of the American Academy of Child Psychiatry 20*, 692–701.

Kootz, J. P., Marinelli, B., & Cohen, D. J. (1982). Modulation of response to environmental stimulation in autistic children. *Journal of Autism and Developmental Disorders, 12*, 185–193.

Larrington, G. G. (1987). A sensory integration based program with a severely retarded/autistic teenager: An occupational therapy case report. In Z. Mailloux (Ed.), *Sensory Integration Approaches* (pp. 101–117). New York: Hawthorn Press.

Le Couteur, A., Rutter, M., Lord, C., Rios, P., Robertson, S., Holdgrafer, M., & McLennan, J. (1989). Autism Diagnostic Interview: A standardized investigator-based instrument. *Journal of Autism and Developmental Disorders, 19*, 363–387.

Levinson, L. J., & Reid, G. (1993). The effects of exercise intensity on the stereotypic behaviors of individuals with autism. *Adapted Physical Activity Quarterly, 10*, (3), 255–268.

Lincoln, A. J., Courchesne, E., Harms, L., & Allen, M. (1995). Sensory modulation of auditory stimuli in children with autism and receptive developmental language disorder: Event-related brain potential evidence. *Journal of Autism and Developmental Disorders, 25*, 521–539.

Linderman, T. M., & Steward, K. B. (1999). Sensory integrative-based occupational therapy and functional outcomes in young children with pervasive developmental disorders: A single subject study. *American Journal of Occupational Therapy, 53*, 207–213.

Link, H. M. (1997). Auditory integration training (AIT): Sound therapy— Case studies of three boys with autism who received AIT. *British Journal of Learning Disabilities, 25*, 106–110.

Masterton, B. A., & Biederman, G. B. (1983). Proprioceptive versus visual control in autistic children. *Journal of Autism and Developmen-*

tal Disorders, 13, 141–152.

McClure, M. K., & Holtz-Yotz, M. (1990). The effects of sensory stimulatory treatment on an autistic child. *American Journal of Occupational Therapy, 45,* 1138–1145.

Minshew, N. J., Goldstein, G., & Siegel, D. J. (1997). Neuropsychologic functioning in autism: Profile of a complex information processing disorder. *Journal of the International Neuropsychological Society, 3,* 303–316.

Mudford, O. C., Cross, B. A., Breen, S., Cullen, C., Reeves, D., Gould, J., & Douglas, J. (2000). Auditory integration training for children with autism: No behavioral benefits detected. *American Journal on Mental Retardation, 105,* 118–129.

Neman, R., Roos, P., McCann, R. M., Menolascino, F. J., & Heal, L. W. (1974). Experimental evaluation of sensorimotor patterning used with mentally retarded children. *American Journal of Mental Deficiency, 79,* 372–384.

Neysmith-Roy, J. M. (2001). The Tomatis method with severely autistic boys: Individual case studies of behavioral changes. *South African Journal of Psychology, 31,* 19–28.

Ohta, M., Nagai, Y., Hara, H., & Sasaki, M. (1987). Parental perception of behavioral symptoms in Japanese autistic children. *Journal of Autism and Developmental Disorders, 17,* 549–563.

Ornitz, E. M., Guthrie, D., & Farley, A. H. (1977). The early development of autistic children. *Journal of Autism and Developmental Disorders, 7,* 207–229.

Ottenbacher, K. (1982). Sensory integration therapy: Affect of effect. *American Journal of Occupational Therapy, 36,* 571–578.

Perez, J. M., & Sevilla, M. (1993). Psychological assessment of adolescents and adults with autism. *Journal of Autism and Developmental Disorders, 23,* 653–664.

Polatajko, H. J., Kaplan, B. J., & Wilson, B. N. (1992). Sensory integration treatment for children with learning disabilities: Its status 20 years later. *Occupational Therapy Journal of Research, 12,* 323–341.

Polatajko, H. J., Law, M., Miller, J., Schaffer, R., & Macnab, J. (1991). The effect of a sensory integration program on academic achievement, motor performance, and self-esteem in children identified as learning disabled. *Occupational Therapy Journal of Research, 11,* 155–176.

Porges, S. W. (1998). Love and the evolution of the autonomic nervous system: The Polyvagal theory of intimacy. *Psychoneuroendocrinology, 23,* 837–861.

Rapin, I. (1997). Autism. *New England Journal of Medicine, 337,* 97–104.

Ray, T. C., King, L. J., & Grandin, T. (1988). The effectiveness of self-initiated vestibular stimulation in producing speech sounds in an autistic child. *Occupational Therapy Journal of Research, 8,* 187–190.

Reilly, C., Nelson, D. I., & Bundy, A. C. (1983). Sensorimotor versus fine motor activities in eliciting vocalizations in autistic children. *Occupational Therapy Journal of Research, 3,* 199–212.

Rimland, B. (1964). *Infantile autism: The syndrome and its implications for a neural theory of behavior.* New York City: Appleton Century Crofts.

Rimland, B., & Edelson, R. (May, 1994). The effects of auditory integration training on autism. *American Journal of Speech and Language Pathology,* 18–24.

Rimland, B., & Edelson, S. (1995). Brief report: A pilot study of auditory integration training in autism. *Journal of Autism and Developmental Disorders, 25,* 61–70.

Rinehart, N. J. Bradshaw, J. L., Brereton, A. V., & Tonge, B. J. (2001). Movement preparation in high-functioning autism and Asperger disorder: A serial choice reaction time task involving motor reprogramming. *Journal of Autism and Developmental Disorders, 31,* 79–88.

Rogers, S. J. (1998). Empirically supported comprehensive treatments for young children with autism *Journal of Clinical Child Psychology, 27,* 138–45.

Rogers, S. J., Bennetto, L., McEvoy, R., & Pennington, B. F. (1996). Imitation and pantomime in high-functioning adolescents with autism spectrum disorders. *Child Development, 67,* 2060–2073.

Scharre, J. E., & Creedon, M. P. (1992). Assessment of visual function in autistic children. *Optometry and Vision Science, 69,* 433–439.

Schleien, S. J., Heyne, L. A., & Berken, S. B. (1988). Integrating physical education to teach appropriate play skills to learners with autism: A pilot study. *Adapted Physical Activity Quarterly, 5,* 182–192.

Schwartz, I. S., Sandall, S. R., Garfinkle, A. N., & Bauer, J. (1998). Outcomes for children with autism: Three case studies. *Topics in Early Childhood Special Education, 18,* 132–143.

Smith, I. M., & Bryson, S. E. (1998). Gesture imitation in autism I: Nonsymbolic postures and sequences. *Cognitive Neuropsychology, 15,* 747–770.

Stagnitti, K., Raison, P., & Ryan, P. (1999). Sensory defensiveness syndrome: A paediatric perspective and case study. *Australian Occupational Therapy Journal, 46,* 175–187.

Stone, W. L., Lemanek, K. L., Fishel, P. T., Fernandez, M. C., & Altemeier, W. A. (1990). Play and imitation skills in the diagnosis of autism in young children. *Pediatrics, 86,* 267–272.

Stone, W. L., Ousley, O. Y., Hepburn, S. L., Hogan, K. L., & Brown, C. (1999). Patterns of adaptive behavior in very young children with autism. *American Journal of Mental Retardation, 104,* 187–199.

Stone, W. L., Ousley, O. Y., Littleford, C. D. (1997). Motor imitation in young children with autism: What's the object? *Journal of Abnormal Child Psychology, 25,* 475–485.

Thelen, E., & Ulrich, B. D. (1991). *Hidden skills. Monograph of the Society for Research in Child Development, 56* (pp. 1–98). Chicago: University of Chicago Press.

Upledger, JE. (1996). An overview of craniosacral therapy: Its origin and its applications for newborns and infants. *Infants and Young Children, 9,* 59–68.

Vargas, S., & Camilli, G. (1999). A meta-analysis of research on sensory integration treatment. *American Journal of Occupational Therapy, 53,* 189–198.

Volkmar, F. R., Cohen, D. J., & Paul, R. (1986). An evaluation of DSM-III criteria for infantile autism. *Journal of the American Academy of Child Psychiatry, 25,* 190–197.

Wainwright, J. A., & Bryson, S. E. (1996). Visual-spatial orienting in autism. Journal of Autism and Developmental Disorders, 26, 423–438.

Watters, R. G., & Watters, W. E. (1980). Decreasing self-stimulatory behavior with physical exercise in a group of autistic boys. *Journal of Autism and Developmental Disorders, 10,* 379–387.

Weber, R. C., & Thorpe, J. (1992). Teaching children with autism through task variation in physical education. *Exceptional Children, 59,* 77–86.

Wilson, B. N., Kaplan, B. J., Fellowes, S., Gruchy, C., & Faris, P. (1992). The efficacy of sensory integration treatment compared to tutoring. *Physical and Occupational Therapy in Pediatrics, 12,* 1–36.

Zentall, S. S., & Zentall, T. R. (1983). Optimal stimulation: A model of disordered activity and performance in normal and deviant children. *Psychological Bulletin, 94,* 446–471.

Zisserman, L. (1991). The effects of deep pressure on self-stimulating behaviors in a child with autism and other disabilities. *American Journal of Occupational Therapy, 46,* 547–551.

Zollweg, W., Palm, D., & Vance, V. (1997). The efficacy of auditory integration training: A double-blind study. *American Journal of Audiology, 6,* 39–47.

The Influence of Vigorous versus Mild Exercise on Autistic Stereotyped Behaviors[1]

Lynn Kern, Robert L. Koegel,[2] and Glen Dunlap

A major problem encountered in many autistic children is their high rate of stereotypic behavior, which has been shown to interfere with on-task responding and other appropriate behaviors. Since the experimental literature indicates that physical exercise can positively influence both appropriate and inappropriate behaviors, including the children's stereotypic behaviors, the purpose of this study was to investigate whether the specific type of exercise (i.e., mild vs. vigorous) would differentially affect subsequent stereotyped behaviors. The results demonstrated that (1) 15 minutes of mild exercise (ball playing) had little or no influence on the children's subsequent stereotyped responding, and (2) 15 minutes of continuous and vigorous exercise (jogging) was always followed by reductions in stereotyped behaviors. These results are discussed in relation to cognitive, physiological, and educational implications.

[1]This research was supported by United States Public Health Service research grants MH 28210 and MH 28231 from the National Institute of Mental Health, and by Research Contract No. 300-82-0362 from the U.S. Department of Education-Special Education Program. The authors are grateful for the contributions of Diane Gilchrist, Julie Martin, Karen Sallus, Lynne Bonngard, Bill Krutzen, Lee Kern, John Burke, and Rob O'Neill. [2]Address all correspondence to Robert L. Koegel, Social Process Research Institute, University of California, Santa Barbara, California 93106.

Numerous studies have suggested that certain highly stereotyped mannerisms (such as hand and arm flapping, body rocking) of autistic and other severely handicapped children may be detrimental to these children's development (cf. Epstein, Doke, Sajwaj, Sorrell, & Rimmer, 1974; Koegel & Covert, 1972; Koegel, Firestone, Kramme, & Dunlap, 1974; Lovaas, Litrownik, & Mann, 1971). Because of this, there have been many attempts to reduce such stereotyped mannerisms. Most of these attempts have involved the manipulation of response consequences (e.g., Baumeister & Forehand, 1973; Bucher & Lovaas, 1968; Foxx & Azrin, 1972; Harris & Wolchik, 1979; Luiselli, 1981; Luiselli & Krause, 1981; Mulhern & Baumeister, 1969; Rincover, 1978; Sachs, 1973).

However, in order to more fully understand the nature of stereotypic responding, researchers have also begun to manipulate antecedent events. One such promising line of investigation involves the use of antecedent physical exercise to assess its influence on subsequent stereotypic responding (cf. Kern, Koegel, Dyer, Blew, & Fenton, 1982; Ohlson, 1978; Watters & Watters, 1980). While many exercise programs have now been shown to have positive influences on a variety of behaviors in numerous populations, there have also been suggestions that certain types and/or amounts of exercise may be more beneficial than others (cf. Allen, 1980; Dodson & Mullens, 1969; Gupta, Sharma, & Jaspal, 1974). Therefore, the purpose of the present investigation was to systematically manipulate two types of physical exercise—a vigorous and continuous exercise (jogging) versus a much less vigorous exercise (ball playing)—and to assess whether these activities would differentially influence the children's subsequent stereotypic (and other) responding.

Method

Subjects

Three children, 7, 11, and 11 years of age, participated in the study. They were diagnosed as autistic by two independent diagnosticians, employing the U.S. National Society for Children and Adults with Autism criteria (NSAC, 1978). They were selected for this experiment because they exhibited especially high levels of stereotypic behaviors. They were formally untestable on standardized intelligence tests. However, they were estimated to have Social Quotients of 80, 60, and 22, respectively, with the Vineland Social Maturity Scale. Prior to treatment, all three children were judged by a physician as being in good physical health, and capable of the physical activities employed in this investigation.

Settings

Two settings were employed in this study: (1) a large open field and (2) a living room. First, following the baseline measures, the physical activity (jogging and ballplaying) periods took place in a large open field, approximately 150 x 150 meters, which was located just outside the building where data were recorded.

Immediately preceding and following each period of physical activity, the children's levels of stereotypic responding were recorded in the second setting. This setting was a 3 x 4-meter room that was furnished as a living room with sofas, chairs, tables, and pictures on the walls. Several age-appropriate toys were scattered around the room, and one adult who was unfamiliar to the child was seated in the room for safety precautions. (No situation occurred that required a response from the adult during the experiment.) The data recorders observed from a separate room, connected by a one-way window and an intercom system.

Experimental Design

A simultaneous-treatments design (Hersen & Barlow, 1976; Kazdin & Hartmann, 1978) was used in which sessions of one condition (e.g., jogging) were alternated with sessions of the other condition (e.g., ball playing). The order was balanced such that the first condition presented per day was alternated across days and across children. Specifically, following the daily baseline condition (1 hour of observation without any antecedent exercise program), one of the two experimental conditions (jogging or ball playing) was implemented. After 15 minutes of one activity (e.g., jogging), the child was observed for a 90-minute period in the experimental setting. Then, the other condition (e.g., 15 minutes of ball playing) was implemented and again followed by 90 minutes of data recording. Finally, the first condition conducted for that child on that day was repeated (e.g., 15 minutes of

Article Reprint Information: Reprinted from Springer/*Journal of Autism and Developmental Disorders*, 14(1), 1984, 57-67, The influence of vigorous versus mild exercise on autistic stereotyped behaviors, Kern, L., Koegel, R. L., & Dunlap, G., with kind permission from Springer Science and Business Media.

Table I.
The Autistic Stereotyped Behaviors Recorded for the Three Children
Who Participated in This Experiment

Autistic stereotyped behaviors

Child 1
   1. Intense staring or gazing (a fixed, glassy-eyed look lasting more than 3 seconds)
   2. Spontaneous loud and repetitive glottal and gutteral vocalizations with hands placed in a
       cupped position next to ears
   3. Loud, high-pitched, repetitive nasal vocalizations
   4. Gazing intently at hand placed within 6" of eye
   5. Repetitive breathy whistles, accompanied by hyperventilation
   6. Flapping hands in air
   7. Repetitive head or body shaking (small rapid movements from side to side)
   8. Repetitive jerking of body
   9. Repetitive saliva fingering
   10. Vigorous forward and backward rocking

Child 2
   1. Prolonged and/or repetitive lip puckering
   2. Repetitive, stereotypic finger flexing and arm waving at shoulder level
   3. Repetitive, continuous babbling of nonsense syllables

Child 3
   1. Repetitive, stereotypic finger flexing (often while simultaneously gazing at them)
   2. Arm and hand flapping
   3. Stereotyped repetitive delayed echolalia (e.g., repeating a command several times)

jogging followed by 90 minutes of observation).

Independent Variable: Type of Physical Exercise

Vigorous Exercise—Jogging. In each (noncontingent) jogging session a randomly selected adult from a pool of eight (naive to the experimental hypothesis) and a child jogged side by side (holding hands if the child began to stray from the area). No direct interventions were made with respect to any of the children's stereotypic behaviors. The jogging pace was adjusted in each session to be mildly strenuous (e.g., child showed increased breathing rate and/or slightly flushed face) but was slowed to a temporary walk (approximately 15 seconds) if the child began to show any observable signs of discomfort (e.g., appearing out of breath or attempting to pull away from the adult's hand). Throughout the sessions the adult occasionally reinforced the child verbally for running (e.g., "Good running"). The total length of the jogging period (not counting the occasional 15-second walks) was 15 minutes.

Mild Exercise—Ball Playing. During each (noncontingent) 15-minute ball-playing session an adult (from the above pool) interacted by gently throwing a large (20 cm) soft rubber ball to the child. A distance of approximately 2 to 3 meters was maintained between the child and the adult during the sessions. In addition, a second adult stood directly behind the child in order to

manually prompt the child to put his/her arms up to catch the ball and to remain in the area, if necessary. The rate of throwing the ball was approximately 10 to 20 times per minute (depending on how quickly the child caught/threw the ball). In instances when the child made no attempt to catch or return the ball, the adult would pick up the ball and gently throw it to the child. Correct ball-playing responses were verbally reinforced by the adult.

Dependent Variable: Stereotypic Behaviors

The term *stereotypic behaviors* was defined as follows: repetitive, stereotypic responses that appeared to be performed for the purpose of providing sensory input, but that did not appear to produce any obvious effects on the child's social environment (Dunlap, Dyer, & Koegel, 1983; Hutt, Hutt, Lee, & Ounsted, 1965; Lovaas, 1967). This category was operationally defined for each individual child on the basis of prior nonexperimental observations (see Table I). These specific behaviors are considered symptomatic of the syndrome of autism and other severe handicaps (cf. Berkson, 1967; NSAC, 1978; Schopler, 1978) and are typically not seen to any large extent in normal populations.

Measurement

Each observation period was divided into 15-minute blocks, with data recorded during the first 5 minutes of each block. Thus,

each 1 hour baseline period contained four blocks and each period following a physical activity contained six blocks. A time-sampling recording procedure was utilized in which 15-second intervals were divided into 5 seconds of observation and 10 seconds of data recording, resulting in 20 intervals per 5-minute block of observation. Observers recorded the presence or absence of stereotypic responding on precoded data sheets with a plus if the behavior category occurred and a minus if it did not occur.

Reliability

Two observers (one naive to the purpose of the experiment) independently recorded occurrences and nonoccurrences of stereotypic behavior during 77 (58.33%) randomly selected sessions. All observers were given lists of the children's behaviors. Then, prior to the first formal reliability session, approximately five practice sessions were held to ensure that each observer was accurately recording the data according to the experimental definitions. Percent agreement was calculated for the formal reliability sessions on an interval-by-interval basis. An agreement consisted of the two observers recording exactly the same response. Percent agreement was calculated for each interval by dividing the number of agreements by the number of agreements plus disagreements. The average percent agreement for recording stereotypic responding across the 77 sessions was 97.70% (range: 90% to 100%).

Results

The results of the simultaneous-treatments analyses with all three children are shown in Figure 1. The graph shows that all three children had high levels of stereotypic responding prior to the exercise. For example, the average baseline level of such responding for Child 1 was 88.75%. A decrease was then evidenced as a result of the jogging sessions. That is, on day 1 Child 1's stereotypic responding decreased from a baseline of 88.75% to 40% following jogging. A similar pattern is evident for each of the other children, and, in fact, in all nine of the instances after jogging was introduced, stereotypic responding decreased below baseline levels.

In contrast, there were no systematic changes following the ball-playing sessions. For example, inspection of Child 2's results for day 1 and day 2 shows that levels of stereotypic responding following ball playing were sometimes lower and sometimes higher than the corresponding baseline levels. This was true for each of the other children with, in total, six of the nine ball-playing conditions showing levels exceeding baseline.

In order to permit examination of individual trends in the data, (e.g., note that stereotypic responding usually reached its low point within about 1 hour following jogging), Table II presents the individual data for each successive 15-minute observational period.

Discussion

These results showing that vigorous exercise (jogging) systematically produced decreases in stereotypic responding are consistent with those in a number of previously reported investigations. In addition, the present data on autistic stereotypies add to the literature by demonstrating that the specific type of physical activity appears to have a differential impact on the subsequent behavior of autistic children.

A number of studies, including those documenting increases in appropriate responding (e.g., Diesfeldt & Diesfeldt-Groenendijk, 1977; Dodson & Mullens, 1969; Kern et al., 1982; Schaney, Brekke, Landry, & Burke, 1976), indicate that fatigue is probably not the mechanism primarily responsible for the positive effects of vigorous exercise (cf. Bachman, 1982) but rather that some other behavioral/physiological mechanism(s) are involved. This seems especially interesting since a number of authors (e.g., Blackstock, 1978; Coleman, 1979; Damasio & Maurer, 1978; Ornitz & Ritvo, 1968; Rutter & Bartak, 1971; Schopler & Reichler, 1971; Student & Sohmer, 1978; Tanguay, 1976; Wetherby, Koegel, & Mendel, 1981) have suggested that physiological mechanisms may be involved in the etiology and behavioral characteristics of autism. It can be speculated that vigorous exercise may directly influence the functioning of such variables as physiological arousal (e.g., Hutt & Hutt, 1968; Ornitz & Ritvo, 1968; Rimland, 1964) or the production and release of neurotransmitters or beta-endorphins (cf. Fraioli et al., 1980; Kline & Lehmann, 1979, VonEuler, 1974).

Whatever the specific mechanism is that underlies the present phenomenon, it may be important to note that many educational programs do not provide even brief periods of physical exercise. Further, of those that do provide some activity, most do not systematically provide for any given type of activity. Thus, further research and programming in this area may be an especially important concern of teachers and other practitioners involved with autistic or other handicapped children.

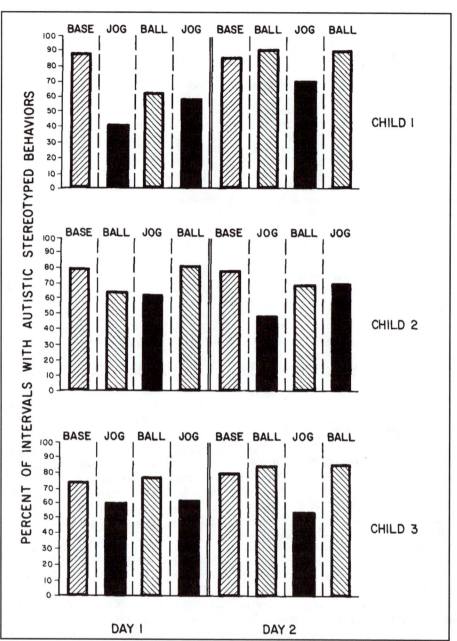

Fig. 1. The percent of intervals with autistic stereotyped responding for children 1, 2, and 3 during the 1-hour baseline conditions, for 90 minutes following the jogging exercise sessions, and 90 minutes following the ball-playing exercise sessions.

References

Allen, J. J. (1980). Jogging can modify disruptive behaviors. *Teaching Exceptional Children, 12*(2), 66-70.

Bachman, J. E. (1982). *Exercise as antecedent control of various inappropriate behavior.* Unpublished master's thesis, Western Michigan University.

Baumeister, A. A., & Forehand, R. (1973). Stereotyped acts. In N. R. Ellis (Ed.), *International review of research in mental retardation* (Vol. 6). New York: Academic Press.

Berkson, G. (1967). Abnormal stereotyped motor acts. In J. Zubin & H. F. Hunt (Eds.), *Comparative psychopathology: Animal and human.* Grune and Stratton.

Blackstock, E. G. (1978). Cerebral asymmetry and the development of early infantile autism. *Journal of Autism and Childhood Schizophrenia, 8,* 339-353.

Bucher, B., & Lovaas, O. I. (1968). Use of aversive stimulation in behavior modification. In M. R. Jones (Ed.), *Miami symposium on the prediction of behavior, 1967: Aversive stimulation.* Coral Gables, Florida: University of Miami Press.

Coleman, M. (1979). Studies of the autistic syndromes. In R. Katzman (Ed.), *Congenital and acquired cognitive disorders.* New York: Raven Press.

Damasio, A., & Maurer, R. (1978). A neurological model for childhood autism. *Archives of*

Table II. Percent of Autistic Stereotyped Responding Behavior during 15-Minute Sessions for Each of the Children

Child 1

Day 1

	1	2	3	4		5	6	7	8	9	10	
% Autistic stereotyped responding	90	85	90	90	Jogging	45	10	45	45	35	65	Ball playing

	11	12	13	14	15	16		17	18	19	20	21	22
% Autistic stereotyped responding	75	55	60	25	80	85	Jogging	75	60	35	55	55	75

Day 2

	1	2	3	4		5	6	7	8	9	10	
% Autistic stereotyped responding	85	90	85	85	Ball playing	85	95	100	100	90	75	Jogging

	11	12	13	14	15	16		17	18	19	20	21	22
% Autistic stereotyped responding	40	40	90	70	85	100	Ball playing	70	95	85	90	100	100

Child 2

Day 1

	1	2	3	4		5	6	7	8	9	10	
% Autistic stereotyped responding	85	75	75	85	Ball playing	75	80	60	35	75	65	Jogging

	11	12	13	14	15	16		17	18	19	20	21	22
% Autistic stereotyped responding	55	25	65	65	90	80	Ball playing	95	90	90	65	70	85

Day 2

	1	2	3	4		5	6	7	8	9	10	
% Autistic stereotyped responding	75	90	75	75	Jogging	20	25	20	60	90	75	Ball playing

	11	12	13	14	15	16		17	18	19	20	21	22
% Autistic stereotyped responding	55	90	45	65	80	85	Jogging	55	75	80	75	70	70

Neurology, 35, 777-786.

Diesfeldt, H. F. A., & Diesfeldt-Groenendijk, H. (1977). Improving cognitive performance in psychogeriatric patients: The influence of physical exercise. Age and Ageing, 6, 58-64.

Dodson, L. C., & Mullens, W. R. (1969). Some effects of jogging on psychiatric hospital patients. American Correctional Therapy Journal, 5, 130-134.

Dunlap, G., Dyer, K., & Koegel, R. L. (1983). Autistic self-stimulation and intertrial interval duration. American Journal of Mental Deficiency, 88(2), 194-202.

Epstein, L. H., Doke, L. A., Sajwaj, T. E., Sorrell, S., & Rimmer, B. (1974). Generality and side effects of overcorrection. Journal of Applied Behavior Analysis, 7, 385-390.

Foxx, R. M., & Azrin, H. H. (1972). Restitution: A method of eliminating aggressive-disruptive behavior of retarded and brain damaged patients. Behaviour Research and Therapy, 10, 15-27.

Fraioli, F., Moretti, C., Paolucci, D., Alicicco, E., Crescenzi, F., & Fortunio, G. (1980). Physical exercise stimulates marked concomitant release of β-endorphin and adrenocorticotropic hormone (ACTH) in peripheral blood in man. Experientia, 36, 987-989.

Gupta, V. P., Sharma, T. R., & Jaspal, S. S. (1974). Physical activity and efficiency of mental work. Perceptual and Motor Skills, 38, 205-206.

Harris, S. L., & Wolchik, S. A. (1979). Suppression of self-stimulation: Three alternative strategies. Journal of Applied Behavior Analysis, 12, 185-198.

Hersen, M., & Barlow, D. H. (1976). Single case experimental designs: Strategies for studying behavior change. New York: Pergamon Press.

Hutt, S., & Hutt, C. (1968). Stereotypy, arousal and autism. Human Development, 11, 277-286.

Hutt, S. J., Hutt, C., Lee, D., & Ounsted, C. (1965). A behavioral and encephalographic study of autistic children. Journal of Psychiatric Research, 3, 181-187.

Kazdin, A. E., & Hartmann, D. P. (1978). The simultaneous-treatment design. Behavior Therapy, 9, 912-922.

Kern, L., Koegel, R. L., Dyer, K., Blew, P. A., & Fenton, L. R. (1982). The effects of physical exercise on self-stimulation behavior and appropriate responding in autistic children. Journal of Autism and Developmental Disorders, 12, 399-419.

Kline, N. S., & Lehmann, H. E. (1979). β-endorphin therapy in psychiatric patients. In Usdin, W. E. Bunney, & N. S. Kline (Eds.), Endorphins in mental health research. New York: Oxford University Press.

Koegel, R. L., & Covert, A. (1972). The relationship of self-stimulation to learning in autistic children. Journal of Applied Behavior Analysis, 5, 381-387.

Koegel, R. L., Firestone, P. B., Kramme, K. W., & Dunlap, G. (1974). Increasing spontaneous play by suppressing self-stimulation in autistic children. Journal of Applied Behavior Analysis, 7, 521-528.

Lovaas, O. I. (1967). Behavior therapy approach to treatment of childhood schizophrenia. Minnesota symposium on child development. Minneapolis: University of Minnesota Press.

Lovaas, O. I., Litrownik, A., & Mann, R. (1971). Response latencies to auditory stimuli in autistic children engaged in self-stimulatory behavior. Behaviour Research and Therapy, 9, 39-49.

Luiselli, J. K. (1981). Behavioral treatment of self-stimulation: Review and recommendations. Education and Treatment of Children, 4(4), 375-392.

Luiselli, J. K., & Krause, S. (1981). Reduction in stereotypic behavior through a combination of DRO, cueing, and reinforced isolation procedures. Behavior Therapist, 4, 2-3.

Mulhern, T., & Baumeister, A. A. (1969). An experimental attempt to reduce stereotypy by reinforcement procedures. American Journal of Mental Deficiency, 74, 69-74.

National Society for Autistic Children. (1978). National Society for Autistic Children definition of the syndrome of autism. Journal of Autism and Childhood Schizophrenia, 8, 162-167.

Ohlsen, R. L. (1978). Control of body rocking in the blind through the use of vigorous exercise. Journal of Instructional Psychology, 5, 19-22.

Ornitz, E. M., & Ritvo, E. R. (1968). Perceptual inconstancy in early infantile autism. *Archives of General Psychiatry, 18,* 76-98.

Rimland, B. (1964). *Infantile autism.* New York: Appleton-Century-Crofts.

Rincover, A. (1978). Sensory extinction: A procedure for eliminating self-stimulating behavior in autistic children. *Journal of Abnormal Child Psychology, 6,* 299-310.

Rutter, M., & Bartak, L. (1971). Causes of infantile autism: Some considerations from recent research. *Journal of Autism and Childhood Schizophrenia, 1,* 20-32.

Sachs, D. A. (1973). The efficacy of time-out procedures in a variety of behavior problems. *Journal of Behavior Therapy and Experimental Psychiatry, 4,* 237-242.

Schaney, Z., Brekke, B., Landry, R., & Burke, J. (1976). Effects of a perceptual-motor training program on kindergarten children. *Perceptual and Motor Skills, 43,* 428-430.

Schopler, E. (1978). On confusion in the diagnosis of autism. *Journal of Autism and Childhood Schizophrenia, 8,* 137-138.

Schopler, E., & Reichler, R. J. (1971). Psychobiological referents for the treatment of autism. In D. W. Churchill, G. D. Alpern, & M. K. DeMyer (Eds.), *Infantile autism.* Springfield, Illinois: Charles C Thomas.

Student, M., & Sohmer, H. (1978). Evidence from auditory nerve and brainstem-evoked responses for an organic brain lesion in children with autistic traits. *Journal of Autism and Childhood Schizophrenia, 8,* 13-20.

Tanguay, P. (1976). Clinical and electrophysiological research. In E. Ritvo (Ed.), *Autism: Diagnosis, current research and management.* New York: Spectrum.

Von Euler, U. S. (1974). Sympatho-adrenal activity in physical exercise. *Medicine and Science in Sports, 6,* 165-173.

Watters, R. G., & Watters, W. E. (1980). Decreasing self-stimulatory behavior with physical exercise in a group of autistic boys. *Journal of Autism and Developmental Disorders, 10,* 379-387.

Wetherby, A., Koegel, R. L., & Mendel, M. (1981). Central auditory nervous system dysfunction in echolalic autistic individuals. *Journal of Speech and Hearing Research, 24,* 420-429.

Table II. Continued

Child 3

Day 1

% Autistic stereotyped responding	1	2	3	4	Jogging	5	6	7	8	9	10	Ball playing
	70	75	85	65		90	40	40	40	80	75	
	11	12	13	14	15	16	Jogging	17	18	19	20	21	22
	65	80	55	85	80	100		50	45	35	75	90	80

Day 2

% Autistic stereotyped responding	1	2	3	4	Ball playing	5	6	7	8	9	10	Jogging
	70	90	75	85		70	85	95	80	95	85	
	11	12	13	14	15	16	Ball playing	17	18	19	20	21	22
	50	30	65	40	45	95		80	90	100	80	80	85

The Effects of Physical Exercise on Self-Stimulation and Appropriate Responding in Autistic Children[1]

Lynn Kern,[2] Robert L. Koegel,[3] Kathleen Dyer, Priscilla A. Blew, and Lisa R. Fenton[4]

A major problem encountered with autistic children is their characteristic self-stimulatory behavior, which frequently interferes with on-task responding and other appropriate behaviors. However, the experimental literature suggests that with many populations, increased physical activity might positively influence subsequent responding. Therefore, the purpose of this study was to investigate the use of increased physical activity (in this experiment, jogging) as a possible method of decreasing subsequent self-stimulatory behaviors as well as increasing subsequent appropriate responding. Seven autistic children with exceptionally high levels of self-stimulatory behavior participated in the investigation. Self-stimulatory and appropriate behaviors were measured both before and after jogging in a repeated-reversal design. The results demonstrated the following: (1) Brief jogging sessions produced decreases in subsequent levels of self-stimulatory behaviors and also produced increases in appropriate play and academic responding; (2) These changes after jogging were evident in three different experimental settings: during academic responding on preschool level tasks" in a clinic; during ball-playing in an outside play area; and in a quiet room, while no other activity was occurring; (3) Supplementary measures obtained in an applied classroom setting showed a similar relationship with both increases in on-task activity and general interest ratings for school tasks following the jogging sessions.

University of California, Santa Barbara, and The May Institute, Inc. [1]This research was supported by Public Health Service research grants MH28210 and MH28231 from the National Institute of Mental Health, and by U. S. Office of Education research grant G007802084 from the Bureau of Education for the Handicapped. We are grateful for the assistance of Stephen C. Luce, Julie Kasanoff, Marie Nugent, Robin Gaines, Gina Deluchi, Rosanna Conti, Carl Bendroff, David Rotholz, Christine Chivas, Katherine Kuba, Linda Diaa, Diane Gilchrist, and Virgina Kostigen. We are especially grateful for the help and comments of Jill Hodgett and Glen Dunlap throughout this investigation. [2]Now at the Carpinteria Unified School District, Santa Barbara, California. [3]Address all correspondence to Robert L. Koegel, Speech and Hearing Center, University of California, Santa Barbara, California 93106. [4]Now at the John F. Kennedy Institute, Johns Hopkins Medical School.

A major problem encountered with autistic children is their characteristic self-stimulatory behavior (Lovaas, 1967). Such behaviors, also referred to in the literature as stereotypic behavior, stereotyped movements, repetitive behavior, or autistic mannerisms, have been studied extensively in a variety of populations (e.g., Berkson & Mason, 1963; Forehand & Baumeister, 1971; Frankel, Freeman, Ritvo, & Pardo, 1978; Hutt & Hutt, 1968; Thelen, 1979). While not all populations behave identically (cf. Hargrave & Swisher, 1975; Klier & Harris, 1977), this type of behavior has often been shown to interfere with learning and the performance of socially appropriate behaviors in many autistic children. For example, Lovaas, Litrownik, and Mann (1971) reported that certain types of self-stimulatory behavior produced abnormally lengthened response latencies to auditory stimuli. Koegel and Covert (1972) and Chock (1979) found that severely autistic children (nonverbal, IQ below 40) had difficulty learning even simple tasks when they were engaged in self-stimulatory behavior. Epstein, Doke, Sajwaj, Sorrell, and Rimmer (1974), Koegel, Firestone, Kramme, and Dunlap (1974), and Glahn (1980) also demonstrated that certain types of self-stimulatory behavior interfered with appropriate play.

In light of the interfering aspects of self-stimulatory behavior, numerous investigators have undertaken efforts to decrease this type of behavior. For example, Koegel and Covert (1972) and Risley (1968) employed physical punishment; Foxx and Azrin (1972) used overcorrection; Koegel et al. (1974) utilized physical restraint; and Rincover (1978) and Rincover, Cook, Peoples, and Packard (1979) employed sensory extinction. While all of these approaches have met with some degree of success, because of limitations pertaining to generalization, maintenance, or applicability to only certain types of self-stimulatory behavior, this behavior still remains a major problem for autistic children and considerable research is being undertaken in this area (Hung, 1978).

One promising avenue of research relates to the fact that self-stimulatory behavior appears to covary with certain other activities. For example, when self-stimulatory behavior is suppressed, appropriate play behaviors typically show an increase (Epstein et al., 1974; Koegel et al., 1974). Because articles such as these suggest that manipulations of one behavior could affect other behaviors, the purpose of this study was to manipulate a preactivity and test the effect of this preactivity on subsequent target behaviors. Also, the literature suggests that physical exercise may be an especially effective preactivity for positively influenc-

ing symptoms of a variety of neurological and psychological disorders (cf. Folkins & Sime, 1981; Ohlsen, 1978; Watters & Watters, 1980). Therefore, this experiment was specifically designed to increase autistic children's physical activity (jogging) and observe the effect this manipulation had on subsequent self-stimulation and appropriate behaviors. During the first portion of the experiment manipulations were made in controlled clinic settings; supplementary classroom measures were also obtained for three additional children. Data were collected over varying periods of time in a repeated-reversal design.

Method

Subjects

Seven children participated in this experiment. Four children, two males and two females, participated as subjects in the controlled clinic (first) portions of the experiment. Their ages were 7 years 6 months, 4 years 9 months, 5 years, and 6 years 11 months, respectively. They were diagnosed as autistic by two independent diagnosticians, each employing U.S. National Society for Autistic Children criteria (National Society for Autistic Children, 1978). They lived at home and attended special education classes in public schools. They were

Article Reprint Information: Reprinted from Springer/*Journal of Autism and Developmental Disorders, 12*(4), 1982, 399-419, The effects of physical exercise on self-stimulation and appropriate responding in autistic children, Kern, L., Koegel, R. L., Dyer, K., Blew, P. A., & Fenton, L. R., with kind permission from Springer Science and Business Media.

Table I.
Complete List of Self-Stimulatory Behaviors Recorded for the Four Children who Participated in the Controlled Portions of the Experiment

Child 1
1. Tongue manipulations (apex of tongue extended outside lips and repetitively moving, without phonation)
2. Spontaneous gutteral and glottal phonemes
3. Rubbing fingers repetitively on hands
4. Waving hands in air
5. Head shaking (small rapid movements from side to side)
6. Staring or gazing (a fixed, glassy-eyed look lasting more than 3 sec)
7. Repetitive rotation of eyes
8. Hands pressing on or twisting ears

Child 2
1. High-pitched, unintelligible vowel phonemes
2. Recognizable words produced repetitively and out of context
3. Repetitively hitting body with hand or fist
4. Rigid tensing of entire body
5. Waving hands in air
6. Gazing (a fixed, glassy-eyed look lasting more than 3 sec)
7. Hand placed in contact with eye or hand placed within 6" of eye in visual field

Child 3
1. Stereotypic phrases that are intelligible but with inappropriate syntax and without recognizable semantic intent (e.g., "Not stew in the air")
2. Hands vigorously and repetitively rubbing clothes
3. Hands vigorously and repetitively rubbing arms
4. Gutteral or glottal phonemes
5. Repetitive rotation of eyes
6. Giggling or laughing (except when adult-elicited)
7. Playing repetitively with eyeglasses while wearing them
8. Yawning repetitively
9. Clucking

Child 4
1. Hand placed in contact with eye or hand placed within 6" of eye in visual field
2. Clicking, clucking, teeth chattering, or audible teeth grinding
3. Inappropriate and rapid inhalation and exhalation at the rate of approximately 2 per sec
4. Repetitive breathy whistles
5. Nasal egressives or snorts
6. Spontaneous gutteral and glottal phonemes
7. Repetitively spitting and rubbing saliva
8. Mouthing of objects (nonedible objects in contact with mouth)
9. Mouthing of body parts (holding shoulder, hand, or finger(s) in mouth)
10. Jabbing or poking body with finger, thumb, or fist
11. Repetitively and vigorously pulling hair
12. Hand vigorously and repetitively rubbing skin or clothing

Table II.
Complete List of Self-Stimulatory and Off-Task Behaviors for Three Additional Children in Their Regular Classroom Setting

Child 5
1. Head shaking (small rapid movements from side to side)
2. Gazing at lights
3. Unintelligible phrases
4. Drawing on desktop
5. Scribbling on paper
6. Hitting or kicking teachers
7. Running around room
8. Out-of-context laughing
9. Banging on furniture

Child 6
1. Spinning objects
2. Gazing at lights
3. Out-of-context phrases
4. Unintelligible vowel phonemes
5. Singing

Child 7
1. Body rocking
2. Hand flapping
3. Out-of-context speech
4. Out-of-context laughing
5. Running around room
6. Tearing papers and books
7. Screaming

hibited by these children in their classroom are listed in Table II.

Prior to treatment, all seven children were diagnosed by a physician as being in good physical health and capable of physical activity (jogging).

Settings

Three experimental settings were randomly used in the first (controlled clinical) portions of the study. (1) In order to assess the influence of jogging on ball-playing and self-stimulation, a large open field approximately 50 x 15 meters was employed, with the child and the therapist playing catch as described below under Ball-Playing. (2) In order to assess the influence of jogging on academic tasks a 2.5 x 3-meter clinic room was employed, with the child and the therapist seated and interacting in a teaching situation (see Academic Responses, below) at a small table containing the stimulus materials. (3) In order to assess the influence of jogging when the child was not subsequently engaging in potentially incompatible behaviors, a quiet room was employed. This latter room was identical to the clinic room except no therapist or task materials were present. One to three data recorders were always present in each of the three settings.

In the second portion of the study, the children were in their regular classroom

selected for participation in this experiment because they had particularly high levels of self-stimulatory behaviors (cf. baseline measurements in Results section). The specific types of self-stimulatory behaviors the children in the first portion of this experiment demonstrated are listed in Table I.

The children's standardized test results represented a wide range of abilities. Children 2 and 4 were considered to be untestable with standardized intelligence testing procedures. They had no functional expressive speech or language skills and limited receptive language abilities. Their social quotients on the Vineland Social Maturity Scale were 48 and 60, respectively. Children 1 and 3 were echolalic but had some appropriate language skills. Child 1's social quotient on the Vineland Social Maturity Scale was 60 and her IQ, measured on the WPPSI, was 48. Child 3's social quotient as measured by the Vineland Social Maturity Scale was 58 and his IQ as measured on the WPPSI was 59.

Supplementary applied classroom measures were also obtained for three additional children. The ages for these children (5, 6, and 7) were 14 years 6 months, 12 years 8 months, and 9 years 2 months, respectively. These children were also diagnosed as autistic by the same criteria listed above and they were functioning academically at the kindergarten/first-grade level. They were selected as subjects because they demonstrated exceptionally high levels on self-stimulatory and related off-task behaviors in their regular classroom setting. The specific self-stimulatory and off-task behaviors ex-

setting. This was a special education classroom for eight developmentally disabled children. Three teachers were present at all times, and they presented the children with their regularly assigned classroom materials, which generally followed a kindergarten/first-grade curriculum format.

Therapists and Therapy Programs

All of the therapists employed in this investigation had a minimum of one course in the behavior modification treatment of autism. During a randomly determined 85% of the experimental sessions and all of the classroom sessions, therapists and teachers who were naive to the experimental questions were employed to interact with the children. Consequences were employed for the children's responses during the various clinical and academic tasks (e.g., saying "good" and smiling for correct responses, and saying "no" for incorrect responses). These contingencies remained constant across all conditions in the experiment. Naturally, in the quiet room (where no therapist was present) no contingencies were in effect for any behavior.

Design

The major portion of the data from this investigation was collected within a repeated-reversal design (cf. Hersen & Barlow, 1976). There were a total of 45 reversals between pre- and postjogging sessions occurring both within and across the 21 days of data collection in this portion of the investigation. Also, data showing longer prejogging (baseline) levels of self-stimulation and data for additional children are included. Child 2 had an extremely long history of exceptionally high levels of self-stimulatory behaviors. These behaviors were typical of those illustrated in her baseline measurements, which were randomly sampled over a 6-month period. During this period no more than three sessions took place per day, and no more than 2 weeks elapsed between sessions. Similar to the other children, Child 2's last baseline sessions and the postjogging sessions were conducted on a single day.

Independent Variable

Jogging. In each jogging session, an adult and the child jogged side by side (holding hands if the child began to stray from the area). No direct interventions were made with respect to any of the children's self-stimulatory behaviors during these sessions. The jogging pace was adjusted in each session to be fast enough to be mildly strenuous (e.g., child showed increased breathing rate or slightly flushed face) but was slowed

to a temporary walk (approximately 15 sec) if the child began to show any observable signs of discomfort (e.g., appearing out of breath or attempting to pull away from the adult's hand). The total length of the jogging period for each child during the initial sessions of the investigation varied between 5 and 10 min (not counting the occasional 15-sec walks). After the initial sessions, the sessions were gradually lengthened to 20 min over the course of the experiment (as the children's endurance increased). The length and pace of each child's jogging sessions were determined in accordance with the recommendations of the children's physicians. In summary, throughout all portions of this investigation, the rule determining the length and pace of the jogging in each session was that the jog be mildly strenuous, with the limitation that it did not become aversive for the child.

Dependent Variables

Measures were obtained for the influence of jogging on three separate dependent variables: (1) self-stimulation, (2) ball-playing, and (3) academic responding. The measurement procedures for recording each of these behaviors are described in detail below.

Self-Stimulation. Throughout all portions of the experiment, data were recorded every 15 min both before and after jogging on the children's self-stimulation. A time-sampling procedure was employed for 5 min at the start of each 15-min session. In each of these 5-min samples, data were recorded during 5-sec intervals, with 10 sec after each interval (one of the two recorders timed these intervals with a stopwatch and verbally signaled the start and finish of each interval). For each of the resulting 20 sessions, self-stimulation (as defined for each child in Table I) was recorded on a precoded data sheet with a plus if it occurred or with a minus if it did not occur. The percentage of intervals with self-stimulation was then computed separately for each child in each session.

Ball-Playing. The influence of jogging on subsequent sessions involving appropriate play (ball-playing) was assessed as follows. During each of these sessions (pre- and postjogging) the therapist and the child interacted by playing catch in the large 50 x 15-meter open field. In order to ensure that it would be possible for the child to catch the ball easily, a maximum distance of 2 to 3 meters was maintained between the child and the therapist, with the therapist saying "catch" and gently throwing a large (20-cm) lightweight plastic ball to the child. The ball

was thrown at a minimum rate of five times per min. The maximum rate of ball-playing was determined by the speed with which the child returned the ball to the therapist (i.e., the therapist would always throw the ball back to the child immediately after receiving it from the child). However, in instances when the child made no attempt to catch or return the ball, the therapist would pick up the ball and gently throw it to the child at the minimum rate of five times per min.

Throughout these sessions ball-playing responses were recorded as correct or incorrect continuously during the time-sampling periods. Self-stimulatory behavior was also recorded during these time-sampling periods, as described above. A correct ball-playing response was recorded each time the child caught the ball and threw it back to the therapist. Because of the relatively simple nature of this task (see above), every time the child attempted (i.e., reached out) to catch the ball, the child was able to catch the ball easily. Incorrect ball-playing responses were recorded each time the child made no attempt to catch the ball (i.e., simply stood still without reaching for the ball at all) or when the child threw the ball in a direction directly away from the therapist (approximately 90 degrees sideways).

Academic Responses. In order to assess the influence of jogging sessions involving both academic responding and self-stimulatory behavior, data were recorded pre- and postjogging for Child 2 in the clinic setting, where she was working on several preschool-level tasks. Self-stimulatory behavior continued to be recorded as described above. In addition, academic responding was recorded continuously on a trial-by-trial basis. The academic responding involved two preschool level tasks: matching colors and shapes, and imitative gross motor activities. No direct manipulation of the child's self-stimulation took place during these sessions, and the pacing of the therapist's instructions was determined by the latency of the child's responding. When a child failed to respond at all within approximately 5 sec of an instruction, the therapist repeated the instruction. The child's response on each trial was recorded as correct if the child responded appropriately to the discriminative stimulus "Where does this go" for matching, or "Do this" (while the therapist modeled the behavior) for gross motor imitation. No response or an incorrect response following the delivery of this discriminative stimulus was counted as an incorrect response.

Reliability

Reliability measures were obtained for each of the three dependent variables (self-stimulation, ball-playing, and academic responding). Two observers (one naive to the purpose of the experiment) independently recorded occurrences and nonoccurrences of self-simulatory behavior during the 20 5-sec intervals in each of 36 randomly selected sessions in the three settings. Percent agreement was calculated on an interval-by-interval basis. An agreement consisted of both the observers recording exactly the same response (e.g., either both recorded the occurrence or both recorded the nonoccurrence of the behavior for that particular interval). Percent agreement was calculated separately for occurrences and nonoccurrences for every session by dividing the number of agreements by the number of agreements plus disagreements. The average percent agreement for recording self-stimulation across the 36 sessions were 88% (range: 50% to 100%). During the ball-playing and academic tasks two additional observers recorded responding for all of the relevant sessions in this experiment. During these sessions the two observers maintained 100% agreement for both correct and incorrect responses.

Supplementary Measures in an Applied Classroom Setting

Given the applied significance of the persent investigation, it also seemed important to gather supplementary measures on related behaviors in an applied classroom setting. Therefore, three additional children were provided with brief periods of jogging during their regular daily classroom activities (at recess time). Data were collected within the context of a repeated-reversal design, comparing no-jogging and jogging recess conditions within and across 6 days of data collection. One or (in 50% of the intervals) two observers independently recorded data on on-task behavior and overall interest during 15-min sessions in each experimental condition.

A child was scored as "on task" when he was (1) sitting quietly, (2) looking at the teacher or classroom materials, or (3) following directions. A child was scored as "off task" when any of the following behaviors occurred: (1) self-stimulation (e.g., flapping, spinning objects, glassy-eyed stare), (2) leaving the chair without permission, (3) aggression (e.g., hitting and kicking), or (4) screaming. If a child took longer than 10 sec to respond to an instruction, he was also scored as off task. Point-by-point interobserver agreement averaged 93% across the

24 sessions in this part of the study.

General interest was also rated by one or (in 50% of the intervals) two observers according to a scale developed by Dunlap and Koegel (1980). This scale numerically rates interest, happiness, and general behavior. Zero to 1.66 indicates disinterest and behavior problems related to escaping the task; 1.67 to 3.33 indicates that the child was involved in the task and exhibited a generally positive level of compliance, and 3.34 to 5 indicates an extremely well-behaved, happy, interested and actively enthusiastic child. The data were recorded in a time-sample technique by observing a child for six consecutive 2½ intervals. At the end of each 15-min session, the ratings from each 2½ interval were added together and divided by the total number of intervals to arrive at a mean rating of child interest for each session. Interobserver agreement on a session-by-session basis for these interest ratings averaged 76%.

Results

The first question asked in this investigation was: Does physical exercise (jogging) decrease autistic children's subsequent self-stimulatory behaviors? The results of the 45 reversals between pre- and postjogging conditions within and across the first 21 days of the experiment are shown in Figure 1 for Children 1 and 2. Percentages of self-stimulation are plotted on the ordinate. Successive 15-min sessions are plotted on the abscissa. The graph shows that: (1) in every instance the children had relatively high levels of self-stimulation prior to jogging, and (2) following jogging there was always a marked decrease in self-stimulatory behavior. This was clearly demonstrated both within and across days. For example, Child 1's initial prejogging level was 75%. Immediately following her first jog her self-stimulation decreased to 70%, and 15 min after the jog a further decrease to 35% was demonstrated. On days 2 and 3 her self-stimulation again returned to the baseline level prior to jogging but again decreased following each respective jogging session. On day 4 this same reversal effect was demonstrated within a single day. That is, on day 4 Child 1's self-stimulatory behaviors averaged 60% during three sessions prior to jogging. Following the jog her self-stimulation rapidly decreased to 20%. Then, 1 hour and 15 min following the jog her self-stimulation again returned to the baseline level.

Child 2's data show this same pattern. For example, on day 1, Child 2's prejogging level was 95%. Immediately following the

jog her self-stimulation decreased to 75%. Similar decreasing trends were replicated across 16 subsequent days. As noted above, to assess whether the jogging effects would occur consistently across settings, Child 2's sessions were randomly assigned to three different settings: a clinic setting where she worked on preschool-level academic tasks, a ball-playing setting in an outside play area, and a quiet room with no people or task materials present. In all instances, self-stimulatory behaviors were always high before the jogging was instituted and always decreased following the jogging, regardless of the setting.

On day 17 four reversal conditions occurred on the same day. Specifically, on day 17 self-stimulation during the initial three prejogging sessions averaged 98.3% (range: 95% to 100%). Following the first jog a rapid decrease was evidenced. Then, 1½ hours later, the child's self-stimulatory behaviors began to increase again. When the child's self-stimulation had returned to baseline levels, a second jogging session was implemented. Following the second jog another decrease in self-stimulation occurred.

In summary, throughout the 45 reversals between pre- and postjogging sessions, the results demonstrated that jogging always produced a decrease in the amount of subsequent self-stimulatory behavior. This was true both within and across days, and in the three different settings.

Figure 2 shows the same decreasing effects after jogging for more children. The figure also includes random samples of Child 2's self-stimulatory behavior obtained over a 6-month period.

The figure shows that in this portion of the investivation, Child 1's prejogging self-stimulatory behaviors were variable but still relatively high (ranging between 45% and 80%) over the initial four prejogging sessions. After jogging her self-stimulatory behavior showed a rapid decreasing trend, with the lowest points being 30% and 35%. Child 1 also showed a replication of the effect when her behavior was measured again (on day 6). On that day, during seven prejogging sessions her self-stimulatory behavior averaged 61% (range 50% to 75%). Following jogging, her self-stimulatory behavior again showed a decreasing trend, with the last session at 30%.

Child 2's prejogging data were measured over a longer period of time. Her self-stimulation was measured on random days over a 6-month period before jogging was instituted. During these 6 months her self-stimulation averaged 93% (range 75% to 100%). Then, on the final day of the 6-

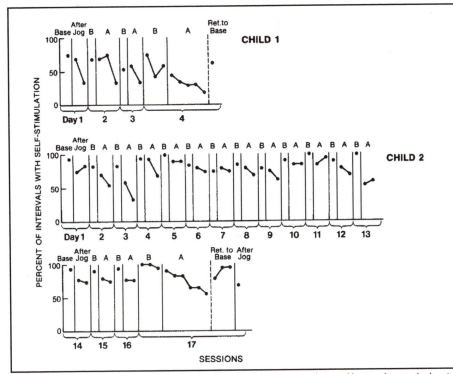

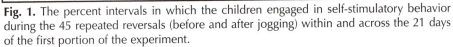

Fig. 1. The percent intervals in which the children engaged in self-stimulatory behavior during the 45 repeated reversals (before and after jogging) within and across the 21 days of the first portion of the experiment.

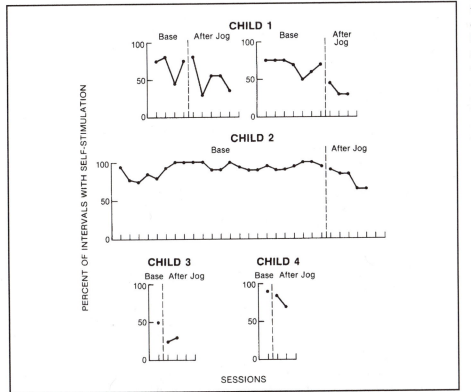

Fig. 2. Additional self-stimulation data with longer baselines, and two additional children.

The other children also showed relatively high levels of self-stimulation before jogging and decreases immediately after jogging. Child 3's prejogging self-stimulation decreased to an average of 27.5%. Child 4's self-stimulation was 95% before he jogged and decreased to 65% by 15 minutes after jogging. In summary, the decreases in self-stimulation after jogging were evidenced in all of the children, including the children whose baseline measurements demonstrated that self-stimulation had been high for long periods of time prior to the initiation of jogging.

Ball-Playing and Academic Responding

Given the above results, it seemed important to determine if decreases such as those shown in Figures 1 and 2 were specific to self-stimulatory behavior, or if some sort of fatigue effect was occurring that might also cause appropriate behaviors such as the children's ball-playing and correct academic responding to decrease. Therefore, additional data were recorded for Child 2 on 12 subsequent days. Figure 3 shows these data. On each of the 12 days there was a replicated inverse relationship between the amount of self-stimulation and the amount of appropriate responding. For example, during Child 1's first prejogging ball-playing session she engaged in self-stimulation 90% of the time and responded 40 times during ball-playing. After jogging, however, her self-stimulation decreased to an average of 75.5% (80% immediately after the jog and 70% 15 min later), while in contrast, her ball-play responding increased to an average of 62.5 times per session (46 and 79 times, respectively). The subsequent sessions over the 12 days of various ball-playing and academic tasks showed essentially the same type of relationship; self-stimulation always decreased and appropriate responding always increased.

Supplementary Classroom Measures

The results for the supplementary classroom measures are shown in Figure 4 for Children 5, 6, and 7. Percentages of intervals with on-task behavior are plotted on the ordinate, and successive 15-min sessions are plotted on the abscissa. The data show higher levels of on-task behavior for each child following jogging sessions relative to no-jogging sessions on days 1, 2, and 4. This is in contrast to minimal or no changes in the levels of on-task behavior on days 3 and 6 when jogging was not implemented.

The results of the interest ratings are presented in Table III. The data show that dur-

month period, jogging was initiated. After jogging her self-stimulatory behavior immediately began to decrease, with the last two sessions at 65%, i.e., 10% lower than her lowest level during any of the 6-month prejogging samples.

Table III.
Summary of General Interest Ratings for Children 5, 6, and 7 Following the No-Jogging and Jogging Recess Conditions[α]

	Enthusiasm ratings	
	No jog	Jog
Child 5	1.06	2.14
Child 6	1.55	2.43
Child 7	1.57	2.77
$\bar{X}$ =	1.39	2.45

[α]Levels between 0 and 1.66 indicate lack of interest and behavior problems related to escaping the task; 1.67 to 3.33 indicates that the child was involved in the task; and exhibited a generally positive level of compliance on the task; and 3.34 to 5.0 indicates an extremely well-behaved, happy, interested, and actively enthusiastic child.

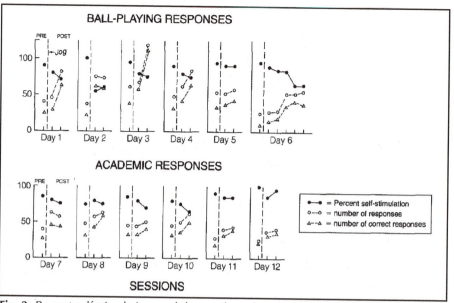

Fig. 3. Percent self-stimulation, and the number of academic and ball-playing responses are plotted on the ordinate for clinic and play sessions in the first portion of the experiment.

ing the no-jogging conditions each child received ratings in the negative category. Specifically, the children were rated as being disruptive, noncompliant, and uninterested in the classroom activities. In contrast, the data from the jogging conditions show that the children typically received ratings indicating that the children were involved in their school tasks and exhibited a generally positive level of compliance.

Discussion

The results showing that jogging decreased self-stimulatory behavior and increased appropriate play and academic responding may be discussed in relation to several issues.

First, it is interesting to consider the results in relation to the possible effects of fatigue. It is notable that fatigue, per se, did not appear to have been an important variable. While self-stimulatory behaviors always decreased after jogging, other appropriate behaviors such as play and academic responding always increased.

Such inverse relationships have been demonstrated in numerous investigations with autistic children (e.g., Epstein et al., 1974; Koegel & Covert, 1972; Koegel et al., 1974). Similarly, body rocking has been reduced in blind children through the use of vigorous exercise (Ohlsen, 1978). Thus, it seems possible that jogging may directly decrease the children's self-stimulatory behavior and therefore indirectly increase the appropriate behaviors.

Another possibility is that jogging, aside from affecting self-stimulatory behaviors, may also directly increase appropriate responding (cf. McKechney, 1972). In areas outside of the field of autism, and among populations of various ages, there are numerous studies that have shown physical

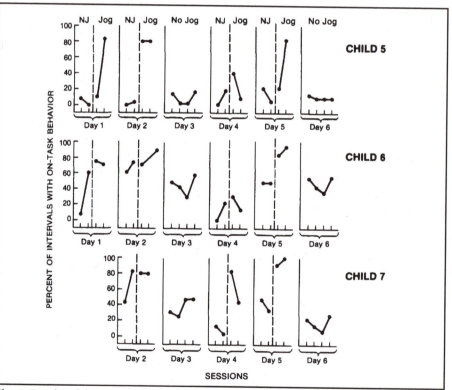

Fig. 4. Results of the repeated-reversal analysis of the influence of no-jogging versus jogging recess conditions on the on-task behavior of Children 5, 6, and 7 during their subsequent classroom activities.

exercise to improve cognitive and physical performance. For example, certain perceptual motor training programs have been shown to cause significant increases in visual-motor function (Schaney, Brekke, Landry, & Burke, 1976). Jogging also has been shown to cause significant improve-

ments in physical fitness and psychological tests of psychiatric hospital patients aged from the teens on into the 50s (Dodson & Mullens, 1969). Similarly, Powell (1974) and Diesfeldt and Diesfeldt-Groenendijk (1977) found significant improvements in two of three cognitive tests in institutionalized geriatric mental patients. In another area, Eickelberg, Less, and Engels (1976) found significant increases in learning in passively exercised muscular distrophic children.

Although some investigations have found that certain types of exercise do not have a favorable effect on learning, there is no consistent evidence in the literature showing that physical exercise is detrimental to learning (cf. Stoner, 1972). However, it is possible that the exact type and duration of exercise may be important. For example, Dodson and Mullens (1969) examined type of exercise (light exercise and jogging) and Gupta, Sharma, and Jaspal (1974) examined the amount of time of exercising. In each case there were differential effects depending on the type or amount of exercise, suggesting that further research in this area may be quite important.

One last issue that should be noted concerns the relative magnitude of the changes in self-stimulatory behavior, and the clinical implications of these changes. In this experiment, while the changes in self-stimulation did seem to have important influences on the children's appropriate responding, the absolute magnitude of the changes in self-stimulatory behavior per se were relatively small. This suggests several possible avenues that may be important for future research. For example, some researchers have discussed the likelihood that various types of self-stimulatory behavior may be differentially influenced by different types of treatment, and that these various subcategories of self-stimulatory behaviors may have important differential influences on the children's behavior (cf. Dunlap, Dyer, & Koegel, Note 1).

Physiological Implications

Although no physiological data were taken in the present investigation, research on the physiological effects of physical activity suggests that strenuous physical activity causes physiological changes, such as the release of beta-endorphins and changes acetylcholine levels (Fraioli, Moretti, Paolucci, Alicicco, Crescenzi, & Fortunio, 1980; VonEuler, 1974). Of particular interest to the present investigation is the fact that other research has shown that such physiological changes seem to positively influence motivation (LeMoal, Koob, & Bloom, 1979), improve attention (Sandman, George, Walker, & Nolan, 1976), facilitate perceptual integration (Sandman, George, McCanne, Nolan, Kaswan, & Kastin, 1977), and counteract effects of mental fatigue (Gaillard & Sanders, 1975). Acetylcholine has also been

associated with emotional conditions (Frankenhaeuser, 1970), including aggression (Ismail & Young, 1977; Sage, 1971). These findings are particularly interesting as children with autism frequently display problems with motivation (Dunlap & Koegel, 1980; Koegel & Egel, 1979), overselective attention (Koegel & Wilhelm, 1973; Lovaas, Schreibman, Koegel, & Rehm, 1971), short-term memory (Hingtgen & Bryson, 1972; O'Conner & Hermelin, 1965), and aggression (Carr, Newsom, & Binkoff, 1980). In view of these and numerous other investigations hypothesizing a physiological etiology of autism (e.g., Blackstock, 1978; Coleman, 1979; Damasio & Maurer, 1979; Hauser, DeLong, & Rosman, 1975; Hier, LeMay, & Rosenberger, 1979; Ornitz & Ritvo, 1976; Rutter & Bartak, 1971; Schopler & Reichler, 1971; Student & Sohmer, 1978; Tanguay, 1976; Wetherby, Koegel, & Mendel, 1981), investigation into the physiological correlates of physical activity in autistic children may be an especially promising area for future research.

Educational Implications

Physical exercise has been demonstrated to decrease self-stimulatory and related off-task behaviors, and has also been shown to improve cognitive functioning in numerous populations. Thus, it is encouraging that many educational programs provide brief periods of physical exercise (e.g., recess) for their students. However, most programs do not systematically provide for any given type or amount of activity. This systematic programming of physical activities into the child's day seems especially important in light of the results of our applied classroom measures. Because the literature suggests that amount, duration, and type of physical activity all appear to be important variables that can affect performance, it seems quite likely that this also may be a particularly profitable area for future research related to classroom curriculum development.

Reference Note

1. Dunlap, G., Dyer, K., & Koegel, R. L. *Autistic versus normal self-stimulation.* Paper submitted for publication, 1982.

References

Berkson, G., & Mason, W. A. Stereotyped movements of mental defectives: III. Situation effects. *American Journal of Mental Deficiency,* 1963, *68,* 409-412.

Blackstock, E. Cerebral asymmetry and the development of early infantile autism. *Journal of Autism and Childhood Schizophrenia,* 1978, 8, 338-353.

Carr, E. G., Newsom, C. D., & Binkoff, J. A. Escape as a factor in the aggressive behavior of

two retarded children. *Journal of Applied Behavior Analysis,* 1980, *13,* 101-117.

Chock, P. N. *Learning and self-stimulation in mute and echolalic autistic children.* Unpublished doctoral dissertation, University of California, Santa Barbara, 1979.

Coleman, M. Studies of the autistic syndromes. In R. Katzman (Ed.), *Congential and acquired cognitive disorders.* New York: Raven Press, 1979.

Damasio, A., & Maurer, R. A neurological model for childhood autism. *Archives of Neurology,* 1979, *35,* 777-786.

Diesfeldt, H. F. A., & Diesfeldt-Groenendijk, II. Improving cognitive performance in psychogeriatric patients: The influence of physical exercise. *Age and Aging,* 1977, 6, 58-64.

Dodson, L. C., & Mullens, W. R. Some effects of jogging on psychiatric hospital patients. *American Correctional Therapy Journal,* 1969, 5, 130-134.

Dunlap, G., & Koegel, R. L. Motivating autistic children through stimulus variation. *Journal of Applied Behavior Analysis,* 1980, *13,* 619-628.

Eickelberg, W. W. B., Less, M., & Engels, W. C. Respiratory, cardiac and learning changes in exercised muscular dystrophic children. *Perceptual and Motor Skills,* 1976, *43,* 66.

Epstein, L. H., Doke, L. A., Sajwaj, T. E., Sorell, S., & Rimmer, B. Generality and side effects of overcorrection. *Journal of Applied Behavior Analysis,* 1974, 7, 385-390.

Folkins, C. H., & Sime, W. E. Physical fitness training and mental health. *American Psychologist,* 1981, 4, 373-389.

Forehand, R., & Baumeister, A. A. Stereotyped body rocking as a function of situation, IQ, and time. *Journal of Clinical Psychology,* 1971, 27, 324-326.

Foxx, R. M., & Azrin, H. H. Restitution: A method of eliminating aggressive-disruptive behavior of retarded and brain damaged patients. *Behaviour Research and Therapy,* 1972, *10,* 15-27.

Fraioli, F., Moretti, C., Paolucci, D., Alicicco, E., Crescenzi, F., & Fortunio, G. Physical exercise stimulates marked concomitant release of B-endorphin and adrenocorticotropic hormone (ACTH) in peripheral blood in man. *Experientia,* 1980, *36,* 987-989.

Frankel, F., Freeman, B. J., Ritvo, E., & Pardo, R. The effect of environmental stimulation upon the stereotyped behavior of autistic children. *Journal of Autism and Childhood Schizophrenia,* 1978, *8,* 389-394.

Frankenhaeuser, M. Catecholamines and behavior. *Brain Research,* 1970, *24,* 541-559.

Gaillard, A. W. K., & Sanders, A. F. Some effects of ACTH 4-10 on performance during a serial reaction task. *Psychopharmacologia,* 1975, *42,* 201-208.

Glahn, T. J. *Play behaviors in autistic children.* Unpublished doctoral dissertation, University of California, Santa Barbara, 1980.

Gupta, V. P., Sharma, T. R., & Jaspal, S. S. Physical activity and efficiency of mental work. *Perceptual and Motor Skills,* 1974, *38,* 205-206.

Hargrave, E., & Swisher, L. Modifying the verbal

expression of a child with autistic behaviors. *Journal of Autism and Childhood Schizophrenia,* 1975, *5,* 147-154.

Hauser, S., Delong, G., & Rosman, N. Pneumographic findings in the infantile autism syndrome. *Brain,* 1975, *98,* 667-688.

Hersen, M., & Barlow, D. H. *Single case experimental designs: Strategies for studying behavior change.* New York: Pergamon Press, 1976.

Hier, D., LeMay, M., & Rosenberger, P. Autism and unfavorable left-right asymmetries of the brain. *Journal of Autism and Developmental Disorders,* 1979, *9,* 153-159.

Hingtgen, J. W., & Bryson, C. Q. Research developments in the study of early childhood psychoses: Infantile autism, childhood schizophrenia, and related disorders. *Schizophrenia Bulletin,* 1972, *5,* 8-54.

Hung, D. W. Using self-stimulation as reinforcement for autistic children. *Journal of Autism and Childhood Schizophrenia,* 1978, *8,* 369.

Hutt, S., & Hutt, C. Stereotypy, arousal and autism. *Human Development,* 1968, *11,* 277-286.

Ismail, A. H., & Young, J. R. Effect of chronic exercise on the multivariate relationships between selected biochemical and personality variables. *Journal of Multivariate Behavioral Research,* 1977, *2,* 49-67.

Klier, J., & Harris, S. L. Self-stimulation and learning in autistic children: Physical or functional incompatibility? *Journal of Applied Behavior Analysis,* 1977, *10,* 311.

Koegel, R. L., & Covert, A. The relationship of self-stimulation to learning in autistic children. *Journal of Applied Behavior Analysis,* 1972, 5, 381-387.

Koegel, R. L., & Egel, A. L. Motivating autistic children. *Journal of Abnormal Psychology,* 1979, *88,* 418-426.

Koegel, R. L., Firestone, P. B., Kramme, K. W., & Dunlap, G. Increasing spontaneous play by suppressing self-stimulation in autistic children. *Journal of Applied Behavior Analysis,* 1974, *7,* 521-528.

Koegel, R. L., & Wilhelm, H. Selective responding to the components of multiple visual cues by autistic children. *Journal of Experimental ChiM Psychology,* 1973, *15,* 442-453.

LeMoal, M., Koob, G. F., & Bloom F. E. Endorphins and extinction: Differential actions on appetite and adversive tasks. *Life Sciences,* 1979, *24,* 1631-1636.

Lovaas, O. I. Behavior therapy approach to treatment of childhood schizophrenia. In *Minesota symposium of child development.* Minneapolis: University of Minnesota Press, 1967.

Lovaas, O. I., Litrownik, A., & Mann, R. Response latencies to auditory stimuli in autistic children engaged in self-stimulatory behavior. *Behaviour Research and Therapy,* 1971, *9,* 39-49.

Lovaas, O. I., Schreibman, L., Koegel, R. L., & Rehm, R. Selective responding by autistic children to multiple sensory input. *Journal of Abnormal Psychology,* 1971, *77,* 211-222.

McKechney, R. G. *The effects of exercise upon learning under psychological stress of rats.* Unpublished doctoral dissertation, University of Minnesota, 1972.

National Society for Autistic Children. National Society for Autistic Children definition of the syndrome of autism. *Journal of Autism and Childhood Schizophrenia,* 1978, *8,* 162-167.

O'Connor, N., & Hermelin, B. Visual analogies of verbal operations. *Language and Speech,* 1965, *8,* 197-207.

Ohlsen, R. L. Control of body rocking in the blind through the use of vigorous exercise. *Journal of Instructional Psychology,* 1978, *5,* 19-22.

Ornitz, E., & Ritvo, E. The syndrome of autism: A critical review. *American Journal of Psychiatry,* 1976, *133,* 609-621.

Powell, R. R. Psychological effects of exercise therapy upon institutionalized geriatric mental patients. *Journal of Gerontology,* 1974, *29,* 157-161.

Rincover, A. Sensory extinction: A procedure for eliminating self-stimulating behavior in autistic children. *Journal of Abnormal Child Psychology,* 1978, *6,* 299-310.

Rincover, A., Cook, R., Peoples, A., & Packard, D. Sensory extinction and sensory reinforcement principles for programming multiple adaptive behavior change. *Journal of Applied Behavior Analysis,* 1979, *12,* 221-223.

Risley, T. R. The effects and side effects of punishing the autistic behaviors of a deviant child. *Journal of Applied Behavior Analysis,* 1968, *1,* 21-34.

Rutter, M., & Bartak, L. Causes of infantile autism: Some considerations from recent research. *Journal of Autism and Childhood Schizophrenia,* 1971, *1,* 20-32.

Sage, G. H. *Introduction to motor behavior: A neuropsychological approach.* Reading, Massachusetts: Addison-Wesley, 1971.

Sandman, D. A., George, J., McCanne, T. R., Nolan, J. D., Kaswan, J., & Kastin, A. J. MSH/ACTH 4-10 influences behavioral and physiological measures of attention. *Journal of Clinical Endrocrine Metabolism,* 1977, *44,* 884-891.

Sandman, D. A., George, J., Walker, B. B., & Nolan, J. D. Neuropeptide MSH/ACTH 4-10 enhances attention in the mentally ret.arded. *Pharmacology, Biochemistry and Behavior,* 1976, *5*(Suppl. 1), 23-28.

Schaney, Z., Brekke, B., Landry, R., & Burke, J. Effects of a perceptual-motor training program on kindergarten children. *Perceptual and Motor Skills,* 1976, *43,* 428-430.

Schopler, E., & Reichler, R. J. Psychobiological referents for the treatment of autism. In D. W. Churchill, G. D. Alpern, and M. K. DeMeyer (Eds.), *Infantile autism.* Springfield, Illinois: Charles C. Thomas, 1971.

Stoner, J. C. *The effects of two levels of pre-task exercise upon the performance of a gross motor task by educable mentally retarded children.* Unpublished doctoral dissertation, University of Georgia, 1972.

Student, M., & Sohmer, H. Evidence from auditory nerve and brainstem-evoked responses for an organic brain lesion in children with autistic traits. *Journal of Autism and Childhood Schizophrenia,* 1978, *8,* 13-20.

Tanguay, P. Clinical and electrophysiological research. In E. Ritvo (Ed.), *Autism: Diagnosis, current research and management.* New York: Spectrum, 1976.

Thelen, E. Rhythmical stereotypies in normal human infants. *Animal Behaviour,* 1979, *27,* 699-715.

VonEuler, U. S. Sympatho-adrenal activity in physical exercise. *Medicine and Science in Sports,* 1974, *6,* 165-173.

Watters, R. G., & Watters, W. E. Decreasing self-stimulatory behavior with physical exercise in a group of autistic boys. *Journal of Autism and Developmental Disorders,* 1980, *10,* 379-387.

Wetherby, A. M., Koegel, R. L., & Mendel, M. Central auditory nervous system dysfunction in echolalic autistic individuals. *Journal of Speech and Hearing Research,* 1981, *24,* 420-429.

The Effects of Exercise Intensity on the Stereotypic Behaviors of Individuals With Autism

Leslie J. Levinson, Greg Reid

The effects of exercise intensity on the stereotypic behaviors of three subjects with autism were examined. Two exercise programs of different intensities were implemented. The mild exercise program involved 15 min of walking, and the vigorous program involved 15 min of jogging. The frequency of stereotypic behavior was measured prior to exercise, immediately following exercise, and 90 min following exercise. The results indicated that significant reductions in stereotypic behaviors occurred as a function of the vigorous exercise condition only. The mean reduction of stereotypic behaviors between prejogging and postjogging was 17.5%. However, the duration of these reductions was temporary. Increases to preexercise levels were noted in stereotypic behaviors 90 min after exercise. The stereotypic behaviors of subjects were categorized into three components: motor, vocal/oral, and other. The motor component was most common. The mild exercise condition had little effect on the motor component; the vigorous condition resulted in a mean reduction of 17%.

Leslie J. Levinson is with the MacKay Center, 3500 Decarie Blvd., Montreal, PQ H4A 3J5. Greg Reid is with the Department of Physical Education, McGill University, 375 Pine Ave. West, Montreal, PQ, Canada H2W 154. Request reprints from Greg Reid.

A large majority of individuals with autism engage in acts of self-stimulation or stereotypic motor patterns (Koegel, Egel, & Dunlap, 1980). As such, self-stimulation is considered to be a defining characteristic of autism (Margolies, 1977). These behaviors are defined as repetitive nonfunctional behaviors (Foxx & Azrin, 1973) and include rhythmic rocking, repetitive jumping, arm flapping, floor pacing, object spinning, hand staring, eye rolling or crossing, and toe walking (Cushings, Adams, & Rincover, 1983).

Stereotypic behaviors prevent appropriate response to the environment. These behaviors have been shown to interfere with previously learned behaviors (Bucher & Lovaas, 1968) and with learning (Koegel & Covert, 1972). Lovaas, Newson, and Hickman (1987) stated in their review article that children with autism who engaged in stereotypic behaviors were hard to reach and oblivious to external stimuli. Because stereotypic behaviors interfere with learning, the elimination or control of these behaviors remains a priority.

A variety of methods have been used to reduce stereotypic behaviors. These range from implementing severe forms of physical punishment such as electrical shock (Baroff & Tate, 1968; Lichstein & Schreibman, 1976; Lovaas, Schaeffer, & Simmons, 1965) and inhalation of ammonia (Baumeister & Baumeister, 1978) to milder methods such as overcorrection (Foxx & Azrin, 1973; Maag, Rutherford, Wolchik, & Parks, 1986). Several researchers have attempted to reduce stereotypic behaviors by altering the physical environment (Duker & Rasing, 1989; Frankel, Freeman, Ritvo, & Pardo, 1978; Runco, Charlop, & Schreibman, 1986), whereas others have varied task variables such as timing (Dunlap, Dyer, & Koegel, 1983) and reinforcement (Haring, Breen, Pitts-Conway, & Gaylord-Ross, 1986).

Physical activity has been used recently to reduce stereotypic behaviors. Several studies have probed the influence of exercise on self-stimulation. Watters and Watters (1980) noted a mean decrease in self-stimulation of 32.7% following exercise. Allen (1980) found that 10 min of jogging was most effective in reducing the number of negative behaviors. Kern, Koegel, Dyer, Blew, and Fenton (1982) showed that jogging decreased self-stimulation and increased appropriate play and academic responding. Kern and colleagues (Kern, Koegel, & Dunlap, 1984) examined the differential effects of mild and vigorous exercise on stereotypic behaviors. They found that the mild exercise condition had little or no influence on the subject's subsequent stereotypic behaviors, whereas the vigorous exercise condition was always followed by reductions in stereotypic behaviors. Bachman and Fuqua (1983) also varied exercise intensity by alternating no jogging, warming up, moderate jogging, and vigorous jogging. They found a mean decrease of 20.8% in the level of inappropriate behaviors whenever exercise occurred, even if the exercise was only warming up.

The present study addresses two important factors concerning the effects of exercise on stereotypic behaviors: the intensity of exercise and the duration of effects. Kern et al. (1984) concluded that vigorous exercise resulted in greater reduction of stereotypic behaviors than mild exercise. However, the process by which the authors differentiated between the intensity of the two exercise conditions was not precise. They assumed that ball catching and throwing activities were less vigorous than jogging. It is necessary to clearly differentiate between mild and vigorous levels of exercise and then examine their relative effects on stereotypic behavior. As well, an examination of the duration of any decrease in stereotypic behaviors is necessary to evaluate its practical utility. Some related evidence indicates that the positive influences of exercise on stereotypic behaviors may be short lived (Allen, 1980; Bachman & Fuqua, 1983).

The conceptual basis for the present study rests on the self-stimulation/feedback theory that stereotypic behaviors are maintained by resulting feedback (Berkson, 1983; Lovaas et al., 1987). Berkson (1983) stated that in order to maintain this sensory input, the behaviors must be repetitive, and the most efficient manner to maintain a behavior is to move in a rhythmic pattern, hence the rhythmic, repetitive nature of stereotypies. Berkson (1983) noted research showing that removal of sensory feedback will eliminate stereotypic behaviors (Rincover, 1978). In one example, the stereotypic behavior of spinning an object on a table was stopped when a cloth was placed on the table, thus silencing the noise. Hence, once the auditory feedback was eliminated, the

Article Reprint Information: Reprinted with permission from Levinson, L. J., & Reid, G. (1993). The effects of exercise intensity on the stereotypic behaviors of individuals with autism. *Adapted Physical Activity Quarterly, 10*(3), 255-268.

stereotypic behavior ceased. Consequently, physical activity may be an effective means to reduce stereotypic behaviors because it provides similar sensory feedback but in a more appropriate manner.

Reid, Factor, Freeman, and Sherman (1988) hypothesized that whole-body movements that imitate the stereotypic movements used by individuals with autism would be effective in reducing the stereotypies. Thus the present study used two forms of exercise differentiated on the basis of intensity (walking and jogging) but involving similar movement patterns. Further, we classified the stereotypic behaviors as motor, vocal/oral, or other, to assess the differential effects of the two exercise conditions on these subdivisions.

Methods

Subjects

The subjects in this study consisted of two males and one female, aged 11 years old, who were enrolled in a special education school specifically designed for the learner with autism, in Montreal, Quebec. All lived at home, had been referred to the school by independent neurologists, and had been classified as autistic based on the criteria outlined in the revised Diagnostic and Statistical Manual of Mental Disorders (American Psychiatric Association, 1987). Also the director of the school confirmed the diagnosis of autism for all three subjects. As the purpose of this study was to examine stereotypic behaviors, the subjects selected were low functioning and preadolescent, because stereotypic behaviors are more frequent in lower functioning individuals, and because stereotypic behaviors tend to decrease with age (Garfin, McCallon, & Cox, 1988; Mesibov, Schopler, Schaffer, & Michal, 1989). A list of the stereotypic behavior patterns exhibited by each subject is shown in Table 1.

Treatment Conditions

There were two treatment conditions, a mild exercise program and a vigorous exercise program. The two programs differed with regard to intensity as measured by the subjects' pre- and postexercise heart rates and the distance covered in 15 min.

The mild exercise program was designed to provide exercise that would be beneficial but would not require vigorous effort; each session lasted 15 min and consisted of walking. The vigorous exercise program, designed to elicit considerably more effort, consisted of a brisk 15-min jog.

Dependent Variables

The main dependent measure in this investigation was the frequency of occurrence of stereotypic behaviors. This was the proportion of recording intervals in which a given subject engaged in stereotypic behavior patterns (Parsonson & Baer, 1978). An interval-sampling procedure was used and each session was videotaped. It was felt that viewing and recording could be done concurrently, so a continuous recording procedure was used. The order of videotaping was randomly selected for each session, but a cyclical pattern was established for that particular session. For example, Subject 1 was videotaped for 1 min, then Subject 2 for 1 min, then Subject 3, then Subject 1, etc. Each minute was divided into four 15-s intervals. The occurrence of a stereotyped behavior was recorded for each subject and frequency of involvement determined.

The stereotypic behaviors were subdivided into three categories: motor, vocal/oral, and other. We achieved this by having an expert in the area of autism review the list of stereotypic behaviors that had been compiled for each subject and categorize each behavior into one of the three categories. To establish the validity of this categorization, an individual who was naive to the purpose of the experiment and to the syndrome of autism repeated the procedure.

We monitored heart rates by obtaining a radial pulse before and after each exercise session. Though radial monitoring is a viable means for determining heart rate (Shephard, Cox, Corey, & Smyth, 1979), the use of a Sport Tester (Polar Vantage Quantum XL) would have been a preferred method of continuously monitoring the subjects' heart rates. However, the use of a Sport Tester was negated, because the subjects refused to wear the device.

Procedure

Two settings were employed: a large open field and a classroom. The physical activity sessions (mild and vigorous) took place in a large open field located just outside the school. For the walking sessions, all subjects, assistants, and the experimenter walked as a group. For the jogging sessions, subjects jogged individually aided by their assistants. The sessions were paced by the assistants, who encouraged the subjects to jog continuously through verbal prompting and, if necessary, physical prompting. Subjects were permitted to walk at a fast pace if they displayed signs of discomfort. Baseline measurements, and all recordings of stereotypic responses preceding and following each exercise period, occurred in

Table 1	
Stereotypic Behavior Profile	
of Subjects	
Differentiation of behavior	
Subject 1	
Intense staring	Other
Gazing at hands	Other
Body rocking	Motor
Finger flexing	Motor
Rotation of eyes	Other
Pulling hair	Motor
Biting hands	Motor
Running	Motor
Spontaneous vocalization	Vocal/oral
Laughing	Vocal/oral
Clucking	Vocal/oral
Subject 2	
Intense staring	Other
Tensing of body	Motor
Shaking of head and body	Motor
Jabbing	Motor
Delayed echolalia	Vocal/oral
Giggling	Vocal/oral
Screaming	Vocal/oral
Repetition of words	Vocal/oral
Biting of hands	Motor
Subject 3	
Intense staring	Other
Flapping of hands	Motor
Body rocking	Motor
Laughing	Verbal
Screaming	Vocal/oral
Snorting	Vocal/oral
Biting	Motor
Hitting	Motor
Kicking	Motor

the classroom. A video camera was set up in the corner of the classroom so as to not distract the students from their work.

Design

This investigation lasted 9 weeks and consisted of three phases. The first was an observational period during which the investigator observed all subjects in the classroom environment for the purpose of establishing a baseline of behaviors. The second part of the study consisted of the administration of the two experimental conditions, the mild and vigorous exercise programs, to all subjects in a counterbalanced, systematic fashion. The third phase was another observational period, identical to the first. The number of sessions for each phase is listed in Table 2.

The initial baseline session lasted 2 weeks and took place over three 2-hr periods, with all observations occurring in the classroom. These observations were on separate days within a 2-week period prior to the commencement of the experimental program.

We began each experimental session (i.e., walking or jogging) with a 45-min pre-

Table 2
Description of Design

Phase	Condition	No. sessions
1	Initial baseline	3
2	Treatment	
	Walking	5
	Jogging	4
3	Final baseline	4

Table 3
Summary of Experimental Sessions

Session	Duration (min)
Preexercise observation	45
Exercise	15
Postexercise observation	45
90-min postexercise observation	30

Table 4
Heart Rates and Distances for the Walking Treatment

	Subject 1		Subject 2		Subject 3		Distance
Session	Pre[a]	Post[b]	Pre	Post	Pre	Post	(m)
1	72	96	84	102	72	90	3401.4
2	78	96	84	108	72	90	3401.4
3	72	108	72	108	72	114	3401.4
4	84	108	108	120	78	120	3401.4
5	78	90	84	120	72	90	3401.4
Mean	78	102	84	114	72	102	3401.4

[a]Pre HR over 1 min immediately prior to exercise. [b]Post HR over 1 min immediately following exercise.

Table 5
Heart Rates and Distances for Jogging Treatment

	Subject 1		Subject 2		Subject 3		Distance
Session	Pre[a]	Post[b]	Pre	Post	Pre	Post	(m)
1	72	126	78	120	66	138	4635.4
2	72	180	90	180	108	168	5620.7
3	78	150	78	180	90	168	6155.1
4	90	126	96	138	----	----	6155.1
Mean	72	144	84	156	90	156	5641.6

Note: Subject 3 was present for only three sessions. [a]Pre HR over 1 min immediately prior to exercise. [b]Post HR over 1 min immediately following exercise.

exercise observational period in order to establish the frequency of stereotypic behavior patterns on that particular day and thus assess the reliability of the baseline. Following this, either the mild or vigorous exercise program was implemented for 15 min. During the postexercise time, the experimenter observed again for 45 min. A final observation session occurred 1-½ hr following the initial implementation of the treatment. This observational period lasted approximately 30 min, occurred after the subjects had eaten their lunch, and was done to establish the duration of any treatment effects. A breakdown of the experimental sessions is described in Table 3.

The experimental sessions were conducted for 5 weeks. The walking and jogging exercise programs were administered alternately once a week, walking occurring on the first day followed by jogging on the second day. Differentiation between walking and jogging was based on pacing and intensity as indicated by the subjects' heart rates. The subjects' preexercise heart rates were determined before they went outside and their postexercise heart rates imme-

diately following exercise. This was done by the experimenter monitoring the radial pulse for 10 s.

A final baseline session occurred following the 5-week exercise sessions and lasted for 2 weeks. Four visits of 2 hr each occurred in the subjects' classroom environment. This final baseline session was included so we could note any changes in stereotypic behavior that might be related to the withdrawal of the exercise intervention.

Data Analysis

Graphs were visually analyzed to determine whether the exercise programs were effective in modifying stereotypic behaviors. We calculated an interrater agreement score by having two observers record the occurrence of stereotypic behaviors. The primary observer recorded each subject's behavior for all 16 sessions. The secondary observer recorded 25% of the sessions, one session from the initial baseline, one session from each treatment, and one session from the final baseline. An agreement consisted of both observers recording the same number of responses. Percent agreement

was calculated by dividing the number of agreements by the number of agreements plus the number of disagreements. In addition, the secondary observer viewed one extra tape to determine the reliability of the classification of the stereotypic behaviors as motor, vocal/oral, or other.

Results and Discussion

Reliability

Percent agreement was calculated separately for each session: initial baseline, walking, jogging, and final baseline. The results were 70%, 85%, 90%, and 95%, respectively; the average was 85%. For the classification of observed stereotypic behavior into motor, vocal/oral, and other, the percent agreement was 75%. Although this agreement is not as high, the differentiation of the stereotypic behavior among subjects was not always clear-cut. Had the secondary observer been familiar with the subjects, but still naive to the purpose of the study, a higher percent agreement might have been achieved.

Intensities of Exercise

The two treatment conditions (walking and jogging) were designed to differ in intensity, measured by heart rate and by distances covered in 15 min. Table 4 includes preexercise and postexercise heart rates (over 60 s) as well as the distance covered in meters for the walking conditions; Table 5 includes the same information for the jogging conditions. The postexercise heart rates of the three subjects as well as the distances covered during the treatment conditions show that the jogging condition was of a higher physical intensity than the walking condition; thus the two treatment conditions were successfully differentiated on the basis of intensity.

Treatment Effects

Figure 1 provides an overall view of changes in frequency of behaviors that occurred throughout the 9 weeks as a result of the two treatments. It can be seen that the walking condition was not associated with decreases in stereotypic behaviors. Rather, in two of three cases, a slight increase in the frequency of behaviors was apparent (Subject 1, 73% to 77.3%; Subject 2, 77.1% to 81.4%). A slight decrease was noted in Subject 3 (70.2% to 66.4%).

However, jogging did result in a reduction of stereotypies, a finding congruent with previous research (Kern et al., 1982, 1984; Watters & Watters, 1980). The present study demonstrated a mean reduction of stereotypic behaviors between prejogging and

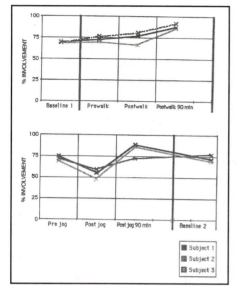

Figure 1. Percent involvement in stereotypic behavior for individual subjects.

postjogging sessions of 17.5% with a range of 12.2% to 20.9% (see Figure 1). Other researchers have noted mean decreases in level of self-stimulation following jogging of 32.7% (Watters & Watters, 1980).

Similar to previous investigations (e.g., Bachman & Fuqua, 1983; Kern et al., 1984), the present study manipulated the intensity of exercise. However, monitoring the heart rate of subjects and the distance covered brought about a more stringent differentiation between the two exercise treatments. The present findings support the notion that exercise must occur at sufficient intensity to reduce stereotypic behaviors in persons with autism.

Might fatigue be an explanation of the present findings? Previous research has shown the effects of fatigue to be negligible because increases in appropriate behaviors have been noted with decreases in stereotypic behaviors as a function of exercise (Kern et al., 1982). This inverse relationship between appropriate behaviors and stereotypic behaviors has also been found in research with persons with visual impairments (Ohlsen, 1978). Thus the present study did not take into account the possible effects of fatigue.

Another important distinction between the present study and previous work centers on the activities chosen to represent the mild and vigorous exercise intensities. We used walking and jogging, two activities involving similar movements, whereas the activities employed by Kern et al. (1984) (ball playing and jogging) required quite different movements. We used walking and jogging to avoid confounding intensity with

type of movement. The data are consistent with Berkson (1983) but are not a direct test of his hypothesis.

Duration of Treatment Effects

To evaluate the duration of the treatment effects in the present study, we filmed the subjects immediately following exercise for 45 min and after lunch for 30 min. For both mild and vigorous treatments the overall frequencies of stereotypic behaviors for each subject (pretreatment, posttreatment and after lunch) are found in Table 6 and are graphically illustrated in Figure 1.

For Subjects 1 and 2, an increase of 4.3% was noted immediately after the walking treatment, with further increases of 10.2% and 10.6%, respectively, 90 min after the walking session. With Subject 3, after an initial decrease of 3.6% following treatment, the level of stereotypic behavior increased 21.1% in the after-lunch session.

Immediately following the jogging treatment, a decrease in stereotypic behaviors was noted for all three subjects (19.3%, 12.2%, and 20.9% for Subjects 1, 2, and 3, respectively), as previously discussed. However, 90 min after jogging, Subjects 1 and 3 exhibited sharp increases in their levels of stereotypic behaviors, 33.3% and 38.4%, respectively, while only a modest increase (12.3%) was noted for Subject 2. Thus, despite the immediate benefits of jogging, subjects returned to or exceeded pretreatment levels of stereotypic behaviors as assessed for 30 min after lunch. These findings concur with the two previous studies that have examined the duration of treatment effects. Allen (1980) analyzed the stereotypic behaviors hourly and found that the least number of disruptive behaviors occurred immediately following 10 min of jogging. Bachman and Fuqua (1983) analyzed the duration of treatment effects immediately following exercise, 1 hr following exercise, and 2 hr following exercise. The authors noted that the lowest level of inappropriate behaviors occurred in the first observational period, immediately following exercise.

The present study found a return to preexercise or greater levels of stereotypic behav-

ior for all three subjects. Due to unavoidable logistics, the time representing 90 min after jogging occurred after their lunch break. During lunch no formal structure existed for the students. Rather they were supervised in their classroom and allowed to engage in any behaviors they wished as long as they were not endangering themselves. Thus, the increase in stereotypic behaviors noted after lunch, in most cases beyond even baseline and pretreatment levels, may be a joint effect of the unstructured nature of lunch and the diminishing positive effects of vigorous exercise with time. The present study was unable to separate these factors.

Larson and Miltenberger (1992) implemented a 15-min jogging program involving six adults with severe mental retardation and failed to replicate decreases in behavior noted in previous studies (Allen, 1980; Bachman & Fuqua, 1983; Kern et al., 1982, 1984; Watters & Watters, 1980). The authors observed their subjects twice during the day. The morning observation period occurred 1 hr after the exercise program was implemented, whereas the afternoon observation period occurred 3-1/2 hr after the exercise session. The present study has shown that decreases occurred immediately following the jogging treatment, but that the duration of these effects may be short-lived. Perhaps the failure by Larson and Miltenberger (1992) to replicate can be attributed to the delay in observing the effects of their exercise program.

Differentiation Between Stereotypic Behaviors

We differentiated stereotypic behaviors to determine if either exercise program was differentially effective in reducing stereotypic behaviors. Behaviors were classified as motor, vocal/oral, or other.

Stereotypic behaviors classified as motor included body rocking, biting, running, tensing and shaking of body, flapping of hands, hitting, and kicking. As seen in Table 7 the motor component of the stereotypic behavior pattern essentially mirrored the findings of stereotypic behaviors in general. There were minimal changes prior to or im-

			Table 6		
		Overall Frequencies (%) of Stereotypic Behaviors Across Subjects for			
		Mild and Vigorous Exercise Treatment			
Experimental phase		**Subject 1**		**Subject 2**	**Subject 3**
Prewalk		73.0		77.1	70.2
Postwalk		77.3		81.4	66.4
90-min walk		87.5		92.0	87.5
Prejog		75.0		72.0	69.0
Postjog		55.7		59.8	48.1
90-min jog		88.8		73.0	86.5

Table 7
Percentage of Motor (M), Vocal/Oral (V), and Other (O)
Stereotypic Behaviors for All Subjects

	Subject 1			Subject 2			Subject 3		
	M	**V**	**O**	**M**	**V**	**O**	**M**	**V**	**O**
Prewalk	51.7	42.1	7.6	42.9	34.7	22.6	48.0	24.2	13.5
Postwalk	53.7	42.1	11.8	56.1	59.5	6.4	45.0	27.7	6.5
Prejog	51.8	40.2	7.1	42.8	25.0	12.0	53.8	21.7	12.0
Postjog	29.9	28.7	7.4	35.5	41.3	2.5	28.8	18.9	10.8

mediately after walking, whereas all three subjects reduced their levels of stereotypic motor behaviors after running, 21.9% for Subject 1, 7.3% for Subject 2, and 25.0% for Subject 3.

Stereotypic behaviors classified as vocal/oral included snorting, screaming, yelling, clucking, laughing, and repetition of words. Stereotyped behaviors considered "other" included intense staring, gazing at hands, and rotating eyes.

As shown in Table 7, the walking condition had inconsistent effects on the subjects' vocal/oral stereotypic behaviors. Subjects 1 and 3 showed no meaningful changes, whereas an increase was noted for Subject 2 (pre, 34.7%; post, 59.5%). In the jogging condition a decrease was noted for Subject 1. With Subject 2 the prejogging vocal/oral level was 25%. This increased to 41.3% in the postjogging session contrary to the overall findings described previously. Subject 3 was not affected by jogging; vocal/oral stereotypic behaviors remained quite constant (pre, 21.7%; post, 18.9%).

Table 7 also shows that the walking condition had very little effect on the subjects' other stereotypic behaviors. The jogging condition did, however, result in reductions for Subjects 2 and 3. For Subject 1, other stereotypic behaviors remained consistent.

Berkson (1983) stated that the alternative activity presented must provide the same sensory input in order to reduce the stereotypic behaviors of an individual. Table 7 and Figure 1 reveal that overall stereotypic behaviors decreased following jogging only, but these reductions occurred primarily in the motor component (mean reduction of 17%). If we follow the argument of Berkson (1983), it is likely that jogging provides sensory input similar to that provided by the motor stereotypic behaviors noted for all subjects.

Conclusion

The vigorous exercise treatment was most effective in reducing stereotypic behaviors immediately after implementation. Treatment effects were no longer evident 1-½ hr following the jogging treatment, as the subjects' levels of stereotypic behaviors returned to or exceeded their preexercise frequencies. Thus vigorous exercise can be viewed as a practical and successful method of temporarily reducing the frequency of stereotypic behaviors of individuals with autism.

The findings also lend credence to the self-stimulatory hypothesis of Berkson (1983). He argued that stereotypic behaviors were maintained by the sensory feedback produced and that they might be eliminated or replaced by activity that produced similar sensory consequences. Our data are consistent with these notions inasmuch as the overall reduction in stereotypic behaviors occurred primarily as a function of a decrease in the motor component, when the alternative activity was of sufficient intensity.

There are several avenues for future research. The effects of other types of exercise on the stereotypic behaviors of individuals with autism should be examined. Specifically, exercises that closely resemble the specific individual's stereotypic behaviors should be used. In the present study it was speculated that the whole-body movements of the vigorous exercise programs imitated the movements that the individuals with autism used to self-stimulate and thus were a possible means of reducing stereotypic behaviors. In addition, if stereotypic behaviors are reduced (even for a short period) due to exercise, does attention or learning improve? Research has shown that a decrease in stereotypic behaviors does not affect appropriate response (Kern et al., 1982).

Other important issues relevant to curriculum planning and research are (a) the feasibility of interspersing exercise throughout the day as a method of decreasing stereotypic behaviors and (b) the amount of vigorous exercise given during each episode. For example, is it more effective to implement a 10-min exercise program three times a day or a 4-min exercise program six times a day?

In sum, the present study supports the effective use of a vigorous exercise program for reducing stereotypic behaviors in individuals with autism. As well, the present study has shown that in addition to intensity, the mode of exercise chosen should mimic the sensory feedback that the individual receives from stereotypic behaviors.

References

Allen, J. (1980). Jogging can decrease disruptive behaviors. *Teaching Exceptional Children, 12*(2), 22-29.

American Psychiatric Association. (1987). *DSM-R-III: Diagnostic and statistical manual of mental disorders* (rev. ed.). Washington, DC: Author.

Bachman, J.E., & Fuqua, R.W. (1983). Management of inappropriate behaviors of trainable mentally impaired students using antecedent exercise. *Journal of Applied Behavior Analysis, 16*, 477-484.

Baroff, G.S., & Tate, B.G. (1968). The use of aversive stimulation in the treatment of chronic self-injurious behavior. *Journal of American Academy of Child Psychiatry, 7*, 454-470.

Baumeister, A.A., & Baumeister, A.A. (1978). Suppression of repetitive self-injurious behavior by contingent inhalation of aromatic ammonia. *Journal of Autism and Childhood Schizophrenia, 8*, 71-77.

Berkson, G. (1983). Repetitive stereotyped behaviors. *American Journal of Mental Deficiency, 88*, 239-246.

Bucher, B., & Lovaas, O. I. (1968). Use of aversive stimulation in behavior modification. In M.R. Jones (Ed.), *Miami symposium on the predication of behavior 1967: Aversive stimulation* (pp. 77-145). Coral Gables, FL: University of Miami Press.

Cushings, P., Adams, A., & Rincover, A. (1983). Research on the education of autistic children. In M. Hensen, R.M. Eisler, & P.M. Miller (Eds.), *Progress in behavior modification* (Vol. 14, pp. 1-49). New York: Academic Press.

Duker, P.C., & Rasing, E. (1989). Effects of redesigning the physical environment on self-stimulation and on-task behavior in three autistic-type developmentally disabled individuals. *Journal of Autism and Developmental Disorders, 19*, 449-460.

Dunlap, G., Dyer, K., & Koegel, R.L. (1983). Autistic self-stimulation and intertrial interval duration. *American Journal of Mental Deficiency, 88*, 194-202.

Foxx, R.M., & Azrin, N.H. (1973). The elimination of autistic self-stimulation behavior by over-correction. *Journal of Applied Behavior Analysis, 6*, 1-14.

Frankel, F., Freeman, B.J., Ritvo, E., & Pardo, R. (1978). The effects of environmental stimulation upon the stereotyped behavior of autistic children. *Journal of Autism and Childhood Schizophrenia, 8*, 389-394.

Garfin, D.G., McCallon, D., & Cox, R. (1988). Validity and reliability of the Childhood Rating Scale with autistic adolescents. *Journal of Autism and Developmental Disorders, 18*, 367-378.

Haring, T.G., Breen, C.G., Pitts-Conway, V., & Gaylord-Ross, R. (1986). Use of differential reinforcement of other behavior during dyadic instruction to reduce stereotyped behavior of autistic students. *American Journal of Mental Deficiency, 90,* 694-702.

Kern, L., Koegel, R.L., & Dunlap, G. (1984). The influence of vigorous versus mild exercise on autistic stereotyped behaviors. *Journal of Autism and Developmental Disorders, 14,* 57-67.

Kern, L., Koegel, R.L., Dyer, K., Blew, P.A., & Fenton, L.R. (1982). The effects of physical exercise on self-stimulation and appropriate responding in autistic children. *Journal of Autism and Developmental Disorders, 12,* 399-419.

Koegel, R.L., & Covert, A. (1972). The relationship of self-stimulation to learning in autistic children. *Journal of Applied Behavioral Analysis, 5,* 381-387.

Koegel, R.L., Egel, A.L., & Dunlap, G. (1980). Learning characteristics of autistic children. In W. Sailor, B. Wilcox, & L. Brown (Eds.), *Methods of instruction for severely handicapped students* (pp. 259-296). Baltimore, MD: Brooks.

Larson, J.L., & Miltenberger, R.G. (1992). The influence of antecedent exercise of problem behaviors in persons with mental retardation: A failure to replicate. *Journal of the Association for Persons with Severe Handicaps, 17,* 40-46.

Lichstein, K.L., & Schreibman, L. (1976). Employing electric shock with autistic children: A review of the side effects. *Journal of Autism and Childhood Schizophrenia, 6,* 163-173.

Lovaas, O.I., Newson, C., & Hickman, C. (1987). Self-stimulatory behavior and perceptual reinforcement. *Journal of Applied Behavior Analysis, 20,* 45-68.

Lovaas, O.I., Schaeffer, B., & Simmons, J.Q. (1965). Building social behaviors in autistic children by use of electric shock. *Journal of Experimental Studies in Personality, 1.* 99-109.

Maag, J.W., Rutherford, R.B., Wolchik, S.A., & Parks, B.T. (1986). Brief report: Comparison of two short overcorrection procedures on the stereotypic behavior of autistic children. *Journal of Autism and Developmental Disorders, 16,* 83-87.

Margolies, P.J. (1977). Behavioral approaches to the treatment of early infantile autism: A review. *Psychological Bulletin, 84,* 249-264.

Mesibov, G.B., Schopler, E., Schaffer, B., & Michal, N. (1989). Use of the childhood Autism Rating Scale with autistic adolescents and adults. *Journal of the American Academy of Child and Adolescent Psychiatry, 28,* 538-541.

Ohlsen, R.L. (1978). Control of body rocking in the blind through the use of vigorous exercise. *Journal of Instructional Psychology, 5,* 19-22.

Parsonson, B.S., & Baer, D.M. (1978). The analysis and presentation of graphic data. In T.R. Kratochwill (Ed.), *Single subject research: Strategies for evaluating change* (pp. 101-162). New York: Academic Press.

Reid, P.D., Factor, D.C., Freeman, N.L., & Sherman, J. (1988). The effects of physical exercise on three autistic and developmentally disordered adolescents. *Therapeutic Recreation Journal, 22,* 42-55.

Rincover, A. (1978). Sensory extinction: A procedure for eliminating self-stimulatory behavior in developmentally disabled children. *Journal of Abnormal Child Psychology, 6,* 299-310.

Runco, M.A., Charlop, M.H., & Schreibman, L. (1986). The occurrence of autistic children's self-stimulation as a function of familiar versus unfamiliar stimulus conditions. *Journal of Autism and Developmental Disorders, 16,* 31-44.

Shephard, R.J., Cox, M., Corey, P., & Smyth, R. (1979). Some factors affecting the accuracy of Canadian Home Fitness Test scores. *Canadian Journal of Applied Sports Science, 4,* 205-209.

Watters, R.G., & Watters, W.E. (1980). Decreasing self-stimulatory behavior with physical exercise in a group of autistic boys. *Journal of Autism and Developmental Disorders, 10*(4), 379-387.

Acknowledgments

The authors gratefully acknowledge the staff and administration at Giant Steps School for their assistance in the data collection of this study. As well the authors would like to thank Jennifer Fiorini for her help with the reliability check.

Decreasing Self-Stimulatory Behavior with Physical Exercise in a Group of Autistic Boys[1]

Robert G. Watters, Wilhelmina E. Watters

Five autistic boys were observed during 27 language training sessions. Each session followed one of three periods: (a) physical exercise, (b) TV watching, or (c) regular academic work. It was found that (a) the lowest levels of self-stimulation followed physical exercise, (b) there were no differences in the levels of self-stimulation following TV watching and following academics, and (c) the levels of correct question answering were not affected by the three different previous periods.

Robert G. Watters, Ottawa University of Ottawa, Wilhelmina E. Watters, M. F. McHugh School. [1]We wish to thank Dora VanStrepen, Alison Lennox, John Rager, Bill Sharkey, and Sheila Connolly for their cooperation and assistance, and Gordon McClure, principal, for providing an environment nurturant to research as well as to children and teachers.

Self-stimulatory behaviors such as rocking, hand flapping, mouthing, and spinning objects are a defining characteristic of autistic children (Rimland, 1964). Reinforcement of incompatible behavior (Luiselli, Helfen, Pemberton, & Reisman, 1977; Mulhern & Baumeister, 1969), overcorrection (Azrin, Kaplan, & Foxx, 1973; Foxx & Azrin, 1973; Freeman, Moss, Somerset, & Ritvo, 1977; Luiselli et al., 1977; Wells, Forehand, Hickey, & Green, 1977), punishment (Baroff & Tate, 1968; Lovaas, Schaeffer, & Simmons, 1965; Risley, 1968; Tate & Baroff, 1966), and time-out (MacDonough & Forehand, 1973; White, Nielson, & Johnson, 1972) are among the behavioral techniques that have been applied to an elimination of self-stimulatory behaviors.

The second author, who teaches autistic children and is familiar with these procedures, noted anecdotally that there seemed to be a decrease in self-stimulatory behavior following gym periods, field trips, and outside excursions. Such an effect, if substantiated, might provide yet another technique for controlling self-stimulatory behavior. However, if the decrease in self-stimulation was accompanied by a general decrease in other behaviors, the technique would be of relatively little use. It was decided, therefore, to assess the effect of exercise on a simple academic performance as well as on self-stimulatory behaviors. To control for the possibility that any observed effects were due simply to a change from the usual academic routine, a second comparison condition (TV watching) was included.

The purpose of the study was, then, to assess the effects of physical exercise on the self-stimulatory behavior of autistic children. This assessment was carried out by monitoring the self-stimulatory behavior and academic performance of a small group of autistic children during a language training session, which was arranged to follow regular academic activity, TV watching, or a period of physical exercise.

Method

Subjects

All five subjects were male and had been diagnosed as autistic by agencies not associated with this study. They ranged in age from 9 years 5 months to 11 years 7 months when the study began, and all had been tested with the Stanford-Binet approximately 1 year before the study began. Each subject had several nonvocal self-stimulatory behaviors that were displayed if no attempt at control was exercised by a teacher. The characteristics of each subject are summarized in Table I.

A sixth and sometimes a seventh child participated in the sessions but no data were collected on these children as they did not display self-stimulatory behaviors.

Setting and Materials

The room where the language training sessions took place was a regular classroom approximately 4 by 5.3 m. The children sat on chairs in a row approximately 3 m long in a cleared area in the center of the room. A piece of cardboard (.7 m by .6 m) was placed on the floor approximately 1.7 m in front of the children. The observer was located at the side of the room and in front of the children, and the teacher not conducting the language training session was located at the other side, also in front of the children.

The picture cards used in the language training sessions were 13 cm by 16.5 cm and were selected from the Language Rehabilitation Program (Hain & Lainer, 1977). A selection of these cards (five or nine) was arranged in a random array on the cardboard on the floor. Each card showed a colored picture representing a descriptive sentence. The cards selected were known to the children, and under optimal conditions they would be expected to do well on the auditory-visual matching task with these cards.

Observation Scheme

The observer rated the children using a 5-second observe/5-second record sampling scheme. The order for observing the children was determined by reference to a randomized sequence. The first 5-second observation interval was directed at the first child, the second 5-second interval at the second child, and so on, until all children had been observed; then the cycle was repeated. Observing and recording continued until the language training session ended. Session length varied from 8 to 13 observation intervals per child (mean = 10.8). During each observation interval, self-stimulatory behavior was monitored. Self-stimulatory behavior was individually defined for each child as the occurrence of any of the behaviors listed for that child in Table I.

A second teacher, not directly involved in the language training session, monitored each child's answers during the language training. Children were asked between three and six questions per session (mean = 4.9). A correct answer was defined as choosing the correct choice card in the auditory-visual matching task that constituted the language training.

Article Reprint Information: Reprinted from Springer/*Journal of Autism and Developmental Disorders*, 10(4), 1980, 379-387, Decreasing self-stimulatory behavior with physical exercise in a group of autistic boys, Watters, R. G., & Watters, W. E., with kind permission from Springer Science and Business Media.

Preconditions

The academic precondition represented the variety of typical academic periods to be found in the school. They ranged from group activities to intensive one-to-one training. No attempt was made to control the duration or content of these periods as this precondition was intended to represent the accumulated recent experience of the child midway through a typical school day.

The TV precondition consisted of seating the children in front of a TV set. The teachers ensured that they remained in their seats but did not control where they looked. These sessions were of 10- to 15-minute duration and the program was always "Sesame Street."

The physical exercise precondition consisted of jogging with the children in the schoolyard for 8 to 10 minutes. Initially, the teachers had to "drag" some of the children along, but by the end of the study the children were jogging along with the teachers with minimal prompting.

During the three preconditions the teachers exerted normal control over the children, including control over self-stimulatory behaviors.

The TV precondition was included as a check for the possibility that any postexercise behavior change would be due to a change from the normal academic routine rather than to exercise per se. If there were changes in behavior following the TV precondition that were similar to changes following the exercise precondition, then it would not be reasonable to attribute the postexercise changes to the exercise. However, it was hard to justify the TV precondition for the school curriculum as it was not part of the regular academic routine for these children. Consequently, the TV precondition was not included throughout the study but was included for five sessions only, the minimum considered necessary to serve as a control function.

There were 5 TV preconditions, 11 academic preconditions, and 11 physical exercise preconditions, for a total of 27 sessions. The first 15 sessions were 5 TV, 5 academic, and 5 physical exercise sessions in randomized order. The remaining 12 were 6 academic and 6 physical exercise sessions in randomized order. There were from 1 to 4 sessions a week with no more than 1 session per day.

During 19 of the 27 sessions a second observer recorded self-stimulatory behavior, and during 19 sessions both teachers conducting the session recorded correct answers. For self-stimulation, reliability for a session was calculated by dividing the

Subject	IQ score	Age (years)	Self-stimulatory behaviors
A	34	11.6	Configuring fingers
			Rocking back and forth
B	73	9.5	Hand flapping
			Mouthing and biting hands
			Rocking back and forth
C	35	11.6	Configuring fIngers
			Biting hands
			Rocking back and forth
D	48	10.2	Rocking back and forth
E	39	9.4	Hand flapping
			Tapping fingers against things
			Rocking back and forth

Table I.
Subject Characteristics

number of observation intervals that had observer agreement by the total number of observation intervals and multiplying by 100. Session reliabilities ranged from 82.5% to 100.0%, with a mean of 95.5% For correct answers reliability for a session was calculated by dividing the number of answers that had observer agreement by the total number of questions asked during the session and multiplying by 100. Session reliabilities ranged from 92.0% to 100% with a mean of 99.1%.

Procedure

The children participated as a group in the language training sessions. The preconditions and language training sessions were conducted by the regular teachers with the assistance of a psychology undergraduate.

Upon completion of the precondition the children were brought to the classroom for the language training session. During this session the teachers made no attempt to control the children's self-stimulatory behaviors.

The general form of the language training was that of auditory-visual matching-to-sample, with which the children were familiar. The teacher said, "I want someone to touch the picture fo X. [Child's name], you touch X." X was a sentence describing the correct choice card. The child named was then expected to leave his seat, go to the cardboard on the floor, and touch the appropriate card from among the array of five picture cards. Correct responses were followed by a verbal reinforcer (e.g., "good"), then by a primary reinforcer (food). Following incorrect responses the child was guided to make the correct response and was then verbally reinforced.

The order in which the children were asked questions was determined by reference to a random sequence. Five to seven times during each session the picture cards were removed and a new set was arrayed on the cardboard. At the end of the language

training session the children were returned to their regular routines.

Results

Each child's self-stimulation data for a session represented the number of intervals during which the child was observed to self-stimulate and the total number of observation intervals. The child's data for sessions following the academic precondition were added together and converted to a percentage. Similarly, for each child the data for sessions following the exercise precondition and the TV precondition were converted to percentages.

Each child's correct answer data for a session represented the number of questions asked of the child during the session and the number of correct answers given by the child. The child's data for sessions following the academic precondition were added together and converted to a percentage, as were data for sessions following the exercise and TV preconditions.

After the first 15 sessions, the percentage of self-stimulation for each child following the 5 TV precondition sessions was compared with the percentage of self-stimulation following the first 5 academic precondition sessions. There were no consistent differences across subjects and a Randomization Test for matched pairs (Siegel, 1956) with $\alpha = .05$ and a two-tailed region of rejection found no statistically significant difference. A similar comparison of the percentage of correct answers for each child following the TV precondition with the percentage of correct answers following the first 5 academic precondition sessions found no statistically significant difference.

Table II presents, for the entire study, the self-stimulation percentages for each child following the academic and the physical exercise preconditions. For all subjects there was a decrease in self-stimulation following the exercise precondition. This decrease expressed as a percentage of the

Table II. Percentage of Self-Stimulation		
Subject	Academic precondition	Physical exercise precondition
A	59.5	28.6
B	25.9	15.6
C	25.0	22.3
D	48.3	20.7
E	76.3	73.5

Table III. Percentage of Correct Answers		
Subject	Academic precondition	Physical exercise precondition
A	88.7	78.0
B	94.3	98.2
C	70.4	56.0
D	94.3	92.9
E	58.5	77.8

level following the academic precondition ranged from a 3.7% decrease for Subject E to a 57.1% decrease for Subject D, with a mean reduction for all subjects of 32.7%. A randomization test for matched pairs (Siegel, 1956) with α = .05 and a one-tailed region of rejection indicated that the observed reduction following the physical exercise precondition was statistically significant.

The percentage of correct answer data for the whole study, presented in Table III, does not show any consistent difference across subjects in the level of correct answers following the academic and the exercise preconditions. A randomization test for matched pairs (Siegel, 1956) with α = .05 and a two-tailed region of rejection found no statistically significant difference in the level of correct question answering following the academic and exercise preconditions.

Discussion

To summarize, the results indicate that (a) there is a decrease in self-stimulation following the physical exercise precondition as compared to the level of self-stimulation following the regular academic precondition, and (b) the levels of correct answering are not different following physical exercise and academics. The lack of a difference in the levels of self-stimulation and question answering following TV watching and academics supports the contention that the decrease in self-stimulation following exercise is due to the exercise rather than to the change from the normal academic routine.

The first finding confirms the anecdotal observation that prompted the study. There is less self-stimulatory behavior following periods of physical exercise and this decrease of 32.7% (on the average) was judged to be a useful reduction by the teachers of these children. The fact that the decrease in self-stimulatory behavior is not accompanied by a decrease in the critical behavior of answering questions correctly means that exercising children is a potentially useful procedure for decreasing self-stimulation.

In addition to the potential health benefit to the child, the physical exercise procedure has two useful characteristics. First,

unlike the usual applications of time-out, overcorrection, punishment, and the reinforcement of incompatible behaviors, the physical exercise intervention occurred before the language training session. Thus the procedure did not interrupt the classroom teaching program. Second, the procedure is relatively undemanding of a teacher's behavior management skills. Holding a child's hand while he jogs across a field requires less preparatory training than does properly administering other behavioral procedures.

A number of questions arise from these results. One concerns the effect of longer or more intensive exercise periods; the present results were obtained with only 8 to 10 minutes of jogging. Another question is about the effect of the physical exercise precondition on a learning task. The task chosen for use in the present study was known to the children and the sessions are best conceptualized as review sessions. The learning of a new task by the children might be influenced differently by the exercise precondition. A third question concerns the role of overlap between the self-stimulatory behavior, the academic task, and the physical exercise.

Self-stimulation, academic tasks, and physical exercise all involve certain responses. In the present study the self-stimulatory behaviors (see Table I) involved finger, hand, arm, mouth, and torso movement. The academic task involved listening, looking, getting up from a chair, walking, bending, and reaching. There was, then, some overlap between the self-stimulation and the academic task (e.g., for some children both involved arm movements), but there were also areas of no overlap (e.g., none of the self-stimulatory behaviors involved looking or walking). The overlap between self-stimulatory behaviors and task requirements has received some attention (Klier & Harris, 1977; Koegel & Covert, 1972; Koegel, Firestone, Kramme, & Dunlap, 1974). A suggestion in this literature is that the greater the degree of overlap, the more the self-stimulatory behavior interferes with the task and the greater is the facilitation of task performance when the self-stimulatory behavior is eliminated. In the present study, the physical exercise precondition resulted in a decrease in self-stimulation with no improvement in task performance. These results might be due to the rather minimal overlap between the self-stimulatory behaviors and the task. For tasks with a greater overlap, the physical exercise precondition might have a facilitating effect on task performance.

The physical exercise of jogging involves leg, arm, and some torso movement. There was, then, some overlap between the exercise and the self-stimulatory behaviors (e.g., for some children the self-stimulation involved arm movement and jogging involved arm movement), but there were also areas of no overlap (e.g., none of the self-stimulatory behaviors involved leg movement). The massed practice or negative practice procedure (Yates, 1970) resembles closely the use of physical exercise to decrease self-stimulatory behaviors in the present study. The procedure proposes to eliminate a behavior by having the patient repeatedly perform the behavior. This exercise is to take place without a break. The major use of the procedure has been to eliminate tics (Jones, 1960; Rafi, 1962; Walton, 1964; Yates, 1958), stuttering (Case, 1960; Yates, 1970), and head banging (Wooden, 1974). The success of the procedure suggests that the greater the overlap between the behavior practiced and the behavior to be eliminated, the greater will be the effect. In the present study, physical exercises chosen to fit each self-stimulatory behavior might have an increased effectiveness in eliminating the self-stimulatory behavior.

References

Azrin, N. H., Kaplan, S. J., & Foxx, R. M. Autism reversal: Eliminating stereotyped self-stimulation of retarded individuals. *American Journal of Mental Deficiency,* 1973, *78,* 241-248.

Baroff, G. S., & Tate, B. G. The use of aversive stimulation in the treatment of chronic self-injurious behavior. *Journal of the American Academy of Child Psychiatry,* 1968, *7,* 454-470.

Case, H. W. Therapeutic methods in stuttering and speech blocking. In H. J. Eysenck (Ed.), *Behavior therapy and the neuroses.* Oxford: Pergamon, 1960.

Foxx, R. M., & Azrin, N. H. The elimination of autistic self-stimulatory behavior by overcorrection. *Journal of Applied Behavior Analysis,* 1973, *6,* 1-14.

Freeman, B. J., Moss, D., Somerset, T., & Ritvo, E. R. Thumbsucking in an autistic child overcome by overcorrelation. *Journal of Behavior Therapy and Experimental Psychiatry,* 1977, *8,* 211-212.

Hain, R., & Lainer, H. *Language rehabilitation program.* New York: Teaching Resources, 1977.

Jones, H. G. Continuation of Yates' treatment of ti-gueur. In H. J. Eysenck (Ed.), *Behavior therapy and the neuroses*. Oxford: Pergamon, 1960.

Klier, J., & Harris, S. L. Self-stimulation and learn-ing in autistic children: Physical or functional incompatibility? *Journal of Applied Behavior Analysis,* 1977, *10,* 311.

Koegel, R. L., & Covert, A. The relationship of self-stimulation to learning in autistic chil-dren. *Journal of Applied Behavior Analysis,* 1972, *5,* 381-387.

Koegel, R. L., Firestone, P. B., Kramme, K. W., & Dunlap, G. Increasing spontaneous play by suppressing self-stimulation in autistic chil-dren. *Journal of Applied Behavior Analysis,* 1974, *7,* 521-528.

Lovaas, O. I., Schaeffer, B., & Simmons, J. Q. Building social behavior in austistic children by use of electric shock. *Journal of Experimen-tal Research in Personality,* 1965, *1,* 99-109.

Luiselli, J. K., Helfen, C. S., Pemberton, B. W., & Reisman, J. The elimination of a child's in-class masturbation by over correction and re-inforcement. *Journal of Behavior Therapy and Experimental Psychiatry,* 1977, *8,* 201-204.

MacDonough, T. S., & Forehand, R. Response-contingent time out: Important parameters in behavior modification with children. *Journal of Behavior Therapy and Experimental Psy-chiatry,* 1973, *4,* 231-236.

Mulhern, T., & Baumeister, A. A. An experimen-tal attempt to reduce stereotypy by reinforce-ment procedures. *American Journal of Mental Deficiency,* 1969, *74,* 69-74.

Rafi, A. A. Learning theory and the treatment of tics. *Journal of Psychosomatic Research,* 1962, *6,* 71-76.

Rimland, B. *Infantile autism*. New York: Apple-ton-Century-Crofts, 1964.

Risley, T. R. The effects and side effects of punish-ing the autistic behaviors of a deviant child. *Journal of Applied Behavior Analysis,* 1968, *1,* 21-34.

Siegel, S. *Nonparametric statistics for the be-havioral sciences*. New York: McGraw-Hill, 1956.

Tate, B. G., & Baroff, G. S. Aversive control of self-injurious behavior in a psychotic boy. *Behaviour Research and Therapy,* 1966, *4,* 281-287.

Walton, D. Massed practice and simultaneous re-duction in drive level--further evidence of the efficacy of this approach to the treatment of tics. In H. J. Eysenck (Ed.), *Experiments in be-havior therapy*. New York: Pergamon, 1964.

Wells, K. C., Forehand, R., Hickey, K., & Green, K. D. Effects of a procedure derived from the over correction principle on manipulated and nonmanipulated behaviors. *Journal of Applied Behavior Analysis.* 1977, *10,* 679-687.

White, G. D., Nielsen, G., & Johnson, S M. Time-out duration and the suppression of deviant behavior in children. *Journal of Applied Be-havior Analysis,* 1972, *5,* 111-120.

Wooden, H. E. The use of negative practice to eliminate nocturnal head banging. *Journal of Behavior Therapy and Experimental Psychia-try,* 1974, *5,* 81-82.

Yates, A. J. The application of learning theory to the treatment of tics. *Journal of Abnormal and Social Psychology,* 1958, *56,* 175-182.

Yates, A. J. *Behavior therapy*. New York: Wiley, 1970.

The Effects of Neurodevelopmental Treatment Versus Practice on the Reaching of Children With Spastic Cerebral Palsy

Linda Fetters and JoAnn Kluzik

Key words: Cerebral palsy, treatment; Neuromuscular disorders; Pediatrics, treatment; Practice.

Background and Purpose. Children with cerebral palsy (CP) are frequently referred for physical therapy, yet the effectiveness of treatment has not been well-documented. In the relatively few available studies, outcomes are divided between support and lack of support for treatment. The purpose of this research was to document and evaluate the effects of a physical therapy program on the reaching movements of children with spastic CP. **Subjects.** Eight children with CP, 10 to 15 years of age, were treated daily for 5 days with a version of neurodevelopmental treatment (NDT) and for 5 days with practice of reaching tasks. **Methods.** Changes in movement time, path, and smoothness of reach were quantified and described using kinematic analysis. **Results.** There were no differences in any of the variables following 5 days of NDT. There was a difference in movement time, but in no other variables, following 5 days of practice. When time in treatment, rather than type of treatment, was the independent variable, the data showed changes. Both movement time and movement units were reduced following 5 days of treatment. Movement time, movement units, and displacement, but not reaction time, were reduced following the completion of both types of treatment. **Conclusion and Discussion.** The two treatments in combination may be necessary to achieve these results. Alternatively, either treatment type alone, when given for at least 2 weeks, may produce similar results. [Fetters L, Kluzik J. The effects of neurodevelopmental treatment versus practice on the reaching of children with spastic cerebral palsy. *Phys Ther.* 1996;76:346-358.]

L Fetters, PhD, PT, is Associate Professor, Department of Physical Therapy, Boston University, 635 Commonwealth Ave. Boston, MA 02215 (USA) (fetters@sarvxl.bu.edu), Research Associate in Pediatrics, Children's Hospital, Boston, MA 02115, and Lecturer in Pediatrics, Harvard Medical School, Boston, MA 02115. Address all correspondence to Dr Fetters at the first address. J Kluzik, PT, is Clinical Assistant Professor, Department of Physical Therapy, Boston University. She was Director of Therapy, Cotting School, Lexington, MA 02173, at the time this research was done. The study was approved by the Institutional Review Board at Boston University. This study was sponsored by a grant from the Foundation for Physical Therapy Inc and a Mary Switzer Research Fellowship from the National Institute on Disability Rehabilitation Research to Dr Fetters. This article was submitted November 14, 1994, and was accepted December 13, 1995.

The purpose of this research was to evaluate the clinical effectiveness of aspects of neurodevelopmental treatment (NDT) and practice on the motor skills of children with spastic cerebral palsy (CP). Cerebral palsy is one of the most common neurologic problems of children referred to physical therapists, with children with spastic CP constituting 60% of this patient population.[1,2] Although NDT is an accepted method of physical therapy practice for children with CP, few data exist to strongly support this approach.[3,4] In this study, we evaluated the short-term effectiveness of both NDT and practice intervention for the improvement of speed and control of reaching.

Neurodevelopmental treatment is the most commonly used approach to treatment of children with CP.[5] This approach focuses on encouraging and building upon normal movement patterns and normal postural reactions, while trying to reduce abnormal movement.[6-9] These treatment outcomes are supposed to be achieved through physical handling of the child during movement, giving the child more normal sensorimotor experiences. As the child gains postural control, the therapist gradually withdraws support. Handling techniques and treatment activities undergo continual change as they are adapted to the responses of a particular child. Traditionally, it has been implicit in NDT that improved postural control will lead to improvement in functional skills without necessarily working on those specific skills. More current interpretations of NDT include the importance of functional skill practice in treatment.[5,10,11] The NDT method used in this study combines treatment of postural control and the functional skill of reaching.

Although NDT is widely used by pediatric therapists in the treatment of children with CP, there is little research evidence regarding its efficacy. This lack of scientific evidence of treatment effectiveness is true not only of the NDT approach but for many types of physical therapy for children with CP.[4,12] Studies of treatment effectiveness in children with CP have varied in research design, selection of subjects, measurement tools, and amount and type of therapy provided. Early studies tended to be descriptive in nature, whereas recent studies have used more rigorous research designs. Researchers face a large number of inherent difficulties when studying treatment efficacy with this particular population.[4,6,12,13] Research on treatment effectiveness in children with spastic CP has varied in terms of the treatments used for intervention as well as the frequency of therapy provided. Numerous studies have focused on the effectiveness of a neurophysiological-based treatment approach, many of which incorporate NDT principles.[6,14-22] Some of these studies[6,15-19] have shown that therapy with an NDT or neurophysiological approach to treatment is effective in improving some measure of motor performance in children with CP. In contrast, some researchers[14,20-22] have found little or no change in motor performance to indicate that therapy with a neurophysiological approach is effective. Noonan[23] found an improvement in postural reactions in only three out of seven subjects following a period of "training." A recent study of the effectiveness of NDT[14] demonstrated no improvement in motor performance and showed a decrement in both motor and mental performance following 6 months of NDT compared with 6 months of infant stimulation.

Meta-analysis offers a method of study-

Article Reprint Information: Reprinted with permission from Fetters, L., & Kluzik, J. The effects of neurodevelopmental treatment versus practice on the reaching of children with spastic cerebral palsy. *Physical Therapy*, 1996, 76(4), 346-358.

ing the cumulative results of a number of studies focused on a specific area. In an excellent review of research of the effectiveness of NDT in children, Ottenbacher et al[4] performed a meta-analysis on studies involving the treatment of children with developmental disabilities or delay. Five criteria had to be met for studies to be included in the meta-analysis. One requirement was that statistical tests had to be sufficient to compute an effect size between treatment and no treatment. Nine studies out of those described in the 37 reviewed research reports met the set criteria, and in those nine studies, greater improvement in the motor area was found in children who had received treatment that utilized NDT techniques in comparison with control subjects. Six of the nine studies analyzed focused on children with CP. The authors concluded that the overall effects of NDT were positive, although small.

A finding of little or no change in motor skills may represent a gain from treatment in older children with spastic CP. Such children are at high risk for developing increasing contractures and deformities, as they tend to assume stereotypic postures and move in stereotypic patterns.[2,6,8,24] Without intervention, they may develop muscle contractures and soft-tissue and joint deformities. These contractures and deformities may make movement even more difficult and eventually lead to a decrease in motor skills. This is an important factor to consider when trying to judge the effectiveness of treatment for children with long-standing motor problems.

The repetition of movement, which we will call "practice," is a fundamental component of any physical therapy approach.[25] Although not always explicitly stated, practice is at least implicit within NDT (see Goodgold-Edwards[26] for a proposed application of motor learning principles to NDT). Practice of motor tasks is explicitly manipulated within a motor learning approach to movement or therapy.[27] Although most research in motor learning has been conducted with nondisabled adults, the principles gleaned from this research may be applicable to the therapeutic setting.[26-28] Motor learning approaches are concerned with how practice affects both performance of a movement task (short-term gain) and retention of the motor skills involved in the task (learning). The variables that affect performance that are measured during or immediately after practice may not continue to show improvement when measured later, after practice has stopped. Thus, the performance of the movement when measured

during therapy may not equate to the learning of that movement for use later in the home or community.

Lee et al[29] have defined movement repetition as being fundamental to the learning of motor skills, yet it is apparent from motor learning research that practice alone does not guarantee learning. These authors suggest that movement repetition actually provides practice at constructing an appropriate action plan for the task.[29] Thus, it is not necessarily the precise rehearsal of muscle patterns or joint combinations that is important in practice, rather it is the construction of a plan of action given the constraints of a particular task that is important. The playing of computer games that require reaching to activate a switch may elicit a variety of movement patterns that have varying degrees of success, as measured by completing the game or beating an opponent. Practice may assist learning by narrowing the field of useful and efficient action plans to successfully complete a functional movement.

The use of feedback during therapy is common in therapy sessions, yet the way in which feedback is given may be crucial to the generalizability of therapeutic gains. Feedback given after every trial may actually be detrimental to learning in comparison with feedback given less often and in a summary format.[27,28]

There is general agreement that movement must be practiced in order to become a part of a movement repertoire, yet the neurological approaches to treatment of children with CP have not emphasized this critical feature of movement acquisition.

A major difficulty in studying the effects of treatment of motor problems resulting from CP is the lack of methods that are sensitive enough to detect changes in motor ability in standardized tests or typical clinical examinations.[6,13,20,30-32] This consideration is particularly important with older children. Such changes in motor function may be in terms of efficiency of movement or quality of movement. The measurement tool used to evaluate motor problems may affect conclusions drawn from a study. The tool used must be appropriate and sensitive enough to detect changes.

Most studies of treatment effectiveness have used some type of motor skill or functional skill checklist to measure motor performance[6,14-17,21,22] changes in motor performance following treatment may involve increments of progress within a skill category, such as changes in quality, ease, smoothness, accuracy, speed, or efficiency of movement. Progress of this nature, however, might not be evident on a skills test.

Older children with spastic CP are particularly likely to exhibit a change in quality of movement as opposed to acquiring new functional skills.[6] Measuring quality of movement is difficult, and there is a lack of objective measurement tools in this area.[13] Therapists often use observation to assess quality of movement, but objectivity, accuracy, and repeatability are limited.

Kinematic analysis offers a means of studying components of a movement in an objective, quantifiable way and is able to detect small changes in movement.[30,33] Kinematic data describe movement irrespective of the forces causing the movement.[34] Movement is described in terms of position and the derivations of position, such as velocity and acceleration. Thus, if reaching is the movement under study, the exact position of the wrist, elbow, and shoulder in three-dimensional space could be specified as well as the rate at which these points change and the angles of the joints as the movement occurs.

Movement Units

Kinematic variables include time, shape of the movement path, velocity, and acceleration. Changes in control of rnovement may result in a shorter reaction time and overall duration of reach. As movement becomes smoother with improved muscle coordination, it may be reflected in the velocity and acceleration profiles, that is, in movement units.

The concept of a movement unit has been described as the portion of a reach between one acceleration and one deceleration[35,36] or the portion of the reach between subsequent points in a curvature-speed relationship.[33] Both methods enable systematic description of the stop-start or jerkiness of a reach. Infant reaches initially include multiple movement units, with the number of movement units decreasing with maturity. As reaching patterns mature, the first movement unit accounts for an increasing percentage of the total duration of the reach.[35] The jerky stop-start action gives way to one smooth, continuous acceleration, followed by a single deceleration. A mature reach includes a single movement unit with only one stop-start action, suggesting that a lower number of movement units reflects greater control of the reaching movement. Thus, counting the number and relative timing of movement units may offer a useful measurement of change of control or coordination.

In our preliminary study of five preadolescent children with CP, we compared reaching for a target before and immediate-

Table 1
Characteristics of Subjects

Subject No.	Age (y)	Gender	First Treatment	Second Treatment	Seating Device
1	13	M	Practice	NDT	Chair without back support
2	15	M	Practice	NDT	Chair with high back
3	12	M	NDT[α]	Practice	Wheelchair, lap belt
4	13	M	NDT	Practice	Wheelchair, side supports and trunk brace
5	13	M	Practice	NDT	Wheelchair, trunk brace
6	11	M	Practice	NDT	Reclined wheelchair, conforming back cushion
7	10	F	Practice	NDT	Reclined wheelchair, lap belt
8	12	F	NDT	Practice	Wheelchair

[α]NDT=neurodevelopmental treatment.

ly after a single NDT treatment.[30] The subjects, aged 7 to 12 years, had moderate to severe spastic CP but normal intelligence. They were asked to reach repeatedly to touch a target placed in front of them at the midline. Each subject participated in one testing session during which performance of the reaching task was recorded immediately before and following a 35-minute NDT-oriented therapy session. A single wrist point represented the movement of the arm in space. All sessions incorporated handling techniques that altered muscle tone during movement and facilitated appropriate weight shifting and postural reactions.

Subjects averaged 3.7 movement units before treatment, and the average duration of reach was 1,692 milliseconds. By comparison, age-matched control subjects without neurological impairment performed this movement in 300 to 600 milliseconds and with a single movement unit (Fetters L, unpublished work). The straightness ratio (the distance the hand traveled compared with the shortest distance to the target) was 1.2. Following treatment, the number of movement units decreased to 2.7 and average duration decreased to 1,267 milliseconds (both findings were statistically significant). The duration of the first movement unit in relation to the entire duration of the reach was greater following treatment. This finding indicates that the reach was becoming characterized by a single movement unit (a single stop-start action), which is typical of mature, well-controlled reaching movements. The length the hand traveled (straightness) and the extent to which associated reactions occurred did not differ after treatment.

This article presents the next logical step in this research program. We used the same operational definitions in a short-term con-

trolled study in which the effects of NDT and practice were studied. We expected that NDT, as applied in this research, would assist in improvement of speed and control of movement, as defined by our measures. Reaching and the postural support necessary for reaching might carry over into a functional task such as sitting in front of a computer and reaching to activate the computer and thus were the focus of treatment. Our measures had supported a change following NDT in our previous research, but change over a more extended period had not been measured. We chose an experimental task that was functionally important for the subjects, namely working with a computer. Because our subjects use computers for communication, schoolwork, and entertainment, it was important for them to improve their performance of this task. Our practice intervention was designed to allow the subjects to repeat the movement necessary for the task and to assess whether this repetition alone was effective in making change in the dependent measures.

The purpose of our study was to investigate the following research questions: (1) Does 5 days of either NDT or practice improve the reaching characteristics of children with spastic CP? and (2) What is the effect of a period of 5 days with no treatment? We hypothesized (1) that following NDT or practice, reaches of children with spastic CP will be smoother and faster and the time to initiate the movement will be less than prior to treatment and (2) that following a period of 5 days of no treatment, effects of treatment will be sustained.

Method

Subjects

Eight children (2 female, 6 male), aged 10 to 15 years, with spastic quadriplegic CP

participated (Tab. 1). This age range extended the ages of the subjects in our previous study, and the number of subjects increased the sample size. Subjects were recruited from the Cotting School, a private school for children with physical disabilities in Lexington, Mass. Subjects were included if, according to their therapist and classroom teacher, they (1) were able to understand and carry out spoken directions included in the reaching task, (2) had sufficient visual skill to localize an object with both eyes, (3) had sufficient passive range of motion to be able to reach the target used in the reaching task, and (4) used computers in the classroom or for schoolwork so that improvement would be functionally useful. Ten subjects were originally tested in the project, but only 8 subjects had sufficient data to be included in the analysis. One subject was eliminated from the analysis because he was available for only 2 days of data collection. The other subject who was eliminated from the study was unable to complete most of the sessions because of fatigue. The children and their parents signed informed consent forms approved by the Institutional Review Board at Boston University and the Cotting School.

The project took place at the Cotting School. A kinematic laboratory was set up in a room adjacent to the physical therapy department at the school. In this way, subjects participated daily at their school with minimum inconvenience. This arrangement was essential to the successful completion of this study.

Instrumentation

Reaching movements were recorded using the WATSMART (Waterloo Spatial Motion Analysis and Recording Technique) motion analysis system.* The WATSMART is a valid and reliable system for reproducing human movement.[37] The reliability values

*Northern Digital Inc, 403 Albert St, Waterloo, Ontario, Canada N21 3V2.

for reproducing a fixed target length (ruler) rotated in three-dimensional space in our laboratory were below 2 mm.[38] This finding means that the WATSMART system reproduced absolute length of the moving ruler with errors of 2 mm or less. The WATSMART was calibrated before every data-collection session using 22 infrared light-emitting diodes (IREDs) from the calibration frame at a sampling rate of 100 Hz. The average error of calibration ranged between 0.7 and 2.7 mm over the entire project period. The tabletop, the computer, and in some cases the chair were covered with an infrared absorbing cloth to minimize reflections. The setup for calibration was kept constant for data collection.

An IRED was attached to the arm used for reaching. The IRED was taped to the skin over the styloid process of the ulna. This limb point was used to represent the arm in space. Two cameras, which were sensitive to the infrared light spectrum, recorded the position of the arm at a sampling rate of 100 Hz. Infrared cameras were fixed to a steel bar mounted across the laboratory. In this way, the camera mounting was rigid and not susceptible to being moved, because moving the sensors after calibration would require recalibration of the system. Cameras were placed with the lines of sight of the lenses forming a 65-degree angle. The skin under the IRED was marked with permanent ink so that the IRED could be placed on exactly the same place for each of the daily sessions. The position of the IRED during each reach was stored as numerical coordinates, which were later converted to three-dimensional numerical values. A Hewlett-Packard Vectra computer[†] was used for collection, storage, and analysis of the positional data. Data missing as a result of obscured IREDs were interpolated only if not more than 5% of the total reach was missing in a continuous segment. This interpolation rule resulted in a loss of approximately 20% of the data.

The decision of how to handle missing data is specific to each laboratory. Obscured data points are always a problem with kinematic data, particularly in the collection of three-dimensional data, where two cameras must view each IRED in order to reconstruct the movement. We have chosen a very conservative approach by not interpolating if more than 5% of the data are missing in any one section of the reach. Our interpolation algorithm uses data points from before and after the missing data. The more data there are both before and after the missing data, the better the estimate will be. In gait data, multiple cycles are usually available in order to make the missing data-point estimates. In a noncyclical movement such as reaching, the data available for estimates are more limited in any given trial. Consequently, estimates are based on fewer data. The biggest problem with this type of decision rule is that a particular class or type of movement may be eliminated from study, restricting study to movements only with certain characteristics. These characteristics may cause obscuring of the IREDs.

Procedures: Pretest-Posttest Tasks

Subjects played an interactive video game (Zigzag[‡]) on an Apple IIe computer[§] before and after each treatment session. The computer game was activated via a light-touch switch (LTS), as many subjects did not have the control to hit the appropriate computer key. Subjects started with their hands on an LTS located in front of them on the tabletop (Fig. 1). The therapist playing the video game with a subject pressed a second LTS simultaneously with a "go" verbal signal for the subject to start. The subject lifted the hand from the tabletop LTS and hit a third LTS positioned at the top of the computer screen, which changed the picture on the computer screen, adding colored lines of varying lengths to the screen. The goal of the game was to fill the screen, and this goal was motivating for the subjects. Zigzag has no time component; thus, there was no time pressure for movement. In addition, there was no wrong response. The change in voltage of the LTS was recorded via the WATSCOPE, an analog-to-digital converter that is synchronized with the WATSMART. In our previous research, we used a touch-to-target task, which proved boring after repeated trials for most subjects. Interacting with a computer was fun and thus more motivating.

Subjects were seated in their wheelchairs or on an appropriately sized straight-backed chair in front of the table. Choice of seating was determined by the typical seating used by each child for computer work. Seating had been determined by the school's occupational therapist or physical therapist in most cases. The LTS that activated the computer was located so that each subject easily touched the pad when the subject's arm was passively extended; thus, the target distance was scaled for each subject. Each

Figure 1. Laboratory setup. C1=camera 1, C2=camera 2, VC=video camera, C=computer, S1=tabletop switch, S2=computer switch.

child performed a minimum of 10 trials of the reaching task using the preferred hand.

Dependent Variables

Movement unit. Smoothness was defined as the number of movement units per reach. A movement unit is the portion of the reach between one acceleration and the following deceleration. An acceleration and a deceleration are defined by a rate of change in velocity of greater than 5 mm/s^2.

Movement time. Duration was determined by the interval between tabletop LTS liftoff and computer-screen LTS touch.

Path. Straightness, or total displacement, was defined as the length of path of the reaching movement between liftoff and computer-screen LTS touch.

Reaction time. Reaction time was the time interval between the signal from the second LTS (activated by the therapist) and the signal from the tabletop LTS indicating liftoff of the hand (beginning reach).

Treatment Conditions

Treatment took place in the physical therapy department, which was adjacent to the laboratory. Subjects were assigned to each of two treatment conditions, NDT and practice, with the order of the two treatments counterbalanced. Slips of paper with "NDT" and "Practice" written on them were placed in a hat, and one slip of paper was drawn. The first subject was assigned to the NDT condition, with subsequent subjects alternately placed in the two treatment conditions. This procedure was followed for all 10 subjects who entered the study. Only data for 8 of the 10 subjects are re-

[†]Hewlett-Packard Co, 3000 Minuteman Rd, Andover, MA 01810.
[‡]Don Johnson Developmental Equipment Inc, PO Box 639, Wauconda, IL 60084.
[§]Apple Computer Inc, 20525 Mariana Ave, Cupertino, CA 95014.

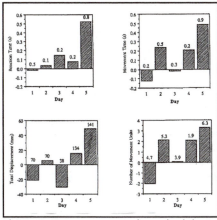

Figure 2. Group means and standard deviations of change scores, by day, for neurodevelopmental treatment condition.

ported here. Five subjects were assigned to the practice condition first and to the NDT condition second; 3 subjects were assigned to the treatment conditions in the opposite order. A no-treatment condition occurred for 1 week between the two treatment conditions. Treatment conditions consisted of five daily sessions of physical therapy for 35 minutes each session. Our previous research demonstrated changes after one session of NDT. We were interested in exploring the effects of treatment after 5 days in order to observe any continued effects of treatment before designing a longitudinal study. Session length was kept to the typical length of treatment during the school day. The subjects received no therapy for 1 week prior to the first treatment session. Another no-treatment week occurred after the first 5 days of treatment and prior to the second 5 days of treatment. With this design, all subjects received both treatments and experienced two no-treatment weeks.

Each day of the study, we measured reaching movements before and after treatment. In our previous research, we measured the effects of treatment only immediately after one treatment session. By recording the movement immediately after treatment and then before treatment on subsequent days, we measured the treatment effects over time. If treatment did not have effects after the first day, this design enabled us to ascertain when, during the 5-day period of daily treatment, effects might be seen. In addition, the week of no treatment followed by measurement provided an opportunity to measure retention of any improvement demonstrated in the first week of treatment.

The NDT sessions were provided by the second author (JK), a physical therapist certified in pediatric NDT.

Although treatment activities varied for each subject, overall goals were the same for all subjects. Goals included improved trunk and shoulder-girdle control during reaching, improved smoothness and efficiency of movement, and improved ability to initiate movement (Appendix).

The practice sessions were also provided by the second author and consisted of repeated reaching to play computer games. During practice, the children could choose from a menu of eight computer games. In each game, the subjects were required to reach to play the game in a way similar to the reach to be measured. The therapist played the computer game with each subject to provide motivation and encouragement, but no feedback about the movement was given. Instead, comments were made occasionally about the subject's video game performance (eg, "You beat me again" or "This is a fun choice"). Although these practice sessions had components of motor learning, they did not strictly adhere to a motor learning framework. Feedback was not planned or manipulated in any systematic way, although to be consistent with the motor learning literature, we restricted feedback about the movement. The amount of practice within a session was controlled by the choices of games made by the subject.

Data Reduction and Analysis

Digitized data were filtered at 5 Hz using a third-order Butterworth filter with forward and reverse passes. The resultant value for the wrist point and the target were computed from the three-dimensional filtered data. The resultant value was used to represent the wrist point in space. The remainder of the IREDs were used for subsequent analyses. Dependent measures were taken from the resultant values of the wrist point over time. Prior to computing means for the pretest and posttest sessions for each subject and each day, a repeated-measures (day x trial) analysis of variance (ANOVA) was performed. There were no main-effect or interaction-effect differences between trials or days for any of the variables. This finding indicated that trials for any given day could be estimated with a mean score, because they were not different. As a consequence, mean values were computed for pretest and posttest scores for each subject, each day. Change scores for resultant values

were computed by subtracting the posttest mean scores from the pretest mean scores for all trials each day. Change scores were then used for the statistical analyses of the dependent measures. A positive change score indicated a decrease in amount of the variable after treatment (ie, improvement), whereas a negative change score indicated an increase in amount of the variable after treatment (ie, worsening).

For various reasons (eg, sickness, death of a family members, school events), none of the subjects completed 5 full days of treatment during either treatment week. Thus, the terms "first day" and "last day" rather than the terms "day 1" and "day 5" are used for analysis. Data were analyzed using an ANOVA for repeated measures and paired t tests. All statistical tests for this project were performed with SAS software[∥] on an IBM RS/6000 950 mainframe computer.[#]

The alpha level was .10 for all statistical tests. This choice was made to avoid a Type II error, that is, assuming that no difference exists when a difference actually does exist. This level of significance is a reasonable choice with a small sample size such as that of our study and in light of the data that will be presented.[39]

Results

Does 5 Days of NDT or Practice Improve the Reaching Characteristics of Children With Spastic CP?

There were no differences between days for change scores of reaction time ($F=0.83$, $df=3$), movement time ($F=1.59$, ($df=3$), total displacement ($F=1.10$, $df=3$), or number of movement units ($F=0.91$, $df=3$) for NDT. Means and standard deviations for the change scores of all subjects, by day, for all variables in the NDT condition are presented in Table 2. The grouped means and standard deviations, by day, for the NDT condition are graphed in Figure 2.

There were no differences between days for the change scores of reaction time ($F=0.95$, $df=2$), movement time ($F=0.78$, $df=2$), total displacement ($F=1.10$, $df=3$), or number of movement units ($F=0.48$, $df=3$) for practice. Means and standard deviations for change scores of all subjects, by day, for all variables in the practice condition are presented in Table 2. The grouped means and standard deviations, by day, for the practice condition are graphed in Figure 3.

The first-day pretreatment values were then compared with the last-day posttreat-

∥SAS Institute Inc, PO Box 8000, Cary, NC 27511.
#International Business Machines Inc, Old Orchard Rd, Armonk, NY 10504.

Table 2
Means, Standard Deviations, and Ranges of Change Scores for All Subjects for All Dependent Measures[α] by Day

	Day 1	Day 2	Day 3	Day 4	Day 5
Neurodevelopmental treatment					
RT (s)					
$\overline{X}$	-0.02	-0.04	-0.15	-0.08	0.53
SD	0.53	0.15	0.20	0.16	0.80
Range	-0.48 to 1.04	-0.13 to 0.26	-0.40 to 0.15	-0.06 to 0.45	-0.28 to 1.37
MT (s)					
$\overline{X}$	-0.12	0.24	-0.02	0.21	0.49
SD	0.22	0.51	0.32	0.23	0.87
Range	-0.60 to 0.07	-0.15 to 1.34	-0.46 to 0.52	-0.06 to 0.56	-0.03 to 1.79
Path (mm)					
$\overline{X}$	-21.30	5.74	-30.48	15.50	48.70
SD	70.43	70.43	38.12	134.03	141.68
Range	-164.77 to 35.52	-136.36 to 64.93	-77.92 to 33.47	-142.86 to 308.05	-62.41 to 255.29
MU					
$\overline{X}$	-2.05	2.10	0.67	2.06	3.30
SD	4.70	5.30	3.90	1.90	6.30
Range	-12.40 to 1.20	-1.15 to 13.86	-5.80 to 5.75	-0.75 to 4.89	-0.40 to 12.67
Practice					
RT (s)					
$\overline{X}$	-0.03	-0.23	-0.13	0.04	-0.24
SD	0.60	0.25	0.22	0.17	0.24
Range	-0.78 to 0.84	-0.67 to 0.02	-0.47 to 0.25	-0.31 to 0.22	-0.41 to 0.07
MT (s)					
$\overline{X}$	0.01	0.19	-0.06	0.04	0.29
SD	0.52	0.24	0.13	0.17	0.30
Range	-0.58 to 0.82	-0.08 to 0.57	-0.20 to 0.12	-0.21 to 0.30	0.08 to 0.51
Path (mm)					
$\overline{X}$	-29.23	-10.68	-21.85	-13.19	7.68
SD	25.35	81.53	68.80	49.63	93.10
Range	-66.77 to 2.89	-131.12 to 89.57	-109.0 to 100.98	-86.75 to 67.56	-58.15 to 73.52
MU					
$\overline{X}$	-0.70	1.30	-0.20	0.02	3.50
SD	7.00	2.10	1.20	2.80	5.20
Range	-12.14 to 9.79	-0.86 to 5.50	-1.33 to 1.47	-2.89 to 6.00	-0.13 to 7.20

[α]RT=reaction time, MT=movement time, path=total displacement, MU=number of movement units.

ment values for each of the variables in the NDT condition. These values are graphed in Figure 4. For example, the pretreatment means after the first day of NDT were compared with the posttreatment means of the last day of NDT. This comparison is equivalent to computing a weekly change score. There were no differences for the variables of reaction time, movement time, total displacement, or number of movement units for the NDT condition. The first-day pretreatment values also were compared with the last-day posttreatment values for the practice condition and are graphed in Figure 5. There was a difference for movement time (*P*<.05) but no difference for reaction time, total displacement, or number of movement units for the practice condition. There was

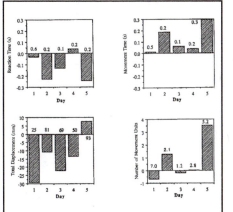

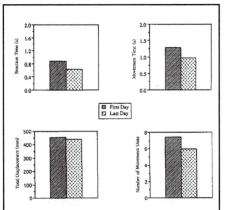

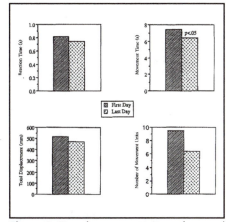

Figure 3. Group means and standard deviations of change scores, by day, for practice condition.

Figure 4. First-day pretreatment values and last-day posttreatment values for neurodevelopmental treatment condition.

Figure 5. First-day pretreatment values and last-day posttreatment values for practice condition.

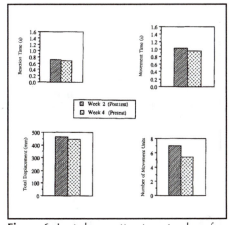

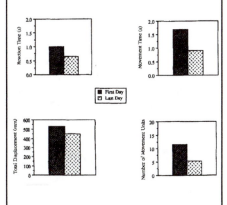

Figure 6. Last-day posttreatment values for first 5-day period of treatment (week 2) and first-day pretreatment values for second 5-day period of treatment (week 4) (comparison with week of no treatment).

Figure 7. First-day pretreatment values for first 5-day period of treatment (week 2) compared with last-day posttreatment values for second 5-day period of treatment (week 4) beginning to end of study.

a decrease in every variable (except reaction time) for each treatment week; however, only the decrease in movement time proved to be statistically significant, even though the alpha level of .10 was used. The decrease was consistently larger for all variables in the practice condition than in the NDT condition.

What Is the Effect of 1 Week With No Treatment?

The posttest scores for the last day of week 2 (end of the first treatment) were compared with the pretest scores for the first day of week 4 (start of second treatment). This analysis allowed us to measure the change after 5 days of treatment coupled with 1 week of no treatment. Means and standard deviations for the pretest-posttest scores for all variables are graphed in Figure 6. There was a continued decrease in the values for all variables, with the exception of reaction

time, which remained unchanged.

Because our original hypotheses were not supported but variables appeared to change, we decided to ask our questions slightly differently. That is, perhaps the type of treatment is less important than the overall amount of time the treatment is given. Thus, we asked: What is the effect of amount of treatment on the reaching variables? The pretest and posttest scores from the beginning to the end of the first treatment (week 2) and also for the second treatment (week 4), regardless of nature of treatment, were compared. This analysis addressed the question of time in treatment rather than the nature of the treatment. The means and standard deviations for all variables are presented in Table 3. At the end of the first week of treatment (three subjects had NDT and five subjects had practice during this week), there was a difference for both movement time ($P<.05$) and number of movement units

($P<.05$). There were no differences for total displacement or reaction time, although the change in both of these variables showed an improvement (total displacement, $P=.12$; reaction time, $P=.14$). There were no differences in any variables after week 4 alone. Inspection of the data in Table 3 reveals the major change in variables occurred during the first week of treatment. During the second week, these changes were maintained or slightly improved.

When the means of the pretest values for the first day of the study were compared with the means of the posttest values for the last day (ie, beginning of the study compared with the end of the study), there was a difference for movement time ($P<.05$), total displacement ($P<.10$), and number of movement units ($P<.01$) but not for reaction time ($P<.12$). The data are graphed in Figure 7.

Discussion

Improvement in the variables under study was not apparent after 5 days of either NDT or practice. The original finding, that these same variables improved after one session of NDT, was not supported in this extended study. This finding may be due to the large variability of response or to an insufficient amount of treatment time. The NDT or the practice given over the entire treatment period may have achieved the improvement in the variables that was seen in this study. It is not possible to ascertain whether 2 weeks of either treatment or both treatments together produced the measured improvements. What is clear is that measuring at the end of the study, rather than the end of each treatment condition, was essential for recognizing change in these variables. A future study should increase the amount of time that each treatment is given. Weekly mea-

Table 3
Means and Standard Deviations by Week From First Day to Last Day[α]

Treatment Week	Reaction Time		Movement Time		Movement Unit		Total Displacement	
	X̄	SD	X̄	SD	X̄	SD	X̄	SD
Week 1								
Day 1	1.00	0.55	1.69	0.84	11.42	6.99	526.34	274.63
Day 5	0.72	0.23	1.02*	0.35	6.95 *	2.95	465.13	246.35
Week 2								
Day 1	0.69	0.35	0.95	0.36	5.43	2.57	446.26	204.87
Day 5	0.66	0.19	*0.90	0.23	* 5.43	1.66	*447.84	208.04

[α]Asterisk (*) indicates significant difference.

sures over multiple weeks might provide the necessary data to sort out the importance of the type of treatment that is most effective for change in these variables. The analysis of the first week of treatment suggests that there may be at least two, and we think perhaps many more, ways to improve a motor skill when treatment is offered with sufficient frequency. The greatest improvement in all variables occurred at the end of the first week of treatment. These improvements however, lasted through a week of no treatment and throughout the second week of treatment. Although a longer study would be necessary to be certain, it may be that once qualitative change has occurred after sufficient frequency of treatment, the change remains. This would be considered learning within a motor learning approach.

The improvements in speed and smoothness of movement that were seen in this study were not measured against a clinical or functional scale of movement. Movement times decreased by 30% for some subjects. Summed over the course of a day, this could certainly be a benefit to the child in terms of energy expenditure and classroom work completed. These measures might be a focus of future studies in which performance in a laboratory setting would be matched to classroom performance.

Each type of treatment (NDT and practice) might be expected to yield different changes in motor performance. Because the NDT approach included goals of decreasing spasticity and improving postural stability, it may be that the treatment effects would be most obvious in the postural set used for reaching. Practice of the task might be expected to affect variables such as movement time, which was the case in this experiment. We are currently evaluating the postural alignment and control in these subjects during the reaching task. Results of this analysis may assist us in understanding the differential effects of treatments on different

parts of a movement.

The importance of time in our research should be emphasized, both time in treatment and the effects of time off. From the motor learning literature, we have learned the value of rest or time off from practice, yet this is not something that therapists typically include when working to improve functional skills. Future research might concentrate more on the effects of high-frequency treatments coupled with "time off," which may encourage the consolidation of the motor skill.

One other feature of our research is the variability between subjects and within each subject's ability. This finding is not new, but analysis and testing of strategies to address this variability are needed. We have suggested elsewhere[40] that subjects might be grouped by movement variables that they have in common rather than by features such as spasticity or body parts involved. We became aware of this possibility more clearly while working on these data. Some children with spasticity may have problems with initiation of movement, whereas others have difficulty with the overall speed of a movement. A new research strategy would be to analyze movement components such as speed, smoothness, cardiorespiratory effort, ability to isolate movement, and so forth prior to treatment and then assign groups for intervention based on these common features of movement. As we outlined in the beginning of this report, the movement problems of children with CP are varied, but children may be grouped based on common features that we have not previously identified.

In future research, additional variables should be assessed following treatment. We had two examples of subjects reporting "tightness" of muscles following their experimental treatment regimen. Five of the subjects experienced 1 week of no treatment followed by 1 week of practice and

Appendix
Neurodevelopmental Treatment-Based Treatment Activities

Improve ability to reach forward and up.

Improve initiation and control of active shoulder flexion with neutral rotation. Increase range of motion between scapula and humerus, strengthen shoulder flexors, and reduce muscle tone or spasticity that may be preventing desired motion.

Improve active elbow extension during a forward reach. Increase range of motion, reduce muscle tone, and strengthen muscles at the elbow.

Improve shoulder and scapular stability during forward reach.

Improve trunk stability and ability to make postural adjustments during reaching tasks so subject can easily reach forward without forward or lateral trunk flexion. If forward or lateral flexion accompanies reaching, then improve ability to regain upright, midline posture.

then another week of no treatment. One subject's mother indicated that if her daughter had not received "real therapy" during the fourth week, she was going to stop participation because she was having so much difficulty helping her daughter put on her shirt in the morning. A second subject reported stiffness in his muscles at the same point in the project. The typical treatment these subjects were receiving was clearly benefiting them in ways we did not measure in this study.

Conclusions

Experimental research on rehabilitation for children with CP is critical for the improvement of our understanding of the nature of change and how it is affected.

Although this study was limited by a small sample size and large variability of the children's movements, we were able to further develop dependent measures that are sensitive to change and features of therapy such as frequency of treatment that should be explored further. The relationship of changeable movement features also must be mapped onto functional abilities. In this study, for example, the improvement in speed and smoothness of reaching may have been accompanied by changes in cardiorespiratory requirements or classroom performance with communication boards. These expanded measures should be included in future research.

References

1 Healy A. Cerebral palsy. In: Blackman JA, ed. *Medical Aspects of Developmental Disabilities in Children Birth to Three.* Rockville, Md: Aspen Publishers Inc; 1984:31-37.

2 Wilson JM. Cerebral palsy. In: Campbell SK, ed. *Pediatric Neurologic Physical Therapy.* New York, NY: Churchill Livingstone Inc; 1984:353-413.

3 Campbell SK. Efficacy of physical therapy in improving postural control in cerebral palsy. *Pediatric Physical Therapy.* 1990;2:135-140.

4 Ottenbacher KJ, Biocca Z, Decremer G, et al. Quantitative analysis of the effectiveness of pediatric therapy: emphasis on the neurodevelopmental treatment approach. *Phys Ther.* 1986;66:1095-1101.

5 Bly L. A historical and current view of the basis of NDT. *Pediatric Physical Therapy.* 1991;3:131-135.

6 Scherrer AL, Tscharmuter I. *Early Diagnosis and Therapy in Cerebral Palsy: A Primer on Infant Development Problems.* New York, NY: Marcel Dekker Inc; 1982.

7 Bobath B, Bobath K. *Motor Development in the Different Types of Cerebral Palsy.* London, England: William Heinemann Medical Books Ltd; 1975.

8 Bobath K, Bobath B. Cerebral palsy. In: Pearson P, Williams C, eds. *Physical Therapy Services in the Developmental Disabilities.* Springfield, Ill: Charles C Thomas, Publisher; 1972:37-185.

9 Keshner EA. Reevaluating the theoretical method underlying the neurodevelopmental theory: a literature review. *Phys Ther.* 1981;61:1035-1040.

10 Olney SJ, Wright MJ. Cerebral palsy. In: Campbell SK, ed. *Physical Therapy for Children.* Philadelphia, Pa: WB Saunders Co; 1994.

11 Horak FB. Assumptions underlying motor control for neurologic rehabilitation. In: Lister MJ, ed. *Contemporary Management of Motor Control Problems: Proceedings of the II Step Conference.* Alexandria, Va: Foundation for Physical Therapy Inc; 1991:11-27.

12 Henderson A. Research in occupational and physical therapy with children. *Advances in Behavioral Pediatrics.* 1981;2:33-59.

13 Parette HP, Hourache JJ. A review or therapeutic intervention research on gross and fine motor progress in young children with cerebral palsy. *Am J Occup Ther.* 1984;38:462-468.

14 Palmer FB, Shapiro BK, Wachtel RC, et al. The effects of physical therapy on cerebral palsy: a controlled trial in infants with spastic diplegia. *N Engl J Med.* 1988;318:803-808.

15 Carlsen PN. Comparison of two occupational therapy approaches for treating the young cerebral palsied child. *Am J Occup Ther.* 1975;29:267-272.

16 Karlsson B, Nauman B, Gardestrom L. Results of physical treatment in cerebral palsy. *Cerebral Palsy Bulletin.* 1960;2:278-285.

17 Kong E. Very early treatment of cerebral palsy. *Dev Med Child Neurol.* 1966;8:198-202.

18 Laskas CA, Mullen SL, Nelson DL, Willson-Broyles M. Enhancement of two motor functions of the lower extremity in a child with spastic quadriplegia. *Phys Ther.* 1985;65:11-16.

19 Mullen SL. *Neurodevelopmental Treatment Techniques and Dorsiflexor Activity in a Child With Spastic Diplegia.* Boston, Mass: Boston University; 1981. Master's thesis.

20 DeCangi GA, Hurley L, Linscheid TR. Towards a methodology of short-term effects of neurodevelopmental treatment. *Am J Occup Ther,* 1983;37:479-484.

21 Footh WK, Kogan KL. Measuring the effectiveness of physical in the treatment of cerebral palsy. *J Am Phys Ther Assoc.* 1963;43:867-873.

22 Wright T, Nicholson J. Physiotherapy for the spastic child: an evaluation. *Dev Med Child Neurol.* 1973;15:146-163.

23 Noonan MJ. Teaching postural reactions to students with severe cerebral palsy: an evaluation of theory and technique. *Journal of Association for Persons With Severe Handicaps.* 1984;9:111-122.

24 Bobath B. The treatment of neuromuscular disorders by improving patterns of coordination. *Physiotherapy.* 1969;55:18-22.

25 Winstrin CJ. Knowledge of results and motor learning: implications for physical therapy. In: *Movement Science.* Alexandria, Va: American Physical Therapy Association; 1991:181-190.

26 Goodgold-Edwards S. Principles for guiding action during motor learning. *Physical Therapy Practice.* 1992;2(4):30-39.

27 Schmidt RA. Motor learning principles for physical therapy. In: Lister MJ, ed. *Contemporary Management of Motor Control Problems: Proceedings of the II STEP Conference.* Alexandria, Va: Foundation for Physical Therapy Inc; 1991:49-63.

28 Winstein CJ. Designing practice for motor learning: clinical implications. In: Lister MJ, ed. *Contemporary Management of Motor Control Problems: Proceedings of the II STEP Conference.* Alexandria, Va: Foundation for Physical Therapy Inc; 1991:65-76.

29 Lee TD, Swanson LR, Hall AL. What is repeated in a repetition? Effects of practice conditions on motor skill acquisition. In: *Movement Science.* Alexandria, Va: American Physical Therapy Association; 1991:191-197.

30 Kluzik J, Fetters L, Coryell J . Quantification of control: a preliminary study of effects of neurodevelopmental treatment on reaching in children with spastic cerebral palsy. *Phys Ther.* 1990;70:65-78.

31 Campbell SK. Measurement in developmental therapy: past, present, and future. In: Miller LJ, ed. *Developing Norm-Referenced Standardized Tests.* Binghamton, NY: Haworth Press; 1989:I-13.

32 Montgomery PC, Halpern D. Quantitative evaluation of upper extremity activity in patients with cerebral palsy. *Phys Ther.* 1972;52:170-175.

33 Fetters L, Todd J. Quantitative assessment of infant reaching movements. *Journal of Motor Behavior.* 1987;19:147-166.

34 Winter DA. *The Biomechanics and Motor Control of Human Gait.* Waterloo, Ontario, Canada: University of Waterloo Press; 1988.

35 von Hofsten C. Development of visually directed reaching: the approach phase. *Journal of Human Movement Studies.* 1979;5:160-178.

36 Brooks VB. Some examples of programmed limb movements. *Brain Res.* 1974;71:299-308.

37 Scholz J. Reliability and validity of the WATSMART™ three-dimensional optoelectric motion analysis system. *Phys Ther.* 1989;69:679-688.

38 Haggard P, Wing AM. *Assessing and Reporting the Accuracy of Developmental Disabilites in Children Birth to Three.* Rockville, Md: Aspen Publishers Inc; 1990:31-37.

39 Stevens J. *Applied Multivariate Statistics for the Social Sciences.* Hillsdale, NJ: Lawrence Erlbaum Associates Inc; 1981.

40 Fetters L. Measurement and treatment in cerebral palsy: an argument for a new approach. *Phys Ther.* 1991;71:244-247.

Parent Reports of Sensory Symptoms in Toddlers with Autism and Those with Other Developmental Disorders

Sally J. Rogers,[1,3] Susan Hepburn,[2] and Elizabeth Wehner

Key words: Autism; developmental delays; sensory; parent report; fragile X syndrome.

The Short Sensory Profile was used to assess parental report of sensory reactivity across four groups of young children (n = 102). Groups were autism (n = 26), fragile X syndrome (n = 20), developmental disabilities of mixed etiology (n = 32), and typically developing children (n = 24). Groups were comparable on overall mental age (x = 22 months), and clinical groups were comparable on chronological age (x = 31 months). Significant differences were detected at alpha <.01 for tactile sensitivity [$F(3,99) = 10.01$], taste/smell sensitivity [$F(3,99) = 11.63$], underreactive/seeks stimulation [$F(3,99) = 4.56$], auditory filtering [$F(3,99) = 19.67$], and low energy/weak muscles [$F(3,99) = 14.21$]. Both children with fragile X syndrome and children with autism had significantly more sensory symptoms overall than the two comparison groups, and children with autism did not differ significantly from children with fragile X syndrome. Both groups were more impaired than developmentally delayed and typically developing children in tactile sensitivity and auditory filtering. Children with autism were more abnormal in responses to taste and smell than all other groups. Children with fragile X syndrome were more abnormal than all other groups in low energy/weak muscles. Sensory reactivity of children with developmental delays was comparable to mental age–matched typically developing toddlers. Correlational analyses indicated that neither overall developmental level nor IQ was related to abnormal sensory reactivity in children with autism or general developmental disorders. However, abnormal sensory reactivity had a significant relationship with overall adaptive behavior.

[1]M.I.N.D. Institute, Department of Psychiatry, University of California, Davis, Sacramento, California. [2]Department of Psychiatry, University of Colorado Health Center, Denver, Colorado. [3]Correspondence should be addressed to Sally J. Rogers, M.I.N.D. Institute, University of California, Davis, 2825 50th Street, Sacramento, CA 95817; e-mail: sally.rogers@ucdmc.udavis.edu.

Introduction

The autobiographical and clinical literatures in autism treat sensory dysfunction as an established core deficit (Grandin & Scariano, 1986). Unusual behavioral responses to sensory stimuli have been described in Autistic Disorder from the 1960s onward and have been incorporated into most systems for diagnosis of autism. Yet compared with the host of studies that have investigated symptoms related to language development, social functioning, and cognitive functioning, the sensory symptom area has been understudied (Goldstein, 2000). A main question regarding sensory responsivity concerns the specificity of this symptom to autism. Wing and Gould (1979) reported unusual sensory responses in other clinical groups, particularly those with severe mental retardation, blindness, and deaf-blindness.

Parent report of children's sensory symptoms has been one of the most frequently used methods for studying sensory responsivity in the autism literature. Studies using parent questionnaires that compare children with autism to chronologically age-matched typically developing children consistently report significantly elevated rates of sensory symptoms in the group with autism, both in preschoolers (Ornitz, Guthrie,

& Farley, 1977) and in school aged children (Kientz & Dunn, 1997). Although Ornitz et al. (1977) reported that only a minority of young children with autism demonstrated abnormalities on the perceptual items on their questionnaire, Kientz and Dunn (1997) reported that children with autism were reported to have widespread difficulties, with significantly more severe or more frequent symptoms reported on 84 of 99 questions on their scale. Similar findings have been published on a comparison of children with Asperger's Syndrome and those with typical development (Dunn, Myles, & Orr, 2002), in which the children with Asperger's differed significantly from the typical comparison group on 22 of 23 items.

Parent questionnaire studies that have compared children with autism to those with other disabilities have also generally reported some autism-specific findings (Dahlgren & Gillberg, 1989; Lord, Rutter, & Le Couteur, 1994; Lord, Storoschuk, Rutter, & Pickles, 1993; Wing & Gould, 1979), though the degree of difference is typically less than in studies using typical age-matched comparison groups. Using the Autism Diagnostic Interview–Revised (ADI-R; Lord et al., 1994) a semistructured parent interview that includes a set of questions on sensory and repetitive behaviors,

Lord and colleagues (Lord, 1995; Lord et al., 1993, 1994) reported elevated levels of sensory symptoms in children with autism compared with children with other kinds of developmental delays in several studies, with children across the age range starting as young as 2 years. Dahlgren and Gillberg (1989) reported that children with autism differed significantly from both delayed and typical comparison groups on only 12 of 130 items.

There are some clinical groups, however, that demonstrate sensory responses quite similar to those seen in autism. Wing and Gould (1979) reported that children with autism and children who were blind and deaf had similarly elevated rates of sensory symptoms on parent report questionnaires. Miller, Reisman, McIntosh, & Simon (2001) found elevated rates in three clinical groups of children—children with fragile X syndrome (FXS), children with sensory modulation disorder (SMD), and children with autism—compared with children with typical development at a mean age of 8.5 years. However, the group with autism did not differ from children with FXS or those with sensory modulation disorder on parent reports of sensory symptoms.

The advantage of using parent questionnaires to study sensory behaviors involves

Article Reprint Information: Reprinted from Springer/*Journal of Autism and Developmental Disorders*, 33(6), 2003, 631-642, Parent reports of sensory symptoms in toddlers with autism and those with other developmental disorders, Rogers, S. J., Hepburn, S., & Wehner, E., with kind permission from Springer Science and Business Media.

the ability to gather cumulative information on a relatively low-frequency behavior across place and time from an observer with great familiarity with the child. However, use of parent questionnaires for studying sensory symptoms raises several questions. Dahlgren and Gillberg (1989) caution that parent responses to questionnaires can be powerfully influenced by the symptoms they know to be associated with their children's diagnosis, and Goldstein (2000) has recently highlighted the methodological problems that occur in many of the studies on sensory functioning in autism—problems including methods and verification of diagnosis, presence of other medical conditions, ranges of age and IQ, and psychometric qualities of the measurement systems.

There are several concerns about external validity of parent questionnaire studies of sensory functioning in autism. Without such validation, it is difficult to interpret the data derived from questionnaires, especially for a symptom that is so widely associated with autism as is sensory responsivity. Miller et al. (1999) addressed many of the questions concerning validity and psychometric qualities of a particular parent questionnaire, The Short Sensory Profile (Dunn, 1999). These authors demonstrated that abnormal scores on the Short Sensory Profile converged with an independent, clinical assessment of sensory modulation disorder. Furthermore, they demonstrated that abnormal scores on the profile converged with abnormal psychophysiological responses to a series of sensory challenges in children with typical development and in those with sensory modulation disorder. Although this work needs to be replicated, this study provides support for the use of this questionnaire as a valid reflection of sensory responsivity in children.

A second question that has come up in recent years concerns the developmental trajectory of sensory symptoms. In a well-designed study of the youngest children with autism thus far reported on, Cox et al. (1999) reported that there were no specific items involving parent reports of repetitive and stereotyped behaviors that differentiated 20-month-old children with autism from those who had language delays, Pervasive Developmental Disorders or typical development, although the children with autism had significantly higher total scores than typical or language-delayed groups. The authors raise the question of whether these symptoms develop somewhat later than the language and social symptoms that differentiate autism by 20–24 months of age. A later-emerging set of symptoms might indi-

cate a different causal mechanism (Bishop, 1997). Lord (1995) similarly suggested that sensory symptoms might increase as children develop through the preschool period.

In addition to the question of relationships between sensory symptoms and age, there is a question concerning relationships with autism severity. Wing and Gould (1979) suggested that sensory symptoms, as one of the two primary symptoms in autism, would co-vary with the severity of autism. However, in perhaps the only study to examine this relationship, Kientz and Dunn (1997) did not find any relationship between autism severity and sensory symptom severity.

To summarize, parent questionnaire studies of sensory symptoms of children with autism have been carried out by a number of authors. This method allows for assessment of a low-incidence behavior over a much greater period of time than an observational study, and the one validation study that has been done demonstrated the congruence between parents' report, clinician report, and psychophysiological measures of sensory responsivity. However, important questions concerning the specificity of these symptoms to autism, the developmental pattern of these symptoms, their relation to severity of other symptoms, and their relevance to the development of adaptive skills have barely been examined.

This study, which is part of a larger longitudinal study of autism early in life, sought to examine the pervasiveness of behaviors thought to reflect sensory abnormalities that parents report in toddlers with autism. The study was designed to replicate the Kientz and Dunn (1997) study, using younger, more developmentally homogeneous children with autism. In addition, two carefully matched clinical control groups, as well as a typical group, were used to examine Wing's (1969) hypothesis that the presence of sensory abnormalities is more related to the severity of disability than to autism per se.

There are four aims to this study: (1) to examine parental reports of sensory symptoms in young children with several different developmental disabilities including autism, in order to examine the presence and specificity of these symptoms in early autism; (2) to examine relationships of sensory symptoms with intellectual ability, age, overall severity of autism, and severity of specific symptom clusters associated with autism; (3) to examine external validity by comparing consistency of parental reports and observer reports of sensory symptoms across several different instruments; and (4) to evaluate the relative contribution of sen-

sory symptoms to the acquisition of adaptive behavior in young children.

Methods

Participants

One hundred two children were included in this study and made up four groups as a function of diagnosis: Autistic Disorder (n = 26), fragile X syndrome (n = 20), developmental delay of mixed/unknown etiology (n = 32), and typically developing children (n = 24). See Table I for participant characteristics. Children in the clinical groups were between the ages of 21 and 50 months (mean age = 31 months). Typically developing children were recruited in an effort to be comparable on mental age to the clinical groups and were, therefore, significantly younger (mean = 19 months). Mental ages were derived via the Mullen Scales of Early Learning (MSEL; Mullen, 1995). There were no significant differences across groups in nonverbal mental age [$F(3,99) = 21.04$, $p = .38$] or overall mental age [$F(3,99) = 1.37$, $p = .26$]; however, there was a significant effect for diagnostic group on verbal mental age [$F(3,99) = 4.32$, $p < .01$]. Post hoc comparisons using a Tukey's correction revealed that typically developing children had higher verbal mental ages than children in the autism group ($p < .01$).

Participants in the clinical groups were recruited from various health and early education agencies, as well as parent support/advocacy groups (e.g., Autism Society of America, National Fragile X Foundation). Children in the fragile X group were also recruited from specialty fragile X clinics across the country (primarily in Denver, Colo.; Oakland, Calif.; and Chapel Hill, N.C.). Children with typical development were recruited from the University of Denver subject pool. The groups were quite similar in ethnic distribution and socioeconomic status (Hollingshead, 1975).

Inclusion criteria for each of the groups were applied in a strict manner. Every child participated in a diagnostic assessment battery designed to identify symptoms of autism in young children. A diagnosis of autism was based on the child meeting four out of five of the following criteria: previous clinical diagnosis of autism, scores above the autism cutoff on the ADI-R (Lord et al., 1994); scores above cutoff on the Autism Diagnostic Observation Schedule (ADOS; Lord, Rutter, DiLavore, & Risi, 1999); endorsements on a DSM-IV checklist; and current clinical diagnosis of autism. Clinical diagnoses were formulated by psychologists with extensive experience in autism.

Table I.
Participant Characteristics (n = 102)

	Autism (n = 26)	Fragile X syndrome (n = 20)	Developmental delay (n = 32)	Typically developing (n = 24)
Chronological age				
Mean (SD)	33.67 (3.6)	36.11 (8.1)	33.23 (6.7)	19.50 (4.8)
Range	26-41	21-50	24-47	12-35
Overall mental age				
Mean (SD)	20.74 (6.3)	20.14 (6.8)	23.13 (6.9)	23.38 (6.3)
Range	12-42	11-34	14-41	14-41
Nonverbal mental age				
Mean (SD)	25.78 (12.0)	21.69 (5.5)	24.35 (7.0)	22.67 (5.6)
Range	16-60	14-35	15-40	15-40
Verbal mental age				
Mean (SD)	17.08 (7.2)	18.77 (8.2)	22.02 (7.2)	24.08 (7.5)
Range	5-37	7-34	12-41	11-43
Developmental quotient (ma/ca) * 100				
Mean (SD)	62 (18)	55 (16)	67 (16)	108 (14)
Range	40-119	35-78	42-78	94-116

Children who met criteria for autism and who presented with extreme prematurity, another medical condition, or a significant illness were excluded from the study. All of the children with autism were free from any other medical condition.

Diagnosis of fragile X syndrome (n = 20) was based on molecular genetic testing, which was completed before the subjects' enrollment in this study. The children with fragile X syndrome were free from another medical condition and had no visual or hearing impairment. Similar to all other participants, subjects with fragile X syndrome were administered an intensive diagnostic protocol to identify children with comorbid fragile X and autism. Seven subjects (35%) with fragile X syndrome met criteria for a diagnosis of autism on two of three diagnostic systems (i.e., DSM-IV, ADI-R, ADOS-Generic [G]) and by clinical judgment.

Children in the developmental delay of mixed or unknown etiology group (n = 32) met the following criteria: developmental delay with an overall standard score on the MSEL (Mullen, 1995) between 35 and 70; absence of a fragile X diagnosis; no past or current diagnosis of autism; and not meeting criteria for autism on two or more of the autism diagnostic measures (e.g., ADOS, ADI-R, DSM-IV). Fifteen of these children (47%) had a diagnosis of Down Syndrome based on chromosomal testing, which was completed before the subjects' enrollment

in this study. Preliminary analyses indicated no significant differences between the children with Down Syndrome and those with other developmental disabilities with respect to developmental functioning or sensory reactivity; thus, the groups were collapsed into one group. In addition to the children with Down Syndrome, three children presented with another known abnormality (on chromosomes 7, 15, and 21). None of the children in the developmentally disabled group had a hearing impairment, but two wore glasses to correct for vision difficulties. Four children (13%) were born prematurely, and four (13%) had a history of significant illness, such as a cardiac problem. None of these subjects had a past or present diagnosis of autism, and none met the criteria for autism on two or more of the autism diagnostic measures (e.g., ADOS, ADI, DSM-IV).

Children in the typically developing group (n = 24) had normal hearing and vision. None were born prematurely. All of these children obtained developmental scores in the average or above-average range across all domains.

Measures

Short Sensory Profile

The Short Sensory Profile is a parent report measure of behaviors associated with abnormal responses to sensory stimuli. The Sensory Profile from which the norms were

established was standardized on 1,200 children; the Short Sensory Profile has reliability of .90 and discriminate validity >95% in identifying children with and without sensory modulation dysfunction (McIntosh, Miller, & Shyu, 1999). Items are scored on a 0–4 scale, with higher scores indicating more impairment. The total score is the best indicator of overall sensory dysfunction. There are also seven factor scores with good internal and external validity: tactile sensitivity, taste/smell sensitivity, movement sensitivity, auditory filtering, low energy/weak, underreactive/seeks stimulation and visual/auditory sensitivity. Internal consistency of factors within the scale ranged from .70 to .90. The instrument takes approximately 10 minutes to complete.

ADI-R

The ADI-R is a structured, standardized parent interview developed to assess the presence and severity of symptoms of autism in early childhood across all three main symptom areas involved in autism: social relatedness, communication, and repetitive or restricted behaviors. The ADI-R has been carefully psychometrically validated across a wide range of ages and severity levels in autism. The interview consists of over 100 questions. Considered the "gold standard" in assessment in autism, this instrument yields an algorithm score and cut offs for a diagnosis of autism. An algorithm has been established that differentiates autism from other developmental disorders at high levels of sensitivity and specificity (over .90 for both) for subjects with mental ages (MAs) of 18 months and older. Dr. Lord trained one author (S.J.R.) to reliability on the ADI-R; this author then trained other raters in her lab to reliability of 80% or better item agreement on three consecutive administrations using the full range of scores (0–3) rather than the truncated scoring usually used (0–2). Interobserver reliability of 80% or better was maintained across the duration of the project and systematically evaluated for more than 20% of subjects. Eleven subjects out of 104 were missing one or more scores for items on the ADI-R. For the purposes of this article, the mean score of the appropriate diagnostic group was substituted for the missing score.

ADOS-G

The ADOS-G is a semistructured standardized interview using developmentally appropriate social and toy-based interactions in a 30–45-minute interview to elicit symptoms of autism in four areas: social interaction, communication, play, and repetitive behaviors. The ADOS-G consists of four different modules, each directed at a particular level of language ability. In this study, all subjects in the clinical groups received Module 1 at the initial visit, for preverbal children or those just beginning to speak. Three typically developing children were administered Module 2, which is for children who are using phrases. The ADOS-G and its predecessors, the ADOS and the PLADOS, have been carefully psychometrically validated across a wide range of ages and severity levels in autism (Lord et al., 1994). In this study, Dr. Lord trained two authors (S.J.R. and E.W.) to reliability on the ADOS-G at the University of Chicago; these authors then trained other raters in the lab to reliability of 80% or better item agreement on three consecutive administrations using the full range of scores (0–3). Reliability was maintained at 85% and checked for 20% of participants across the period of data gathering. The ADOS-G was administered to all subjects in the study as part of the diagnostic qualification process.

MSEL

The MSEL (Mullen, 1995) is a standardized developmental test for children ages 3 months to 60 months that yields five subscale scores representing developmental ages: gross motor, fine motor, visual reception, expressive language, and receptive language. The MSEL allows for separate standard verbal and nonverbal summary scores to be constructed. The MSEL demonstrates strong concurrent validity with other well-known developmental tests of motor, language, and cognitive development. The MSEL was administered to all subjects according to standard instructions by raters with advanced degrees who were trained in assessing young children with autism and other developmental disorders. Reinforcers for all subjects in all groups were used at times to reward cooperation and attention.

Vineland Scales of Adaptive Behavior, Interview Edition

The Vineland (Sparrow, Balla, & Cicchetti, 1984) is a standardized parent interview that yields adaptive behavior scores and developmental ages across four domains: social, communication, daily living, and motor skills. The domain age equivalents, standard scores, and adaptive behavior composite were used in these analyses. The interview was administered by a graduate student or psychologist to the primary caregiver of the child during a laboratory visit.

Procedures

The entire study was carried out under institutional review board approval. Consent forms were reviewed with each family, and all questions were answered before consent was obtained and before any measures were gathered. Mothers completed the Short Sensory Profile before the first visit with the research staff, which was usually conducted at the family's home. During this initial visit, a psychologist or Master's-level clinician administered the ADI-R and the Vineland to the mother of the child. The ADOS-G and the MSEL were administered in the lab over several visits, along with other measures not reported here. For children living in other states, clinicians from the team administered a brief assessment battery in a clinic within an hour of the family's home. Follow-up medical information was obtained from pediatricians and other medical personnel who treated the children. The lead psychologist then reviewed all diagnostic and medical information and assigned each child to one of the clinical groups or excluded them from the study. In addition, other data were gathered that are not being reported here.

Results

Group Differences in Parent Report of Sensory Symptoms

Preliminary Analyses. Before conducting analyses of variance across the four groups (i.e., autism, fragile X syndrome, developmental delay of mixed etiology, and typically developing children), normality of the data and homogeneity of the variances across groups were examined. Total sensory scores were normally distributed (with values of skewness and kurtosis statistics ranging from -1 to +1) for all of the clinical groups but were slightly kurtotic (value = -1.93) for the typical group. This indicates that the distribution of scores for the typical group was rather flat, although the skewness approached zero. Examination of scores by domain area (e.g., taste, tactile, etc.) revealed that the distributions were normal across groups for tactile sensitivity, taste/smell sensitivity, underreactive, and visual/auditory sensitivity domains. The scores of the fragile X group were positively skewed and highly kurtotic for auditory filtering (indicating a tendency for scores to cluster at the low end of the distribution, revealing few auditory filtering symptoms). Scores for all other groups were normally distributed for this variable. The domain of low energy/weak muscles revealed non-normal distributions across groups: The autism and typical groups evidenced flat, positively skewed scores (indicating few abnormalities), and the fragile X and DD groups evidenced kurtotic, negatively skewed scores (indicating a tendency toward abnormality within a subset of children). Examination of normality of distributions indicates that parametric techniques can be employed for the total sensory score, tactile sensitivity, taste/smell sensitivity, underreactive, and visual/auditory. Corrections for non-normality will be applied to examine group differences in auditory filtering, and low energy/weak muscles.

Standard deviations of scores by group are presented in Table II. Levene's homogeneity of variances test was applied across groups, and results were nonsignificant, indicating that the groups are fairly comparable in the variances of key variables.

One-Way Analyses of Variance: Sensory Symptoms by Diagnostic Group. Four groups were compared (autism, fragile X syndrome, developmental delays of mixed etiology, and typically developing children) on the overall sensory score and the seven summary scores of the Short Sensory Profile with post hoc tests of multiple comparisons using Tukey's test. Because of the number of tests, alpha was set at .01; see Table II. Significant differences by group were detected for the total score and for five of the seven domains. Post hoc comparisons revealed that children in the autism and fragile X groups obtained significantly higher scores than children with developmental delays or those who were developing typically, with overall mean score 2 SD above the typical

Table II.
Mean Scores on Short Sensory Profile Domains and Autism Diagnostic Observation Schedule (ADOS)/Autism Diagnostic Interview (ADI) Summary Scores by Diagnostic Group (n = 102)

	Autism	Fragile X syndrome	Developmental delay	Typically developing	F	p
Total sensory score						
Mean (SD)	50.29 (13.7)	55.82 (21.1)	38.32 (16.7)	23.23 (11.1)	13.01	.000
Range	27-75	15-97	5-70	8-36		
Tactile						
Mean (SD)	9.09 (4.8)	8.26 (5.3)	5.22 (2.9)	3.22 (2.4)	10.01	.000
Range	2-20	1-19	1-13	0.7		
Taste and smell						
Mean (SD)	8.91 (4.8)	5.21 (4.4)	4.19 (3.6)	2.42 (2.5)	11.63	.000
Range	0-16	0-12	0-13	0-8		
Underreactive						
Mean (SD)	9.44 (4.0)	12.12 (4.6)	7.97 (4.1)	8.45 (3.7)	4.55	.005
Range	2-17	4-25	1-18	1-14		
Auditory filtering						
Mean (SD)	9.78 (3.0)	10.14 (4.7)	6.03 (3.0)	3.29 (2.3)	19.67	.000
Range	3-16	4-25	0-13	1-9		
Visual and auditory sensitivity						
Mean (SD)	6.91 (2.7)	5.88 (3.2)	5.75 (3.2)	5.15 (2.2)	1.54	.211
Range	3-13	2-14	0-14	1-8		
Low energy and weak muscles						
Mean (SD)	4.32 (4.8)	10.59 (6.5)	6.84 (5.1)	.84 (1.4)	14.21	.000
Range	0-12	0-21	0-17	0-5		
ADI-Revised repetitive behavior algorithm score						
Mean (SD)	3.00 (1.6)	2.75 (1.19)	1.28 (1.2)	0.50 (.59)	18.16	.000
Range	1-6	0-6	0-4	0-2		
ADI-Revised repetitive total score						
Mean (SD)	13.96 (9.1)	7.68 (4.7)	4.24 (3.6)	1.58 (2.1)	24.21	.000
Range	3-43	1-20	0-14	0-10		
ADOS repetitive behavior algorithm score						
Mean (SD)	4.73 (2.1)	3.65 (2.1)	1.78 (1.7)	.82 (8)	24.68	.00
Range	0-8	0-8	0-7	0-2		

group mean and .5 *SD* above the developmentally delayed group mean. Children with autism obtained significantly higher scores on taste/smell sensitivity than children in all of the other groups and obtained significantly higher scores on tactile sensitivity and auditory filtering than children in the developmental delay and typical groups. Children with fragile X syndrome obtained significantly higher scores than children in all of the other groups in low energy/weak muscles and obtained higher scores than the developmental delay and typical groups in tactile sensitivity, underreactive/seeks stimulation, and auditory filtering (see Fig. 1).

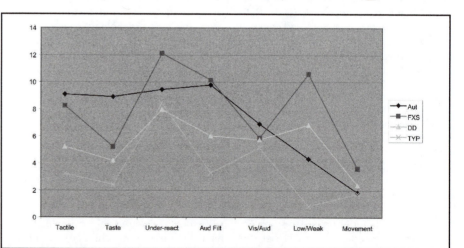

Fig. 1. Mean scores of sensory profile domains by diagnostic group (n = 102).

Table III.
Sensory Symptoms within Subgroups of Fragile X Syndrome: With and Without Autism

	Fragile X with autism (n = 7)	Fragile X without autism (n = 14)
Total sensory score		
Mean (SD)	66.28 (9.6)	50.03 (22.6)
Range	53-81	15-97
Tactile		
Mean (SD)	10.66 (5.2)	7.11 (4.9)
Range	2-18	1-19
Taste and smell		
Mean (SD)	5.17 (4.3)	5.14 (4.5)
Range	0-11	0-12
Underreactive		
Mean (SD)	13.49 (2.3)	10.64 (5.9)
Range	9-17	1-25
Auditory filtering		
Mean (SD)	11.37 (1.6)	9.16 (5.5)
Range	10-14	4-25
Visual and auditory sensitivity		
Mean (SD)	6.41 (3.6)	6.01 (3.5)
Range	3-14	2-14
Low energy and weak muscles		
Mean (SD)	15.11 (4.6)	8.42 (6.0)
Range	10-21	0-19
Movement sensitivity		
Mean (SD)	4.01 (3.7)	3.49 (2.2)
Range	0-9	0-8

Because of the small numbers of subjects within the subgroups of children with fragile X syndrome (with autism: n = 7; without autism: n = 14), it was not feasible to compare statistically the sensory profile scores between subgroups. Further examination of these two subgroups with more subjects is warranted. Preliminary examination of the data indicates that children with comorbid fragile X syndrome and autism may demonstrate more unusual sensory responses and have a tendency toward low energy and weak muscles when compared with children with fragile X syndrome who do not meet criteria for autism (see Table III for means and standard deviations). However, these data must be considered preliminary because of the small numbers of subjects in each cell.

One-Way Analyses of Variance: Repetitive/Restrictive Symptoms by Diagnostic Group.

All four diagnostic groups were compared on Restricted/Repetitive Total Algorithm Scores of the ADI-R and ADOS-G with post hoc tests of multiple comparisons using Tukey's test. Significant differences by group were detected for both scores: ADI-R Restricted/Repetitive Total Algorithm Score [$F(3,98) = 18.15$, $p < .001$] and ADOS-G Restricted/Repetitive Total Algorithm Score [$F(3,98) = 24.68$, $p < .001$]. Post hoc comparisons on the ADI-R score revealed that both the group with autism and the group with fragile X syndrome did not differ from each other, and both had significantly higher scores ($p < .001$) than the typical and developmental delay groups. Post hoc comparisons on the ADOS-G were similar, with the groups with autism and fragile X syndrome not differing significantly from each other. The group with autism differed significantly from the typical and developmental delay groups ($p < .001$ for both), as did the group with fragile X syndrome ($p < .002$ for the developmental delay group, $p < .001$ for the typical group).

It was possible that the elevated Sensory Profile scores for the autism and fragile X

syndrome groups were caused by a general increase in repetitive and restrictive behaviors, which are known to characterize those two groups. To examine that question, all four groups were compared on the summed scores of all the ADI-R Repetitive/Restrictive Behavior questions, numbers 70–85. There was a significant difference by group [$F(3,98) = 24.21$, $p < .001$]. Post hoc comparisons revealed that the group with autism had significantly higher scores than all other groups ($p < .001$). As reported in Table II, their mean scores were triple the mean scores of the developmental delay group and almost twice as large as the fragile X syndrome group.

Relations among Sensory Symptoms, Developmental Variables, and Symptoms of Autism.

Correlations among total sensory scores, IQ, mental age, and algorithm scores on the ADI-R and the ADOS-G were conducted to examine the relations among sensory symptoms, overall developmental level, and symptoms of autism per group. Patterns of correlations were different across groups, perhaps as a function of the restricted range of autism symptom scores in the developmental delay and typical groups. Correlations are displayed for diagnostic groups in Table IV. For the group with autism, total sensory score was significantly and moderately correlated with the ADOS repetitive/restrictive behavior algorithm score, but not with the social/communicative score, indicating some independence among the symptom sets. In the group with fragile X syndrome, ratio IQ and ADI-R total symptom score were moderately associated with sensory symptoms, perhaps indicating that the children with fragile X syndrome who also had autism had more severe sensory symptoms and more severe developmental delays. Neither ratio IQ nor MSEL mental age was associated with sensory score in the other three groups, indicating that neither the severity of mental retardation nor cognitive immaturity was associated with severity of unusual sensory responses reported by the parents.

Convergent Validity of Parental Report of Sensory Symptoms.

As shown in Table IV, there was a significant and moderate correlation between parent report of sensory symptoms using the Short Sensory Profile and clinician observation of repetitive/restricted behavior symptoms on the ADOS for the group with autism ($r = .43$, $p = .03$).

Sensory Symptoms and Adaptive Behaviors

To assess the relative effects of unusual sensory responses on children's general be-

Table IV.
Correlations among Sensory Symptoms, Autism Symptoms, and IQ

Sensory total score	ADI total algorithm score	ADI social and communicative score	ADI restricted activities algorithm score	ADOS social and communicative score	ADOS restricted activities algorithm score	IQ	Overall mental age
Autism (n = 26)	.32	.32	-.14	-.21	.43*, p = .03	-.25	-.09
Fragile X syndrome (n = 20)	**.50*** p = .03	**.50*** p = .03	.25	.34	.35	**-.48,** p = .06	-.30
Developmental delay (n = 32)	.04	.05	-.12	-2.1	.06	.02	.16
Typically developing (n = 24)	-.08	-.09	.14	.14	-.11	-.06	-.18

Note: ADI, Autism Diagnostic Interview; ADOS, Autism Diagnostic Observation Schedule.

havioral functioning, a regression analysis was conducted with the Vineland adaptive behavior composite score as the dependent variable. The predictors entered into the model in a stepwise fashion were overall standard score from the Mullens (i.e., Early Learning Composite), severity of autism symptoms (total from the ADI algorithm), and the total sensory score. As expected, the standard score on the Mullens was the best predictor of adaptive behavior, yielding an adjusted R^2 of .77. Severity of autism symptoms did not add to the prediction of adaptive behavior; however, total scores on the sensory profile did add to the model, accounting for an additional 4% of the variance in Vineland composite scores as shown in Table V.

Table V.
Predictors of Adaptive Behavior Composite Scores from Vineland in Young Children with Various Developmental Disabilities (n = 102)

Variable	Standardized B	t	p	Adjusted
Mullens standardized score (early learning composite)	.88	17.28	.00	.77
Severity of autism symptoms (Autism Diagnostic Interview total score)	-.16	-3.09	ns	Excluded from model
Total sensory score	-.24	-4.31	.00	.04

Discussion

Although repetitive and restricted behaviors are part of the autism phenotype, the relationships among abnormal sensory reactivity, repetitive and restricted behaviors, and core social-communicative symptoms have not often been examined. Sensory and perceptual abnormalities in autism were seen as a primary symptom in earlier decades, but a convincing empirical base for this view was not well established, because of both methodological problems and lack of consistent results. Over the last 20 years, this orientation to autism has been replaced to a large extent with a focus on primary abnormalities in social communicative and social cognitive processes, given the often replicated empirical findings of impairments in joint attention and affective, pragmatic, and theory-of-mind impairments in autism. Yet the autobiographical literature on autism emphasizes the sensory area, findings of abnormal responses to auditory stimuli have been consistently reported, and parent questionnaire–based studies have consistently reported elevated sensory symptoms in older children with autism compared

with other well-matched clinical groups.

This study was undertaken to examine some inconsistencies in the field in terms of how early and how well sensory symptoms differentiate autism from other developmental disorders. We examined one of the youngest groups of children with autism thus far reported on (mean age of 34 months), and we compared these children to several different comparison groups, both with children with typical development matched on developmental level and with children with other kinds of developmental delays, including children with fragile X syndrome, children with Down Syndrome, and children with other developmental disorders, all matched on both chronological and developmental age. Multiple measures of sensory symptoms were used, including two parent report measures (The Short Sensory Profile and the ADI-R) and one clinician observation (the ADOS), designed to allow for observation of sensory related behaviors. All the children were examined on quantitative measures of autism symptoms, allowing us to examine relationships between sensory behaviors and the various core symptoms of autism. In addition, several developmental measures were used to examine the relationships between mental age, IQ, and number and intensity of parent-reported sensory symptoms in this

group of 2- and 3-year-old children.

The first question to be examined had to do with the presence and specificity of sensory symptoms in 2-year-old children with autism. Consistent with most other studies using parent report, we found significantly elevated levels of sensory symptoms in these children with autism compared with both children with typical development and those with delayed development of the same mental ages. There has been a recent suggestion that the repetitive and restrictive symptom set in autism may develop later than the social communicative symptoms (Cox et al., 1999). This has also led to the question of whether this symptom set may be secondary, rather than primary. These data, as well as the other studies of 20–35–month–old children with autism, indicate that both sensory symptoms and other kinds of repetitive and restrictive behaviors are already present and differentiate children with autism from other clinical groups by age 2.5 years, though they may continue to increase in frequency or intensity over time. The sensory symptoms of the group with autism were elevated on some (roughly half), but not all, of the sensory subscales.

However, we also found increased level of sensory symptoms in children with fragile X syndrome, but not Down Syndrome, compared with typical and mixed developmentally delayed groups. Thus, we replicated Wing's findings that, although sensory symptoms are increased in autism compared with some clinical groups, other clinical groups show similar elevations. Children with fragile X syndrome had increased symptoms as a group as well, and the correlations in the fragile X syndrome group between sensory symptoms and other autism symptoms indicated that those children with fragile X syndrome who had more symptoms of autism in other areas also had greater sensory symptoms as well, further underlining the relationship between autism and sensory symptoms.

Although the children with autism and the children with fragile X syndrome had similar levels of sensory behaviors, the children with autism had markedly higher scores (more than 1 SD) than the children with fragile X syndrome on the total score from the repetitive behavior domain of the ADI-R. These findings indicate that what differentiates autism in this sample is not the reported abnormal sensory responses but, rather, the high level of repetitive behaviors and the restricted behavioral repertoire. Furthermore, contrary to clinical lore, the presence of abnormal sensory responses in the children with autism does not appear to explain the elevation in repetitive behaviors, as the children with fragile X syndrome have equally elevated sensory scores but much lower repetitive behavior scores.

The second main question had to do with the relationship between severity of abnormal sensory responses and relationships with mental retardation and developmental immaturity. Higher levels of stereotypic behavior have often been associated with more severe mental retardation, and Thelen (1996) has documented increased levels of repetitive behaviors early in life. However, in this study, neither sensory scores nor repetitive behavior scores demonstrated significant associations with either developmental levels or with ratio IQ scores for any group except the children with fragile X syndrome. Increased sensory scores were associated with clinical diagnosis, either autism or fragile X syndrome, rather than with low IQ or immature developmental levels.

The next important finding from this study had to do with the relationships between sensory symptoms and the social and communicative symptoms of autism. There were no meaningful or significant relationships between social-communicative scores on either the ADI or the ADOS and sensory scores in the children with autism, the children with mixed developmental delays, or

the typically developing children. Thus, in these young children with autism, the symptoms in the social-communicative domain were independent of their symptoms in the sensory domain. Because increased sensory symptoms were not related to the other social-communicative impairments in autism, and as sensory symptoms are not specific to autism, it may be that the sensory impairment is an additional primary impairment, but not an autism-specific impairment. Efforts to find one overall psychological explanation that accounts for all three symptom groups in autism may be in vain.

However, this was not true in fragile X syndrome, in which there were moderate and significant relationships between sensory scores, social-communicative behavior on the ADI, overall ADI score, and IQ. Because the fragile X group includes children with and without autism, this positive relationship appears to reflect the increased severity of sensory symptoms in those children who had comorbid fragile X and autism. On the basis of visual comparison of the data, the children with comorbid fragile X and autism appeared to have the most severe sensory symptoms. This observation is based on only seven children with both fragile X and autism, however, so it is a very preliminary observation and needs to be tested with a group of reasonable size.

Another important finding from this study was the relationship between adaptive behavior and sensory symptoms. A regression analysis revealed that sensory responsivity contributed significantly to adaptive behavior and, indeed, had more influence on adaptive behavior scores than did autism severity scores. However, overall developmental level accounted for most of the variability in adaptive behavior, with sensory symptoms accounting for only 4% of the variance.

The final finding of note involves convergence of findings across differing methods. The substantial correlation between the sensory scores and the ADOS repetitive and restrictive algorithm score provides independent validation of the parent questionnaire data, which has seldom been examined in other studies of parent reports of sensory symptoms.

Strengths of this study involved reasonably sized groups, the use of several well-matched comparison groups, and multiple measures of the constructs being examined. However, a real understanding of the sensory symptoms in autism and other disorders will require information about psychophysiological responses to sensory stimuli in addition to behavioral observations. Miller

et al.'s (1999) preliminary report of parent reports of elevated sensory symptoms and physiological data demonstrating underresponsiveness to sensory stimuli in autism demonstrate the complexity of this symptom. As in many other areas of research in autism, understanding this symptom will require the integration of data from a variety of sources.

In summary, this study found elevated levels of sensory behaviors as reported by parents on two different measures in a group of 2–4-year-old children with autism and children with fragile X syndrome, compared with two other groups: children with developmental delays resulting from other causes and children with typical development of the same developmental levels as the clinical groups. The reported sensory symptoms in the children with autism co-occurred with, but appeared unrelated to, the social-communicative features of autism. Parent reports of sensory symptoms correlated with clinician observation of sensory and repetitive behavior symptoms. Children with fragile X syndrome had similarly elevated levels of sensory behaviors as the children with autism. Thus, abnormal sensory responses did not appear to be specific to autism. However, overall sensory scores correlated with severity of autism symptoms and IQ in the group with fragile X syndrome. Level of sensory symptoms was unrelated to overall mental age or IQ in children with autism or in the group with developmental delays, counter to expectations. This would appear to rule out the presence or level of mental retardation as an explanation for increased sensory symptoms in groups of children similar to those being reported on here. Finally, there were significantly higher scores for repetitive behavior seen in the children with autism than any of the other groups, and this does not seem to be the result of their sensory abnormalities, as the children with fragile X syndrome, equivalent in their sensory score, demonstrated no such elevation in overall repetitive scores.

Acknowledgments

The Definition and Development of the Phenotype in Autism is an ongoing study supported by the following: National Institutes of Child Health and Human Development PO1 HD35468, A Collaborative Program of Excellence in Autism. Dr. Rogers is also supported by National Institute of Deafness and Communication Disorders R21 DC05574. The ongoing help of the Developmental Psychobiology Research Group is gratefully acknowledged.

References

Bishop, D. V. M. (1997). Cognitive neuropsychology and developmental disorders: Uncomfortable bedfellows. *The Quarterly Journal of Experimental Psychology, 50A,* 899–923.

Cox, A., Klein, K., Charman, T., Baird, G., Baron-Cohen, S., Swettenham, J., Drew, A., Wheelwright, S., & Nightingale, N. (1999). The early diagnosis of autism spectrum disorder: Use of the autism diagnostic interview-revised at 20 months and 42 months of age. *Journal of Child Psychology and Psychiatry, 40,* 719–732.

Dahlgren, S. O., & Gillberg, C. (1989). Symptoms in the first two years of life: A preliminary population study of infantile autism. *European Archives of Psychiatry and Clinical Neurosciences, 238,* 169–174.

Dunn, W., Myles, B. S., & Orr, S. (2002). Sensory processing issues associated with Asperger syndrome: A preliminary investigation. *The American Journal of Occupational Therapy, 56,* 97–102.

Dunn, W. (1999). Development and validation of the short sensory profile. In W. Dunn (Ed.), *The sensory profile examiner's manual.* San Antonio, TX: The Psychological Corporation.

Goldstein, H. (2000). Commentary: Interventions to facilitate auditory, visual, and motor integration: "Show me the data." *Journal of Autism and Developmental Disorders, 30,* 423–425.

Grandin, T., & Scariano, M. M. (1986). *Emergence, labeled autistic* (1st ed.). Novato, CA: Arena Press.

Hollingshead, A. B. (1975). *Four factor index of social status.* New Haven, CT: Author.

Kientz, M. A., & Dunn, W. (1997). A comparison of the performance of children with and without autism on the sensory profile. *The American Journal of Occupational Therapy, 51,* 530–537.

Lord, C. (1995). Follow-up of two-year-olds referred for possible autism. *Journal of Child Psychology and Psychiatry, 36,* 1365–1382.

Lord, C., Rutter, M., DiLavore, P., & Risi, S. (1999). *Autism Diagnostic Observation Schedule-WPS Edition.* Los Angeles, CA: Western Psychological Services.

Lord, C., Rutter, M., & Le Couteur, A. (1994). Autism diagnostic interview-revised: A revised version of a diagnostic interview for caregivers of individuals with possible pervasive developmental disorders. *Journal of Autism and Developmental Disorders, 24,* 659–685.

Lord, C., Storoschuk, S., Rutter, M., & Pickles, A. (1993). Using the ADI-R to diagnose autism in preschool children. *Infant Mental Health Journal, 14,* 234–252.

McIntosh, D. N., Miller, L. J., & Shyu, V. (1999). Development and validation of the short sensory profile. In W. Dunn (Ed.), *The sensory profile examiner's manual.* San Antonio, TX: The Psychological Corporation.

Miller, L. J., McIntosh, D. N., McGrath, J., Shyu, V., Lampe, M., Taylor, A. K., Tassone, F., Neitzel, K., Stackhouse, T., & Hagerman, R. J. (1999). Electrodermal responses to sensory stimuli in individuals with fragile X syndrome: A preliminary report. *American Journal of Medical Genetics, 83,* 268–279.

Miller, L. J., Reisman, J., McIntosh, D. N., & Simon, J. (2001). An ecological model of sensory modulation: performance of children with fragile X syndrome, autism, attention deficit disorder with hyperactivity and sensory modulation dysfunction. In S. Smith-Roley, E. Imperatore-Blanche, & R. C. Schaaf (Eds.), *Understanding the nature of sensory integration with diverse populations.* San Antonio, TX: Therapy Skill Builders.

Mullen, E. M. (1995). *Mullens scales of early learning.* (AGS ed.). Circle Pines, MN: American Guidance Service.

Ornitz, E. M., Guthrie, D., & Farley, A. H. (1977). The early development of autistic children. *Journal of Autism and Childhood Schizophrenia, 7,* 207–229.

Sparrow, S. S., Balla, D. A., & Cicchetti, D. (1984). *Vineland Adaptive Behavior Scales.* Circle Pines, MN: American Guidance Service.

Thelen, E. (1966). Normal infant stereotypes: A dynamic systems approach. In R. L. Sprague & K. M. Newell (Eds.), *Stereotyped movements: Brain and behavior relationships.* Washington, DC: American Psychological Association.

Wing, L. (1969). The handicaps of autistic children: a comparison study. *Journal of Child Psychology and Child Psychiatry, 10,* 1–40.

Wing, L., & Gould, J. (1979). Severe impairments of social interaction and associated abnormalities in children: epidemiology and classification. *Journal of Autism and Developmental Disorders, 9,* 11–29.

The Effect of Training Older Adults With Stroke to Use Home-Based Assistive Devices

Cindy W. Y. Chiu, David W. K. Man

Key words: bathing devices, usage rate, functional independence

Abstract: This study evaluated whether an additional home training program on bathing devices would improve the rate of use, personal independence, and service satisfaction of older adults who had experienced strokes. A prospective pretest and posttest randomized control trial design was adopted. Fifty-three older adults who had experienced strokes were randomly assigned to either the intervention group or the control group. The prescription of and training in the use of devices was conducted with both groups while they were in the hospital. The intervention group received additional home-based intervention in the use of devices immediately after discharge, but the control group did not. All of the subjects were assessed before discharge and 3 months after discharge using the Functional Independence Measure and the Quebec User Evaluation of Satisfaction with Assistive Technology. The results showed that the intervention group improved significantly in functioning ($t = 3.89$; $df = 51$; $P = .01$) and satisfaction ($t = 69.8$; $df = 29$; $P = .01$) after intervention. The rate of use of bathing devices was relatively higher in the intervention group (96.7%) than in the control group (56.5%). Further studies with extended follow-up services are needed to evaluate the long-term effects of training in the use of assistive devices.

Cindy W. Y. Chiu, MS, BscOT, HKROT, is Staff Occupational Therapist, Tuen Mun Hospital, Hong Kong, China. David W. K. Man, PhD, MS, PDOT, HKROT, is Associate Professor, Program in Occupational Therapy, The Hong Kong Polytechnic University, Hong Kong, China.

Cerebral vascular accident, or stroke, is the third leading cause of death in the United States and the leading cause of disability involving physical and cognitive impairment. A reported 550,000 people experience strokes every year and nearly 150,000 die of strokes. Three million people survive after their strokes with varying degrees of neurological impairment (U.S. Department of Health and Human Services, 1995). The situation is similar in Hong Kong, where approximately 22,000 individuals have been admitted to hospitals. Among them, 3,000 die of strokes each year. Reports have also shown that the incidence of stroke is increasing and that more stroke survivors are younger (Hong Kong Department of Health, 1999; Hong Kong Hospital Authority, 1998; Geddes, Fear, Tennant, Pickering, Hillman, & Chamberlain, 1996). Hong Kong is also experiencing growth in its population of older adults. Figures provided by the Hong Kong Census and Statistics Department (1999) show that the life expectancy of older adults has increased. However, there has also been an increase in disability in terms of activities of daily living due to morbidity and a decline in function and physical inactivity.

In view of these problems, a cost-effective rehabilitation measure to maximize independence is urgently needed. One of the issues to be addressed is related to the use of assistive devices, which is reportedly effective in assisting with the daily function-ing of older adults. These devices can help overcome impairments, prevent accidents, and promote independence and comfort (Mann, Hurren, & Tomita, 1993). Therefore, the purpose of this study was to evaluate whether additional home-based intervention in the use of bathing devices would affect the rate of use, improvement in personal independence, and service satisfaction of older adults who had experienced strokes.

The application of and training in the use of assistive devices is thought to have a significant influence on body function and occupational performance in activities of daily living, work, and leisure. This can enhance a person's daily independence. The Technology-Related Assistance to Individuals with Disabilities Act of 1988 defined assistive devices as "any item, piece of equipment, or product system, whether acquired commercially, modified or customized, that is used to increase, maintain or improve the functioning capacities of individuals with disabilities" (Technology-Related Assistance for Individuals with Disabilities Act of 1988; Gitlin, Luborsky, & Schemm, 1998).

Reports have detailed the use of assistive devices to improve the functioning and personal independence of individuals. Manton, Corder, and Stallard (1993) showed a significant increase in the use of assistive devices. The use of assistive devices also decreased the amount of personal assistance required by older adults and could reduce some of the burdens experienced by caregivers (Chen, Mann, Tomita, & Nochajski, 2000). In addition, assistive devices can potentially compensate for disabilities and reduce participation restrictions, and thus promote independence and improve quality of life (Edwards & Jones, 1998). Not only can such devices help individuals to become personally independent at home, they can also reduce the strain on informal caregivers, social services, and healthcare professionals (Edwards & Jones, 1998). Bynum and Rogers (1987) found that approximately 80% of older adults who received care in their home environment were using assistive devices. Such devices can help minimize the effects of age-related changes such as the weakening of coordination, vision, and strength. Therefore, the use of assistive devices can improve many of the problems associated with occupational performance and functioning in older adults.

Stroke is an early clinical sign of focal disturbance in cerebral functions, presumably of vascular origin, and of more than 24 hours' duration. Stroke brings on a sudden and possibly complete change in cognitive functioning and physical ability. These changes can be minimal, moderate, or severe, and typically require a process of rehabilitation during which people who have had a stroke must learn how to function using a range of compensatory mechanisms and assistive devices. During rehabilitation, some older adults who have had a stroke frequently use assistive devices to reduce or

Article Reprint Information: Reprinted with permission from Chiu, C. W. Y., & Man, D. W. K. (2004). The effect of training older adults with stroke to use home-based assistive devices. *Occupational Therapy Journal of Research: Occupation, Participation and Health, 24*(3), 113-120.

compensate for the loss of functions. Smith, Walton, and Garraway (1981) found that patients in stroke units used almost twice as many assistive devices as did those in medical units. The use of such devices can better assist a person who has been discharged to achieve personal independence with regard to self-care. In addition, using such devices may enable them to engage in the activities of daily living to achieve a sense of well-being and to see meaning in life.

Bathing devices are among the most frequently prescribed assistive devices. The reported rate of use for bathing devices ranges from 48% (Chamberlain, Thornely, & Wright, 1978) to 84% (Hollings & Haworth, 1978). Bathing devices are worthy of attention because they are significant in maintaining quality of life and personal independence (Parker & Thorslund, 1991). However, most older adults experience problems in bathing and many accidents that involve falls occur in the bathroom. To overcome these problems, a variety of assistive devices are available that make bathing safer and more comfortable. Personal independence in bathing and in the use of the toilet have been found to be important for a person's self-esteem and crucial in maintaining a person in the community (Chamberlain et al., 1978; Clemson & Martin, 1996). In addition, bathing devices that offer support and security can increase safety in bathing (Mann, Hurren, Tomita, & Charvat, 1996).

However, an international study has found that up to 56% of older adults do not comply with such devices and up to 15% stopped using the devices. One of the reasons why older adults do not use assistive devices after they are discharged is that occupational therapists have been unable to provide follow-up services (Finlayson & Havixbeck, 1992). Moreover, occupational therapists might not know whether their interventions have been adequate and effective in raising the level of personal independence unless the older adults make inquiries or return unwanted devices. A low rate of use and inconsistency of use occur during the first 3 months after patients are discharged (Gitlin, Levine, & Geiger, 1993; Phillips & Zhao, 1993). A review of the literature has shown that the abandonment of assistive device use can be related to four significant factors: (1) lack of consideration of the user's opinion in selection, (2) inability to procure device easily, (3) poor device performance, and (4) change in a user's needs or priorities (Phillips & Zhao, 1993). The rate of abandonment is highest for the first year and after 5 years. For the first year,

however, abandonment is highest in the first 3 months. Another indication of the high rate of abandonment is the poor follow-up that determines the performance of such devices and the level of satisfaction of the older adults (Demers, Weiss-Lambrou, Wessels, Ska, & Dewitte, 1996).

Home-based demonstration services in occupational therapy and physiotherapy programs have been reported to increase the rate of assistive device use by people who have experienced hip replacement and those with disabilities that have resulted from a stroke, arthritis, and neurological or orthopedic difficulties (Gitlin & Levine, 1992). The use of bathing devices after home training programs were provided has also resulted in a higher rate of use, improved satisfaction, and safer bathing practices (Bynum & Rogers, 1987). The percentage of assistive devices in use increases when instructions are given on the use of such devices (Bynum & Rogers, 1987; Gilbertson & Langhorne, 2000; Stowe, Thornely, Chamberlain, & Wright, 1982). This also increases the satisfaction and personal safety rating of older adults.

However, assistive devices are not suitable in every environment. Such devices may be useful in hospitals but not necessarily in the homes of older adults. Without follow-up services, older adults may find it difficult to translate skills learned from an institutional setting to a home setting. To reduce problems and improve satisfaction, routine follow-up services for the use of assistive devices are recommended as part of service delivery (Kohn, LeBlanc, & Mortola, 1994).

Method

Subjects

Fifty-three older adults participated in this study. The number of subjects was decided by changes in the outcome measures scores of two groups (intervention and control) using the software program Power Analysis and Sample Size (NCSS Statistical Software, Kaysville, UT). Using the total Functional Independence Measure (FIM) score as an example and by aiming at a power of 0.8 and setting the significance level at .05, the calculated sample size was 25 for both the intervention and the control groups. A single-center approach was adopted, in which the subjects were mainly drawn from the inpatient and outpatient services of the Geriatric and Medicine Unit of Tuen Mun Hospital in Hong Kong. The majority of subjects were from the inpatient services and only a small number (approximately 5%) came

from the outpatient services. To minimize the recruitment of heterogeneous groups, the outpatients were those who had been discharged from the hospital for 2 weeks or less. Subjects who were eligible included those (1) who were 55 years or older; (2) with a primary diagnosis of stroke; (3) able to follow instructions; (4) able to communicate using speech; (5) living at home with family support; and (6) who were assessed by occupational therapists in the hospital as needing a bathing device. Individuals with acute or terminal diseases were excluded from the study.

Procedures

The pretest and posttest randomized control trial design was used to compare the intervention group and the control group. Subjects in need of bathing devices were randomly assigned to the two groups. The occupational therapists, who were involved in the random assignment procedures, were blind to the study's purpose. The prescription of and training in the use of assistive devices were demonstrated to both groups while they were in the hospital. The intervention group received additional home-based training in the use of assistive devices by occupational therapists immediately after being discharged.

The total number of follow-up home services was at least two but not more than three. The first follow-up service took place within 10 days of the first assessment. At this time, an occupational therapist demonstrated and explained the use of assistive devices and safety techniques to the subjects and caregivers (Finlayson & Havixbeck, 1992). The second visit was related to bathing practices, and time was allowed for the subject and the caregiver to express the problems and difficulties encountered in using such devices. The subjects were encouraged to use the bathing devices every time they bathed. In addition, the devices were checked for correct fit and safety. The third visit was optional and depended on the patients' proficiency in device use skills. The control group was provided a pre-discharge home visit for preparing a suitable environment for the client's living and conventional training in the hospital, but did not receive any treatment post-discharge. All of the subjects in the control group and the intervention group were assessed during a follow-up home visit after 3 months for data collection.

Ethical approval was sought before implementation of the study from both the Chief of Service of the Geriatric and Medicine Unit of Tuen Mun Hospital and the Departmental Research Committee at the Department of Rehabilitation Sciences of the Hong Kong Polytechnic University, Hong Kong.

Instrumentation

The instruments used for the assessment were the FIM (Mann et al., 1993; Daving, Andren, Nordholm, & Grimby, 2001) and the Quebec User Evaluation of Satisfaction with Assistive Technology (QUEST) (Demers, Weiss-Lambrou, & Ska, 2000). The measures of functional independence included two subsections, cognitive and motor. The FIM motor measured areas of self-care, sphincter control, mobility, and locomotion, whereas the FIM cognition included the areas of communication and social cognition (Granger, Hamilton, Linacre, Heinemann, & Wright, 1993). It was developed as an instrument to determine the severity of disabilities. The FIM was selected due to its sensitivity and relatively short administration time. The maximum score of the FIM motor was 91 for 13 sub-items. A higher score indicated a better level of function and independence, a lower score reflected an increased need for personal assistance. The scale was rated from 7 to 1, and each score level was defined (e.g., 7 = completely independent or 3 = moderate assistance). The FIM motor included items of self-care (eating, grooming, bathing, dressing, and toileting), locomotion (walk/wheelchair, stairs), sphincter control (bladder management, bowel management), and transfers (bed/chair, toilet, tub, and shower). The maximum score of FIM cognition was 35 for 5 sub-items: communication (comprehension and expression) and social cognition (social interaction, problem solving, and memory). The reliability and validity of the instrument have been extensively investigated and reported in the literature (Dodds, Martin, Stolo, & Deyo, 1993; Pollak, Rheault, & Stoecker, 1996).

The QUEST is an instrument that measures outcomes. It was designed to evaluate a person's satisfaction with assistive technology devices. The QUEST consists of 12 satisfaction items and is divided into two parts: devices (8 items) and services (4 items). The characteristics of the items under devices are dimension, weight, adjustment, safety, durability, simplicity of use, comfort, and effectiveness. The satisfaction items for services are related to service delivery, repairs and servicing, professional services, and follow-up. Each item was scored using a 5-point satisfaction scale, with a score of 1 denoting "not satisfied at all" and 5 indicating that the person was "very satis-

fied." A checklist with the 12 satisfaction items was subsequently presented on the QUEST form, and the user was required to select the three most important items. Regarding the psychometric properties of the QUEST, good test–retest stability, interrater reliability, and internal consistency have been demonstrated (Demers, Ska, Gironx, & Weiss-Lambrou, 1999). A questionnaire was designed to inquire about the subjects' rate of use and bathing independence after training in the intervention and control groups. In addition, evidence of training effect was based on the findings of FIM motor–bathing subscores.

Data Analysis

All of the data in the study were analyzed on a personal computer using the Statistical Package for the Social Sciences (SPSS for Windows version 11.0; SPSS Inc., Chicago, IL). Descriptive statistics were first generated for the sociodemographic variables, rate of use, level of satisfaction, and functional performance of the older adults with stroke. A t test was used to compare the mean differences in the level of independence and satisfaction of the users between and within the two groups.

Results

The 30 intervention and 23 control group participants were equivalent on all measures at the start of the trial. The groups showed no significant differences in age, martial status, educational level, and social and living environment. The average age of the subjects was 72.1 years. The standard deviation was 7.81 years and the range was 55 to 92 years. The majority of the subjects had suffered first from stroke (75%) and then from infarction (80%). Male subjects constituted 66% of the two groups. The prescription of bathing devices to the intervention group and to the control group was similar. However, occupational therapists made more home visits to the intervention group (mean = 2.74) than to the control group (mean = 1.39). Table 1 summarizes the characteristics of the groups.

Functional Performance

There were significant improvements in the mean FIM motor score and the total score (motor and cognition) in both the intervention group and the control group.

As mentioned earlier, both the FIM motor and FIM cognition include several items. In the intervention group, the mean FIM total score of items increased from 97.6 (standard deviation [SD] = 10.7) to 108.9 (SD = 11.6). In the control group, however, the mean FIM total score increased from 97.7 (SD = 11.8)

to 104.9 (SD = 12.0). The mean difference between the pretest and posttest scores was higher in the intervention group (mean total FIM difference = 11.4, SD = 4.2, $P < .001$) than in the control group (mean total FIM difference = 7.0, SD = 3.7, $P < .001$). The mean FIM motor score in the intervention group (motor difference = 10.8, $P < .001$) was higher than in the control group (motor difference = 7.0, SD = 3.7, $P < .001$). All of the mean differences showed a tendency toward a higher score. This indicated better functioning in the intervention group than in the control group (Table 2).

In contrast, there was no significant difference in the FIM cognition score between the two groups. In the intervention group, the mean FIM cognition score increased slightly from 29.8 (SD = 5.55) to 30.7 (SD = 5.58) ($P = .398$). In the control group, the mean FIM cognition score increased from 30.7 (SD = 5.58) to 31.35 (SD = 5.3) ($P = .447$).

There was also a significant improvement in the mean FIM motor score between the intervention group and the control group. In the intervention group, the mean FIM motor score at 3 months after discharge was 78.6 (SD = 7.42). In the control group, the mean FIM motor score at 3 months after discharge was 73.5 (SD = 10.9). The pooled t test was used, because Levene's test for the FIM motor was 0.177. The P value for the pooled t test was .051, which indicated that the mean FIM motor score for the two groups was significantly different (Table 3).

Demographic variables such as age, educational level, diagnoses, and living environment were found to be similar between the intervention and control groups. Because there was a gender imbalance in both groups, analysis of covariance was used to test whether gender had a confounding effect on the outcome. The results were negative. In other words, the difference in FIM scores between the intervention group and the control group still existed.

The QUEST

The evaluation of assistive technology for devices and services, as measured by the QUEST, is provided in Table 4. The total mean score (devices and services) was 4.63 in the intervention group ($P < .01$), but it was only 3.72 in the control group ($P < .01$). The mean score of the devices was 4.59 (SD = 0.4) in the intervention group, but 3.58 (SD = 0.78) in the control group. For services, the mean score was 4.62 (SD = 0.39) in the intervention group, but 3.72 (SD = 0.35) in the control group. These results indicated that there was greater satisfaction with using assistive devices in the intervention group. Moreover, the top three most important satisfaction items for subjects were safety, professional services, and the arrangement of services (Figure).

The rate of bathing device use was higher in the intervention group (96.7%) than in the control group (56.5%). Moreover, the intervention group performed better in functional performance and achieved a higher independent level. The findings also indicated that, in the intervention group, 25 subjects could bathe independently 3 months after being discharged. Only nine subjects could do so in the control group.

Discussion

The results of this study support the findings from studies in Canada (Finlayson & Havixbeck, 1992) by indicating that the non-use of assistive devices can be prevented through home visits. It was also found that instruction and practice in the use of devices had the potential to further improve the level of independence, as indicated in better FIM scores. In fact, a higher level of functioning and independence can be achieved by prescribing and training older adults in the use of assistive devices. Personal independence and functioning were found to be better in the intervention group. Twenty-five subjects in the intervention group could bathe independently 3 months after being discharged. However, only nine subjects could do this in the control group. In addition, the relatively poorer rate of use of such devices by the control group (56.5%) might suggest a need for training services similar to those given to the intervention group (96.7%). These clinically significant findings indicate that home training in the use of bathing devices could promote safer bathing practices.

It may be crucial to provide ongoing assessment and follow-up services to older adults, because the need for assistive devices will change over time. Follow-up services should be provided to identify any problems with the use, compliance with, or abandonment of such devices, although there has always been a need to consider reimbursement of such services over time. Because the subjects were subjectively satisfied with the home visit provided, and were able to demonstrate the proper use of devices on follow-up, occupational therapists should give careful consideration to the inclusion of a home visit in the intervention procedure.

The findings of the QUEST study (satisfaction with assistive device) suggest that occupational therapists may play an important role in the delivery of knowledge and promote acceptance and use of assistive devices by older adults. An occupational therapist might consider conducting relevant assessments or home visits before the prescription of assistive devices to determine related accessibility or the need to environmentally modify the home. This suggests the need for occupational therapists to spend more time determining the importance of such types of treatment activity for individual patients (structuring intervention

Table 1
Characteristics of Subjects

Characteristics	Intervention Group (N = 23) No. (%)	Control Group (N = 23) No. (%)	Overall (N = 53) No. (%)
Demographic			
Gender			
Female	13 (43)	5 (22)	18 (34)
Male	17 (57)	18 (78)	35 (66)
Age, years (mean ± SD)	72.1 ± 6.36	72.2 ± 9.53	72.1 ± 7.81
Having care	30 (100)	23 (100)	53 (100)
Marital status (M or D)	30 (100)	23 (100)	53 (100)
Education			
Illiterate	15 (50)	12 (52)	27 (50.9)
Literate	15 (50)	11 (48)	26 (49.1)
Diagnoses			
Stroke			
First stroke	21 (70)	19 (82.4)	40 (75.5)
Recurrent stroke	9 (30)	4 (17.4)	13 (24.5)
Lesion type			
Infarction	24 (80)	20 (87)	44 (83)
Hemorrhage	6 (20)	3 (13)	9 (17)
Social/living environment			
Type of housing			
Public	7 (23.3)	3 (13)	10 (18.9)
Rental	4 (13.3)	5 (21.7)	9 (17)
Private	19 (63.4)	15 (65.2)	34 (64.2)
Type of bathing facilities			
Bathtub (high)	19 (63.4)	10 (43.5)	29 (54.7)
Bathtub (low)	7 (23.3)	5 (21.7)	12 (22.6)
Shower area	4 (13.3)	8 (34.8)	12 (22.6)
Type of bathing devices			
Bathboard	20 (66.7)	10 (43.5)	30 (56.6)
Stool	3 (10)	2 (8.7)	5 (9.7)
Bathtub transfer bench	1 (3.3)	0 (0)	1 (1.9)
Bathseat	0 (0)	1 (4.3)	1 (1.9)
Shower chair	6 (20)	10 (43.5)	16 (30.2)
Environmental modification			
On-site alteration	8 (26.7)	8 (34.8)	16 (30.2)
Minor modification	20 (66.6)	14 (60.9)	34 (64.2)
Major modification	2 (6.7)	1 (4.3)	3 (5.7)
Financial			
Receiving government subsidy	9 (30)	3 (13)	12 (22.6)
Supported by family	21 (70)	20 (87)	41 (77.4)

SD = standard deviation; M = married; D = divorced.

Table 2
Pretest and Posttest Difference in FIM Scores Between the Intervention Group and the Control Group

	Intervention Group (N = 30)				Control Group (N = 23)			
Outcome	Pretest Mean (SD)	Posttest Mean (SD)	Difference Mean (SD)	P	Pretest Mean (SD)	Posttest Mean (SD)	Difference Mean (SD)	P
Motor	67.7 (7.0)	78.6 (7.4)	10.8 (3.8)	.001	66.5 (10.8)	73.5 (10.9)	7.0 (3.7)	.001
Cognitive	29.8 (5.55)	30.7 (5.30)	0.47 (2.0)	.398	30.7 (5.58)	31.35 (5.3)	0.13 (0.63)	.447
Total	97.6 (10.7)	108.9 (11.6)	11.4 (4.2)	.001	97.7 (11.8)	104.9 (12.0)	7.0 (3.7)	.001

FIM = Functional Independence Measure; SD = standard deviation.

Table 3
Comparison of 3-Month Post-Discharge FIM Motor Outcome Measures Between the Intervention Group and the Control Group

FIM Motor Score	Mean	SD	No.	F value 2-tail Prob.	t	df	Pooled Variance Estimate 2-tail Prob.
Intervention Group	78.6	7.42	30				
				0.177	2.002	51	0.051
Control Group	73.5	10.9	23				

FIM = Functional Independence Measure; SD = standard deviation.

Table 4
Evaluation of Satisfaction With Assistive Technology by Users, as Measured by the QUEST

Score	Intervention Group Mean ± SD	Control Group Mean ± SD
Devices	4.59 ± 0.4	3.58 ± 0.78
Services	4.63 ± 0.39	3.73 ± 0.35
Total	4.62 ± 0.36	3.72 ± 0.28

QUEST = Quebec User Evaluation of Satisfaction with Assistive Technology; SD = standard deviation.

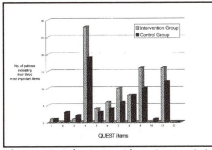

Figure. Satisfaction with using assistive devices as measured by the Quebec User Evaluation of Satisfaction with Assistive Technology (QUEST) for the intervention and control groups. 1 = dimensions, 2 = weight, 3 = adjustments, 4 = safety, 5 = durability, 6 = easy to use, 7 = comfort, 8 = effectiveness, 9 = service delivery, 10 = repair/servicing, 11 = professional service, 12 = follow-up service.

during on-site home training and education). Occupational therapists should also consider whether the need for assistive devices is temporary or permanent, based on the disability of the patients. Loan services for some assistive devices may be necessary for short-term use.

As gatekeepers of technology, occupational therapists must train older adults and their caregivers to use and take care of assistive devices. They should also provide instructions to promote the health and safety of patients who are using such devices. Follow-up services and training in the use of the devices could increase the efficiency of device prescription. The findings of the current study also support the importance of the involvement of caregivers in the use of assistive devices by older adults who experience strokes. Patients and caregivers could subsequently achieve a higher level of personal independence and service satisfaction.

However, the generalizability of the results is limited by the period of the follow-up services. A 3-month follow-up period may not be adequate, because some of the older adults were still in the stage of recovering from their strokes. Moreover, the subjects were recruited solely from the Tuen Mun Hospital. The results cannot be generalized to the entire stroke population without further multicenter studies. Furthermore, the resources and costs involved were higher for the intervention group. This is not consistent with the government's suggestion of promoting the use of limited resources with better results. Nevertheless, the use of devices can reduce the stress on caregivers, social services, and healthcare professionals (Edwards & Jones, 1998). Although the intervention may have cost more to deliver, the cost benefits in the reduced need for formal or informal caregiver assistance should also be determined, and explored in a future study. To some extent, it is anticipated that the costly option of residential care can thus be postponed (Finlayson & Havixbeck, 1992). Hence, future studies should examine patient satisfaction with the use of prescribed equipment, the rate of use of devices after patients have been discharged, and the importance of activity to the patients. The use of evidence to underpin practice in occupational therapy service will therefore be ensured.

Conclusions

The use of devices and other technology will promote the quality of life of older adults who have experienced strokes. The prompt and correct use of assistive devices and the provision of follow-up services in device use training after discharge could ensure safer bathing in all intervention groups.

Acknowledgments

The authors thank Mr. Joseph Poon, Departmental Manager, Occupational Therapy Department, for his advice and Dr. Mok Chun Keung, Consultant Geriatrician, Geriatric Department of Tuen Mun Hospital, for his support in performing this study.

References

Bynum, H. S., & Rogers, J. C. (1987). The use and effectiveness of assistive devices possessed by patients seen in home care. *Occupational Therapy Journal of Research, 7,* 181-191.

Chamberlain, M. A., Thornley, G., & Wright, V. (1978). Evaluation of aids and equipment for bath and toilet. *Rheumatology and Rehabilitation, 17,* 187-194.

Chen, T.-Y. A., Mann, W. C., Tomita, M., & Nochajski, S. (2000). Caregiver involvement in the use of assistive devices by frail older persons. *Occupational Therapy Journal of Research, 20,* 179-199.

Clemson, L., & Martin, R. (1996). Usage and effectiveness of rails, bathing and toileting aids. *Occupational Therapy in Health Care, 10*(1), 41-59.

Daving, Y., Andren, E., Nordholm, L., & Grimby, G. (2001). Reliability of an interview approach to the Functional Independence Measure. *Clinical Rehabilitation, 15,* 301-310.

Demers, L., Ska, B., Gironx, F., & Weiss-Lambrou, R. (1999). Stability and reproducibility of the Quebec User Evaluation of Satisfaction with Assistive Technology (QUEST). *Assistive Technology, 3,* 42-52.

Demers, L., Weiss-Lambrou, R., & Ska, B. (2000). *Quebec User Evaluation of Satisfaction with Assistive Technology (QUEST) version 2.0: An outcome measure for Assistive Technology Devices.* Webster, NY: Institute for Matching Person & Technology.

Demers, L., Weiss-Lambrou, R., Wessels, R. D., Ska, B., & Dewitte, L. (1996). An international content validation of the Quebec User Evaluation of Satisfaction with Assistive Technology (QUEST). *Occupational Therapy International, 6,* 159-175.

Dodds, T. A., Martin, D. P., Stolo, W. C., & Deyo, R. A. (1993). A validation of the Functional Independence Measurement and its performance among rehabilitation inpatients. *Archives of Physical Medicine & Rehabilitation, 74,* 531-536.

Edwards, N. I., & Jones, D. A. (1998). Ownership and use of assistive devices amongst older people in the community. *Age & Aging, 27,* 463-468.

Finlayson, M., & Havixbeck, K. (1992). A post-discharge study on the use of assistive devices. *Canadian Journal of Occupational Therapy, 59,* 201-207.

Geddes, J. M. L., Fear, J., Tennant, A., Pickering, A., Hillman, M., & Chamberlain, M. A. (1996). Prevalence of self reported stroke in a population in northern England. *Journal of Epidemiology and Community Health, 50*, 140-143.

Gilbertson, L., & Langhorne, P. (2000). Home-based Occupational Therapy: Stroke patients' satisfaction with occupational performance and service provision. *British Journal of Occupational Therapy, 63*, 464-468.

Gitlin, L. N., & Levine, R. E. (1992). Prescribing adaptive devices to the elderly: Principles for treatment in the home. *International Journal of Technology & Aging, 5*, 107-120.

Gitlin, L. N., Levine, R., & Geiger, C. (1993). Adaptive device use by older adults with mixed disabilities. *Archives of Physical Medicine & Rehabilitation, 74*, 149-152.

Gitlin, L. N., Luborsky, M. R., & Schemm, R. L. (1998). Emerging concerns of older stroke patients about assistive device use. *The Gerontologist, 38*, 169-180.

Granger, C. V., Hamilton, B. B., Linacre, J. M., Heinemann, A. W., Wright, B. D. (1993). Performance profiles of the Functional Independence Measure. *American Journal of Physical Medicine & Rehabilitation, 72*, 84-89.

Hollings, E. M., & Haworth, R. J. (1978). Supply and use of aids and appliances. *British Journal of Occupational Therapy, 41*, 336-339.

Hong Kong Census and Statistics Department. (1999). *Hong Kong population projections 1997-2016.* Hong Kong: Government Printer.

Hong Kong Department of Health. (1999). *Annual report for the financial year 1997-98* (p. 182). Hong Kong: Department of Health.

Hong Kong Hospital Authority. (1998). *Statistical report 1997/98.* Hong Kong: Hospital Planning and Development Section, Hospital Authority.

Kohn, J. G., LeBlanc, M., & Mortola, P. (1994). Measuring quality and performance of assistive technology: Results of a prospective monitoring program. *Assistive Technology, 6*, 120-125.

Mann, W. C., Hurren, D., & Tomita, M. (1993). Comparison of assistive device use and needs of home-based older persons with different impairments. *American Journal of Occupational Therapy, 47*, 980-987.

Mann, W. C., Hurren, D., Tomita, M., & Charvat, B. (1996). Use of assistive devices for bathing by elderly who are not institutionalized. *The Occupational Therapy Journal of Research, 16*, 261-285.

Manton, K. G., Corder, L., & Stallard, E. (1993). Changes in the use of personal assistance and special equipment from 1982 to 1989: Results from the 1982 & 1989 NLTCS. *The Gerontologist, 33*, 168-176.

Parker, M. G., & Thorslund, M. (1991). The use of technical aids among community-based elderly. *American Journal of Occupational Therapy, 45*, 712-718.

Phillips, B., & Zhao, H. (1993). Predictors of assistive technology abandonment. *Assistive Technology, 5*, 36-45.

Pollak, N., Rheault, W., & Stoecker, J. L. (1996). Reliability and validity of the Functional Independence Measures for persons aged 80 years and above from a multilevel continuing care retirement community. *Archives of Physical Medicine & Rehabilitation, 77*, 1056-1061.

Smith, M. E., Walton, M. S., & Garraway, W. M. (1981). The use of aids and adaptations in a study of stroke rehabilitation. *Health Bulletin, 39*, 98-106.

Stowe, J., Thornely, G., Chamberlain, M. A., Wright, V. (1982). Evaluation of aids and equipment for bathing. *British Journal of Occupational Therapy, 45*, 92-95.

Technology-Related Assistance for Individuals with Disabilities Act of 1988. *Catalogue No. 850* (Senate Rpt. 100-438). Washington, DC: U.S. Government Printing Office.

U.S. Department of Health and Human Services. (1995). *Clinical practice guideline* (No. 16) (p. 248). Rockville, MD: The Agency for Health Care Policy and Research.

Incorporating or Resisting Assistive Devices: Different Approaches to Achieving a Desired Occupational Self-Image

Maria Larsson Lund, Louise Nygård

Key words: understanding, disability experience, occupations, self-image

Abstract: The purpose of this study was to enhance the understanding of how people with disabilities experience the meaning of their assistive devices in their occupations and how they act on their experiences. Seventeen participants were interviewed and data were analyzed using a qualitative approach. The participants' experiences showed that they reacted differently to the manifold and often contradictory meaning of assistive devices. The analysts organized the participants' reactions into three categories: pragmatic users, ambivalent users, and reluctant users. The differences between the participants were understood as representing different adaptive approaches to achieve desired occupational self-images. Thus, the assistive devices were not in themselves important, but were merely a means to achieve a desired self-image. The findings reflect that the participants' experiences of using assistive devices reveal meanings about their use that go beyond the traditional medical perspective that focuses on the role of assistive devices as compensation for physical impairment.

Maria Larsson Lund, MSc OT, Leg OT, is a Doctoral Candidate, Division for Occupational Therapy, Department of Health Sciences, Luleå University of Technology, Boden, and Department of Community Medicine and Rehabilitation, Umeå University, Umeå, Sweden. Louise Nygård, PhD, Leg OT, is Associate Professor, Division of Occupational Therapy, Department of Neurotec, Karolinska Institutet, Stockholm, Sweden.

The use of assistive devices is linked to the overall experience of adapting to disability and can therefore be seen as an important component in the rehabilitation process of people with disabilities (Gray, Quatrano, & Lieberman, 1998). In Sweden, the concept of assistive devices encompasses a wide variety of equipment for people with disabilities financed through public sources (Blomqvist & Nicolaou, 2000), such as hand reachers, bath benches, crutches, wheelchairs, and power-driven wheelchairs. The purpose of assistive devices is to enable and enhance an individual's engagement in activities and participation in society through bridging the discrepancy between the individual's abilities and the demands of the environment in which he or she exists (Baum, 1998; Trefler & Hobson, 1997).

The incorporation and use of assistive devices in everyday life is especially complicated because the devices are closely associated with the user's appearance and functioning in everyday settings (Brooks, 1990). The process of incorporating assistive devices into everyday life takes place gradually (Bates, Spencer, Young, & Rintala, 1993; Gitlin, 1998). Furthermore, different aspects influence the process of incorporation in complex ways (i.e., if the assistive devices are accepted and used or if they are rejected and not used) (Bates et al., 1993; Gray et al., 1998). More specifically, the willingness of a person to accept assistive devices as a part of his or her life has been suggested to be influenced by interactions between the person, the settings in which the assistive devices are used, the device itself (Bain, 1998; Cook & Hussey, 1995), and the goals the person wants to accomplish (Bain, 1998; Baum, 1998; Cook & Hussey, 1995). Research indicates that the influence of the personal and sociocultural meanings of assistive devices is of fundamental importance to whether people incorporate assistive devices in their lives (Bates et al., 1993; Cole Spencer, 1998). However, in clinical practice, the person's actual skills in using the devices are often emphasized.

Assistive devices can be described as objects that are given meaning through the activities in everyday life in which they are used (Cole Spencer, 1998; Kielhofner, 1995). This implies that the meaning of assistive devices is associated with certain activities and with the context in which the devices are used. Consequently, the meaning of an assistive device can vary greatly with the activity and its context for a single user, between users, and between users and groups of nonusers such as professionals. Research has also confirmed that the meanings attributed to assistive devices vary (Bates et al., 1993; Gitlin, Luborsky, & Schemm, 1998).

Accordingly, a meaning-centered view of the incorporation of assistive devices emphasizes the users' experiences of the meaning that assistive devices have in any given context. In both research and clinical practice, it is important to understand why some people incorporate assistive devices and others do not. This can provide occupational therapists and other health care professionals with important insights into how potential users can be helped (Cole Spencer, 1998).

Several studies examining assistive devices have concentrated on whether they are used and the reasons for these circumstances. Consequently, the research has revealed reasons for not using assistive devices (Gitlin, Levine, & Geiger, 1993; Hastings Kraskowsky & Finlayson, 2001; Sonn, Davegårdh, Lindskog, & Steen, 1996) and benefits of using them (Nordenskiöld, 1996; Sonn et al., 1996), but has not yet provided a means to understand these opposing circumstances. Further, research indicates that the variety of aspects influencing how assistive devices are included in the user's daily life (Bain, 1998, Cook & Hussey, 1995) have seldom been considered in the same empirical study. Finally, the personal and sociocultural meanings of using assistive devices have not been studied exhaustively (Brooks, 1990; Gray et al., 1998; Luborsky, 1993).

Thus, a review of the literature emphasizes the importance of understanding how people with disabilities experience the meaning of their assistive devices and how

Article Reprint Information: Reprinted with permission from Lund, M. L., & Nygård, L. (2003). Incorporating or resisting assistive devices: Different approaches to achieving a desired occupational self-image. *Occupational Therapy Journal of Research: Occupation, Participation and Health, 23*(2), 67-75.

this meaning influences their use of such devices in everyday life. However, only limited empirical research concerning this area is available, suggesting that further exploration is warranted. A better understanding of these matters could be useful to health care professionals in supporting people with disabilities, thereby facilitating their participation in society. Knowledge about the meaning associated with assistive devices and how they influence the users' interaction with their environment is important in occupational therapy because it contributes to an understanding of human engagement in occupations. Therefore, the purpose of this study was to enhance the understanding of how people with disabilities experience the meaning of their assistive devices in their occupations and how they act on this experience.

Methods

Design

The study was guided by a qualitative and explorative approach that allowed a flexible research design. The approach was selected in an attempt to inductively uncover the meanings people with disabilities assigned to their experiences with assistive devices.

Participants and Data Collection

Nonstandardized, open-ended interviews were performed with 17 participants. Potential participants were identified by primary care providers and associations for people with disabilities in two municipalities in the north of Sweden. The selection of participants was guided by the principles of purposive sampling (Patton, 1990). The predefined set of inclusion criteria was that the participants should (1) have a physical disability, (2) live in their own home (i.e., not in an institution), (3) have several assistive devices, and (4) be able to actively participate in an interview dialogue. Accordingly, a heterogeneous sample was favored because we sought to obtain a broad understanding of the use of assistive devices (i.e., understand the experiences that participants shared rather than focus on the experiences related to any particular disease or injury) (Conrad, 1987; Strauss et al., 1984). The participants were selected as the analysis of data proceeded. This allowed a search for a rich variety of experiences involving assistive devices. The selection of new participants terminated when saturation (Strauss & Corbin, 1990) was achieved in the coding of data.

The mean age of the participants (10 women and 7 men) was 50 years (range, 25

to 73 years). The participants used from 4 to approximately 20 assistive devices each, including some kind of mobility aid and aids for self-maintenance. All participants had used assistive devices for 5 or more years, except two who had begun to use devices 3 months to 1 year before the interviews. The need for assistive devices had changed over time and the participants had used them for different lengths of time (i.e., some devices were rather new for the users, whereas most had been used for several years). The study participants had a wide range of impairments related to spinal cord injury (6), rheumatoid arthritis (4), traumatic brain injury (2), multiple sclerosis (2), muscular dystrophy (1), osteoarthritis (1), and fractures (1). All participants received support from other people in their daily lives; twelve of them received informal support and nine received formal support. Nine participants lived with someone, whereas eight lived alone.

An interview guide (Patton, 1990) was designed with broadly defined questions that gave the participants the opportunity to freely express their experiences with assistive devices. Nine of the participants were interviewed once and eight were interviewed twice because of a need to further clarify certain related experiences. The themes that were explored in more detail in the second interview differed among participants depending on which experiences, from their first interview, needed to be developed further. The first interview took between 45 and 120 minutes and the second took between 25 and 45 minutes. The first author conducted the interviews in the home of each participant. All interviews were tape recorded and transcribed verbatim. The local ethical committee at Umeå University approved the study.

Data Analysis

In the initial analysis, the guidelines for the constant comparative method provided by Strauss and Corbin (1990) were used. The method was selected because it focuses on the nature of humans' interactions, how they take actions and engage in processes (e.g., when they use assistive devices), and how they interpret these interactions. This analysis began with repeated readings of the interview transcripts to obtain general information about the participants' experiences. In the line-by-line analysis, the first author coded data reflecting the meaning of using assistive devices. The codes were then compared to find similar experiences that could be grouped together into higher-order concepts. The emerging concepts were constantly discussed and reviewed by the

two authors. From these comparisons, we found that the meanings related to assistive devices were experienced in terms of desirable versus undesirable consequences.

In the next step of the analysis, we examined how the participants acted on these desirable and undesirable consequences and what the overall consequences were. This analysis indicated that the participants acted differently on the consequences of using assistive devices, and we realized that their different approaches could be organized into three categories, identified as pragmatic users, ambivalent users, and reluctant users.

However, this level of the data analysis did not provide an understanding of why participants experienced and acted differently on the meaning of assistive devices. With the intention of further understanding these circumstances, an additional analysis was performed using a hermeneutic approach (Ödman, 1979). During this phase of the analysis, possible interpretations were considered before a final interpretation was determined. This process led us to explore the participants' adaptive approaches to achieve a desired image of the occupational self (Nygård, Borell, & Gustavsson, 1995) and the consequences that followed from these, as reflected in the three themes.

The interpretation was considered to be valid because it corresponded to all essential data and was the only one that explained the essential data in a reasonable manner (Ödman, 1979). In enhancing the credibility (Lincoln & Guba, 1985), the emerging categories and themes were presented and discussed in peer debriefing sessions with researchers in the field.

Results

The Double-Edged Meaning of Assistive Devices

The participants' experiences showed that their use of assistive devices had double-edged meanings for them, which at the first level of analysis was broadly conceptualized by the participants as desirable and undesirable consequences for their occupations. These mixed feelings were expressed to the extent that the participants reported that the assistive devices made it easier to engage in activities because the devices saved them substantial time and energy. At the same time, the assistive devices were experienced as cumbersome to use, which made it difficult to engage in activities.

Some of the participants described the devices as natural objects in their daily lives, but at the same time, they were experienced as unnatural, bulky, and space consuming. Because the assistive devices enabled many occupations and provided the participants with the opportunity to continue to live in their own home, they believed that the use of the devices enriched their lives. Simultaneously, the assistive devices were experienced as obvious signs of a future that was not unfolding according to their plans and therefore made their lives slightly less rich. The assistive devices made the participants independent or at least less dependent on others, but at the same time, the devices served to increase feelings of dependency. When the assistive devices enabled participants to engage in occupations, the participants reported a feeling of normality. On the other hand, because the assistive devices were highly visible to others, they advanced a handicap identity and stigmatization.

Participants' Weighing of the Desirable and Undesirable Consequences of the Assistive Devices for Their Occupations

The participants' parallel experiences of the meaning of their assistive devices as being manifold and often contradictory suggest that these conflicting consequences for their occupations were weighed. The weighing of the importance of these consequences varied among the participants (i.e., some of the desirable or undesirable consequences seemed to become a determining factor for their occupations), and three categories were identified: pragmatic users, ambivalent users, and reluctant users.

Pragmatic Users. The desirable consequences of the assistive devices appeared to become particularly decisive for some of the participants when they weighed the desirable consequences against the undesirable ones. These participants took a practical view of their situation and wanted their everyday occupations and events to run smoothly. The assistive devices were seen as a prerequisite for the realization of this goal. The overall consequences of using assistive devices for the participants in this category were thus characterized by their continued engagement in occupations considered important (e.g., self-care, cooking, and going to the movies). The participants reported that they did not mind using assistive devices, apart from the fact that they sometimes were cumbersome as mobility aids in inaccessible places.

The pragmatic users' experiences with assistive devices over time reflected that the desirable aspects had been of decisive importance already when they received the assistive devices. This observation is illustrated by the following quote: "When I became seriously ill, I had to understand that this new situation was how things would be. It was then that one began to think about how life would be at home... how one would have to learn to adjust to living at home with a wheelchair and other aids."

Ambivalent Users. For some participants, the overall consequence of weighing was that they explicitly expressed their continuous ambivalence toward the desirable and undesirable consequences of the devices as being of decisive importance for their occupations. The ambivalent users believed that it was important to engage in the same occupations as before their disability, although they found it difficult to come to terms with having to use assistive devices. For these participants, the ambivalence associated with the devices represented a continuous dilemma, which can be illustrated by one participant's comment: "One is well aware that the aids are very helpful and thus it feels good that one has access to these devices; yet, this is precisely the problem—one doesn't want to acknowledge that they are needed." The overall consequences for their occupations, as exemplified in their experiences, were that their engagement in occupations continued but was experienced as being plagued by deep-rooted conflict.

The ambivalent users' experiences of assistive devices indicated that their mixed feelings had changed over time. The participants tried to manage all of their occupations without using the devices when they were recommended to them. One participant stated: "A rather long period passed before I accepted that my disability would be visible to others and that I was different because of this disorder. I couldn't handle my condition and thus I did not want too many assistive devices because they are so obvious." Later, the desirable consequences took precedence over the undesirable ones, which seemed to come about because the participants realized they could not manage without the assistive devices. The participants therefore began to use them, but convinced themselves that they were only going to use them temporarily. With the passing of time, the status of the undesirable consequences decreased as these participants found they could continue to engage in occupations that would otherwise not have been possible without using the assistive devices. However, the resistance toward assistive devices remained and manifested in the form of ambivalence.

Reluctant Users. When some participants weighed the desirable and undesirable consequences of using assistive devices, the undesirable consequences took precedence, although they admitted that the devices also had desirable consequences. They described a strong resistance to many of their aids, and especially to their wheelchairs, despite having used them in numerous occupations for several years. One of the undesirable consequences important for their occupations was that the assistive devices had strong negative symbolic value. The participants described emotional difficulties associated with using the devices in activities taking place in public settings because they believed that they were treated differently from other people. In addition, they experienced strong feelings of exclusion from society and as people of less worth. One participant expressed the following observation: "One feels less worthy when sitting in a wheelchair: somehow one feels that people are looking down the whole time when one is sitting there and being always forced to look up. Even if one is rather large, one still has the feeling of being small and beneath others."

The participants reported that the repeated experiences of the negative attitudes of other, inaccessible environments, and also their own convictions made them feel that they had no options: they neither could nor wanted to adapt to a life in a wheelchair, because such a life would be less meaningful in their mind. They therefore reported using their assistive devices only unwillingly, and those who could do so avoided using them in public places by staying at home. Consequently, the participants systematically avoided or even gave up occupations they had once considered important, such as shopping, social activities, and car maintenance. This led to seclusion and feelings of isolation. The overall consequences, as reflected in the participants' experiences, were that their engagement in occupations became increasingly difficult, filled with stress and conflict.

In retrospect, the reluctant users' experiences show that their weighing of the desirable versus undesirable consequences of using aids had changed. When the participants first started to employ assistive devices in the hospital, they tended to concentrate primarily on the desirable consequences of the devices. Later, when the participants realized that they had to learn to live with their disability, the undesirable consequences of the assistive devices were increasingly experienced as important.

Interpretation of the Differences Found in the Three Categories of Users

When we compared the three categories of users (pragmatic users, ambivalent users, and reluctant users), it was clear that the analysis thus far failed to provide a means to understand the marked differences between the disparate meanings of the assistive devices and the participants' responses to their devices. The three categories were therefore compared in a new analysis to more fully understand these circumstances. In doing so, different interpretations were made and examined to discover one that could support our understanding of the differences.

A plausible interpretation examined was that the differences among the different categories of users had to do with their self-image in daily life. Because the participants' self-image concerned how they perceived themselves as performers in daily life and how they tried to achieve satisfying images of themselves when they incorporated or resisted assistive devices, and how they were perceived by others when engaged in various pursuits, we came to use the concept "images of the occupational self" (Nygård et al., 1995). This interpretation was close to the participants' experiences because their descriptions reflected the images the participants held of themselves in certain situations (Charon, 1998; Mark, 1998; Mead, 1967) and how they tried to achieve and present a desired self-image. Consequently, concepts that are more comprehensive, such as "self" and "identity" (Charon, 1998; Mead, 1967), were seen as less preferable because they were only partly reflected in the participants' experiences. Thus, the difference between the three categories of users could be understood as different adaptive approaches to achieve a desired image of the occupational self.

Pragmatic Users. The general attitudes of the pragmatic users were understood as an adaptive approach to achieve a desired self-image. The pragmatic users' experiences suggested that they did not consider themselves as people with disabilities when they were able to continue to engage in occupations through assistive devices. Their continued engagement in occupations therefore seemed to influence their interactions and relations with others, where they saw themselves as "whole" individuals with lives no different from those of people without disabilities. This view can be understood as a confirmation of the images they wanted to have of themselves in their occupations. Occasionally, when the use of

assistive devices in certain public locations was cumbersome and they had to either receive support from others or abandon the activities, their self-image seemed to be challenged. Yet, overall, the pragmatic users were able to achieve desired images of their occupational self as they continued to perform occupations through the incorporation of assistive devices.

Ambivalent Users. The reaction of the ambivalent users to both the desirable and undesirable consequences of assistive devices was interpreted as another adaptive approach in their efforts to achieve desired images of the occupational self as capable. This adaptive approach was characterized by the individual's hesitation in using assistive devices. Because ambivalent users initially avoided using assistive devices, even if this meant a reduction in performance, we understood this avoidance behavior to imply that their occupational self-image would be weakened because of the need for assistive devices. This seemed to be influenced by disparaging social and cultural values. Later, when the participants actually experienced the benefits of assistive devices, the desirable consequences became more evident.

Thus, the participants' image of a person who is highly capable seemed to be strengthened through engaging in occupations requiring assistive devices. Nonetheless, the participants still hoped that their use of the devices would be temporary so that they would be able to attain a more desirable self-image. Overall, their occupational self-image was understood as partly unsatisfied because it was a conflicting situation for them to be engaged in occupations requiring assistive devices. Still, their experiences reflected that the self-image they achieved through engaging in divergent occupations with assistive devices was the best possible image attainable in their present situation.

Reluctant Users. The reluctant users tended to experience the undesirable consequences of assistive devices as extremely important and thus resisted the opportunity to use them. This attitude resulted in withdrawal from many of their earlier occupations and represents yet another adaptive approach in building a desired image of the occupational self. This adaptive approach was understood to arise from the reluctant users' own convictions, but also from their experiences of others not perceiving them the way they wanted to be perceived when they used assistive devices. They were concerned that others would see them as inferior when they used assistive devices.

Thus, these users attempted to conceal their limitations, difficulties, and dependency by withdrawing from occupations. Their withdrawal from activities was therefore understood and recognized as a way of influencing the impression they made on other people to protect themselves against negative attitudes and feelings of shame. In this way, they could preserve a more secure and desired occupational self-image.

Thus, for reluctant users, the negative attitudes of others influenced the sociocultural meaning of assistive devices and their effect on interactions with others to be more important than the pleasure and personal meaning of actually engaging in occupations. However, such an approach in seeking confirmation of a desired self-image seemed to bring about an undesirable self-image, because they were not as actively engaged as they would have preferred. Still, their experiences reflect that their desired self-image was achieved to a greater extent when they chose not to perform occupations requiring assistive devices. The fact that they first experienced the benefit of assistive devices as extremely important can be interpreted as a means of giving them an acceptable occupational self-image when they were in the hospital. However, when they returned home, their urge to assume another, more valued image of the occupational self in this context forced them to resist using the assistive devices rather than changing their ideal self-image.

Discussion

The present findings suggest that the participants' different approaches of incorporating or resisting assistive devices in their occupations represent three adaptive approaches for the same objective (i.e., to enhance the image of the occupational self). However, these different approaches had dissimilar consequences for the participants' occupations and influenced their experiences of their self-image differently. Consequently, the assistive devices were not themselves the most important component. They were merely a means that the participants incorporated or resisted in their struggle to achieve and present the most desired occupational self-image. This suggests that the reason assistive devices are used or not used goes beyond aspects related to the actual performance of activities, which has been the focus of research (Gitlin et al., 1993; Hastings Kraskowsky & Finlayson, 2001; Sonn et al., 1996), and thus reflects another dimension.

Accordingly, our findings imply that the medical perspective, which focuses on the role of assistive devices as preventing and compensating for impairment, fails to explain the meaning of assistive devices for people with disabilities and how they act on these experiences. By searching for the meaning, we gained a possible understanding that goes beyond the medical perspective and a new insight into the use of assistive devices. Other researchers in the field of occupational therapy (Mattingly & Fleming, 1994) have also emphasized that more attention needs to be given to the subjective disability experience rather than to the individual's physical problem in enhancing engagement in occupations.

The participants' experiences reflected that others in society identified them through a medical understanding (Shakespeare, 1996) based on normality. Consequently, when the participants used assistive devices they were considered by others as different (i.e., not normal), eliciting stigmatizing attitudes and embarrassment. The participants' experiences of these attitudes, combined with inaccessible settings, affected their willingness and ability to engage in occupations using assistive devices and therefore to form and present a positive self-image. These findings suggest that the occupational context and particularly the attitudes in the social environment influenced what kind of occupational self-image the participants wanted to achieve and present to others.

In addition, the participants' own convictions and their interpretations of their experiences also seemed to influence their desired image of the occupational self. Thus, the disability itself did not seem to influence their occupational self-image; rather, it was the entire occupational context. Moreover, the self-image that the participants wanted to achieve affected those occupations that they engaged in when using assistive devices. Concerning these findings, the presentation of who the participants were seemed to be more important to them than what they actually did. Additionally, the different approaches to achieve a desired occupational self-image, as reflected in the three categories of users, may be viewed as approaches to avoid a poor occupational self-image as a person with a disability and instead be seen as a capable performer in the occupational realm of life.

The consequences of the participants' adaptive approaches were closely related to the meaning that they ascribed to their disability. Therefore, their struggle with their self-image seems to be part of the ongoing adaptation to the disability. Consistent with our findings, research has shown

that the strategies used in everyday occupations influence how people with disabilities view themselves and experience the disability (Magnus, 2001; Nygård et al., 1995; Thorén-Jönsson & Möller, 1999).

The occupational self-images of the participants in our study provide a possible means of understanding why they responded as they did regarding the use of assistive devices in everyday situations. In agreement with our findings, Bates, Spencer, Young, and Rintala (1993) found that adaptation to using a wheelchair implied an emotional adaptation to a new self-image that includes the assistive device. Theories state that the self arises and changes continuously through social interaction even if individuals develop a stable self-concept over time (Charon, 1998; Mead, 1967). Through their self-image, individuals are able to see and understand themselves in relation to various situations. Moreover, a self-image is a part of the creation of the individual's identity (Charon, 1998).

In line with our findings, Charmaz (1983) found that becoming a person with a chronic illness implies that the meanings and experiences that constituted the former positive self-image no longer exist. Consequently, our findings suggest that if the assistive devices are to be incorporated into the users' daily activities they must be incorporated into their self-image, suggesting remolding of the earlier self-images. Hence, occupational therapists enhancing engagement in occupations play an important role in supporting the clients' task of remolding their occupational self-image when prescribing assistive devices.

The experiences of using assistive devices among the participants in our study reflect the complexity when the different meanings of assistive devices are weighed. Therefore, we concur with Cole Spencer (1998) and others (Gitlin et al., 1998) who emphasize that an understanding of the meaning of assistive devices ascribed by the users in their activities is important if we wish to improve our support to the users. Professionals who embrace a rehabilitation perspective that emphasizes the functional benefits of using assistive devices may interpret the behavior of people with disabilities (e.g., reluctant and ambivalent users) as uncooperative or unmotivated. Our findings provide a means to understand the users' perspectives and possible reasons for their approaches. However, further studies are needed to examine how people with disabilities with similar attitudes can be supported to achieve an enhanced self-image.

The participants' adaptive approaches

could be understood in part from other frameworks, including coping (Lazarus & Folkman, 1984), adaptation (Schultz & Schkade, 1997), the course of adaptation to disability (Cullberg, 1992), and notions related to stigma (Goffman, 1963). Because these standpoints did not provide a means of understanding the difference in the participants' adaptive approaches, they were not used in the analysis of the present data. For example, although all participants experienced some form of stigma, they related to this in different ways.

The concept of the images of the occupational self was found to be a reasonable interpretation in understanding the participants' adaptive approaches. The concept has been used previously (Nygård et al., 1995), and thus our study can be viewed as a step toward further development and understanding of the concept. However, our study suggests only one possible way to understand the users' responses to their assistive devices. We focused on the individuals' experiences. Another possible way to understand the use of assistive devices would be by focusing on the influence of the environment on the occupations for which individuals require assistive devices.

A methodologic limitation in this study is the trustworthiness of the data collection (Kvale, 1997), because we had to rely completely on the participants' accounts of their experiences. It is important to be cognizant of the fact that the interviews captured the participants' subjective interpretation of events (Kvale, 1997). Events far removed in time are limited to retrospective interpretation. Furthermore, the use of assistive devices is a complex phenomenon. Although some of the participants were interviewed twice to increase validity, it is only possible to capture the experiences the participants chose to share with us. Therefore, it is possible that data collected under other circumstances could have provided our understanding with other dimensions. It is also reasonable to contemplate whether the participants expressed how the circumstances appeared to them or whether they presented them in a certain way (e.g., to give a positive view of their circumstances) (Krefting, 1991). However, in our data, participants revealed both desirable and undesirable consequences of using assistive devices, suggesting good validity of the data.

Considering the interpretation that was accepted, it could be described as an interpretation close to the data (i.e., the participants' experiences). The interpretation captures the participants' "insider" perspective in contrast to an interpretation that goes beyond what they meant, implying an "outsider" perspective (Gustavsson, 2000). This can also be regarded as an aspect of validity.

Our findings present one possible way to understand the participants' intentions underlying their approaches toward assistive devices. The incorporation of or resistance to assistive devices represents adaptive approaches used in achieving and presenting a desired occupational self-image. Professional health care providers can bring this understanding of occupational self-images of people with disabilities into the process of rehabilitation.

Acknowledgments

The authors express their gratitude to the participants who shared their experiences with us. The authors are also grateful to Staffan Josephsson for his creative and constructive suggestions on the manuscript and to Birgitta Bernspång and members of the "Kreativa Konditoriet" for their comments and for improving the English. We thank Maare Tamm for her comments on an earlier draft of the findings. The study has been financially supported by the Swedish Foundation for Health Care Sciences and Allergy Research and the Norrbotten County Council.

References

Bain, B. K. (1998). Assistive technology in occupational therapy. In M. E. Neistadt & E. Blesedell Crepeau (Eds.), *Occupational Therapy* (9th ed., pp. 498-517). Philadelphia: Lippincott-Raven.

Bates, P. S., Spencer, J. C., Young, M. E., & Rintala, D. H. (1993). Assistive technology and the newly disabled adult: adaptation to wheelchair use. *American Journal of Occupational Therapy, 47,* 1014-1021.

Baum, C. M. (1998). Achieving effectiveness with a client-centered approach: A person–environment interaction. In D. B. Gray, L. A. Quatrano, & M. L. Lieberman (Eds.), *Designing and using assistive technology: The human perspective* (pp. 137-147). Baltimore: Paul H. Brookes.

Blomqvist, U.-B., & Nicolaou, I. (2000). *Förskrivningsprocessen för hjälpmedel till personer med funktionshinder* [Prescribing assistive devices for people with disabilities]. Stockholm: Hjälpmedelsinstitutet.

Brooks, N. A. (1990). Users' perceptions of assistive devices. In R. V. Smith & J. H. Leslie (Eds.), *Rehabilitation engineering* (pp. 496-511). Boca Raton, FL: CRC Press.

Charmaz, K. (1983). Loss of self: A fundamental form of suffering in the chronically ill. *Sociology of Health and Illness, 5,* 168-195.

Charon, J. M. (1998). *The nature of the self, symbolic interactionism: An introduction, an interpretation, an integration* (6th ed., pp. 72-97). Upper Saddle River, NJ: Prentice-Hall.

Cole Spencer, J. (1998). Tools or baggage? Alternative meanings of assistive technology. In D. B. Gray, L. A. Quatrano, & M. L. Lieberman (Eds.), *Designing and using assistive technology: The human perspective* (pp. 89-97). Baltimore: Paul H. Brookes.

Conrad, P. (1987). The experience of illness: recent and new directions. *Research in the Sociology of Health Care, 6,* 1-31.

Cook, A. M., & Hussey, S. M. (1995). *Assistive technologies: principles and practice*. St. Louis, MO: Mosby-Year Book.

Cullberg, J. (1992). *Kris och utveckling* [Crises and development] (3rd ed.). Stockholm: Natur och Kultur.

Gitlin, L. N. (1998). From hospital to home: Individual variations in experience with assistive devices among older adults. In D. B. Gray, L. A. Quatrano, & M. L. Lieberman (Eds.), *Designing and using assistive technology: The human perspective* (pp. 117-135). Baltimore: Paul H. Brookes.

Gitlin, L. N., Levine, R., & Geiger, C. (1993). Adaptive device use by older adults with mixed disabilities. *Archives of Physical Medicine and Rehabilitation, 74,* 149-152.

Gitlin, L. N., Luborsky, M. R., & Schemm, R. L. (1998). Emerging concerns of older stroke patients about assistive device use. *The Gerontologist, 38,* 169-180.

Goffman, E. (1963). *Stigma: Notes on the management of spoiled identity*. Englewood Cliffs, NJ: Prentice Hall.

Gray, D. B., Quatrano, L. A., & Lieberman, M. L. (Eds.). (1998). *Designing and using assistive technology: The human perspective*. Baltimore: Paul H. Brookes.

Gustavsson, A. (2000). *Tolkning och tolkningsteori 1: Introduktion* [Interpretation and interpretation theory 1: An introduction]. Stockholm: Pedagogiska Institutionen, Stockholm Universitet.

Hastings Kraskowsky, L., & Finlayson, M. (2001). Factors affecting older adults, use of adaptive equipment: review of the literature. *American Journal of Occupational Therapy, 55,* 303-310.

Kielhofner, G. (1995). *A model of human occupation: Theory and application* (2nd ed.). Baltimore: Williams & Wilkins.

Krefting, L. (1991). Rigor in qualitative research: The assessment of trustworthiness. *American Journal of Occupational Therapy, 45,* 214-222.

Kvale, S. (1997). *Den kvalitatva forskningsintervjun* [InterWievs]. Lund, Sweden: Studentlitteratur.

Lazarus, R. S., & Folkman, S. (1984). *Stress, appraisal and coping*. New York: Springer.

Lincoln, Y. S., & Guba, E. G. (1985). *Naturalistic inquiry*. Newbury Park, CA: Sage Publications.

Luborsky, M. R. (1993). Sociocultural factors shaping technology usage: Fulfilling the promise. *Technology and Disability, 2,* 71-78.

Magnus, E. (2001). Everyday occupations and the process of redefinition: A study of how meaning in occupation influences redefinition of identity in women with disability. *Scandinavian Journal of Occupational Therapy, 8,* 115-124.

Mark, E. (1998). *Självbilder och jagkonstitution.* [Self-images and the constitution of self]. Doctoral dissertation, Acta Universitatis Gothoburgensis, Göteborg, Sweden.

Mattingly, C., & Fleming, M. H. (1994). *Clinical reasoning: forms of inquiry in a therapeutic practice*. Philadelphia: F. A. Davis.

Mead, G. H. (1967). *Mind, self & society from the standpoint of a social behaviorist*. Chicago: University of Chicago Press.

Nordenskiöld, U. (1996). *Daily activities in women with rheumatoid arthritis*. Doctoral dissertation, Göteborg University, Göteborg, Sweden.

Nygård, L., Borell, L., & Gustavsson, A. (1995). Managing images of occupational self in early stage of dementia. *Scandinavian Journal of Occupational Therapy, 2,* 129-137.

Ödman, P. J. (1979). *Tolkning, förståelse, vetande: Hermeneutik i teori och praktik.* [Interpretation, understanding, knowing: Hermeneutics in theory and practice]. Stockholm: Almqvist & Wiksell.

Patton, M. Q. (1990). *Qualitative evaluation and research methods* (2nd ed.). Newbury Park, CA: Sage Publications.

Schultz, S., & Schkade, J. (1997). Adaptation. In C. H. Christiansen & C. M. Baum (Eds.), *Enabling function and well-being* (2nd ed., pp. 458-481). Thorofare, NJ: SLACK Incorporated.

Shakespeare, T. (1996). Disability, identity, difference. In C. Barnes & G. Mercer (Eds.), *Exploring the divide: Illness and disability* (pp. 94-113). Leeds, England: The Disability Press.

Sonn, U., Davegårdh, H., Lindskog, A.-C., & Steen, B. (1996). The use and effectiveness of assistive devices in an elderly urban population. *Aging Clinical and Experimental Research, 8,* 176-183.

Strauss, A., & Corbin, J. (1990). *Basics of qualitative research: Grounded theory procedures and techniques*. Newbury Park, CA: Sage Publications.

Strauss, A. L., Corbin, J., Fagerhaugh, S., Glaser, B. G., Maines, D., Suczek, B., et al. (1984). *Chronic illness and the quality of life* (2nd ed.). St. Louis, MO: C. V. Mosby.

Thorén-Jönsson, A.-L., & Möller, A. (1999). How the conception of occupational self influences everyday life strategies of people with poliomyelitis sequelae. *Scandinavian Journal of Occupational Therapy, 6,* 71-83.

Trefler, E., & Hobson, D. (1997). Assistive technology. In C. H. Christiansen & C. M. Baum (Eds.), *Enabling function and well-being* (2nd ed., pp. 483-506). Thorofare, NJ: SLACK Incorporated.

Frail Older Adults' Self-Report of Their Most Important Assistive Device

William C. Mann, Catherine Llanes, Michael D. Justiss, Machiko Tomita

Key words: older adults, assistive devices, adaptive equipment

Abstract: The increasing number of older individuals, especially those in the oldest-old age group, has resulted in a significant increase in the number of people with disabilities. Assistive technology offers the potential of increasing independence and quality of life for older individuals with disabilities, as well as reducing health-related costs. To increase our understanding of the value older individuals themselves place on their assistive devices, this study interviewed 1,016 home-based older individuals in western New York and northern Florida, specifically asking them what they considered their "most important" assistive device and why. Not considering the number of users, the top five most important devices were eyeglasses, canes, wheelchairs, walkers, and telephones. Controlling for the number of people using the device, the top five most important devices were oxygen tanks, dentures, 3-in-1 commodes, computers, and wheelchairs. This study suggests that older individuals with disabilities view certain assistive devices as important in maintaining independence.

William C. Mann, OTR, PhD, is Chair and Professor, and Catherine Llanes, OTR/L, is Master's Student, Department of Occupational Therapy, University of Florida, Gainesville, Florida. Michael D. Justiss, MOT, OTR/L, is Research Assistant, RERC-Tech-Aging, Rehabilitation Science Doctoral Program, University of Florida, Gainesville, Florida. Machiko Tomita, PhD, is Clinical Associate Professor, Department of Occupational Therapy, University at Buffalo, Buffalo, New York.

The number of frail older adults is increasing as a result of advances in medicine and lifestyle. More people are living with age-related impairments that impact their independence and functional performance as a consequence of living longer (Chen, Mann, Tomita, & Burford, 1998). Assistive devices can help older individuals maintain or increase levels of independence and autonomy (Hammel, 2000; Mann, Ottenbacher, Fraas, Tomita, & Granger, 1999), and can reduce the need for personal assistance, which in turn could reduce caregiver burden. The use of assistive technology by older individuals not only reduces their cost of care by maintaining independence, but also enhances quality of life (Haber, 1986). Older individuals view assistive devices as useful in energy and time conservation, reducing the amount of frustration, and providing a sense of security (Chen, Mann, Tomita, & Nochajski, 2000). To increase our understanding of the value older individuals place on their assistive devices, the current study explored the perceptions of frail older adults toward the assistive device they considered "most important."

Review of Literature

Mann et al. (1999) investigated the effectiveness of assistive devices and environmental interventions in maintaining independence and reducing home care costs for frail older adults. One hundred four frail older adults recently referred to home health care were randomly assigned to a treatment group or a control group. Individuals in the treatment group received a functional assessment, a home assessment, and any necessary assistive devices and environmental interventions. The control group received usual care services. Eighteen months later, both groups showed a decline in functional status, but the control group declined significantly more. Costs related to hospitalization and nursing home stays were more than three times higher for the control group. This randomized control trial provided strong evidence that appropriate and necessary assistive devices can slow the rate of functional decline and reduce health-related costs.

Allen, Foster, and Berg (2001) explored the effects of replacing human assistance with mobility equipment and found that the use of canes and crutches decreased the amount of personal assistance required by caregivers and the out-of-pocket cost to fund trained caregivers. Mann, Hurren, and Tomita (1993) compared assistive device use by non-institutionalized older individuals with different impairments and found that overall they owned an average of 13.7 devices. Older individuals with physical impairments had the most devices (average, 15.0), whereas older individuals with cognitive impairments had the fewest devices (average, 5.7). A strong correlation was found between the type of impairments and the type of devices used.

Sonn and Grimby (1994) conducted a longitudinal study with older individuals at 70 and 76 years of age. They found that one-fifth of the participants had assistive devices at 70 years of age and assistive device ownership jumped to approximately half of the participants at 76 years of age. Most of the devices participants used were related to mobility and bathing. Gitlin, Levine, and Geiger (1993) examined 13 subjects 60 years and older who were discharged from a rehabilitation unit in a hospital and found the most commonly prescribed devices were those used for dressing and bathroom tasks.

Mann, Hurren, and Bentley (1993) studied assistive device use by individuals with visual impairments living at home and found the mean number of devices used was 14.5. Mann, Kuruza, Hurren, and Tomita (1992) studied assistive device use among individuals with cognitive impairments and found that these older individuals used a mean of 5.8 devices, but most devices addressed physical impairments rather than cognitive impairments. The cognitive devices that were used related to short-term memory problems and safety.

Chen et al. (1998) studied the use of reachers by elderly individuals with disabilities who lived at home. The study identified the top eight activities for which older individuals use a reacher: picking up remote controls, getting a newspaper from the floor, placing cans in the cupboard, taking cans

Article Reprint Information: Reprinted with permission from Mann, W. C., Llanes, C., Justiss, M. D., & Tomita, M. (2004). Frail older adults' self-report of their most important assistive device. *Occupational Therapy Journal of Research: Occupation, Participation and Health*, 24(1), 4-12.

Table 1

Demographic Information for Older Individuals With Disabilities Who Reported Their Most Important Assistive Device (n = 1,016)

Variable	No.	(%)
Mean age, y	75.4	(8.0)
Gender		
Female	743	(73.2)
Male	272	(26.8)
Missing	1	(0.1)
Race		
Black	187	(18.5)
White	815	(80.2)
Hispanic	5	(0.5)
Asian	2	(0.2)
Native American	2	(0.2)
Other	1	(0.1)
Missing	4	(0.4)
Education		
Less than high school	241	(23.9)
High school	378	(37.5)
Some college	224	(22.2)
College	95	(9.4)
Masters degree	50	(5.0)
Doctorate	20	(2.0)
Missing	8	(0.8)
Marital status (n = 1,015)		
Married	320	(31.5)
Widowed	494	(48.6)
Divorced	106	(10.4)
Single	79	(7.8)
Other	16	(1.7)
Living status		
Live alone	546	(53.8)
Live with someone	468	(46.2)
Missing	2	(0.2)
Housing status		
Own	555	(54.6)
Rent	389	(38.3)
Other	72	(7.1)

Table 2

Health, Functional, Psychosocial, and Mental Status of Participants (n = 1,016)

Variable	No.	(%)
Health		
Mean no. of physician visits in the past 6 months (SD)	5.7	(5.9)
No. of sick days in the past 6 months		
None	537	(52.9)
Less than a week	150	(14.8)
1 week to 1 month	130	(12.8)
1 month to 3 months	117	(11.5)
Mean no. of days in a hospital (SD)	2.6	(8.0)
Mean no. of medications (SD)	5.4	(3.8)
Mean no. of chronic illnesses (SD)	6.3	(3.2)
Eyesight		
Excellent/good	587	(57.8)
Fair	256	(25.2)
Poor	153	(15.1)
Hearing ability		
Excellent/good	600	(59.1)
Fair	255	(25.1)
Poor	138	(13.6)
Mean pain score (Jette) (SD) (range, 10 to 40)[a]	4.6	(6.7)
Mean functional status score (SD)		
FIM (range, 18 to 126)[b]	106.3	(19.5)
IADL–OARS (range, 0 to 14)[b]	9.3	(3.8)
Sickness Impact Profile (range, 0 to 100)[a]	26.9	(15.4)
Mean psychosocial and mental status score (SD)		
Mental status–MMSE (range, 0 to 30)[b,c]	26.0	(6.5)
Self-esteem–Rosenberg (range, 10 to 40)[b]	32.3	(5.1)
Depression–CESD (range, 0 to 60)[a,c]	2.51	(0.2)

SD = standard deviation; FIM = Functional Independence Measure; IADL = instrumental activities of daily living; OARS = Older Americans Research and Service Center Instrument; MMSE = Mini-Mental Status Examination; CESD = Center for Epidemiologic Studies–Depression.
[a]Higher scores reflect more impairment or pain. [b]Higher scores reflect less impairment or pain. [c]Cutoff scores: MMSE < 24 indicates cognitive impairment (N = 178), CESD > 16 indicates "depression" (N = 269).

out of the cupboard, dressing and pulling up socks, opening and closing drawers, getting dishes out of the cupboard, and putting dishes into the cupboard. Reachers provide a simple solution for older individuals who have difficulty with bending and reaching.

Edwards and Jones (1998) studied types of assistive devices that 1,405 elderly people in the community owned and used. Ninety-seven percent of the sample had eyeglasses, but only 16% had a hearing aid. The most commonly owned devices were nonslip bath mats, canes, and grab bars.

Several studies have addressed the use of assistive devices by frail older adults. These studies relate assistive device use to common themes such as mobility, balance, safety, vision, and activities of daily living. However, there has been little study of the importance older individuals place on their assistive devices (Demers, Weiss-Lambrou, & Ska, 1996). The inclusion of user input as a factor in determining retention and use of devices has been suggested by several re-

searchers and has led to the development of tools to measure these factors (Demers, Weiss-Lambrou, & Ska, 2002; Jutai & Day, 2002).

Although "importance" is a general construct, it embodies the perception of "usefulness" and impact on ability to do tasks and participate in activities. The current study asked frail older adults to name their most important assistive device and to explain why they considered it most important.

Method

Sample

This article is based on the Rehabilitation Engineering Research Center on Aging Consumer Assessments Study (CAS), a longitudinal study of the coping strategies of older individuals with disabilities. From 1991 to 2001, 26 senior service agencies and hospital rehabilitation programs referred to the CAS individuals they currently served or, in the case of hospital rehabilitation programs, individuals discharged home. A comparison of initial interviews of the CAS sample with the 1986 National Health Interview Survey (Prohaska, Mermelstein, Miller, & Jack,

1992) and the 1987 National Medical Expenditure Survey (Leon & Lair, 1990) reported that the CAS sample closely resembled the approximately 8% to 12% of the elderly population who have difficulty with at least one activity of daily living or instrumental activity of daily living (Mann, Hurren, Tomita, & Charvat, 1997).

The CAS was initiated in western New York, where 791 older individuals were interviewed. In the final 2 years, the CAS was replicated with 312 study participants in northern Florida. For the current study, we combined the northern Florida and western New York samples (n = 1,103), and selected those participants who responded to the question asking them to name their most important device (1,016 of 1,103 or 92.1%).

Demographic information on these 1,016 subjects is presented in Table 1. Subjects' ages ranged from 60 to 106 years, with a mean of 75 years. Seven hundred forty-three participants were women, and 80.2% were white. Thirty-seven percent had completed high school, 31% of subjects were married, 53% lived alone, and 54% owned their own home. Eighteen percent of the sample had incomes under $10,000 per year. Table 2

Table 3

Number and Percentage of Subjects With Chronic Diseases or Conditions (n = 1,016)

Condition	No.	(%)
Musculoskeletal disorders	848	(83.5)
Heart disease	837	(82.4)
Eye disease	544	(53.3)
Nervous system disorders	421	(41.4)
Glandular disorders	387	(38.1)
Urinary disease	369	(36.3)
Stomach or intestinal disorders	363	(35.7)
Lung disease	271	(26.7)
Other[a]	715	(70.3)

[a]Includes cancer, affective or anxiety disorders, skin disorders, hearing impairment, speech impairment, foot problems, and gout.

Table 5

Ranked List of Devices Participants Stated as Most Important (n = 1,016 subjects)

Rank	Device	No.	(%)
1	Eyeglasses	159	(15.6)
2	Cane	149	(14.7)
3	Wheelchair	114	(11.2)
4	Walker	112	(11.0)
5	Telephone	52	(5.1)
6	Grab bar	38	(3.7)
7	Television remote control	30	(3.0)
8	Magnifying glass	27	(2.7)
9	Microwave oven	26	(2.6)
10	Bathroom equipment	25	(2.5)
11	Hearing aid	24	(2.4)
12	Raised toilet	21	(2.1)
13	3-in-1 commode	20	(2.0)
14	Dentures	18	(1.8)
15	Hospital bed	14	(1.4)
16	Reacher	13	(1.3)
17	Scooter	11	(1.1)
18	Print enlargement system/closed-circuit television	9	(0.9)
19	Crutches	9	(0.9)
20	Computer	7	(0.7)
21	Hand-held shower hose	6	(0.6)
22	Incontinence briefs	6	(0.6)
23	Oxygen tank	5	(0.5)
24	Bath mat	4	(0.5)
25	Answering machine	2	(0.2)

Table 4

Instruments in the Consumer Assessments Study Interview Battery

Dimension	Instrument(s)	Developed By
Demographic information	Older Americans Research and Service Center	Duke University[a]
	RERC–Aging	RERC–Aging
Health status		
Physical health	Older Americans Research and Service Center	Duke University
Pain	Functional Status Index–Modified	A. Jette
Impairment status		
Vision and hearing	Older Americans Research and Service Center	Duke University
Cognition	Mini-Mental Status Examination	M. Folstein, S. Folstein, P. McHugh
Motor	Sickness Impact Profile	Gilson et al.
Functional status		
IADL	Older Americans Research and Service Center	Duke University
Functional independence	Functional Independence Measure	C. Granger
Psychosocial status		
Depression	Center for Epidemiologic Studies–Depression	L. Radloff
Self-esteem	Rosenberg Self-Esteem Scale	R. Rosenberg
Assistive technology	Assistive Technology Used	RERC–Aging

RERC–Aging = Rehabilitation Engineering Center on Aging–Aging Demographic Survey; IADL = instrumental activities of daily living.
[a]Duke University Center for the Study of Aging and Human Development.

presents information on measures of health, functional, and psychosocial status. Participants averaged 5.7 physician visits per month and 2.6 days hospitalized during the 6 months prior to the study interview. They were taking an average of 5.4 medications, and had a mean of 6.3 chronic diseases or conditions. Table 3 lists the frequencies of the chronic diseases and conditions faced by the subjects. On average, study participants were 26.9% physically disabled (Sickness Impact Profile score). Participants scored a mean of 9.3 of 14 for instrumental activities of daily living, and 106.3 of 126 on Functional Independence Measure total

scores. Subjects' mean Mini-Mental State Examination score was 26.0; 24 is typically the cutoff point for separating samples into cognitively or noncognitively impaired groups (Braekus, Laake, & Engedal, 1992).

Instruments

The CAS uses a battery of instruments to measure multiple dimensions, including instruments developed by other investigators and instruments developed to meet the unique requirements of this study. The CAS Interview Battery includes several parts from the Older Americans Research and Service Center Instrument, including the Physical Health Scales and Instrumental Activities of Daily Living Scale (Borchelt & Steinhagen-Thiessen, 1992). A summary of the instruments included in the CAS Interview Battery is presented in Table 4. Each of the instruments is described in detail in an earlier article from the Consumer Assessment Study (Mann, Hurren, Charvat, & Tomita, 1996a).

Data Collection

Research staff who were nurses or occupational therapists collected all data in face-to-face interviews in study participants' homes, with interview time averaging 2.5 hours. Appointments were scheduled at times convenient for study participants. In a few cases, two visits were necessary due to participant fatigue.

Analysis

Descriptive statistics were used to report sample characteristics. Within the Assistive Technology Used Survey, we asked an open-ended question: "Among the devices

you use, which is the most important to you? Why?" We first determined the top 25 most frequently reported important assistive devices (Table 5). The open-ended responses were then categorized by the type of devices (Table 6). Several typical responses are listed for each category.

There were significant differences in the total number of each type of assistive device used by study participants. To control for differences in number of devices study participants were using, we divided the number of devices used (e.g., total number of canes) into the number of these devices older individuals reported as their most important device. For example, 114 people identified a wheelchair as the most important device; there were 357 wheelchairs used by the study participants. We divided 114 by 357 and found that 31.9% of those wheelchairs used were considered to be the most important device. Results of this analysis are reported in Table 7.

To relate the type of impairments that older individuals experienced to their report of most important device, we first grouped study participants into one of 16 impairment groups: vision, hearing, neuromotor/musculoskeletal, cognitive, a combinations of these four impairment categories, and a group of "minimally impaired" individuals who had limitations in activities of daily living but did not reach the threshold score for assignment to one of the other impairment-based groups. The procedure for determining group assignment has been described previously (Mann, Lehman, Wu, & Tomita, manuscript submitted for publication). We categorized the assistive devices into device

Table 6
Reasons Stated for Why Devices Were Most Important

Item Identified	Reason Why Most Important
Eyeglasses, magnifying glass, and print enlargement system/closed-circuit television	Vision
	Sight
	Reading
	Enlarge print
	Money management (write own bills)
Cane, wheelchair, walker, and crutches	Safety
	Balance
	Mobility (ambulation)
	Stability
	Fall prevention
Telephone	Communication
	Socialization
	Safety and emergency purposes
Bathroom equipment, bath mat, and grab bar	Stability
	Balance
	Safety while bathing
	Fall prevention
Television remote control	Leisure
	Entertainment
	Convenience
Microwave oven	Independence in meal preparation
	Eases meal preparation
	Helps to conserve energy
Hearing aid	Hearing
	Communication
3-in-1 commode and raised toilet	Independence in toileting
	Decreases safety hazards
	Makes toileting easier
	Hygiene
Hospital bed	Adjustable
	Comfort
Reacher	Easy access to items
	Access to items without standing up
	Access to items without bending down
Scooter	Mobility
	Access to different places
	Enables long-distance mobility
Computer	Access to information
	Allows person to run business
	Writing
	Means of correspondence
	Aids in maintaining mental health
	Communication and socialization
Hand-held shower hose	Self-care
	To bathe self
	Allows person to bathe while sitting, to reduce fatigue

Table 7
Most Important Device, Considering Number of Devices Used (n = 1,016)

Rank	Device	No. of Times Identified as Most Important	No. of Devices Used	% Who Use Device Who List It as Most Important
1	Oxygen tank	5	6	83.3
2	Dentures	18	31	58.1
3	3-in-1 commode	20	44	45.5
4	Computer	7	20	35.0
5	Wheelchair	114	357	31.9
6	Print enlargement system/closed-circuit television	9	30	30.0
7	Eyeglasses	159	732	21.7
8	Walker	112	532	21.1
9	Scooter	11	55	20.0
10	Cane	149	837	17.8
11	Crutches	9	56	16.1
12	Hearing aid	24	166	14.5
13	Hospital bed	14	101	13.9
14	Raised toilet	21	186	11.3
15	Television remote control	30	650	8.3
16	Telephone	52	679	7.7
17	Magnifying glass	27	361	7.5
18	Microwave oven	26	448	5.8
19	Bathroom equipment	25	508	4.9
20	Reacher	13	267	4.9
21	Grab bar	38	847	4.5
22	Incontinence briefs	6	137	4.4
23	Answering machine	2	78	2.6
24	Hand-held shower hose	6	357	1.7
25	Bath mat	4	238	1.7

types by the type of impairment they were designed to address. For example, a cane would be a neuromotor/musculoskeletal device and a magnifying glass would be a vision device. We developed a grid (Table 8) to show the number and percentage of participants in each impairment group who chose each type of assistive device.

All analyses were completed using SPSS version 11.0 (SPSS, Inc., Chicago, IL).

Results

Table 5 provides a ranked list (by frequency of response) of assistive devices that study participants stated were their most important assistive device. The first ten include eyeglasses, canes, wheelchairs, walkers, telephones, grab bars, television remotes, magnifying glasses, microwave ovens, and bathroom equipment (e.g., tub bench, chair, and stool). Seventy-one subjects reported two devices, and 12 subjects reported three devices as "most important," not being able to list one as "most important." Their additional devices are included in the ranked list (Table 5). Eight subjects stated that all of their devices were equally important. We did not include their devices in the analysis. The reasons why frail older adults chose these devices are summarized in Table 6. Common themes included safety and fall

prevention, balance, mobility, communication and socialization, and independence.

In looking at the top 25 "most important" devices (Table 5), we placed each into one of five impairment categories that they address and report the number that appears in each category: mobility (13 devices), vision (3 devices), hearing (1 device), cognitive (0 devices), and other (8 devices). Other devices included telephones, television remote controls, microwave ovens, dentures, computers, incontinence briefs, and oxygen tanks. The mobility and other impairment categories were the most frequently reported device categories for most important assistive device. Table 7 provides a ranked list of "most important devices" considering the number of participants who owned the device. We divided the number of people who owned the device into the number of times the device was listed as most important. Table 8 considered the type of impairments that the older individuals had, and looked at the number of people in that impairment group who selected each type of device.

Discussion

Four assistive devices (eyeglasses, canes, wheelchairs, and walkers) accounted for more than 50% of the responses to the ques-

Table 8
Most Important Devices by Impairment Groups (n = 1,004 subjects)

Group[a]	Motor (n = 865)		Hearing (n = 41)		Vision (n = 249)		Cognitive (n = 36)		Other (n = 11)		Total (n = 1,202)	
	No.	(%)	No.	(%)	No.	(%)	No.	(%)	No.	(%)	No.	(%)
Minimal (n = 237)	165	(19.1)	7	(17.1)	86	(34.5)	8	(22.2)	3	(27.3)	269	(22.4)
NM (n = 377)	412	(47.6)	3	(7.3)	33	(13.3)	11	(30.6)	3	(27.3)	462	(38.4)
V (n = 44)	13	(1.5)			37	(14.9)	5	(13.9)			55	(4.6)
H (n = 42)	13	(1.5)	17	(41.5)	15	(6.0)	2	(5.6)			47	(3.9)
C (n = 24)	9	(1.0)			12	(4.8)	3	(8.3)			24	(2.0)
V, NM (n = 60)	52	(6.0)			14	(5.6)	2	(5.6)			68	(5.7)
H, NM (n = 53)	49	(5.7)	5	(12.2)	8	(3.2)					62	(5.2)
C, NM (n = 86)	94	(10.9)	1	(2.4)	11	(4.4)	1	(2.8)	3	(27.3)	110	(9.2)
V, H (n = 10)	2	(0.2)	4	(9.8)	9	(3.6)	1	(2.8)			16	(1.3)
V, C (n = 5)	3	(0.3)			2	(0.8)					5	(0.4)
H, C (n = 5)	3	(0.3)	1	(2.4)	2	(0.8)					6	(0.5)
NM, V, H (n = 22)	14	(1.6)	1	(2.4)	9	(3.6)	1	(2.8)			25	(2.1)
NM, V, C (n = 17)	10	(1.2)			7	(2.8)	2	(5.6)	2	(18.2)	21	(1.7)
NM, H, C (n = 10)	11	(1.3)			2	(0.8)					13	(1.1)
V, H, C (n = 2)	1	(0.1)			2	(0.8)					3	(0.2)
NM, V, H, C (n = 10)	14	(1.6)	2	(4.9)							16	(1.3)

Minimal = minimally impaired; NM = neuromotor/musculoskeletal; V = vision; H = hearing; C = cognitive.
[a]No. of subjects in each group is listed in parenthesis.

tion, "What is your most important assistive device?" These four devices are among the most common assistive devices, and we could explain the findings as a reflection of the large numbers of older individuals who use eyeglasses and mobility devices. However, study participants owned an average of 14 assistive devices, and used an average of 12, but still selected those four as their "most important devices." We might hypothesize that the reason there are so many older individuals who use these devices relates to their perception of how important they are. The importance of these devices would certainly be a reflection of the importance of the activities with which they assist, and the effectiveness of the assistance they provide. Eyeglasses can make it possible for many older individuals with impaired vision to see well enough to read, drive, and "watch" (e.g., television, games, and grandchildren). Canes and walkers provide support in walking, and wheelchairs make it possible to get places without walking. Vision and mobility rank high in importance, and for many people, eyeglasses, canes, and walkers adequately address their vision and mobility impairments.

These results also provide an alternative view to a previous report from the CAS that found high rates of nonuse and dissatisfaction with canes, walkers, and wheelchairs (Mann, Hurren, & Tomita, 1993). In follow-up studies of canes (Mann, Granger, Hurren, Tomita, & Charvat, 1995), walkers (Mann, Hurren, Tomita, & Charvat, 1995), and wheelchairs (Mann, Hurren, Charvat, & Tomita, 1996b) the problems were largely related to issues associated with service de-

livery: failure to follow up on the effectiveness of devices as the person's condition changed, lack of maintenance, and lack of professional involvement in the selection of the mobility device. In the current study, participants affirmed their belief that these mobility devices are important, a finding of greater significance given that a significant number of them reported some level of dissatisfaction.

Telephones ranked fifth on the list of most important devices. Although all study participants had access to a telephone, we listed as assistive devices only those telephones that had special features to assist with impairments, such as enlarged buttons for a person with vision or fine motor impairment. Communication, socialization, and safety and emergency use were cited as reasons for considering the telephone the most important assistive device. Previous reports describe the importance of the telephone to older individuals with disabilities (Mann, 1997; Mann, Hurren, Charvat, & Tomita, 1996c).

Table 7 provides an alternate way of summarizing the results on most important device, by taking into consideration the number of people using the device. Oxygen tanks are most important for five of six (83.3%) people who use oxygen, and rank first under this analysis, whereas they ranked 23rd when not considering the number of people who use the device. Dentures move from 14th place to second place when considering actual number of devices used. Without considering number of devices used, three mobility devices appear in the top five, whereas when consid-

ering number of devices used, this drops to one. Clearly, it is important to consider number of devices used when looking at older individuals' perceptions of their "most important" assistive device.

The results (Table 7) also raise questions about the definition of the terms "assistive device" and "assistive technology," which are typically used interchangeably. Perhaps because oxygen and dentures are provided by specially trained professionals focused on one area (e.g., respiratory therapists and dentists) they are not usually listed as assistive devices. Yet dentures provide assistance with a basic activity of daily living—eating—just as a cane provides assistance with mobility. From the perspective of older individuals with disabilities, dentures and oxygen are assistive devices, with a high percentage of those who have them rating them as "most important."

Table 8 provides a breakdown of the type of device listed as most important by the type of impairments the person had, by assigning study participants to impairment groups. Although there were relatively fewer "most important" devices that addressed hearing and cognitive impairment, the distribution of responses by impairment group is also somewhat unexpected. Twenty-four of 36 of the most important cognitive devices were listed by participants in the minimal, neuromotor/musculoskeletal, or vision groups. Only six of these cognitive devices were listed by people who scored at the threshold for assignment to one of the cognitive groups: less than 24 on the Mini-Mental State Examination.

It is also possible that people with more

involved cognitive impairments were not offered many cognitive devices or were not able to obtain them, which could reflect a service delivery or incorrect needs assessment issue more than whether people thought the technology was useful. Assistive devices for people with cognitive impairment are few, and these results would suggest that cognitive devices are found to be most useful by people with relatively minimal cognitive impairment. As primary providers of assistive devices, occupational therapists recognize that assistive technology is considered "important" by the older individuals they serve. This research suggests that the concept of importance is an individual perception and is related to impairment status.

This study focused on older individuals' perspective of their most important assistive device. More than 90% of the study participants in the CAS listed at least one device as "most important." Participants listed devices that provided assistance with walking, eating, and communication, that compensated for limitations in vision and mobility, and that served as tools for leisure activities as well as activities of daily living and instrumental activities of daily living. Although advanced age brings many age-related changes and age-related chronic conditions, older individuals do rely on, and consider important, their assistive devices.

Acknowledgment

This is a publication of the Rehabilitation Engineering Research Center on Aging, funded by the National Institute on Disability and Rehabilitation Research of the Department of Education under grant number H133E60006.

References

Allen, S. M., Foster, A., & Berg, K. (2001). Receiving help at home with the interplay of humans and technological assistance. *The Journals of Gerontology Series B: Psychological Sciences and Social Sciences, 56,* S374-S382.

Borchelt, M. F., & Steinhagen-Thiessen, E. (1992). Physical performance and sensory functions as determinants of independence in activities of daily living in the old and the very old. *Annals of New York Academy Sciences, 673,* 350-361.

Braekus, A., Laake, K., & Engedal, K. (1992). The Mini-Mental State Examination: Identifying the most efficient variables for detecting cognitive impairment in the elderly. *Journal of the American Geriatrics Society, 40,* 1139-1145.

Chen, L. K., Mann, W. C., Tomita, M. R., & Burford, T. E. (1998). An evaluation of reachers for use by older persons with disabilities. *Assistive Technology, 10,* 113-125.

Chen, T. Y., Mann, W. C., Tomita, M., & Nochajski, S. (2000). Caregiver involvement in the use of assistive devices by frail older persons. *Occupational Therapy Journal of Research, 20,* 179-199.

Demers, L., Weiss-Lambrou, R., & Ska, B. (1996). Development of the Quebec User Evaluation of Satisfaction with Assistive Technology (QUEST). *Assistive Technology, 8,* 3-13.

Demers, L., Weiss-Lambrou, R., & Ska, B. (2002). The Quebec User Evaluation of Satisfaction with Assistive Technology (QUEST 2.0): An overview and recent progress. *Technology and Disability, 14,* 107-111.

Edwards, N. I., & Jones, D. A. (1998). Ownership and use of assistive devices amongst older people in the community. *Age and Ageing, 27,* 463-468.

Gitlin, L. N., Levine, R., & Geiger, C. (1993). Adaptive device use by older adults with mixed disabilities. *Archives of Physical Medicine and Rehabilitation, 74,* 149-152.

Haber, P. A. L. (1986). Technology in aging. *Gerontologist, 26,* 350-357.

Hammel, J. (2000). Assistive technology and environmental intervention impact on the activity and life roles of aging adults with developmental disabilities: Findings and implications for practice. *Physical and Occupational Therapy in Geriatrics, 18*(1), 37-58.

Jutai, J., & Day, H. (2002). Psychosocial impact of assistive devices scale. *Technology and Disability, 14,* 101-105.

Leon, J., & Lair, T. (1990). *Functional status of the non-institutionalized elderly estimates of ADL and IADL difficulties, National Medical Expenditure Survey Research Findings 4* (DHHS Publication No. 90-3462). Rockville, MD: Public Health Service, Department of Health and Human Services.

Mann, W. (1997) An essential communication device: The telephone. In R. Lubinski, & J. Higginbotham (Eds.), *Communications technologies for the elderly: Hearing, vision, and speech conference* (pp. 323-339). San Diego: Singular Publishing Group, Inc.

Mann, W., Granger, C., Hurren, D., Tomita, M., & Charvat, B. (1995). An analysis of problems with canes encountered by elderly persons. *Physical & Occupational Therapy in Geriatrics, 13*(1/2), 25-49.

Mann, W. C., Hurren, D., & Bentley, D. (1993).

Needs of home-based older visually impaired persons for assistive devices. *Journal of Visual Impairment and Blindness, 87,* 106-110.

Mann, W. C., Hurren, D., Charvat, B., & Tomita, M. (1996a). Changes over one year in assistive device use and home modifications by home-based older persons with Alzheimer's disease. *Topics in Geriatric Rehabilitation, 12*(2), 9-16.

Mann, W. C., Hurren, D., Charvat, B., & Tomita, M. (1996b). Problems with wheelchairs experienced by frail elders. *Technology and Disability, 5,* 101-111.

Mann, W. C., Hurren, D., Charvat, B., & Tomita, M. (1996c) The use of phones by elders with disabilities: Problems, interventions, costs. *Assistive Technology, 8,* 23-33.

Mann, W. C., Hurren, D., & Tomita, M. C. (1993). Comparison of assistive device use and needs of home-based older persons with different impairments. *American Journal of Occupational Therapy, 47,* 980-987.

Mann, W., Hurren, D., Tomita, M., & Charvat, B. (1995). An analysis of problems with walkers encountered by elderly persons. *Physical & Occupational Therapy in Geriatrics, 13*(1/2), 1-23.

Mann, W., Hurren, D., Tomita, M., & Charvat, B. (1997). Comparison of the UB-RERC-Aging Consumer Assessments Study with the 1986 NHIS and the 1987 NMES. *Topics in Geriatric Rehabilitation, 13*(2), 32-41.

Mann, W. C., Kuruza, J., Hurren, D., & Tomita, M. (1992). Assistive devices for home-based elderly persons with cognitive impairments. *Topics in Geriatric Rehabilitation, 8*(2), 35-52.

Mann, W. C., Lehman, L. A., Wu, S., & Tomita, M. *Comparison of assistive device ownership among elders with different impairments.* Manuscript submitted for publication.

Mann, W. C., Ottenbacher, K. J., Fraas, L., Tomita, M., & Granger, C. V. (1999). Effectiveness of assistive technology and environmental interventions in maintaining independence and reducing home care costs for the frail elderly: A randomized controlled trial. *Archives of Family Medicine, 8,* 210-217.

Prohaska, T., Mermelstein, R., Miller, B., & Jack, S. (1992). Functional status and living arrangements. In J. F. Van Nostrand, S. E. Furner, R. Suzman (Eds.), *Vital health statistics, health data on older Americans: United States, 1992* (pp. 23-37). Hyattsville, MD: National Center for Health Statistics, U.S. Department of Health and Human Services.

Sonn, U., & Grimby, G. (1994). Assistive devices in an elderly population studied at 70 and 76 years of age. *Disability and Rehabilitation, 16,* 85-92.

Removing Environmental Barriers in the Homes of Older Adults With Disabilities Improves Occupational Performance

Susan Stark

Key words: environment, home modifications, occupational performance

Abstract: The current study examines the effectiveness of an occupational therapy home modification intervention program by examining differences in self-reported occupational performance before and after intervention in a population of community-dwelling older adults with disabilities. An occupational therapy intervention was provided in the homes of 16 older adults with functional limitations. The intervention included changing the existing space by the provision of adaptive equipment and making architectural modifications (including major remodeling) to the home. No remediative treatment was provided. The Canadian Occupational Performance Measure was used to measure satisfaction and performance in daily activities in the home before and after home modification intervention. Overall, the mean scores on the satisfaction and performance subscales indicated an improvement in performance and satisfaction with occupational performance. The average number of barriers in each home was 4.7. An average of only 2.5 barriers were solved during the intervention. The removal of environmental barriers from the homes of older adults who have functional limitations can significantly improve their occupational performance and their satisfaction with their ability to perform everyday activities.

Susan Stark, PhD, is Instructor, Washington University School of Medicine, Program in Occupational Therapy, St. Louis, Missouri.

Community-dwelling adults advancing in age and experiencing increased physical and cognitive impairments are at significant risk for disability in activities of daily living (Fried & Guralnik, 1997; Gill, Williams, & Tinetti, 1995; Guralnik, Ferrucci, Simonsick, Salive, & Wallace, 1995). As the population of aging adults continues to grow at rates never experienced before in the United States (Administration on Aging, 2001), this cohort will without question make increasing demands on medical and social services. Critical gaps continue to exist in knowledge of how to manage the health needs of aging adults with disabilities. The Centers for Disease Control and Prevention (2002) notes that there are currently no effective measures to prevent the onset of functional losses associated with chronic diseases and conditions.

Despite promising findings that environmental interventions can influence health and function (Gitlin, Corcoran, Winter, Boyce, & Hauck, 2001; Mann, Ottenbacher, Fraas, Tomita, & Granger, 1999), most studies of prevention continue to focus on the notion that disability is an individual characteristic (Gill, Williams, Robison, & Tinetti, 1999). A shift in perspective regarding the cause of functional decline in older adults may provide valuable insight regarding potential intervention strategies. By using an ecological rather than a medical perspective, the decline in functional abilities associated with the process of disablement will

shift from an emphasis on impairments to a focus on the environmental demands that may exceed an individual's capacity (Lawton & Nahemow, 1973; Verbrugge & Jette, 1994; World Health Organization, 2001). To date, little attention has been given to the influence of the environment on health and functioning in studies that focus on preventing disability (Satariano, 1997). This lack of evidence regarding the effectiveness of environmental modifications has resulted in no formal healthcare policy or payment system to provide home modifications, even though environmental modifications may forestall the need for more costly traditional medical services (Mann et al., 1999).

When asked, aging adults state that they prefer to live out their later years in their own homes (American Association of Retired Persons, 2000). Aging in place is an important aspect of quality of life for older adults with disabilities because people generally have strong emotional ties to their homes (Fogel, 1992). Successful aging in place is often threatened by the high number of environmental barriers that are present in the homes of older adults. These barriers occur as a result of a mismatch between the environment and changing functional abilities that accompany the aging process. Mismatches between the home environment and the physical capacity of community-dwelling older adults are estimated to be as high as 80% in the homes of older adults (Gill et al., 1999). Things that cause

barriers in the home include items that are located out of reach, stairs, and controls that are difficult to manage (Mann, Hurren, Tomita, Bengali, & Steinfeld, 1994; Stark, 2001; Steinfeld & Shea, 1993). The number of barriers in the homes of older adults is approximately four per household (Mann et al., 1994; Stark, 2001).

These barriers often exist despite evidence that older adults are willing to accept and use home modifications (Trickey, Maltais, Grosselin, & Robitaille, 1993). Although the notion of compensation for functional loss by providing accessible modifications to existing homes is promising, fewer than 10% of the 100 million homes in the United States currently contain these modifications (Center for Universal Design, 1997). The barriers in home environments of aging adults with functional limitations in the United States could contribute to the extent and impact of their disability, yet outcome studies seldom consider the environmental factors that influence performance in the home.

Preliminary work supports the use of environmental modifications as an important intervention strategy to help manage chronic healthcare conditions, maintain or improve functioning, increase independence, ensure safety, reduce the need to relocate to institutional facilities, and even reduce the costs of personal care services. For example, Connell and Sanford (2001) found that people with disabilities who modified

Article Reprint Information: Reprinted with permission from Stark, S. (2004). Removing environmental barriers in the homes of older adults with disabilities improves occupational performance. *Occupational Therapy Journal of Research: Occupation, Participation and Health, 24*(1), 32-40.

their homes had little to moderate difficulty or dependence in the conduct of daily activities. Gitlin and Corcoran (1993) and Gitlin et al. (2001) concluded that home modifications slowed the rate of functional dependency and enhanced caregiver self-efficacy. Mann et al. (1999) reported that the rate of decline in independence of older adults decreased and costs for personal assistance and health care were also reduced with an increased use of assistive technology and environmental interventions.

Current models of occupational therapy practice support maintaining occupational performance by providing environmental modifications. According to the Person–Environment Occupational Performance model (Christiansen & Baum, 1997), occupational performance is the result of the transaction between personal characteristics and environmental characteristics during the performance of occupations. By ensuring the match between the capacity of individuals with disabilities and the environment in which they perform their occupations, improved occupational performance can result (Christiansen & Baum, 1997). Assisting older adults to age in place by providing environmental modifications that remove barriers and increase safety is an important aspect of the continuum of rehabilitation services (Law, Cooper, Strong, Stewart, Rigby, & Letts, 1996; Trickey et al., 1993). Although the need for home modification services for older adults with functional limitations is clear, the efficacy is yet undocumented.

This preliminary study examines the effect of a home modification intervention program that includes architectural modification and adaptive equipment by examining differences in self-reported occupational performance before and after intervention in a population of community-dwelling older adults with disabilities. This study was conducted using a Person–Environment Occupational Performance approach (Christiansen & Baum, 1997). We hypothesized that the provision of modifications using a client-centered approach would result in improved perceived performance and satisfaction with performance using a client-centered measure, the Canadian Occupational Performance Measure (COPM) (Law, Baptiste, Carswell, McColl, Polatajko, & Pollock, 1994). Unlike other home modification studies, this program was designed to be client centered and to use individual occupational performance goals as the outcome measure of the program.

Methods

Subjects and Setting

The sample of low income older adults with disabilities was identified by a not-for-profit agency that provides free or low cost architectural modifications in partnership with an occupational therapist. Prior to working with the occupational therapist, the services offered by this agency included minor home repairs such as installing security locks or providing roof repair. This accessibility modification program was initiated after the agency was contacted by former clients and asked to provide ramps, grab bars, and bathroom modifications. Recognizing their limited resources, the agency determined that they would need assistance in ascertaining which modifications would maximize the independence of their clients. The agency contacted an occupational therapist who specializes in home modifications for individuals with disabilities, and a program that included a client-centered assessment (Fearing, Clark, & Stanton, 1998) and a barrier removal plan was developed.

A total of 30 individuals who reported impairments affecting their ability to perform daily activities were enrolled in a home modification program between July 1999 and June 2001. Each individual who met the inclusion criteria was invited to participate in the study. Subjects were included in the study if they reported a problem in one or more areas of the Functional Independence Measure (FIM) motor subscale and indicated a need for environmental modifications to support their ability to physically function in their home. Potential subjects or their family members were also required to own a private home to comply with agency regulations.

Individuals with cognitive dysfunction as indicated by a score of 25 or less on the cognitive subscale of the FIM were excluded from this study due to the need for subjects to respond to questions regarding their goals for intervention. Of the sample population, one individual was excluded from the study due to significant cognitive impairment. Each of the remaining 29 individuals gave written informed consent to participate in this study and permission to complete the modifications to their home. For comparison, descriptive characteristics of the population are provided in Table 1. The study was approved by the Washington University Human Subjects Committee.

Baseline Data Collection

Each participant underwent a baseline interview and assessment in his or her

Table 1
Characteristics of Subjects Enrolled in the Study (n = 29)

Sample Characteristics	Frequency
Gender	
Male	6
Female	24
Age, y (SD)	67.3 (9.9)
Ethnicity	
White	5
African American	22
Asian	1
Other	1
Marital status	
Married	9
Divorced	5
Widowed	11
Never married	4
Work status	
Currently employed part time	1
Seeking work	1
Retired	26
Homemaker	1
Education	
8th grade or less	1
Some high school	8
High school diploma	12
Some college	6
College degree	2

SD = standard deviation.

home by a trained occupational therapist. Demographic information including age, gender, ethnicity, living situation, education, primary medical diagnoses, and work status was collected in addition to a battery of standardized assessments. Severity of patient disability was determined by administration of an interview version of the FIM. The FIM is an 18-item instrument developed to assess the severity of patient disability and functional outcomes of rehabilitation (Keith, Granger, & Hamilton, 1987). The tool consists of a motor domain examining client performance in self-care tasks, sphincter control, transfers, and locomotion, and a cognitive domain that assesses comprehension, expression, social interaction, memory, and problem-solving abilities. The examiner rates all items on an ordinal scale ranging from 1 to 7. A score of 7 denotes "complete independence" on a particular task, whereas a score of 1 signifies "total assistance," with the subject performing less than 25% of the effort. A score below 6 represents the need for supervision or physical assistance from another individual. Hamilton, Laughlin, Fiedler, and Granger (1995) reported the inter-rater reliability of the FIM as .96. The interview version of the FIM has been validated as an acceptable method of obtaining FIM scores in a population of community-dwelling older adults (Chang, Chan, Slaughter, & Cartwright, 1997; Petrella, Overend, & Chesworth, 2002).

Occupational performance was assessed using the COPM (Law et al., 1994). It was used to identify change in clients' self-perceptions of their occupational performance. For this study, individuals were asked to identify problems that occurred within the home. The COPM consists of a semistructured interview and structured scoring method. Clients are asked to list occupational performance problems they encounter in self-care, work, and leisure. These problems are rated in terms of importance, satisfaction, and performance on a 10-point Likert-type scale. McColl, Paterson, Davies, Doubt, and Law (2000) demonstrated that COPM construct validity was supported by multivariate analysis, criterion validity was established, and community utility was high. Two studies established test–retest reliability of the COPM among adults in rehabilitation. The first demonstrated an intraclass correlation of .63 for performance and .84 for satisfaction, and the second reported an intra-class correlation of .80 for performance and .89 for satisfaction.

To identify and quantify the environmental barriers that impacted participants' occupational performance goals, the Environmental Functional Independence Measure (Enviro-FIM) (Steinfeld & Danford, 1997) was used. On completion of the COPM interview, a room by room walk through of the home was conducted to identify safety issues and to observe the areas in the home where the occupational problems currently occurred. Environmental barriers that prevented the performance of occupational performance areas were identified and rated using the Enviro-FIM. The Enviro-FIM is derived from the 7-point FIM; it expands the score from 7 to 10 points. The additional 3 points account for safety, assistive technology, and environmental modifications. The Enviro-FIM provides a method of determining the influence of environmental features on the occupational performance of an individual (Steinfeld & Danford, 1997). It is designed to quantify a mismatch between an environment's demand character and a subject's performance (Steinfeld & Danford, 1997).

Each environmental barrier was photographed for the community agency and for follow-up to determine if or how the barrier was solved. During this phase of the study, two occupational therapists completed the assessment and intervention plans. In all cases, the author reviewed the assessment results and barrier removal plan prior to modifications. The therapists completed training in the use of the assessments and were certified to administer the FIM.

Procedure

Based on the occupational goals and priorities of the participant (as indicated by the COPM), a home modification plan was developed by the occupational therapist to eliminate the environmental barriers. Home modifications included a range of possible strategies such as the provision of adaptive equipment (e.g., reachers and tub benches), architectural modifications (e.g., ramps, stair rails, and bathroom modifications) and major home renovations (e.g., roll-in shower and accessible bathroom). For the purposes of this study, interventions were limited to compensatory strategies. No remediative interventions (e.g., range of motion or strengthening) provided in traditional occupational therapy treatment were used. With the exception of safety risks identified during the evaluation, all of the intervention modifications were designed to address the occupational performance issues identified by the participant. If safety issues (e.g., loose railings on stairs) were identified, they were discussed with the subject and were addressed in the modification plan with the subject's approval.

After completion of the baseline assessment and the development of a barrier removal plan by the participant and the occupational therapist, the plan was supplied to the home modification construction team. The agency provides home modifications based on a sliding payment scale. For this program, if subjects were able to pay for a portion of the modifications, they did so. If subjects were unable to afford the fee, the modifications were provided at no cost. The average time between initial evaluation and follow-up was 6 months due to the length of the agency's waiting list. The occupational therapist provided supervision during construction to ensure that the modifications were installed according to the barrier removal plan. The occupational therapist provided training in the use of the modifications and made follow-up visits to the subject's home as needed during and immediately after the construction phase.

Posttest Data Collection

The occupational therapist scheduled a follow-up visit with each subject between 3 and 6 months after the home modifications were in place. The agency was not able to complete all of the adaptations recommended by the occupational therapist for various reasons. In some cases, the numerous work requests and limited funding prohibited an extensive architectural modification, and in several cases the home modification was not possible given the structure of the home (e.g., not enough space for a ramp).

The barrier status was noted at the time of follow-up via photographs. Of the 29 individuals initially enrolled in the study, seven of the modification jobs were not completed by the agency, three individuals moved to more accessible housing or to live with family, two of the modification plans were unable to be completed or modified due to poor structural integrity of the home, and one individual refused to have home modifications and withdrew from the program. During the follow-up visit, the COPM was repeated on the remaining 16 subjects who received home modifications. Photographs of the barriers and solutions were taken to verify the changes that had been made.

Data Analysis

Data were analyzed using the SAS program (version 6.12 for Windows; SAS, Inc., 1996). Descriptive statistics were calculated to characterize the sample. Mean outcome measures at baseline and change scores from baseline were determined. Paired t tests were used to examine the differences between pretest and posttest scores for both satisfaction and performance.

Results

The analysis is based on the sample of 16 subjects who had home modifications completed. The baseline characteristics of the final sample are provided in Table 2. Of the 16 subjects included in the final analysis, most were African American (n = 12) and women (n = 12). Subjects' ages ranged from 57 to 82 years, with a mean age of 70.69 years. Most of the subjects were retired (n = 14). Six subjects were married, whereas five were widowed. Two subjects had never married and three were divorced. Eight of the subjects lived alone. Three subjects had some college experience, whereas most (n = 12) had attended high school. One subject had only a grade school education. Eight of the subjects were currently receiving personal assistance during daily activities and 12 had received some type of accommodation (e.g, walkers or grab bars) in the past. Functional disability (as measured by the motor subscale of the FIM) indicated mild to moderate disability, with a mean score of 70.12 (range, 34 to 88). Enviro-FIM scores were taken as an average (rather than a total score) to account for the different number of barriers between subjects. Enviro-FIM scores ranged from 1 (totally dependent) to 6.4 (safety risk), with an average score of 3.67 for the group.

A total of 75 barriers were identified in the homes of the participants. The average number of barriers per person was 4.7, with a range of 1 to 7 barriers per person. Each individual was provided with an average of 2.5 modifications, ranging from 1 to 7 modifications for each individual. Safety and accessibility modifications such as the installation of handrails, grab bars, and ramps were the most frequent environmental modifications. Less common solutions included providing bed rails, widening doors, relocating laundry facilities from the basement to the living floor, and providing additional lighting. Sixty percent of the modifications were completed. Only 45 of 75 identified barriers were resolved due to various difficulties encountered by the agency (e.g., funding, staffing shortages, and structural problems with home) or refusal by the client. The type and frequency of modifications, in descending order of frequency, are reported in Table 3.

Paired t tests were used to examine the differences between pretest and posttest scores for both satisfaction and performance scores. The sample means, displayed in the figure, show that subjects demonstrated an improvement in scores in both satisfaction and performance. The mean pretest performance score rose from 3.19 to 7.81 points on posttest. Scores on the COPM satisfaction subscale increased from pretest to posttest, with an initial mean score of 2.25 and a posttest mean score of 7.69, which was significant. The analysis revealed a significant difference between the two groups for both occupational performance ($t = -8.23$; $p = .0001$) and for satisfaction with performance ($t = -9.54$; $p = .0001$).

Discussion

In the current study, the occupational performance of older adults with disabilities was examined before and after an intervention program that was implemented to remove environmental barriers from their homes. Only 45 of the 75 identified barriers (an average of 2.5 per subject) were resolved during the course of the study. Of the 16 subjects, most were African-American women, all were considered low income according to the agency guidelines to qualify for service, and all were community-dwelling adults with disabilities living in an urban environment. All subjects reported a positive change from before to after intervention with regard to their occupational performance (as measured by the COPM). After receiving home modifications, participants experienced statistically significant increases in both participation and satisfaction scores. The results of this study support the hypothesis that occupational performance of older adults with functional limitations improves after home modifications are provided.

Table 2 Characteristics of Subjects Retained in the Study ($n = 16$)	
Sample Characteristics	**Frequency**
Gender	
Male	4
Female	12
Age, y	
57 to 64	3
65 to 70	6
71 to 82	7
Ethnicity	
White	2
African American	12
Asian	1
Other	1
Marital status	
Married	6
Divorced	3
Widowed	5
Never married	2
Work status	
Currently employed part time	1
Seeking work	1
Retired	14
Education	
8th grade or less	1
Some high school	6
High school graduate	6
Some college	3
Receiving services (aide, nursing, chore worker, family help, paid help)	
Yes	8
No	8
Previous accommodations	
Yes	12
No	4

These findings support the current literature that suggests that the removal of barriers in the home will result in improved occupational performance (Mann et al., 1999; Steinfeld & Shea, 1993). This study also validated the frequency of barriers previously reported in the literature (Mann et al., 1999; Stark, 2001). In addition, the types of barriers identified through the client-centered approach were similar to those in previous studies using experts to identify barriers (Mann et al., 1994; Trickey et al., 1993).

By eliminating environmental barriers in the homes of individuals with occupational performance problems, satisfaction with performance and perception of performance improved. This ecological approach validates current models of occupational performance that include the environment (e.g., Christiansen & Baum, 1997) by demonstrating the outcome of an intervention targeted only at the environmental features that influenced the occupational performance of an aging adult with a disability.

The results of this study are meaningful for several reasons. To our knowledge, this is the first study to report outcomes of

Table 3 Frequency and Types of Home Modifications Provided	
Item	**Frequency of Installation**
Handrails	14
Grab bar	7
Ramps	4
Provide additional lighting	4
Provide hand-held shower	3
Raised toilet	3
Shower retrofit (provide roll-in shower)	2
Widen door	2
Relocate laundry facilities to first floor	1
Provide bed rail	1
Adaptive equipment	1
Safety features (deadbolts, smoke detectors)	1
Lever handles on doors	1
Provide designated parking area on street	1

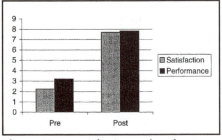

Figure. Mean satisfaction and performance scores before and after intervention.

a home modification study based on a client-centered approach to problem identification and intervention. Although other studies have included utilization rates of modifications (Trickey et al., 1993) and healthcare costs (Mann et al., 1999) as outcome measures of environmental interventions, this study employed subjective measures of occupational performance in an attempt to maintain the client-centered or individualized approach to improving performance that is relevant to occupational therapy practice. With the exception of safety concerns, the entire plan was based on the goals of the individual. Similarly, the outcome measures are also based on individual goals for each subject.

An additional reason to note the outcome of this study is the level of disability of this group (operationalized by the FIM motor subscale score in this study). Although the study sample did represent a group with relatively mild functional impairment, they demonstrated a significant response to the removal of barriers. They also identified a greater overall influence of the environmental barriers than was expected given their level of impairment. The severity of barrier rating (using the mean Enviro-FIM score) was 3.67, which means that the individual required minimal to moderate assistance from a caregiver to complete tasks in the home. The individuals in this study reported a significant impact of the barriers in their homes on their daily living performance prior to intervention and suggested a significant change in satisfaction and performance of daily living activities after intervention. Although the Enviro-FIM was not completed at follow-up, this finding suggests that further study of the influence of barriers on performance is warranted, especially in light of the poor rate of barrier removal on the part of the home modification agency.

Limitations of the Study

Several limitations of this study warrant consideration. First, the preliminary nature of this study, small sample size, and limited follow-up demand caution when interpreting the results. The group clearly does not represent the general population of older adults with disabilities because they were primarily African-American women. They do represent a population that has been identified in the literature as at risk for decreased activities of daily living performance (Lysak, MacNeill, Neufield, & Lichtenberg, 2002; Miller et al., 1996). This study may provide valuable insight regarding the types of interventions that may result in disability prevention within this cohort.

Due to limitations of the agency providing the modifications, the time lapse from enrollment to completion of the modifications was in some cases lengthy. Although this was not desirable given the likely changes in physical status that occurred during the waiting period (in some cases 12 months), this was a naturalistic study of an existing program for low income urban residents and likely represents the reality of how home modifications will be delivered to this population of individuals. Although other programs may have more efficient results, this program provides interesting insight into a sample of low income, urban older adults.

The limited follow-up assessment also leaves unanswered questions regarding what impact a change of physical status may have on the occupational performance of individuals dealing with chronic conditions. In the study conducted by Mann et al. (1999), there was little improvement in functional abilities but significant decline in impairment during the course of the study. A characterization of the postmodification impairment status might yield important information about health status changes over time and the influence of environmen-

tal modifications on changing impairment status. In addition, a more rigorous longitudinal approach could yield important information about the impact of the modifications long term.

There may also be reason to suspect that the change from pretest to posttest would have been more robust had the entire barrier removal plan been completed across the groups. Because approximately 40% of the recommendations were not implemented during this program due to various reasons, it is unknown what effect those modifications would have had on the satisfaction and performance scores. The significant expense of home modifications and the length of time that it takes to complete each intervention contributed to the low numbers of completed intervention programs. The results of this study suggest the potential reasons for the low number of accessibility modifications currently in place in the homes of individuals with disabilities. The problems associated with construction of the modifications greatly influenced the outcome of the study. In addition, a more in-depth understanding of the types of modifications that were not made and reasons why may provide further insight into the barriers faced by this population. This information could have consequences for future studies of this nature.

The results of this preliminary study offer support to the theoretical models of person–environment fit (Lawton & Nahemow, 1973) and underscore the importance of environmental factors in contributing to occupational performance (Christiansen & Baum, 1997). Although preliminary in nature, the success of this small exploratory study points to the necessity of a larger study of the outcome of home modifications on occupational performance. A controlled, longitudinal study with cost analysis and additional assessments reflecting the personal characteristics of the individual, caregiver support, and other environmental characteristics would be important to inform policy makers about the value of interventions that include home modifications. Despite the sample size and poor rate of retention in the sample, this investigation yields important preliminary data to permit estimation of power and a primary outcome measure for future studies of environmental interventions. This study provides evidence that an environmental modification intervention using a client-centered approach is an effective method for improving occupational performance.

References

Administration on Aging. (2001). *A profile of older Americans: 2001.* Washington, DC: Administration on Aging.

American Association of Retired Persons. (2000). *Fixing to stay: A national housing survey on housing and home modification issues.* Retrieved October 13, 2003, from the AARP Research web site: http://research.aarp.org/il/home_mod_1.html.

Center for Universal Design. (1997). *A blueprint for action: A resource for promoting home modifications.* Retrieved October 13, 2003, from http://www.homemods.org/library/blue.

Centers for Disease Control and Prevention. (2002). *Healthy aging: Preventing disease and improving quality of life among older Americans.* Atlanta, GA: Author.

Chang, W. C., Chan, C., Slaughter, S. E., & Cartwright, D. (1997). Evaluating the FONE FIM: Part II. Concurrent validity and influencing factors. *Journal of Outcome Measurement, 1,* 259-285.

Christiansen, C. H., & Baum, C. M. (1997). Person–environment occupational performance: A conceptual model for practice. In C. H. Christiansen & C. M. Baum (Eds.), *Occupational therapy: Enabling function and well-being* (2nd ed., pp. 47-70). Thorofare, NJ: SLACK Incorporated.

Connell, B. R., & Sanford, J. A. (2001). Difficulty, dependence, and housing accessibility for people aging with a disability. *Journal of Architecture and Planning Research, 18,* 234-242.

Fearing, G., Clark, J., & Stanton, S. (1998). The client-centered occupational therapy process. In M. Law (Ed.), *Client centered occupational therapy* (pp. 67-87). Thorofare, NJ: SLACK Incorporated.

Fogel, B. S. (1992). Psychological aspects of staying at home. *Generations, 16*(2), 15-19.

Fried, L. P., & Guralnik, J. M. (1997). Disability in older adults: Evidence regarding significance, etiology, and risk. *Journal of the American Geriatrics Society, 45,* 92-100.

Gill, T. M., Williams, C. S., Robison, J. T., & Tinetti, M. E. (1999). A population-based study of environmental hazards in the homes of older persons. *American Journal of Public Health, 89,* 553-556.

Gill, T. M., Williams, C. S., & Tinetti, M. E. (1995). Assessing risk for the onset of functional dependence among older adults: The role of physical performance. *Journal of the American Geriatrics Society, 43,* 603-609.

Gitlin, L., & Corcoran, M. (1993). Expanding caregiver ability to use environmental solutions for problems of bathing and incontinence in the elderly with dementia. *Technology and Disability, 2*(4), 12-21.

Gitlin, L. N., Corcoran, M., Winter, L., Boyce, A., & Hauck, W. W. (2001). A randomized, controlled trial of a home environmental intervention: Effect of efficacy and upset in caregivers and on daily function of a person with dementia. *Gerontologist, 41*(1), 4-14.

Guralnik, J. M., Ferrucci, L., Simonsick, E. M., Salive, M. E., & Wallace, R. B. (1995). Lower-extremity function in persons over the age of 70 years as a predictor of subsequent disability. *New England Journal of Medicine, 332,* 556-561.

Hamilton, B. B., Laughlin, J. A., Fiedler, R. C., & Granger, C. V. (1995). Interrater reliability of the 7-level Functional Independence Measure (FIM). *Scandinavian Journal of Rehabilitation Medicine, 26*(3), 115-119.

Keith, R. A., Granger, C. V., & Hamilton, B. B. (1987). The Functional Independence Measure: A new tool for rehabilitation. In M. G. Eisenberg & R. C. Grzesiak (Eds.), *Advances in Clinical Rehabilitation* (pp. 6-18). New York: Springer.

Law, M., Baptiste, S., Carswell, A., McColl, M. A., Polatajko, H., & Pollock, N. (1994). *Canadian Occupational Performance Measure* (2nd ed.). Toronto, Ontario, Canada: Canadian Association of Occupational Therapists.

Law, M., Cooper, B., Strong, S., Stewart, D., Rigby, P., & Letts, L. (1996). The person-environment-occupation model: A transactive approach to occupational performance. *Canadian Journal of Occupational Therapy, 61*(1), 9-23.

Lawton, M. P., & Nahemow, L. (1973). Ecology and the aging process. In C. Eisdorfer & M. P. Lawton (Eds.), *The psychology of adult development and aging* (pp. 619-674). Washington, DC: American Psychological Association.

Lysack, C., MacNeill, S., Neufield, S., & Lichten-berg, P. (2002). Elderly inner city women who return home to live alone. *OTJR: Occupation, Participation and Health, 22,* 59-69.

Mann, W. C., Hurren, D., Tomita, M., Bengali, M., & Steinfeld, E. (1994). Environmental problems in homes of elders with disabilities. *Occupational Therapy Journal of Research, 14,* 191-211.

Mann, W. C., Ottenbacher, K. J., Fraas, L., Tomita, M., & Granger, C. V. (1999). Effectiveness of assistive technology and environmental interventions in maintaining independence and reducing home care costs for the frail elderly: A randomized controlled trial. *Archives of Family Medicine, 8,* 210-217.

McColl, M. A., Paterson, M., Davies, D., Doubt, L., & Law, M. (2000). Validity and community utility of the Canadian Occupational Performance Measure. *Canadian Journal of Occupational Therapy, 67*(1), 22-30.

Miller, D. K., Carter, M. E., Miller, J. P., Fornoff, J. E., Bentley, J. A., Boyd, S. D., et al. (1996). Inner-city blacks have high levels of functional disability. *Journal of the American Geriatrics Society, 44,* 1166-1173.

Petrella, R. J., Overend, T., & Chesworth, B. (2002). FIMTM after hip fracture: Is telephone administration valid and sensitive to change? *Physical Medicine and Rehabilitation, 81,* 639-644.

SAS, Inc. (1996). SAS (Version 6.12) [Computer Software]. Cary, NC: Author.

Satariano, W. (1997). The disabilities of aging: Looking to the physical environment. *American Journal of Public Health, 87,* 331-332.

Stark, S. (2001). Creating disability in the home: The role of environmental barriers in the United States. *Disability and Society, 16*(1), 37-49.

Steinfeld, E., & Danford, G. S. (1997). Environment as a mediating factor in functional assessment. In S. Dittmar & G. Gresham (Eds.), *Functional assessment and outcome measures for the rehabilitation health professional* (pp. 37-56). Gaithersburg, MD: Aspen.

Steinfeld, E., & Shea, S. (1993). Enabling home environments: Identifying barriers to independence. *Technology and Disability, 2*(4), 69-79. Retrieved October 13, 2003, from http://www.arch. buffalo.edu/~idea/publications/free_pubs/ pubs_eheb.html.

Trickey, F., Maltais, D., Gosselin, C., & Robitaille, Y. (1993). Adapting older persons' homes to promote independence. *Physical & Occupational Therapy in Geriatrics, 12*(1), 1-14.

Verbrugge, L. M., & Jette, A. M. (1994). The disablement process. *Social Science and Medicine, 38,* 1-14.

World Health Organization. (2001). *International classification of functioning disability and health.* Geneva, Switzerland: Author.

Randomized Controlled Trial of the Use of Compensatory Strategies to Enhance Adaptive Functioning in Outpatients with Schizophrenia

Dawn I. Velligan, PhD, C. Christine Bow-Thomas, PhD, Cindy Huntzinger, BA, Janice Ritch, MA, Natalie Ledbetter, MA, Thomas J. Prihoda, PhD, Alexander L. Miller, MD

Objective: Cognitive adaptation training is a novel psychosocial treatment approach designed to improve adaptive functioning by using compensatory strategies in the home or work environment to bypass the cognitive deficits associated with schizophrenia. The authors tested the effect of cognitive adaptation training on level of adaptive functioning in outpatients with schizophrenia. **Method:** Forty-five patients with DSM-IV schizophrenia or schizoaffective disorder were randomly assigned for 9 months to one of three treatment conditions: 1) standard medication follow-up, 2) standard medication follow-up plus cognitive adaptation training, and 3) standard medication follow-up plus a condition designed to control for therapist time and provide environmental changes unrelated to cognitive deficits. Comprehensive assessments were conducted every 3 months by raters who were blind to treatment condition. **Results:** Significant differences were found between the three treatment groups in levels of psychotic symptoms, motivation, and global functioning at the end of the 9-month study period. Patients in the cognitive adaptation training group overall had higher levels of improvement, compared with those in the remaining treatment conditions. In addition, the three groups had significantly different relapse rates over the 9-month study: 13% for the cognitive adaptation training group, 69% for the group in which therapist time and environmental changes were controlled, and 33% for the group who received standard follow-up only. **Conclusions:** Compensatory strategies may improve outcomes for patients with schizophrenia. (*Am J Psychiatry* 2000; 157:1317–1323)

Received Oct. 19, 1999; revision received Jan. 31, 2000; accepted Feb. 4, 2000. From the Department of Psychiatry, The University of Texas Health Science Center at San Antonio. Address reprint requests to Dr. Velligan, Department of Psychiatry, Mail Stop 7792, Division of Schizophrenia and Related Disorders, The University of Texas Health Science Center at San Antonio, 7703 Floyd Curl Dr., San Antonio, TX 78229-3900; velligand@uthscsa.edu (e-mail).

Schizophrenia is often characterized by deficits in adaptive functioning ranging from difficulties in performing basic activities of daily living to problems maintaining competitive employment (1). Impairments in neurocognitive functioning are believed to underlie the problems in instrumental and role functioning observed in this illness (1, 2). In a recent study using path analysis, we found that cognitive deficits rather than the positive or negative symptoms of schizophrenia predicted poor performance in basic activities of daily living (3). In fact, several investigations have found that neurocognitive deficits predict approximately half of the variance in measures of adaptive functioning (3, 4). In a comprehensive review of 17 studies, Green (2) found measures of verbal memory, executive functions, and attention to predict multiple domains of community outcome for patients with this disorder. Furthermore, cognitive deficits have been seen as rate-limiting factors in the ability of patients to benefit from psychosocial rehabilitation (5).

Recent studies have found that treatment with atypical antipsychotic medications can improve neurocognitive performance (6–8).

However, even with these newer treatments, significant cognitive deficits remain (6). Thus, the development of strategies to compensate for residual cognitive impairment is important to pursue. One promising approach is the use of compensatory strategies—environmental adaptations designed to bypass lingering neurocognitive impairments and improve adaptive functioning. Compensatory strategies include the use of signs, labels, and electronic devices designed to cue and sequence appropriate behaviors. These techniques have been used successfully for years to treat patients with head injuries and mental retardation but have only recently been applied to schizophrenia in a systematic manner (9).

Cognitive adaptation training is a manual-driven group of compensatory strategies used to address impairments in the adaptive functioning of patients with schizophrenia. The study reported here examined the effect of cognitive adaptation training in medicated outpatients recently discharged from a state psychiatric facility. We hypothesized that rates of relapse and levels of positive and negative symptoms for patients in cognitive adaptation training would be lower

at the end of 9 months than for patients in control conditions. In addition, we hypothesized that patients participating in cognitive adaptation training would have higher levels of adaptive functioning than patients participating in control conditions.

Method

Design

Forty-five patients were randomly assigned to one of the three treatment conditions: 1) standard medication follow-up, 2) standard follow-up plus cognitive adaptation training, or 3) standard follow-up plus a condition that controlled for therapist contact time and for changes in the patient's environment. Each group included 15 patients. The treatment groups are described below. Patients in groups 2 and 3 were seen weekly for a 9-month period. Therapist contact time for these two groups was equivalent. In addition, the same individuals (bachelor's-level psychology and social work practicum students) provided treatment for both groups. Patients were assessed on entrance into the study and at 3-month intervals throughout the study by research personnel who were unaware of

Article Reprint Information: Velligan, D. I., Bow-Thomas, C. C., Huntzinger, C., Ritch, J., Ledbetter, N., Prihoda, T. J., & Miller, A. L. (2000). Randomized controlled trial of the use of compensatory strategies to enhance adaptive functioning in outpatients with schizophrenia. *American Journal of Psychiatry, 157*(8), 1317-1323. Reprinted with permission from the *American Journal of Psychiatry*, Copyright 2000. American Psychiatric Association.

subjects' treatment groups. Patients who relapsed were assessed at the point of relapse and dropped from the study. Their last observation was used for an endpoint data analysis.

Subjects

Subjects were 45 patients recruited at discharge from a state psychiatric facility after treatment for an acute exacerbation of their psychosis. After providing written informed consent, subjects were interviewed by a master's-level research assistant to ensure that they met the following entry criteria: 1) diagnosis of schizophrenia or schizoaffective disorder based on the Structured Clinical Interview for DSM-IV (SCID) (10), 2) age between 18 and 55, 3) no history of seizure disorder, head trauma, organic brain disorder, or mental retardation, 4) history of compliance with antipsychotic medication and clinic visits, 5) no history of substance abuse or dependence in the past 3 months, and 6) discharge destination to an apartment, family home, or boarding facility within 70 miles of the hospital. All patients received standard follow-up care, including medications, through public outpatient clinics throughout the 9 months of the study. Medication was prescribed in doses in the recommended therapeutic range for all but two patients. One patient in the cognitive adaptation training group received 3 mg daily of risperidone (lower than the recommended dose), and one patient in the control condition received 1000 mg of clozapine daily (higher than the recommended dose).

Eighty-four percent of subjects participating in the study had a diagnosis of schizophrenia (N=38), and the remainder met criteria for schizoaffective disorder (N=7). Seventy-five percent (N=34) were men. Forty-eight percent of subjects were Mexican American (N=22), 37% were Anglo (N=17), and the remainder were African American, Asian, or of mixed ethnicity (N=6). The mean age of all subjects was 37.12 years (SD=8.99). Mean age at onset of psychosis was 22.35 years (SD=4.74). The majority of patients had at least a high school education. Socioeconomic status was in the range of lower-middle to low income. The length of the index hospitalization ranged from 4 weeks to 48 months, with a mean of 6 months (SD=9.9).

Treatment Groups

Cognitive adaptation training group. Cognitive adaptation training is a manual-driven series of compensatory strategies based on neuropsychological, behavioral, and occupational therapy principles (9).

Cognitive adaptation training procedures include a comprehensive behavioral assessment utilizing the Frontal Lobe Personality Scale (11) to quantify the level of apathy and disinhibition in overt behavior. Furthermore, a neuropsychological assessment is conducted to examine the level of executive functioning (i.e., problem-solving, cognitive flexibility, and the ability to plan and carry out goal-directed activity), attention, and memory. Adaptive functioning is assessed by using the Functional Needs Assessment (12), which identifies specific areas of impairment in activities of daily living. Finally, an environmental assessment is conducted in the patient's home environment to identify triggers that may promote maladaptive behavior, the presence of safety hazards, the availability of needed equipment or supplies, and the organization of belongings. These assessments have been described in detail elsewhere (9).

Treatment plans that include cognitive adaptation training are based on two dimensions: 1) the patient's level of apathy versus disinhibition, and 2) the patient's level of impairment in executive functions. Behaviors characterized by apathy can be altered by providing prompting and cueing that help the patient initiate each step in a sequenced task. Examples of environmental alterations for apathetic behavior include: using checklists for tasks that involve complex behavioral sequencing, placing signs and equipment for daily activities directly in front of the patient (e.g., placing a toothbrush, toothpaste, and a sign summarizing steps in brushing teeth in a basket attached to the bathroom mirror), using labels, and using electronic devices (e.g., tape recorders and menu-driven electronic cooking instructions) to cue and sequence behavior. Individuals who exhibit disinhibited behavior respond well to the removal of distracting stimuli and behavioral triggers and to redirection. For disinhibited behavior, supplies are organized to minimize inappropriate use (e.g., placing complete outfits with one shirt, one pair of pants, etc., in separate boxes in the patient's closet to prevent him or her from putting on multiple layers of clothing; providing different colored bins for sorting laundry to help prevent patients from mixing clean and soiled clothing). Individuals with mixed behavior (both apathy and disinhibition) are offered a combination of these strategies.

Individuals with greater degrees of executive impairment are provided a greater level of structure and assistance and more obvious environmental cues (larger, more brightly colored, and more proximally

placed cues). Individuals with less impairment in executive function can perform instrumental skills adequately with less structure and more subtle cues. These general plans are adapted for individual strengths or limitations in verbal/visual attention, memory, and fine motor coordination. For example, the color of signs may be changed frequently to capture the individual's attention, or Velcro may be used instead of buttons on clothing to help individuals with fine-motor problems. Interventions are explained and maintained or altered as necessary by means of brief weekly visits from a cognitive adaptation training therapist.

Control group. The control condition was designed to account for some of the nonspecific effects of cognitive adaptation training. Subjects assigned to this condition were seen on the same schedule as those assigned to cognitive adaptation training and were given adaptations for their environment that were unrelated to cognitive or adaptive functioning (e.g., posters, plants). They were allowed to choose two items per month. Contact time was equivalent to that in the cognitive adaptation training group, and the same therapists provided treatment for both the cognitive adaptation training and control conditions.

Follow-up only group. Subjects assigned to this condition were assessed on the same schedule as those in the other two treatment conditions, but they did not receive any additional interventions besides standard follow-up care.

Assessments

Symptoms. The expanded version of the Brief Psychiatric Rating Scale (13) is a 24-item scale that is used for assessing a wide range of psychopathology on a series of Likert-type scales from 1 to 7. The psychosis factor score, composed of items assessing hallucinations, unusual thought content, suspiciousness, and conceptual disorganization, was used as a measure of positive symptoms. Higher scores indicate higher levels of symptoms.

Negative symptoms were assessed by using the Negative Symptom Assessment (14). The Negative Symptom Assessment is a 26-item scale assessing multiple domains of negative symptoms, including communication, social behavior, emotion, motivation, cognition, and psychomotor retardation. Higher scores indicate more negative symptoms. As described by Eckert et al. (15), a total score for the Negative Symptom Assessment, calculated by determining the mean of the six subscales, was used as a measure of negative symptoms. The mo-

Table 1.
Demographic and Clinical Characteristics of Outpatients With Schizophrenia or Schizoaffective Disorder Who Received Cognitive Adaptation Training, Control Treatment, or Standard Follow-Up Only[a]

Characteristic	Cognitive Adaptation Training (N=15)		Control (N=15)		Follow-Up (N=15)	
	N	%	N	%	N	%
Male	12	80.0	11	73.3	11	73.3
Schizophrenia diagnosis	12	80.0	13	86.7	13	86.7
Taking atypical anti-psychotic medication	10	66.7	9	60.0	14	93.3
	Mean	SD	Mean	SD	Mean	SD
Age (years)	36.15	10.55	36.33	8.20	39.00	8.62
Age at onset (years)	22.36	4.67	22.50	6.05	22.17	3.30
Education (years)	11.78	2.36	11.54	2.02	12.67	2.27
Length of index hospitalization (months)	7.33	15.29	7.08	12.98	5.33	1.58

[a]All three groups received standard outpatient follow-up treatment, including medications. The cognitive adaptation training group also received home visits and compensatory interventions to address impairments in adaptive functioning. The control group received home visits but no compensatory interventions.

tivation subscale of the Negative Symptom Assessment was used to assess involvement in productive activities. Increased involvement in productive activity is a particular focus of cognitive adaptation training.

Global functioning was assessed by using the Global Assessment of Functioning scale (DSM-IV). This instrument assesses the overall level of functionality on a scale from 1 to 100 on the basis of the clinician's judgment about the patient's social and occupational functioning and the impact of symptoms on functionality. Higher scores indicate better adaptive functioning. Midway through the study we added an additional, more comprehensive measure of functionality, the Multnomah Community Ability Scale (16). The Multnomah Community Ability Scale is a 17-item instrument that is rated by the clinician on the basis of an interview with the patient. To increase the validity of ratings, collateral information was obtained from caregivers and relatives. The total score on the Multnomah Community Ability Scale reflects the overall level of community functioning; higher scores indicate better functioning. The numbers of subjects in each group are smaller than 15 for analyses that include this variable.

Relapse. Relapse was considered to have occurred if the patient was rehospitalized during the study or if the patient experienced a significant exacerbation of positive symptoms, defined as an increase of 2 points or more to a score of 4 or greater on at least two of the four BPRS items composing the positive symptom subscale. In all but two cases of relapse, both of these criteria were met. In one of those cases, the relapse of a patient in the control condition

was characterized by a return of hallucinations and delusions. However, the patient was not hospitalized due to an intense effort by family members to provide 24-hour supervision. In the second case, the evidence for the relapse of a patient in the cognitive adaptation training condition consisted of suicidal behavior rather than a worsening of psychosis.

Data Analysis

Group differences in symptoms and functionality at the end of 9 months were examined by using a series of analyses of covariance (ANCOVAs). For each variable, scores on assessments obtained at study entry were used as covariates. We plotted residuals versus predicted scores and residuals versus the covariate for each variable to verify that the assumptions for the model were correct. For each variable, we verified that the slopes of the covariate were the same for the three groups. On one measure (the Multnomah Community Ability Scale), where the variances between groups were unequal, we verified that after adjusting for the covariate, the residuals from the model had homogeneous variances for the three groups. We examined planned comparisons between the cognitive adaptation training condition and each of the two remaining conditions (control and follow-up only) by using Dunnett's procedure to correct for experiment-wise error rate. In each comparison, the means at the end of the study, corrected for the covariate, were compared.

In addition to endpoint analyses (with the last observation used as endpoint) described above, we did an additional series of repeated measures analyses of variance (ANOVAs). These ANOVAs were conduct-

ed by using the SAS GLM procedure (17) on only the data collected in an effort to examine the time (a within-subjects factor) at which groups (a between-subjects factor) began to diverge with respect to dependent variables. (These analyses were adjusted for time points for which data were missing on some subjects.) We examined planned comparisons of the interaction of group and time between the cognitive adaptation training group and the remaining groups by using Dunnett's procedure at each time point.

Results

The demographic and clinical characteristics of the three treatment groups are presented in Table 1. There were no statistically significant differences between groups on any of these variables at the time of initial assessment. However, 14 of 15 subjects in the follow-up only group (93.3%), but only 9 of 15 subjects in the control group (60.0%), were taking atypical antipsychotic medications ($x^2=4.0$, df=1, p<0.07). Ten of 15 subjects in the cognitive adaptation training group (66.7%) were taking atypical antipsychotic medications.

The three treatment groups' mean scores and standard deviations on measures of symptoms and adaptive functioning at the initial and final assessments are presented in Table 2.

Symptom scores

ANCOVA revealed a significant difference among the three treatment groups in positive symptom scores at the end of the 9-month study period (F=8.31, df=2, 41, p<0.001). Planned comparisons were conducted to examine differences between the cognitive adaptation training group and the two remaining groups (control and follow-up only). Only the mean difference in positive symptom scores between the cognitive adaptation training group and the control group was statistically significant, when the analysis was corrected for multiple comparisons. An inspection of means indicated improvement of symptoms in the cognitive adaptation training group and worsening in the other treatment groups. Differences in positive symptom scores between the initial and final assessments for the three treatment groups are presented in Figure 1.

Repeated measures ANOVA for positive symptoms revealed a nonsignificant main effect for group (F=2.59, df= 2, 42, p<0.09), a significant main effect for time (F=3.38, df=3, 100, p<0.02), and a significant interaction of group and time (F=2.89, df=6, 100, p<0.02). Significant differences

Table 2.
Scores for Positive and Negative Symptoms and Adaptive Functioning at Initial Assessment and 9 Months of Outpatients With Schizophrenia or Schizoaffective Disorder Who Received Cognitive Adaptation Training, Control Treatment, or Standard Follow-Up Only[a]

Measure and Treatment Group	Initial score		Score at 9 Months	
	Mean	SD	Mean	SD
Positive symptoms[b]				
Cognitve adaptation training (N=15)	2.53	1.36	2.05	1.00
Control (N=15)	2.55	0.81	3.47	1.07
Follow-up (N=15)	2.83	1.32	2.97	1.11
Negative symptoms[c]				
Cognitive adaptation training (N=15)	13.83	2.22	11.84	3.11
Control (N=15)	15.04	3.75	14.62	3.20
Follow-up (N=15)	14.41	3.17	14.30	3.45
Global Assessment of Functioning[d]				
Cognitive adaptation training (N=15)	43.81	2.22	54.47	15.68
Control (N=15)	38.93	9.39	30.40	12.05
Follow-up (N=15)	42.53	11.91	41.80	10.54
Multnomah Community Ability Scale[d,e]				
Cognitive adaptation training (N=8)	61.37	9.16	68.12	3.72
Control (N=8)	67.37	11.06	59.50	12.91
Follow-up (N=14)	60.00	9.01	60.64	11.11

[a]All three groups received standard outpatient follow-up treatment, including medications. The cognitive adaptation training group also received home visits and compensatory interventions to address impairments in adaptive functioning. The control group received home visits but no compensatory interventions.
[b]Brief Psychiatric Rating Scale (13) psychosis factor score. Higher scores indicate more severe symptoms.
[c]Negative Symptom Assessment (14) total score. Higher scores indicate more severe symptoms.
[d]Higher scores indicate better adaptive functioning.
[e]After adjustment for unequal variances, the residuals from the model had homogeneous variances for the three groups (variance=7.8, 8.1, and 6.1 for the cognitive adaptation training, control, and follow-up only groups, respectively).

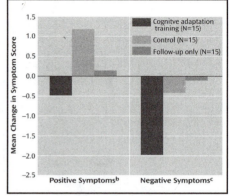

Figure 1. Change at 9 Months in Scores for Positive and Negative Symptoms of Outpatients With Schizophrenia or Schizoaffective Disorder Who Received Cognitive Adaptation Training, Control Treatment, or Standard Follow-Up Only.[a]
[a]All three groups received standard outpatient follow-up treatment, including medications. The cognitive adaptation training group also received home visits and compensatory interventions to address impairments in adaptive functioning. The control group received home visits but no compensatory interventions.
[b]Brief Psychiatric Rating Scale (13) psychosis factor score. Higher scores indicate more severe symptoms. Significant difference between treatment groups (F=8.31, df=2, 41, p<0.001).
[c]Negative Symptom Assessment (14) total score. Higher scores indicate more severe symptoms.

in positive symptom scores between the cognitive adaptation training group and the control group emerged at 3 months and continued throughout the follow-up period. Differences between the cognitive adaptation training group and the follow-up only group were significant at 9 months. Mean positive symptom scores by group and assessment period are presented in Figure 2.

With respect to negative symptom scores, ANCOVA results showed no significant difference between the three treatment groups at the end of the 9-month study period (F=2.73, df=2, 41, p<0.08). Differences in negative symptom scores between the initial and final assessments for the three treatment groups are presented in Figure 1.

As for motivation subscale scores, the ANCOVA results showed significant differences among the three treatment groups (F=6.78, df=2, 41, p<0.003). In addition, planned comparisons that used Dunnett's procedure to correct for multiple comparisons showed that the differences between the cognitive adaptation training group and both the control group and follow-up only group were statistically significant. An inspection of means indicated that the motivation problems of patients in the cognitive

adaptation training group decreased to a greater extent than those of patients in other treatment conditions. Differences in motivation scores between the initial and final assessments for the three treatment groups are presented in Figure 3.

Repeated measures ANOVA for the total Negative Symptom Assessment score revealed a nonsignificant main effect for group (F=2.69, df=2, 42, p<0.08), a significant main effect for time (F=2.82, df=3, 100, p<0.05), and a significant interaction of group and time (F=3.47, df=6, 100, p<0.005). Comparisons between the cognitive adaptation training group and the two remaining treatment groups at each time period, with corrections for multiple comparisons, revealed that the negative symptom scores of the cognitive adaptation training group were significantly different from those of the control group at 3 and 6 months. At 9 months, the negative symptom scores of the cognitive adaptation training group differed significantly from those of the follow-up only group. Results for the motivation subscale from the Negative Symptom Assessment were more consistent. Significant main effects were found for group (F=4.69, df=2, 42, p<0.02) and time (F=4.87, df=3,

100, p<0.004), and there was a significant interaction of group and time (F=3.17, df=6, 100, p<0.007). Significant differences in motivation were apparent between the cognitive adaptation training group and the control group by 3 months and remained significant throughout the study. Significant differences between the cognitive adaptation training group and the follow-up only group appeared at the 9-month assessment. In the interest of space, these data are not presented in figure form.

Level of Functioning

We used an ANCOVA, with the initial Global Assessment of Functioning score as a covariate, to examine whether Global Assessment of Functioning scores differed between groups at the end of treatment. The results indicated a main effect for treatment group (F=13.12, df=2, 44, p<0.0001). In addition, planned comparisons that used Dunnett's procedure showed that the score for the cognitive adaptation training group was significantly different from the score for both the control group and the follow-up only group. Differences in scores for level of functioning between the initial and final assessments for the three treatment groups are presented in Figure 4.

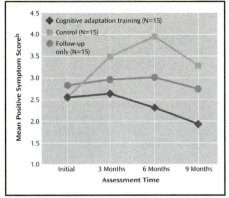

Figure 2. Positive Symptom Scores Over 9 Months of Outpatients With Schizophrenia or Schizoaffective Disorder Who Received Cognitive Adaptation Training, Control Treatment, or Standard Follow-Up Only.[a]

[a]All three groups received standard outpatient follow-up treatment, including medications. The cognitive adaptation training group also received home visits and compensatory interventions to address impairments in adaptive functioning. The control group received home visits but no compensatory interventions. Nonsignificant difference between treatment groups (F=2.59, df=2, 42, p<0.09). Significant difference between assessment times (F=3.38, df=3, 100, p<0.02). Significant interaction of treatment group and assessment time (F=2.89, df=6, 100, p<0.01).

[b]Brief Psychiatric Rating Scale (13) psychosis factor score. Higher scores indicate more severe symptoms.

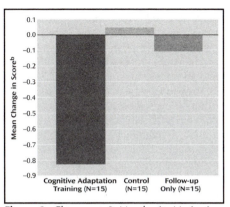

Figure 3. Change at 9 Months in Motivation Scores of Outpatients With Schizophrenia or Schizoaffective Disorder Who Received Cognitive Adaptation Training, Control Treatment, or Standard Follow-Up Only.[a]

[a]All three groups received standard outpatient follow-up treatment, including medications. The cognitive adaptation training group also received home visits and compensatory interventions to address impairments in adaptive functioning. The control group received home visits but no compensatory interventions. Significant difference between treatment groups (F=6.78, df=2, 41, p<0.003).

[b]Score on the motivation subscale of the Negative Symptom Assessment (14). Higher scores indicate more severe symptoms.

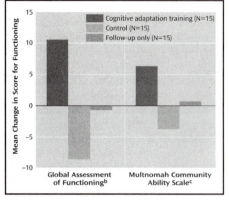

Figure 4. Change at 9 Months in Scores for Adaptive Functioning of Outpatients With Schizophrenia or Schizoaffective Disorder Who Received Cognitive Adaptation Training, Control Treatment, or Standard Follow-Up Only.[a]

[a]All three groups received standard outpatient follow-up treatment, including medications. The cognitive adaptation training group also received home visits and compensatory interventions to address impairments in adaptive functioning. The control group received home visits but no compensatory interventions.

[b]Higher scores indicate better adaptive functioning. Significant difference between treatment groups (F=13.12, df=2, 44, p<0.0001).

[c]Higher scores indicate better adaptive functioning. N=8 for the cognitive adaptation training group and the control group; N=14 for the follow-up only group. Significant difference between treatment groups (F=4.46, df=2, 26, p<0.02)

With respect to individual subjects, scores on the Global Assessment of Functioning indicated that all but two of the 15 subjects in the cognitive adaptation training group improved in level of adaptive functioning over the 9-month study period. In the control group, 12 of 15 individuals got worse or experienced no change in adaptive functioning. Finally, in the follow-up only group, 10 of 15 individuals got worse or experienced no change in adaptive functioning.

Results of a repeated measures ANOVA for the Global Assessment of Functioning score indicated a significant main effect for group (F=7.71, df=2, 42, p<0.002), a nonsignificant main effect for time (F=2.63, df=3, 100, p<0.06), and a significant interaction of group and time (F=3.87, df=6, 100, p<0.002). Differences between the cognitive adaptation training group and the control group were significant at 3 months and were sustained throughout the study. Significant differences between the cognitive adaptation training group and the follow-up only group appeared at 9 months.

An ANCOVA indicated that the scores on the Multnomah Community Ability Scale of

the three treatment groups were significantly different (F=4.46, df=2, 26, p<0.02). (Eight patients in the cognitive adaptation training group, eight patients in the control group, and 14 patients in the follow-up only group participated in this assessment.) The results of planned comparisons between the cognitive adaptation training group and both the control group and the follow-up only group were significant after the analysis corrected for multiple comparisons. An inspection of means indicated a clinically significant improvement of 10 points in the cognitive adaptation training group, compared to a worsening of symptoms and almost no change in the control group and the follow-up only group, respectively (Figure 4).

The results of the repeated measures ANOVA for scores on the Multnomah Community Ability Scale were essentially the same as those for Global Assessment of Functioning scores.

Relapse rates

Number of relapses by treatment group was examined by using chi-square analysis. Relapse rates for the cognitive adaptation training, control, and follow-up groups were 13.33%, 67.67%, and 33.33%, respectively. The difference between groups was significant (x^2=9.27, df=2, p<0.01).

Discussion

This is the first randomized, controlled study we are aware of that has demonstrated the benefit of compensatory strategies for outpatients with schizophrenia. Although these strategies have been used successfully for patients with other disorders, they have not been applied in a systematic way to the treatment of patients with schizophrenia.

Patients who received cognitive adaptation training did better than those in the control and follow-up only conditions with respect to level of symptoms and level of adaptive functioning. Improvements in functioning seen in patients participating in cognitive adaptation training were not observed in the vast majority of patients assigned to other treatment conditions. In addition, relapse rates were better for those participating in cognitive adaptation training. Compensatory strategies appear to help individuals with their transition from inpatient status to living in the community.

The control condition, which included a therapist's weekly visits to patients and manipulation of the environment in nonspecific ways, did not lead to better outcomes. In fact, patients in the control condition did worse than those in the follow-up only group. We examined whether the poor outcomes for individuals in the control condition relative to the follow-up only group may have been due to the almost universal use of atypical antipsychotic medications in the follow-up only group. When we examined data for only those patients in each group who were taking atypical antipsychotic medications, the results were unchanged.

An alternative explanation for the difference may be that whenever the therapists who made the home visits observed problems that needed the attention of clinic staff, they asked patients to contact their clinic or case manager. These contacts may have resulted in a higher level of intervention (and accompanying clinic chart documentation) for patients in the control condition. Because these patients were seen every week, any serious problems they experienced were more likely to be identified, compared with those of patients in the follow-up only group. However, the therapists who visited the subjects in the cognitive adaptation training group and the control group, as well as the raters who assessed the subjects, did not make determinations about the need for hospitalization but rather referred subjects to clinic treatment team members who were blind to the subjects' treatment groups.

Differences in rates of medication compliance between the groups could possibly explain some of the differences in symptom scores between the cognitive adaptation training group and the other treatment groups. Although we selected patients who were compliant with medication treatment and we had evidence from chart review that the subjects had regularly attended clinic appointments as outpatients before their index hospitalization, these factors may not guarantee that medication compliance was equivalent between groups. However, all patients had a history of willingness to take medications. If patients in the cognitive adaptation training group had better compliance, it may have been due to the compensatory strategies used in cognitive adaptation training to cue patients to take medications at appropriate times. This result would support the use of compensatory strategies. Previous research has indicated that medications are not sufficient for improving functional outcomes in patients with schizophrenia (18). It is therefore somewhat unlikely that differences in medication compliance alone would have produced differences in levels of functioning between groups.

Additional research will be needed to examine whether cognitive adaptation training is as effective as other currently available treatments, such as Assertive Community Treatment teams. Certainly, compensatory strategies could be used by Assertive Community Treatment teams to help focus interventions.

The study reported here has several methodological weaknesses, including a small sample size and the lack of a therapeutically active control condition. These limitations will need to be addressed in future studies. In addition, the subjects included only patients who were recently hospitalized in a state hospital. The results may not apply to more stable outpatients. However, in an ongoing study with stable outpatients, preliminary results have been similar to those presented here (19).

Despite the limitations mentioned above, the results of this study suggest that the use of compensatory strategies may add to the growing repertoire of interventions that can help patients with schizophrenia and schizoaffective disorder lead more productive and satisfying lives. Continued development and study of compensatory strategies for this population may identify which approaches are best for which patients.

References

1. Velligan DI, Bow-Thomas CC: Executive function in schizophrenia. *Semin Clin Neuropsychiatry* 1999; 4:24–33
2. Green MF: What are the functional consequences of neurocognitive deficits in schizophrenia? *Am J Psychiatry* 1996; 153: 321–330
3. Velligan DI, Mahurin RK, Diamond PL, Hazleton BC, Eckert SL, Miller AL: The functional significance of symptomatology and cognitive function in schizophrenia. *Schizophr Res* 1997; 25: 21–31
4. Harvey PD, Howanitz E, Parrella M, White L, Davidson M, Mohs RC, Hoblyn J, Davis KL: Symptoms, cognitive functioning, and adaptive skills in geriatric patients with lifelong schizophrenia: a comparison across treatment sites. *Am J Psychiatry* 1998; 155:1080–1086
5. Green MF: Cognitive remediation in schizophrenia: is it time yet? *Am J Psychiatry* 1993; 150:178–187
6. Green MF, Marshall BD Jr, Wirshing WC, Ames D, Marder SR, McGurk S, Kern RS, Mintz J: Does risperidone improve verbal working memory in treatment-resistant schizophrenia? *Am J Psychiatry* 1997; 154:799–804
7. Velligan DI, Newcomer JW, Pultz J, Csernansky JG, Hoff AL, Mahurin RK, Miller AL: Changes in cognitive function with quetiapine fumarate versus haloperidol, in *1999 Annual Meeting New Research Program and Abstracts*. Washington, DC, American Psychiatric Association, 1999, p 247
8. Meltzer H: Dimensions of outcome with clozapine. *Br J Psychiatry Suppl* 1992; 17:46–53
9. Velligan DI, Bow-Thomas CC: Two case studies of cognitive adaptation training for schizophrenic outpatients. *Psychiatr Serv* 2000; 51:25–29
10. First MB, Spitzer RL, Gibbon M, Williams JBW: *Structured Clinical Interview for DSM-IV Axis I Disorders (SCID)*. New York, New York State Psychiatric Institute, Biometrics Research, 1994
11. Grace J, Stout JC, Malloy PF: Assessing frontal behavioral syndromes with the Frontal Lobe Personality Scale. *Assessment* 1999; 6:269–284
12. Dombrowski SB, Kane M, Tuttle NB, Kincaid W: *Functional Needs Assessment Program for Chronic Psychiatric Patients*. Tucson, Ariz, Communication Skill Builders, 1990
13. Ventura J, Lukoff D, Nuechterlein KH, Liberman RP, Green MF, Shaner A: Manual for the expanded Brief Psychiatric Rating Scale. *Int J Methods in Psychiatr Res* 1993; 3:227–244
14. Alphs LD, Summerfelt A: The Negative Symptom Assessment. *Psychopharmacol Bull* 1989; 25:159–163
15. Eckert SL, Diamond PM, Miller AL, Velligan DI, Funderburg LG, True JE: A comparison of instrument sensitivity to negative symptom change. *Psychiatry Res* 1996; 63:67–75
16. Barker S, Barron N, McFarland B, Bigelow D: A community ability scale for chronically mentally ill consumers, part I: reliability and validity. *Community Ment Health J* 1994; 30:363–383
17. SAS, Version 6.12. Cary, NC, SAS Institute, 1990
18. Liberman RP, Kopelowicz A, Young AS: Biobehavioral treatment and rehabilitation of schizophrenia. *Behavior Therapy* 1994; 25:89–107
19. Velligan DI, Bow-Thomas CC, Ritch J, Ledbetter N, Miller AL: Preliminary evidence that compensatory strategies improve adaptive function and quality of life in stable outpatients (abstract). *Schizophr Res* 2000; 41:299–300

Use of Environmental Supports Among Patients With Schizophrenia

Dawn I. Velligan, PhD, Janet Mueller, MA, Mei Wang, MS, Margaret Dicocco, MS, Pamela M. Diamond, PhD, Natalie J. Maples, MA, Barbara Davis, MA

Objective: Cognitive adaptation training is a psychosocial treatment that uses individually tailored environmental supports, such as signs, calendars, hygiene supplies, and pill containers, to cue and sequence adaptive behavior in the client's home environment. Generic environmental supports offer a less costly treatment that provides a predetermined package of helpful supports to clients at the time of their routine clinic visit. Previous studies have demonstrated the efficacy of cognitive adaptation training. The study reported here examined the extent to which environmental supports are used by clients. **Methods:** As part of an ongoing study, persons with schizophrenia were randomly assigned to one of three conditions: cognitive adaptation training, generic environmental supports, or assessment only. Rates of use of supports for the first three months of treatment were examined for the first 64 patients assigned to the first two groups. **Results:** Rates of overall use averaged approximately 80 percent for cognitive adaptation training and 44 percent for generic environmental supports. Specific categories of supports were also significantly more likely to be used by patients who were receiving cognitive adaptation training. More than 66 percent of patients in cognitive adaptation training were classified as high users of supports (used more than 75 percent of supports provided appropriately), compared with only 13 percent of those who were receiving generic environmental supports. **Conclusions:** Environmental supports have been found to improve functional behaviors for patients with schizophrenia. However, supports are not likely to be used unless they are customized for individual clients and set up in the home environment. (*Psychiatric Services* 57:219–224, 2006)

The authors are affiliated with the department of psychiatry of the University of Texas Health Science Center at San Antonio, 7703 Floyd Curl Drive, MSC 7792, San Antonio, Texas 78229 (e-mail, velligand@uthscsa.edu). Ms. Mueller is also with the Center for Health Care Services in San Antonio.

Schizophrenia is characterized by cognitive deficits that predict the ability of afflicted individuals to perform basic activities of daily living and how well they will function in their social and occupational roles (1–5). A number of psychosocial treatments have been devised to address the cognitive impairments exhibited by persons with schizophrenia. Cognitive remediation seeks to directly improve cognitive functions that require attention, planning, problem solving, and memory skills (6–10). Rather than attempting to alter cognitive function per se, compensatory strategies attempt to bypass cognitive deficits by establishing supports in the person's environment that cue and sequence adaptive behavior. Our research group has applied environmental supports to persons with schizophrenia, with very encouraging results in a treatment we call cognitive adaptation training.

Cognitive adaptation training is a manual-driven series of environmental supports—such as signs, checklists, supplies, and organization of belongings—designed for each individual on the basis of cognitive strengths and weaknesses, specific functional problems, environmental barriers, and behavioral styles (11–13). These supports are offered to the client during home visits on a weekly basis to address specific problems, including in the areas of hygiene, care of the person's living quarters, adherence to

medication regimens, and social or leisure activities. Although cognitive adaptation trainers use behavioral techniques, such as positive reinforcement, shaping, and antecedent control, unlike cognitive-behavioral therapy, cognitive adaptation training does not seek to change the emotions attached to thoughts.

The treatment is described in a series of articles (11–13), and the manual is available from the first author. Examples of some of the specific environmental supports used in cognitive adaptation training are listed in Table 1. We found that persons who received cognitive adaptation training were hospitalized less often and had better community outcomes than those in a control group or a treatment-as-usual group (12,13).

Although cognitive adaptation training is effective, a program that involves weekly home visits may be prohibitively expensive for underfunded, understaffed community agencies that serve persons with serious mental illnesses. Cognitive adaptation training has been shown to be less expensive than assertive community treatment but shares the problem that caseloads fill quickly (14). There is a great need to develop lower-cost treatments that use environmental supports to cue and sequence adaptive behavior.

With this goal in mind, our research group developed strategies for using environmental supports in a more cost-effective

manner. One strategy, generic environmental supports, provides environmental supports such as calendars and pill containers to clients at the time of their regular clinic visits. Clients are expected to set up the supports on their own, using a tape recording of the trainer's and client's discussion of how and where to use the supports in the home environment. The intensity of treatment varies between cognitive adaptation training and generic environmental supports. However, in previous studies we demonstrated that an intensive control condition involving weekly home visits by a therapist did not improve outcomes for persons with schizophrenia (13,14). Thus the intensity of cognitive adaptation training is not enough to account for improvements identified in previous studies. Differences between cognitive adaptation training and generic environmental supports, shown in Table 2, go beyond intensity. The comparatively higher cost of home visits makes it important to examine the extent to which a generic package of supports offered at clinic visits will be used by patients.

Although it is assumed that improvement in symptoms and adaptive functioning in cognitive adaptation training results from the use of environmental supports, few data are available on the use of these supports among persons with schizophrenia. Previous studies have not examined the use

Article Reprint Information: Velligan, D. I., Mueller, J., Wang, M., Dicocco, M., Diamond, P. M., Maples, N. J., & Davis, B. (2006). Use of environmental supports among patients with schizophrenia. *Psychiatric Services, 57*(2), 219-224. Reprinted with permission from the *Psychiatric Services*, Copyright 2006. American Psychiatric Association.

Table 1

Examples of environmental supports used in cognitive adaptation training among persons with schizophrenia

Area	Environmental supports
Medication adherence	Pill containers, alarm clocks set specifically for medication times, checklists, reminder signs, memo pads to record questions for the psychiatrist, placing medication and water by the bed for evening dose, supports for dealing with side effects (for example, lotion for dry skin)
Transportation	Bus passes, tape-recorded messages in real time to ensure getting on and off the bus at the correct stop, list of neighbors who may provide transportation to appointments, car parts
Leisure skills	Games to involve the patient with others (for example, cards), art or recreational supplies (for example, paints or a basketball). Daily checklist to remind the patient to engage in leisure activity
Orientation and scheduling	Watch, alarm clock, calendar with attached marker for keeping track of the date and appointments (the participant is trained to cross the day off before going to bed), day planner
Grooming and hygiene	Shampoo, soap, toothpaste, mirror, checklist attached to the mirror for reviewing specific problem areas, appropriate clothing
Care of living quarters	Cleaning products, daily checklist of household tasks, file boxes, labels for drawers and cupboards, tape-recorded instructions for specific chores

---

Table 2

Differences between cognitive adaptation training and generic environmental supports for clients with schizophrenia

Dimension	Cognitive adaptation training	Generic environmental supports
Frequency of visits	Weekly	Monthly
Visit location	Home	Clinic plus a tape recorder and instruction tape
Areas addressed by supports	All domains of adaptive functioning	Medication adherence, orientation and scheduling, grooming and hygiene
Level of customization of supports	All supports set up for the patient's individual level of cognitive functioning, level of adaptive functioning, behavioral style, and environment	Same supports given to all patients regardless of need
Therapeutic relationship	More intense	Less intense

---

of environmental supports in a systematic manner (12,13). The extent to which individuals use the supports that cognitive adaptation training therapists set up in their homes and the extent to which individuals will use generic environmental supports that have been given to them at clinic visits remains unclear.

The purpose of this study was to examine rates of use of supports offered to persons with schizophrenia in these two treatments. Given the fact that supports in cognitive adaptation training are individually tailored and set up in the home environment, and their use is reinforced on weekly home visits, we hypothesized that patients in the cognitive adaptation training group would use a greater proportion of the environmental supports than those in the generic environmental supports group.

Methods

Participants

The study sample comprised 64 participants in an ongoing study, funded by the National Institute of Mental Health, of the use of environmental supports. The sample was recruited from February 2002 to September 2003. Outpatients with schizophrenia or schizoaffective disorder who were receiving medication and routine follow-up care at community clinics were approached about participating in this study at the time of their clinic visit and were asked to sign

an informed consent document approved by the university's institutional review board. Participants met the following inclusion criteria: diagnosis of schizophrenia or schizoaffective disorder according to the Structured Clinical Interview for DSM-IV (15), age between 18 and 60 years, receipt of a second-generation antipsychotic medication other than clozapine, an absence of hospitalizations in the past three months, ability to provide evidence of a stable living environment for the past three months, and no current plans to move out of the area within the next two years. Individuals were excluded if substance abuse would have interfered with their study participation (for example, with assessment or treatment); if they had a documented history of significant head trauma, seizure disorder, neurologic disorder, or mental retardation; if they were currently being seen by an assertive community treatment team; or if they had engaged in violent behavior in the previous year.

After a baseline assessment, participants who were monitored by community clinics for standard medication management were randomly assigned to one of three additional treatments: cognitive adaptation training, generic environmental supports, or assessment only. Among the first 68 participants who were assigned to either cognitive adaptation training (N=34) or generic environmental supports (N=34), three-month data were available for 29 and 31 patients,

respectively. Three patients in the cognitive adaptation training group dropped out of the study, one withdrew after signing the informed consent form, one could not be contacted after completing initial assessments, and one moved out of the area. Of the remaining 31 patients, two could not be contacted by the utilization researcher during the first three months after repeated attempts, leaving 29 for whom utilization data were available in the cognitive adaptation training group. One patient who was receiving generic environmental supports withdrew consent to participate, and two patients could not be contacted by the utilization researcher after repeated attempts, leaving 31 patients for whom utilization data were available in the generic environmental supports group.

Assessments

Baseline assessments included the Expanded Version of the Brief Psychiatric Rating Scale (16), the Negative Symptom Assessment (17), and the Social and Occupational Functioning Scale (15).

Treatment groups

Cognitive adaptation training. Cognitive adaptation training is a manual-driven series of compensatory strategies based on neuropsychological, behavioral, and occupational therapy principals (11). Before participating in cognitive adaptation training, patients receive comprehensive behavioral, neuropsychological, functional, and environmental assessments. These assessment procedures are described in detail elsewhere (11). Treatment plans are based on two dimensions: level of apathy (poor initiation) versus disinhibition (distracted by irrelevant cues and information in the environment) and level of impairment in executive functions (the ability to plan and carry out goal-directed activities). Behaviors characterized by apathy can be altered by providing prompting and cueing to initiate each step in a sequenced task. For example, therapists may provide checklists for tasks that involve complex behavioral sequencing or place signs and equipment for daily activities directly in front of the patient, such as a checklist for medication placed on the refrigerator. Individuals who exhibit disinhibited behaviors respond well to the removal of distracting stimuli and behavioral triggers and to redirection. For example, a therapist may help to discourage taking of multiple doses of medication at the same time by placing pills in single-dose containers, or remove outdated medications to be stored elsewhere. Individuals with mixed behavior (apathy and disinhibition) are offered a combination of these strategies.

Individuals with greater degrees of executive impairment are provided with a greater level of structure and assistance and more obvious environmental cues (larger and more proximally placed). Individuals who have less impairment in executive functioning can perform instrumental skills adequately with less structure and more subtle cues. These general plans are adapted for individual strengths or limitations in other cognitive areas. Interventions are explained, maintained, and altered as necessary during brief (30-minute) weekly visits from a cognitive adaptation trainer. Detailed progress notes list all supports provided and their intended target behaviors.

Generic environmental supports. Generic environmental supports is a manual-driven series of environmental supports offered to patients at their regular clinic visit. The generic package is composed of the supports that were frequently used and described as helpful by clients in the cognitive adaptation training program on the basis of progress notes and store receipts. Supports selected for the generic package required minimal training and were designed to address three primary problems: medication adherence, orientation and scheduling, and grooming and hygiene. Supports included an alarm clock, a watch, bus passes, a checklist of everyday activities such as taking medication and showering, hygiene products such as shampoo and toothpaste,

pill containers, and reminder signs—for example, "Did I take my medication?" or "Did I remember to brush my teeth?" A bookstore gift card is given to participants in an effort to promote leisure activity, and one of the items on the checklist is intended to prompt social behavior. However, these areas of functioning are not well addressed by generic environmental supports.

Therapists offered the same supports to all participants and provided instructions on how to use each item. The therapist discussed with the client where to place signs to get maximum benefit and how to use watches, alarms, and pill containers. The session was audiotaped, and the client was given both the tape and the tape recorder to replay the instructions any time. Once a month, the therapist called the client to ask whether the client needed any replacement supplies. If supplies were needed, the client picked them up from the clinic. For some patients, for the purposes of the study, supports were delivered to the client's home.

Utilization. Each month, a utilization researcher telephoned each client. The utilization reviewer used treatment notes and store receipts to determine all supports provided during the preceding one-month period for patients in cognitive adaptation training. From the therapist notes, the utilization researcher determined the intended function of each support offered. For patients who were receiving generic environmental supports, the utilization researcher used the original item list for the package and the therapist's notes regarding which items were supplied in the previous month. The researcher asked the participant whether he or she had used each support over the past seven days and exactly how the support was used. In an effort to prevent the participant from trying to make his or her therapist "look good," the participant was told at the beginning of each call that the information provided would not be shared with the cognitive adaptation training therapist or the generic environmental supports therapist.

On the basis of the information provided, the utilization researcher calculated a percentage use based on the intended use of the support. For example, if an item was intended to be used daily and it was used four out of seven days, the percentage use would be 57 percent. A mean percentage use for each contact was generated by averaging the percentages for each item, and then the contacts for the three-month period were averaged. Supports provided were also placed into categories, and a mean utilization percentage by category was calculated. Categories common to both treat-

ments included medication adherence, orientation and scheduling, and grooming and hygiene. Categories were not mutually exclusive, and the same support could have been counted in more than one category. For example, a calendar may have been used to keep track of medication appointments as well as to keep oriented to day and date.

Data analysis

The three primary behavioral targets addressed in generic environmental supports—medication adherence, orientation and scheduling, and grooming and hygiene—were examined in both treatment groups. Differences in percentage use between the cognitive adaptation training group and the generic environmental supports group at three months were compared by using t tests for overall use of supports as well as for specific categories. To correct for multiple comparisons, we set the significance level conservatively at .01. Data were also examined by using nonparametric statistics, because the distributions of the individual categories of supports were not always normal. Because nearly identical results were obtained with both approaches, we report the results of the t tests below.

We used the intraclass correlation coefficient to examine whether the individual categories of supports could be combined into a meaningful composite score for overall percentage use.

Results

Descriptive and baseline data

Demographic characteristics of the two treatment groups are listed in Table 3. No statistically significant baseline differences were observed between groups in terms of age, gender, or ethnicity. Furthermore, clinical variables, such as level of psychotic symptoms, negative symptoms, and social and occupational functioning, did not differ significantly between groups at baseline. Baseline characteristics of participants for whom utilization data were available and those for whom data were not available did not differ significantly.

Rates of utilization

Mean utilization rates for overall supports and by categories are shown in Figure 1. Participants who received cognitive adaptation training had a higher mean percentage use of supports than those who received generic environmental supports. The differences between groups were statistically significant for overall supports

Table 3
Baseline characteristics of a sample of patients with schizophrenia who received cognitive adaptation therapy or generic environmental supports

Variable	Cognitive adaptation training N	%	Generic environmental supports N	%
Age (mean±SD years)	40.76±7.49		41.41±9.30	
Male	20	59	18	53
Race				
Hispanic	15	44	16	47
White	14	41	11	32
BPRS[a] psychosis factor score (mean±SD)	2.97±1.11		2.85±1.43	
Negative Symptom Assessment global score (mean±SD)	3.00±1.17		2.94±.92	
Social and Occupational Functioning score (mean±SD)	46.42±12.00		45.29±12.64	

[a]Brief Psychiatric Rating Scale

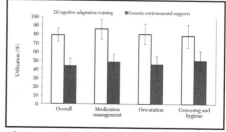

Figure 1. Use of environmental supports in cognitive adaptation training and generic environmental supports.

(t=5.75, df=58, p<.001) and for each category (orientation and scheduling, t=4.78, df=56, p<.001; medication adherence, t=5.43, df=56, p<.001; and grooming and hygiene, t=3.23, df=46, p<.001). Degrees of freedom differ for specific utilization categories because cognitive adaptation training is customized for the individual, so not all participants in that group received all types of supports.

The intraclass correlation coefficient for the categories was .87, which suggests that the categories of support could be meaningfully combined into a composite score reflecting overall use. We classified participants as high or low utilizers on this overall utilization composite score on the basis of a cutoff of 75 percent. This is a commonly used cutoff in the medication adherence literature for schizophrenia, reflecting the idea that in a negotiated treatment, a person who is taking between 70 percent and 80 percent of the recommended dosage has good adherence to the treatment (18,19).

We found that more than 66 percent of patients in the cognitive adaptation training group (19 of 29) were high utilizers, compared with less than 13 percent of patients in the generic environmental supports group (four of 31) (Fisher's exact test, p<.001). Thus only a small percentage of patients in the generic supports group actually received a recommended "dose" of the treatment.

Clinical observations

Utilization problems in the generic environmental supports group appeared to have several origins. Some clients forgot to use the kit provided. Others did not like the brands or styles of products provided. Moreover, very limited social reinforcement

was provided for the use of items. Clients undergoing cognitive adaptation training receive regular praise and other social reinforcement during weekly in-home visits.

Discussion and conclusions

Several methodologic limitations should be kept in mind. By necessity, the utilization researchers were aware of participants' treatment group assignment when asking about the use of supports provided. It is possible that participants exaggerated their use in an effort to make their therapist look good. However, store receipts for replacement of environmental supports and progress notes kept by therapists are consistent with the notion that use of supports was high among patients who received cognitive adaptation training. Generic environmental supports target primarily basic activities of daily living. An analysis of utilization or supports for higher-level behaviors for patients receiving cognitive adaptation training will be conducted once the study has been completed. It is also possible that supports may be used less frequently over the course of cognitive adaptation training treatment. This possibility will be investigated in follow-up studies.

High utilization levels in cognitive adaptation training suggest that the use of supports may be the key to the improvements in adaptive functioning that have been observed in previous studies. Future studies will need to examine this process-outcome relationship specifically. Generic supports provided in a clinic setting may improve behavior if the supports are used. Unfortunately, supports are unlikely to be used if they are not individualized, set up, trained, and maintained in the patient's home environment. It is unclear whether the higher

rate of use in the cognitive adaptation training group was due to the individualization of supports; the training in the use of the supports in the home environment; the weekly visits that prompt, reinforce, and check the use of supports; or a combination of these procedures.

Future research is needed to tease out each of these factors. It is conceivable that weekly telephone calls in the generic environmental supports group may be enough to stimulate use by providing the social reinforcement and prompting necessary to form habits around the use of supports. In addition, offering a limited range of choice of item brand may prompt higher use. Additional research will be necessary to test these hypotheses.

Although previous studies have suggested that patients participating in cognitive adaptation training improved in terms of adaptive functioning more than those in the control conditions, ours is the first study to formally examine the degree of use of specific supports. Even though findings lend credence to the continued study of supportive environments for persons with schizophrenia, process-outcome relationships between the use of supports and adaptive functioning need to be specifically examined.

Acknowledgment

This study was funded by grant R01-MH-61775-04 from the National Institute of Mental Health. During manuscript preparation, Dr. Velligan was supported in part by grant R01-MH62850-08 from the National Institute of Mental Health.

References

1. Saykin AJ, Gur RE, Gur RC, et al: Neuropsychological function in schizophrenia: selective impairment in memory and learning. *Archives of General Psychiatry* 48: 618–622, 1991

2. Gold JM, Harvey PD: Cognitive deficits in schizophrenia. *Psychiatric Clinics of North America* 16:295–312, 1993

3. Velligan DI, Bow-Thomas CC: Executive

function in schizophrenia. *Seminars in Clinical Neuropsychiatry* 4:24–33, 1999

4. Velligan DI, Mahurin RK, Diamond PL, et al: The functional significance of symptomatology and cognitive function in schizophrenia. *Schizophrenia Research* 25:21–31, 1997

5. Green MF: What are the functional consequences of neurocognitive deficits in schizophrenia? *American Journal of Psychiatry* 153:321–330, 1996

6. Benedict R, Harris AE, Markow T, et al: Effects of attention training on information processing in schizophrenia. *Schizophrenia Bulletin* 20:537–546, 1994

7. Pilling S, Bebbington P, Kuipers E, et al: Psychological treatments in schizophrenia: II. meta-analyses of randomized controlled trials of social skills training and cognitive remediation. *Psychological Medicine* 32:783–791, 2002

8. Medalia A, Revheim N, Casey M: The remediation of problem-solving skills in schizophrenia. *Schizophrenia Bulletin* 27:259–267, 2001

9. Spaulding W, Reed D, Storzbach D, et al: The effects of a remediational approach to cognitive therapy for schizophrenia, in *Outcome and Innovation in Psychological Treatment of Schizophrenia*. Edited by Lewis S. West Sussex, England, Wiley, 1998

10. Wykes T, Reeder C, Corner J, et al: The effects of neurocognitive remediation on executive processing in patients with schizophrenia. *Schizophrenia Bulletin* 25:291–307, 1999

11. Velligan DI, Bow-Thomas CC: Two case studies of cognitive adaptation training for outpatients with schizophrenia. *Psychiatric Services* 51:25–29, 2000

12. Velligan DI, Bow-Thomas CC, Huntzinger CD, et al: A randomized controlled trial of the use of compensatory strategies to enhance adaptive functioning in outpatients with schizophrenia. *American Journal of Psychiatry* 157:1317–1323, 2000

13. Velligan DI, Prihoda TJ, Maples N, et al: A randomized single-blind pilot study of compensatory strategies in schizophrenia outpatients. *Schizophrenia Bulletin* 28:283–292, 2002

14. Korell SC, Velligan DI, DiCocco M, et al: *Assertive community treatment versus cognitive adaptation training: a cost comparison.* Poster presented at the Winter Workshop on Schizophrenia, Davos, Switzerland, Feb 24 to Mar 1, 2002

15. *Diagnostic and Statistical Manual of Mental Disorders.* Washington, DC, American Psychiatric Association, 1994

16. Ventura J, Lukoff D, Nuechterlein KH, et al: Manual for the Expanded Brief Psychiatric Rating Scale. *International Journal of Methods Psychiatric Research* 3:227–244, 1993

17. Alphs L, Summerfelt A, Lann H, et al: The Negative Symptom Assessment: a new instrument to assess negative symptoms of schizophrenia. *Psychopharmacology Bulletin* 25:159–163, 1989

18. Adams J, Scott J: Predicting medication adherence in severe mental disorders. *Acta Psychiatrica Scandinavica* 101:119–124, 2000

19. Kamali M, Kelly L, Gervin M, et al: Psychopharmacology: insight and comorbid substance misuse and medication compliance among patients with schizophrenia. *Psychiatric Services* 52:161–163,166, 2001

Caregiving and Autism: How Does Children's Propensity for Routinization Influence Participation in Family Activities?

Elizabeth Larson

Key words: human activity and occupation, occupational science, parenting

Abstract: Children with autism characteristically prefer routinization, yet their mothers seem to experience greater parenting stress orchestrating family life than mothers parenting children with other disabilities. This qualitative study examined the development and use of routines for nine mothers parenting children with autism spectrum diagnoses. Interview transcripts were coded by sorting data into categories and searching for variations within the category and the relationships between categories. Findings describe: (1) development of routines, (2) child's comfort or discontent in routines, (3) child's fluctuations in participation in routines, (4) effects of irregular routines on participation, (5) maternal strategies to manage irregular routines, (6) mothers' selective modification of routines, and (7) alterations in family activities and rituals. The implications of these findings for practice are discussed.

Elizabeth Larson, PhD, OTR, is Assistant Professor, Occupational Therapy Program, Department of Kinesiology, University of Wisconsin–Madison, Madison, Wisconsin. Accepted for publication May 9, 2005. Address correspondence to Elizabeth Larson at blarson@education.wisc.edu.

There has been a shift in focus and emphasis in disability research from studying maternal stress and family dysfunction to studying maternal management of daily family routines. Gallimore, Bernheimer, and Weisner (1999) suggest that researchers should not focus on crises, but rather on how mothers develop functional family routines that manage the demands presented by a child with special needs and accommodate the demands and needs of other family members. This tactic is aimed at diminishing a heretofore prominent pathological orientation to disability research and emphasizing the strengths of families (Gallimore et al., 1999).

Family routines are believed to organize family activities, sustain and propagate the family's cultural beliefs, and provide stability and continuity in daily life (Boyce, Jensen, James, & Peacock, 1983). Routines, crafted by design or default, create predictability, organization, and order through structural, temporal, and action matrices (Boyce et al., 1983). For parents of children with disabilities, sustaining daily routines that are responsive to the family constraints, responsive to individual family members' characteristics, and in line with values is the focus of daily efforts (Gallimore et al., 1999).

Family routines are built from the interlocking of individual family members' routines, of which the mother is often the major orchestrator or organizer (Larson, 2000). The structure of these routines is determined by forces outside the family such as work and school schedules, the need to meet basic functions of food, safety, and shelter, and the preferences and desires of the family for discretionary time (Segal & Frank, 1998). There are indications that families of children with autism may experience more difficulty orchestrating smooth functional family routines. In fact, the sustainability of functioning routines was viewed as a gauge of the achievement of a sense of normalcy in family life (Gray, 1997).

Compared to other families of children with disabilities, parents of children with autism report more family stress and adjustment problems in daily life (Sanders & Morgan, 1997; Wolf, Noh, Fisman, & Speechley, 1989). Daily tasks such as teaching the child, keeping the child safe, and managing his or her behavior in social situations, during play, and during self-care activities were rated as moderately difficult to manage by parents in Tel-Aviv, Israel (Milgram & Atzil, 1988). Fifty percent of Australian parents rated daily parenting stressors at high to very high levels, with 80% feeling "stretched beyond their limits" at some time (Sharpley, Bitsika, & Efremidis, 1997). Greater disruptions and decreased spontaneity in daily schedules and greater caretaker burden were reported by mothers of children with autism (Gray, 1997; Rodrigue, Morgan, & Geffken, 1990). Factor, Perry, and Freeman (1990) suggest that it is the chronicity of autism that leaves parents exhausted, pessimistic, and at risk for burnout.

Perhaps due to this chronicity of demands, mothers parenting children with autism report spending 50% more time with their children than parents of typical children, an average of 9.7 waking hours per day compared to 6.1 hours (Tunali & Power, 2002). Although this implies that mothers construct significantly different routines when parenting a child with autism, it does not address how and why mothers are spending this additional time. Families with children with autism spend significantly less time in recreational, sporting, social, or cultural activities than typical families (Sanders & Morgan, 1997), so it appears this additional time is not used in greater family leisure. How does parenting a child with autism alter the construction and implementation of daily family routines?

Certain features of autism are likely suspects in accounting for the greater daily demands and for the accommodations in daily routines that mothers must make for a child with autism. These may include social and language impairments (Milgram & Atzil, 1988; Myles & Southwick, 1999), delays in self-care abilities (Dalrymple & Ruble, 1992; Koegel et al., 1992), sleep dysomnias (Schreck & Mulick, 2000), and sensory processing difficulties (VerMaas-Lee, 1999) that may impede participation.

Routines ideally should assist mothers in managing their children's participation in daily activities by fostering skill acquisition

Article Reprint Information: Reprinted with permission from Larson, E. (2006). Caregiving and autism: How does children's propensity for routinization influence participation in family activities? *Occupational Therapy Journal of Research: Occupation, Participation and Health, 26*(2), 69-79.

Table
Participants' Ages, Self-identified Ethnicity, and Children's Ages and Diagnoses[a]

Mother	Age (Y)	Self-identified Ethnicity	Marital Status	Child	Age (Y)	Diagnoses Reported by Mothers	No. of Siblings
Elena	42	African American & Puerto Rican	Married	Randall	10	High functioning autism, ADHD, mental health issues	0
Helen	41	White	Married	Ned	14	PDD/high functioning autism, nonverbal learning disability, ADHD, OCD	1
Juliana	27	Mexican	Married	Andrew	8	Autism	1
Kay	28	Chinese	Married	Simon	3	Autism	0
Lesley	43	Scandinavian German/ English	Married	Matt & James	13 & 9	Autism spectrum disorder, PDD-NOS–High functioning	0
Mary	46	White, European descent	Married	Darien	6	Autism, dyspraxia	0
Sarah	47	Jewish	Married	Nathan	9	Autism, epilepsy, mild cerebral palsy, & soft neurological	2
Yvette	41	White, French, & Austrian	Married	Lance	9	Autism	1
Wanda	37	White–Ashkenazi	Married	Danny	6	Autism	1

ADHD = attention-deficit hyperactivity disorder; PDD = pervasive developmental disorder; OCD = obsessive–compulsive disorder; PDDNOS = pervasive developmental disorder–not otherwise specified.
[a]Names have been changed to protect anonymity.

to address developmental delays, providing regularity in expectations for performance, and assisting in the development and refinement of workable strategies for managing the child's autistic symptoms. However, is this the case? Children with autism are often diagnosed in part by their characteristic preference to engage in repetitive actions and routines (American Psychiatric Association, 1994). However, some of the children's behaviors may in fact be ritualistic nonfunctional actions that interfere with participation in daily family routines. Although it would seem that this willingness to participate in repetitive patterns could facilitate sustainability of family routines, the inflexibility of the children to deviate from their own routines when circumstances demand it may be a barrier to the family group's routines and the external demands of work and school schedules. How do the preferences of children with autism for specific routines and their participation in these routines alter family life and create greater time demands and parenting stressors for mothers? This study examined how routines were used and implemented by mothers parenting boys with autism, and the challenges mothers faced in constructing sustainable daily routines.

Methodology

The nine mothers in this study were volunteers recruited to participate in a larger study examining maternal well-being when parenting children with disabilities. Culturally diverse participants who were parenting a child with a disability that according to previous research could be identified as high demand were recruited. Child characteristics such as being nonverbal, having dependence in self-care, possessing more severe intellectual impairments, and exhibiting behavior problems have been demonstrated to increase perceived maternal burden (Dunst, Trivette, & Cross, 1986; Floyd & Zmick, 1991; Friedrich, Cohen, & Wilturner, 1987; Frey, Greenberg, & Fewell, 1989; Mercer & Chavez, 1989). Children needed to have only one of these characteristics for mothers to participate in the larger study.

Initial analyses of the whole data set indicated significant differences in the responses of mothers parenting children with autism compared to other groups. Therefore, additional mothers of children with autism were recruited through brochures in occupational therapy clinics and colleague referrals, and a separate analysis was undertaken. The procedures and informed consent for this study were reviewed by the University of Wisconsin Human Subjects Review Board and approved. In addition, approval was obtained through collaborating clinics; their procedures for review of research studies were followed before brochures and signs were posted in the clinics. In the case of referrals, potential participants were first contacted by the referring colleague. If they expressed interest in participating, they were then contacted by the researcher to discuss the study.

Participants' ages ranged from 27 to 47 years. Participants varied in self-identified ethnicity and had educations ranging from several years of high school to a doctoral degree. Family size ranged from one to three children. One family had two boys with autism spectrum diagnoses. In two families, brothers of the child with autism had a diagnosis of dyspraxia or attention-deficit hyperactivity disorder. Three other families included typical younger siblings, and the child with autism was an only child in the final three families. Families resided in cities on the East Coast, in the Midwest, and on the West Coast. Income ranged widely from $16,000 to $30,000 for families in low-income inner city areas to $36,000 to $250,000 for the remaining families residing in urban areas. This diversity of informants allowed the researcher to examine the specific influence of autism on family routines despite differences in ethnicity, and in relation to the family's resources (maternal education and socioeconomic). The table provides a detailed description of mothers and their children. Names have been changed to protect anonymity.

Nearly half of the boys had additional diagnoses besides autism. Although this may suggest that the participating group included children with specific developmental delays or more complex diagnoses than other children with autism, clinical accounts suggest multiple diagnoses are common (Myles & Southwick, 1999). All mothers described significant delays in some aspect of their son's self-care skills compared to typical milestones. For example, this included toilet training beyond 6 years of age and assistance with aspects of dressing and showering through adolescence. This was similar to children in other studies, where only 28% to 50% of adolescents and young adults with autism were found to be independent in the most basic self-care skills (Green, Gilchrist, Burton, & Cox, 2000; Howlin, Mawhood, & Rutter, 2000). The caregiving demands presented by these particular children appear to be common to many children with autism. Although these boys varied on their skills, they all continued to require maternal assistance or monitoring in the majority of daily routines.

As far as current services, four of the mothers were receiving counseling and taking psychotropic drugs for depression. All boys had received or were receiving occupational therapy services.

This study employed an interpretive interactionist approach (Denzin, 1989). This approach aims to articulate how individuals explicate the meaning of everyday life situations. This is achieved by framing and critically analyzing the phenomenon within current knowledge, capturing multiple instances of the phenomenon, bracketing the phenomenon by examining only the essential elements, assembling these essential elements, and contextualizing the phenomenon in the real world through thick descriptions (Denzin, 1989).

In-depth interviews were guided by questions from two semi-structured interview guides. Mothers participated in two to four interviews each ranging from 90 minutes to 4 hours in length to address all of the questions on these two interview guides for the length of time convenient for the mothers. Interviews were conducted over several months in the mother's home (6 of 9 participants) or by telephone, if necessary due to the distance (3 of 9 participants). Both in-person and telephone interviews yielded similar detail and number of pages of data transcripts. Questions and probes asked mothers about their typical daily routines, holiday and family celebrations, and parenting stressors.

A redundancy in information about participation in routines and parenting stress was gathered by the ninth participant and saturation of data was achieved. In addition, both negative and positive cases on different dimensions were noted in the analysis. Data integrity was ensured through: (1) mul-

tiple in-depth interactions with participants; (2) verbatim transcription of all interviews and a systematic comparison of transcripts to taped interviews, correcting for accuracy; (3) triangulation of information across interviews—comparing earlier statements with later explanations and elaborations; (4) verbatim use of quotes to support the analysis; and (5) member checking of data analysis.

Two of the informants reviewed the preliminary findings in written form and provided critiques or confirmations of the analysis during an interview. Data collection and analysis included: (1) reviewing current theory and research on routines in families of children with autism; (2) identifying all references to routines in transcripts; (3) sorting and grouping of data segments into categories; (4) examining variations within categories and between participants; and (5) generating a description of the relationship of categories and of exemplars of the categories.

Findings

Routines were essential building blocks in creating lifestyles for these families and a regularity that supported the family's emotional environment. Order and structure in daily routines assisted in integrating the child into family activities. Although some mothers initially did not have difficulty managing routines or find a need for highly structured routines because their boys were "easy babies," all mothers eventually experienced challenges in developing workable routines when the symptoms of autism became prominent.

In the most extreme example, one mother revisited that challenging time when functioning routines were not in place and the child disrupted all of family life. She remembered wondering, "Would [we] be able to live with this child? Can he live with us? [We all expect] a certain life style, everybody eats, everybody sleeps...a social life, work. This child didn't want to do any of this...none." Lacking even the most rudimentary sleep/wake patterns, the mother described the child's years between 3 and 5 years of age as "hell." An overall structure with some predictable activity patterns was necessary to coordinate a reasonable life for family members.

Developing routines required considerable skill and focused on orderliness and the emotions of those participating. The mother of one of the youngest boys described the improvisation necessary to develop workable routines respectful of her son's daily variations in mood:

Now there is structure [but I] show a greater...respect for his individuality.... I'm not, this is the way we do it...because that doesn't work. My kid is screaming right back at me so it's not working.... Next time see [what] happens. It goes different....I'm going to be a smooth operator. Slide in there and...study the situation. The kid is screaming [his] head off...so, I just learn it like that...learning what works for him, and me, and how can we best solve the situation.

Successful routines took time to develop and needed to be responsive to the child's emotional and developmental needs and create a livable family life for other family members.

The Comfort of Daily Routines

Once in place, routines aided mothers in providing predictable expectations for the child that smoothed the way for participation: "The whole day is routines...their food, their lunches, getting them off to school, when they come home...if you find something that works [you keep doing it]...they're comfortable with routines so we try to keep as much of them in the day." Routines helped children feel content: "Danny, with his routine stuff, it's gotta be in the same cup and it has to have the same top and it has to have the same straw, and then he knows all is well with the world." The children often adhered to or enforced participation in routines, perhaps due to the comforting predictability: "Every day we drive in the car to his therapy appointment and...[he] tells me the whole route on the way back. He's full of routines....I can change it if there's really strong reason to. But he definitely wants it to be the same."

Despite the age of the children, none of the boys went to bed independently or without parental oversight. Parents used bedtime routines similar to those for preschoolers to assist them in transitioning to sleep. Mothers seemed to suggest that regularity of routines provided a sense of security. This was deemed more necessary for the boys with autism than for their siblings. Deviations from routine—changes in the timing or form of the activity or objects used—often led to anxiety:

When a kid like Danny is thrown off his schedule, any kid its [sic] hard, but with him, the consequences are much more dire...and they leave a longer mark of anxiety...even if regular kids get anxiety ridden about the changes [when] they're tired and they're hungry...but with him it's like it build[s] up in his nervous system into this big mean anxiety blob.

His father...hadn't poured his glass of milk yet [for breakfast] and Nathan just decided that [his dad] had ruined his whole day....He [didn't understand that he needs a glass of milk....You have to ask [Nathan] if he wants a glass of milk and let him say "yes." Because if you don't ask him, then he gets mad when you give it to him....It's like a dance.

The absolute adherence to some routines was a barrier to the improvisation required in daily life, such as when there was an alternate caregiver or schedule change. For example:

The problem about him throwing tantrums is when he doesn't know the routine. If he knows he is going to go to therapy at a particular time...he understands that on a [therapy day] he watches Teletubbies....That's all he cares about because it is always the same....I turn off the TV, he knows...he's going to get his shoes on and get out of there....One time I wanted him to eat [instead]...[but] he started putting his socks on [because] he wanted to go...[I said] "I didn't want your [socks on" but that's] what he's expecting. When he's expecting, it's OK. But when he doesn't expect...

Routines were used to provide regular expectations, ease transitions, and manage the child's anxiety. Finding what worked was a dance between creating a structure and then improvising depending on the child's responses, while minimizing the child's need to change in instances of anxiety. Once routines worked, several mothers challenged whether they or their child insisted on the maintenance of these sequences: "And I realize part of that now is me. Because like in the morning I don't function well so like I know that dah, dah, dah...it's such a routine. I don't know if we don't change it because they won't change it or because I won't."

Difficulties and Discontent in Daily Routines

In contrast, when children had difficulties in performance, participation in daily routines was frustrating rather than comforting. The expected performance may routinely be expected, but homework, chores, or unmastered self-care tasks often led to children resisting participation, directive assistance, or both. Maternal insistence on a challenging task was not well received: "He never performs under pressure....Once he senses that he's expected to do something, he will deliberately not do it....When the pressure is gone, he suddenly does it." An-

other mother said, "I had wanted Ned to do some chores. It's really tough....He's got to be in the mood or you're just in for a huge battle to get it to happen."

Nathan's chore appeared too difficult for him despite the everyday repetition:

His job is to peel the carrots and the cucumbers before dinner....He has trouble with the methodicalness of it....He'll load his arms up with carrots and cucumbers and then he won't get the idea that like if he puts them down first, he'll be able to carry the chopping board or the knife. ...You have to walk through step by step...sometimes it seems as though he has figured them out and then it just isn't there.

These routines did not smoothly facilitate participation or, for Nathan, help in learning the task. Task qualities such as the complexity or novelty, performance anxiety, and perhaps dyspraxia, may underlie these difficulties in participation (Page & Boucher, 1998).

For some activities, mothers sometimes offered assurances and options, giving the child greater control of the circumstances to facilitate his attempts at difficult tasks: "Because what I found with Matt, he's so routine oriented...with homework [I expected we'd] have to do it the same time and same place every day. And it was a disaster. And finally when he could pick when he wanted to do his homework, and he likes to go outside and do it...it turned out to be a totally opposite thing than I expected." This was also true of other children; homework provided a challenge that upset even set routines: "When he gets home...the thing that will throw things off sometimes is the homework. [Especially if he feels] that it's too much." At those points in time, when the activity was too much, mothers needed to intervene and provide one-to-one assistance.

One mother recognized this time as volatile: "After dinner, homework time is generally going to be a hot spot." Mothers relaxed evening routines to decrease time and performance pressures on themselves and the family. Some mothers avoided fixed dinner times and allowed children to graze or eat on their own. This flexibility of dinner strategy has been used in healthier typical families at points in routine when time pressure is likely due to the multiple family needs and demands to minimize instances of family flare-ups, containing emotional brushfires where negative emotions spread among family members (Larson & Richards, 1999).

The Wild Card in Daily Routines: The Child With Autism

The boys were often the "fickle factor" waylaying maternal efforts to create peaceful family environments and smooth daily routines. This unpredictability of responses undermined maternal confidence in caregiving:

We try to stay within the routines to keep the unpredictability to a minimum. Because they're the unpredictable factor... you never know....There are some days James is going to have a bad [day] and then he's going to look to cause problems...other days he could care less.

If you can tailor your day...in a known territory, you know what your child needs at different times of the day, you can function that way....But when it's always the unknown...that causes anxiety....I was not depressed, I was just very anxious. Am I doing the right thing? What's going to happen next?

Within the home environment, mothers felt they could more predictably manage a narrower set of circumstances that might trigger disruptions or discontent. Yet even with this foresight, mothers frequently questioned their efficacy in doing the right thing for the child in the right circumstance at the right time. Because of the children's unpredictability despite carefully constructed routines, and their inability to clearly communicate feelings, frustrations, and pleasures, even if the boys were verbal, mothers were often anxious about whether they took the right tack.

Effects of Irregularity of Routines on Children's Participation

There are frequent cyclic variations that alter daily schedules, such as changes from weekends to weekdays, school schedules to summer schedules, or intermittent holidays. Mothers recognized that these changes often brought difficulties for their sons. Even for an adolescent, the change from weekend to weekday schedules often led to a refusal to attend school or therapy:

Mondays are always hard coming off the weekend. If you have two days off for anything, not even just school, like getting him to therapy appointments when the schedule changes, like when school was ending and summer was starting. I had a heck of a time getting him to therapy appointments. The time hadn't changed, it was the same after school time. But because his whole schedule changed he had trouble going. And there were a couple days when he just wouldn't.

The inability to tolerate change in weekly routines severely restricted any changes in schedules or participation in spontaneous or infrequent activities outside the home. Attempted weekly schedule changes were examined in terms of the cost–benefit ratio of such alterations:

I spent all this energy getting him an 8:30 in the morning appointment so that I could drop those two off at school and then just loop right around, but autistic child that he is, not being able to have his regular morning routine was so disruptive to him, that he just couldn't deal with it. [So, he'd go to school and less than an hour later you'd go pick him up?] Right. Because if I didn't do that, then he'd flip out.

The weekend–weekday variations in routines were taxing for families when the boys did not easily adapt to the differences in routines, and also because the boys did not organize their own activities but were dependent on the mother. Weekends lacked a predictable structure and left large blocks of unfilled time. For the family with two boys who had autism spectrum diagnoses, both presented challenges in this regard: "The weekends [are stressful because] they're home!...James when he's been out of school for too long, it's very stressful. Matt we can do things with, we can plan. [His dad] takes him to his mother's [house] and they can go to church together. And James it's just hard...he needs that much of his day filled up."

In another family with an adolescent boy, the mother also felt the burden of weekends: "[Weekends are stressful when they're] totally open...I feel like I'm the entertainment committee for the kids." Under normal circumstances, adolescents typically spend the majority of their free time with their peers, but mothers of children with autism were orchestrating the free time of or participating in activities with their adolescent children.

Strategies to Manage Irregularity in the Schedule

Infrequent weekly occurrences presented challenges to ensuring smooth transitions from one activity to the next and the child's willingness to participate. Mothers sometimes attempted to impose participation in irregular events that were especially important activities, such as therapy sessions, medical appointments, family birthday parties, or holiday celebrations. Despite mothers' efforts, the child's participation was unpredictable over time and mothers had to rely on a trial-and-error approach rather than systematic strategies. Mothers

found these periods stressful and fatiguing because they wrestled with understanding the child's reasons for refusal to participate that day and finding a workable strategy to facilitate participation.

Scheduled transitions could be persistently problematic. Despite the consistent schedule and use of strategies that eased the transition—dealing with hunger and reminding the child of the irregular event—one mother suggested that the child's capacity or tolerance was reached and led to a meltdown:

It's stressful [when I pick him up and he has] a tantrum.... We've tried to mitigate it different ways...bringing something cold for him to drink and something to eat, but sometimes he's really tired, and the minute he hears he has to go to therapy, even if I've reminded him in the car in the morning, he's just held it together for the whole day and he lets loose in the car. Once he goes he has a great time. But he's tired.

Mothers used strategies such as foreshadowing the event, tricking the child into agreement or compliance, appealing to a specialized interest, or offering desired activities after completion of the infrequent one that ensured compliance. Foreshadowing included informing the child of the specifics of what was going to happen. This reassured the child, even if the event did not unfold exactly the way described:

I don't tell the kids unless I'm absolutely sure it's going to happen. I always warn [them] before we're leaving. There are all these little clues and tips that I do just to make [it] easier....He need[s] to know all the specifics of it. So we found that even if you make it up, it's better, even if you change it....He's not upset if it doesn't work out that way.

Another mother described the invitation she considered the "special ed" mother's dream; it contained all of the details that she needed to prepare her children for the event:

Matt just got invited to a birthday...[it was] the perfect special needs invitation...it gave the usual information and then it says, "Put on your comfy clothes and have fun dancing to our DJ." And I'm like, OK there's going to be a DJ. And they said "pizza and hoagies will arrive at 4." OK, I know what the food is and what time it's coming...this is perfect... because my kids are better if they know [the times and menu] ahead of time....[It helps to know] if there's going to be a TV available or where they're allowed to go...[to prepare them]. It's doing my best and then if we go somewhere then

it's...adapting....We never really relax when we go anywhere...nothing we do is ever easy.

A few mothers confessed to occasionally tricking their children to manage their behavior or facilitate participation. Helen said that to get her child to go to a doctor's appointment, "You try to pull every trick you can think of." James' mother reset her older son's alarm on vacations and weekends to get more sleep, because he would only get up when the clock read 7:00.

Sometimes mothers wove in, albeit tangentially, an interest of the child to motivate him to participate:

[He was sleeping.] I tried, "Dad's waiting for us, we're going to go on this great bike ride," anything I could think of to make him get out of bed....When I said "You know, Ned, we're going...right past the 147...where there are buses," well, he popped out of bed....If I can relate everything to a bus line...I can get him out of bed.

Getting the child to agree to go to the event was often half the battle; once the boys agreed, parents often found that the prior discontent did not affect their participation at the event unless additional circumstances provoked them. However, if the boys did not agree, their participation continued to be difficult.

Another strategy that worked was to offer a preferred activity after the irregularly scheduled event:

I'm constantly [fatigued trying] to figure out what in the world is going on and what...to do about [it]....Nathan needed to get a blood test. I have realized that if you say let's go get a blood test that that doesn't work. So the last time he needed one, I said, "Well, Nathan, would [you] rather have an eating treat or a buying treat after you have your blood test?" And he said, "Oh, a buying treat" and he was like, "Oh, let's go get the blood test." And I'm going, "Yes, it worked."

Strategizing was fatiguing for mothers. Regardless of their efforts, mothers could not predictably manage the child in home and social situations despite their large repertoire of strategies.

Modifying Daily Routines: Pick Your Battles

Mothers used the metaphor "you have to pick your battles" when describing times they chose to alter daily routines. Because changes had significant consequences, mothers made decisions based on their energy, their judgment of the need for change, and the child's readiness for new skills. Because of the child's slow piecemeal progress, mothers often talked about cyclic instructional attempts at mastering activities of daily living and other skills. Partly successful initial instruction was often terminated when the child resisted, but mothers later returned to teaching the task when they had the energy and believed it a "battle" worth choosing:

I've tried to get Ned to do his own laundry, which I've had limited success with, but I've come to know that the little bit I've tried in the past is going to help me when I try it again, when I'm ready for him to try it again...it's not just one training session and you walk away and you're done. Not with Ned anyway. He's got to let it go when he's not doing it and try it again in a month or two and keep at it.

In toilet training, once committed, mothers dedicated large blocks of time to develop this skill:

I waited a really long time [to push the toilet training] because he has very severe apraxia...his little body just wasn't ready to do that kind of motor sequencing....This summer...we'll push through the bowel movements and it has not been easy...He was probably about 50% or 60% successful doing it in the potty.... He doesn't speak but we have a communication medium....I write out multiple-choice answers for him and he very grossly can scribble through the correct answer....I wrote "I don't poop on the potty because" [and his choice of answers was] "I don't care"....[Later I said] "There are some things in life that [are] part of being a family....This pooping in the potty thing, I know you don't care about it, but maybe just because I care about it, do you think you could work a little harder toward it?"...Now he's like 90%...just from that conversation.

Like this 6 year old, other boys' independence in self-care, chores, and leisure activities were moderately or severely delayed compared to typical developmental milestones. Lesley viewed it as a miracle that her 13-year-old son was finally showering independently; this gave the family hope that his younger brother eventually could achieve the same skill. The boys' independence in simple activities was often partial, still required supervision, and continued to develop well into the teenage years.

Alterations in Family Activities and Rituals

As in other studies (Gray, 1997; Rodrigue et al., 1990), families participated less often than they desired in activities such as shopping, going out to eat, family day trips, or vacationing. This was due to the special and arduous accommodations required and mothers' assessment that the cost was greater than the benefit. For instance, this shopping trip was traumatic:

[At the mall] he started acting difficult because it was Friday 4:30...the worst possible time to go....It just ended up being an awful time...they were doing all the things I told them not to do....If I had gone there by myself, I would have been in and out....Daniel [wouldn't have picked the gift], I would just say, "Here, give this to your teacher," and it would [be a] piece of cake....Sometimes [I have to] drag them around to do my chores and it's the worst thing to do with a kid like him.

In addition, spontaneity of family life was constrained:

We couldn't pick up and suddenly decide to go to a restaurant or something like that or a movie because there was no guarantee that he would go or that once he went if he would go in. So we began to have to start a lot earlier to prepare him for where we were going to go and make contingency plans and avoid certain places.

Several families made focused and repeated efforts to take their child on occasional outings, such as to grocery stores or restaurants, so that the child could accompany the family, or, alternatively, made different accommodations for the child during these events. The training sessions described below required several months or years before success. Yvette was assisted in this success by using strategies suggested by her child's occupational therapist:

Two years ago, we couldn't go to the beach....[He screamed] like you were skinning him...he couldn't deal with the sensory things, the sand, the sun, the noise of the waves. He would literally hide under a blanket....So we would have to take him home....I knew it was torture for him, but [gradually we'd go back] for just a half hour [and then] go home....Now he loves the beach...we can go to the beach.

Another mother placated the child by minimizing his waiting time eating out:

We've actually worked it so we can all go [to dinner together]. It was a little rough at first, but ...as long as they can bring [French fries for James while we wait it's easier]....It took a while to [do]...like six months.

After traumatic experiences, mothers did not attempt some events again. The costs were too high or the risks to the child too great. This curbed participation in special events, sometimes creating distance from extended family, or limited the number of family events attended. The decision to no longer participate or limit participation in family birthday parties or holidays was often done to minimize the child's emotional turmoil during such social events:

I couldn't take [Randall to parties]. He freaked out around...so many people....[Once he was literally] in a corner, scared to death! [The psychiatrist said,] "Ask if he wants to go. If he doesn't want to go, don't take him!" So there's this distance now between [us and our family], they want you to come [to parties], and you say "no."... [So] there's this chasm.

These withdrawals from family events were uneasy compromises between the child's needs and family togetherness.

Holiday traditions were often restructured to allow the child to partially participate in a way that was comfortable but often tangential. One mother said, "Last Christmas was pretty horrid... [We had family for four days]...Lance can take one day. Four days was really hard....Christmas day, when he saw more people coming, he just couldn't take it anymore [and he locked himself in his room]." Sarah's complicated plan to include Nathan as he was able to participate was waylaid by a forgetful babysitter:

I had hired someone to be with him all day [at the bar mitzvah] so he could stay and leave as he needed to. She didn't show. As we're leaving, Nathan won't leave the house. So I went first with stuff to bring over [to the hall] and Gary stayed home trying to get Nathan to go and calling various sitters....Finally he got our across the street neighbors just as they were [leaving] for our bar mitzvah...to stay home and watch him....He didn't come at all, which was not what we expected.

Mothers felt a loss of tradition, but also felt the alternative of fitting the child into the expected traditions was too costly:

[You] do Christmas as you remember... most of the time, James could care less [about opening presents] so I stopped insisting....[I] just let them open what they want to open when they want to....Now in my family, everybody opened one gift at a time and everybody watched. That's just not going to happen in any shape or form [for us]. Sometimes it's kind of a let down but they know the holidays... even if it's little things, at least we try to

keep some routine or tradition that they know.

These difficulties with outings were noticeably less problematic for the family with the most parental education and resources, which afforded them the "BMW" of child-focused intervention services. On family holidays, Darien also became undone by extended visits, becoming tired and needing to be reigned in to avoid playing too roughly with cousins. Yet the majority of the time, these parents and their only child participated frequently in child-focused outings, choosing places he liked to go, allowing Darien to actively engage in bouncing or other calming strategies at any time, and taking their cues from him when deciding to terminate an activity. They frequently took plane trips with their son. Successful travel required a team—the parents and another caregiver and a strategic plan that included locating the closest McDonald's restaurant and scouting all of the local activities of interest to the child.

Irregularly experienced events, especially holidays and family outings, were particularly difficult to manage for most families, although these difficulties could be overcome by repeated step-by-step exposure to facilitate participation over time. Still, extended and nuclear family togetherness was limited due to the child's difficulties in participating in these events. The symbolic form of routines, family rituals, were often modified, yet mothers attempted to continue threads of family traditions while addressing the child's needs.

Discussion

It appears that achieving a routinization of daily life is an exceptionally challenging project for families of boys with autism. Similar to other studies (Gray, 1997, 2002a, 2002b; Rodrigue et al., 1990), mothers restructured family life in circumscribed ways largely due to the child's unpredictable and difficult behaviors, including: (1) creating and maintaining highly structured regular family routines, often devoid of spontaneity, especially to manage basic care tasks (eating, bathing, dressing, and grooming); (2) restricting family social events and home visitors, and keeping the social environment as predictable as possible; (3) carefully selecting family activities and organizing plans and contingencies to accommodate the child's needs in staying (or leaving the event while the family stayed); and (4) re-forming family holidays and rituals to include the child in a limited way.

Constructing functioning daily routines was impeded by impairments common in autism, including poor social skills, impaired communication skills, poor attentional focus related to attention-deficit hyperactivity disorder, and increased dependency in activities of daily living and free-time use. In addition, the boys' episodic capriciousness in participating in the same daily, cyclic, or periodic routines presented considerable challenges for the mothers. Even in the most regular weekday routines, frequent behavioral disruptions occurred during transitions between activities or during difficult activities, especially homework and chores. Mothers' sense of competence was undermined by these persisting challenges despite their large repertoire of parenting strategies.

Irregularity and disruptions in daily routines produced anxiety for both mothers and children for different reasons. The boys often demanded regularity in timing, form, and sequence of daily activities except when doing tasks difficult for them. When tasks were difficult, even if mothers attempted to routinize the activity, low levels of mastery or changes in form (e.g., a new type of homework) led to refusals to participate, attempts by the child to control aspects of activity participation such as changing the timing or place, and demands for assistance. In addition, the children's inflexibility and inability to improvise when daily events required it, intolerance of additional demands, or fatigue evoked emotionally charged responses or behavioral meltdowns. These behavioral disruptions, as well as the children's resistance and inability to participate in simple activities, were a difficult element in daily routines for mothers that provoked anxiety. Despite the careful structuring and insurance of regularity in routines, mothers could not assume that similar strategies to facilitate participation produced similar results on different days.

For occupational therapists, this research points out an important focus for family-centered care provision and future research. This was highlighted by one mother, who articulated her frustration in not being able to turn to experts for assistance in managing these daily challenges and anticipating future ones. Due to the highly contextual nature of children's problems, participation in daily routines needs to be investigated in situ and over time as the children's skills and preferences change. Although in-home observations and parent–professional collaborations are common in early intervention services, later practitioners may not engage in this situated problem solving due to the different demands or requirements of service provision systems (i.e., school-based).

Even after early intervention services had addressed basic problems and current intervention services assisted the children in school, there remained many other problems in home life that the mothers in this study accommodated by changing routines or components of the activity or giving in to a child's particular preference regardless of whether these changes were desired or always positive. Most of these children still had difficulties with many of the following activities: selecting, donning, and tolerating appropriate clothing; bathing or showering; toileting; doing chores; independently occupying themselves during leisure time; eating diverse foods and food textures necessary for a balanced diet; taking medications; and tolerating haircuts and other grooming activities.

These mothers often felt alone in making decisions and strategizing about how to modify daily routines and foster development of self-care and other daily living skills. They desired sensitive professional assistance in managing the child's participation in daily life as the child grew. Suggested strategies needed to consider the child's emotional needs and the targeted behaviors or skills. Careful consideration of the impact and costs of change on the child's and family's routine was a crucial consideration for mothers.

This identified gap in services aimed at developing self-care, leisure, and other skills for children with autism until they achieve a reasonable level of independence is one that occupational therapists can clearly fill. Longitudinal research can assist by describing the developmental skill trajectories that children with autism, and sub-groups within autism, may follow to guide families and practitioners in service provision.

Conclusion

This study identifies mothers' use of routines and specific maternal strategies to facilitate participation for their sons with autism, as well as the impediments to the creation of smooth family routines. It also points to a need for further in-home collaborative consultation services that extend over a longer period of time (at least through adolescence) and address the child with autism's problems of participation in in-home and community occupations such as self-care, free-time activities, and family outings. For mothers, this intervention ideally would focus on enhancing the child's participation in family life by providing strategies that respect the child's emotional well-being and are tuned to the specifics of the family situation.

The knowledge from this study can assist the occupational therapist in designing interventions that address the identified service gap and in making recommendations to families. In addition, this study points to the need for research that describes common developmental trajectories of skills for children with autism to assist families in preparing for the children's future needs and to assist in the development of services that "improve 'real world' functioning of individuals with autism" (Zerhouni, 2004, p. 19).

Acknowledgments

This research was supported by funding from the University of Wisconsin–Madison Graduate School and School of Education. The author also thanks the two anonymous reviewers for their thoughtful comments.

References

American Psychiatric Association. (1994). *Diagnostic and statistical manual of mental disorders* (4th ed.). Washington, DC: Author.

Boyce, W. T., Jensen, E. W., James, S. A., & Peacock, J. L. (1983). The family routines inventory: Theoretical origins. *Social Science and Medicine, 17*, 193-200.

Dalrymple, N. J., & Ruble, L. A. (1992). Toilet training and behaviors of people with autism: Parent views. *Journal of Autism and Developmental Disorders, 22*, 265-275.

Denzin, N. (1989). *Interpretive interactionism.* Newbury Park, CA: Sage Publications.

Dunst, C., Trivette, C., & Cross, A. H. (1986). Mediating influences of social support: Personal, family and child outcomes. *American Journal of Mental Deficiency, 90*, 403-417.

Factor, D. C., Perry, A., & Freeman, N. (1990). Stress, social support, and respite care use in families with autistic children. *Journal of Autism and Developmental Disorders, 20*, 139-146.

Floyd, F. J., & Zmick, D. E. (1991). Marriage and the parenting partnership: Perceptions and interactions of parents with mentally retarded and typically developing children. *Child Development, 62*, 1434-1448.

Frey, K. S., Greenberg, M. T., & Fewell, R. R. (1989). Stress and coping among parents of handicapped children: A multidimensional approach. *American Journal of Mental Retardation, 94*, 240-249.

Friedrich, W. N., Cohen, D. S., & Wilturner, L. S. (1987). Family relations and marital quality when a mentally handicapped child is present. *Psychological Reports, 61*, 911-919.

Gallimore, R., Bernheimer, L. P., & Weisner, T. S. (1999). Family life is more than managing crisis: Broadening the agenda of research on families adapting to childhood disability. In R. Gallimore, S. Vaughn, D. L. Speece, D. L. MacMillian, & L. P. Bernheimer (Eds.), *Developmental perspectives on children with high-incidence disabilities* (pp. 55-80). Mahwah, NJ: Lawrence Erlbaum Associates.

Gray, D. E. (1997). High functioning autistic children and the construction of "normal family life." *Social Science and Medicine, 44*, 1097-1106.

Gray, D. E. (2002a). 'Everybody just freezes. Everybody is just embarrassed': Felt and enacted stigma among parents of children with high functioning autism. *Sociology of Health & Illness, 24*, 734-749.

Gray, D. E. (2002b). Ten years on: A longitudinal study of families of children with autism. *Journal of Intellectual & Developmental Disability, 27*, 215-222.

Green, J., Gilchrist, A., Burton, D., & Cox, A. (2000). Social and psychiatric functioning in adolescents with Asperger syndrome compared with conduct disorder. *Journal of Autism and Developmental Disorders, 30*, 279-293.

Howlin, P., Mawhood, L., & Rutter, M. (2000). Autism and developmental receptive language disorder: A follow-up comparison in early adult life: II. Social, behavioural, and psychiatric outcomes. *Journal of Child Psychology and Psychiatry and Allied Disciplines, 41*, 561-578.

Koegel, R. L., Schriebman, L., Loos, L. M., Dirlich-Wilhelm, H., Dunlap, G., Robbins, F. R., et al. (1992). Consistent stress profiles in mothers of children with autism. *Journal of Autism and Developmental Disorders, 22*, 205-216.

Larson, E. A. (2000). The orchestration of occupation: The dance of mothers. *American Journal of Occupational Therapy, 54*, 269-280.

Larson, R., & Richards, M. (1999). Healthy families: Toward convergent realities. In A. Skolnick & J. H. Skolnick, *Family in transition* (10th ed., pp. 202-208). New York: Longman.

Mercer, J., & Chavez, D. (1989). *Families coping with disability: Study of California families with developmentally disabled children.* Riverside, CA: University of California Riverside.

Milgram, N., & Atzil, M. (1988). Parenting stress in raising autistic children. *Journal of Autism and Developmental Disorders, 18*, 415-424.

Myles, B. S., & Southwick, J. (1999). *Asperger syndrome and difficult moments: Practical solutions for tantrums, rage and meltdowns.* Shawnee Mission, KS: Autism Asperger Publishing Company.

Page, J. B., & Boucher, J. (1998). Motor impairments in children with autistic disorder. *Child Language Teaching & Therapy, 14*, 233-259.

Rodrigue, J. R., Morgan, S. B., & Geffken, G. (1990). Families of autistic children: Psychological functioning of mothers. *Journal of Clinical Psychology, 19*, 371-379.

Sanders, J. L., & Morgan, S. B. (1997). Family stress and parent adjustment as perceived by parents of children with autism or Down syndrome: Implications for intervention. *Child and Family Behavior Therapy, 19*, 15-32.

Schreck, K. A., & Mulick, J. A. (2000). Parental report of sleep problems in children with autism. *Journal of Autism and Developmental Disorders, 30*, 127-135.

Segal, R., & Frank, G. (1998). The extraordinary construction of ordinary experience: Scheduling daily life in families of children with attention deficit hyperactivity disorder. *Scandinavian Journal of Occupational Therapy, 5*, 141-147.

Sharpley, C. F., Bitsika, V., & Efremidis, B. (1997). Influence of gender, parental health, and perceived expertise of assistance upon stress, anxiety and depression among parents of children with autism. *Journal of Intellectual & Developmental Disability, 22*, 19-28.

Tunali, B., & Power, T. G. (2002). Coping by redefinition: Cognitive appraisals in mothers of children with autism and children without autism. *Journal of Autism and Developmental Disorders, 32*, 25-34.

VerMaas-Lee, J. R. (1999). *Parent ratings of children with autism on the evaluation of sensory processing (ESP).* Unpublished master's thesis, University of Southern California, Los Angeles, California.

Wolf, L. C., Noh, S., Fisman, S. N., & Speechley, M. (1989). Psychological effects of parenting stress on parents of autistic children. *Journal of Autism and Developmental Disorders, 19*, 157-166.

Zerhouni, E. A. (2004). *Congressional Appropriations Committee Report on the state of autism research.* Bethesda, MD: U.S. Department of Health and Human Services, National Institutes of Health.

Mothers of Children With Disabilities: Occupational Concerns and Solutions

Brianna K. McGuire, Terry K. Crowe, Mary Law, Betsy VanLeit

Key words: well-being, occupational balance, support group

Abstract: Mothers of children with disabilities have identified multiple challenges associated with achieving occupational balance in their lives. Occupational therapists are just beginning to explore the occupational and time use strategies that mothers use to successfully care for their children and get through the day in a positive manner. The Person–Environment–Occupation model was used to guide an occupational therapy intervention program called "Project Bien Estar," which was designed to increase the satisfaction, time use, and occupational performance of mothers of school-aged children with disabilities. This article focuses on the rich content of the group discussions and individual reflections, providing insight into the world of women caring for children with disabilities. Thematic analysis was used to identify person, environment, and occupation factors that contribute positively and negatively to the mothers' well-being, and the effects of the occupational therapy intervention are discussed.

Brianna K. McGuire, MSc (OT), is Occupational Therapist, Regional Municipality of Halton Children's Resource Services, and Mary Law, PhD, FCAOT, is Professor and Associate Dean, School of Rehabilitation Sciences, McMaster University, Hamilton, Ontario, Canada. Terry K. Crowe, PhD, OTR/L, FAOTA, is Director and Professor, and Betsy VanLeit, PhD, OTR/L, is Assistant Professor, Occupational Therapy Graduate Program, Department of Orthopaedics, University of New Mexico, Albuquerque, New Mexico.

Mothers of children with disabilities have their "hands full." These women spend extensive amounts of time performing physical caregiving activities such as bathing, dressing, and feeding their children (Barnett & Boyce, 1995; Crowe, 1993; Eisner, 1993), and time for sleep and other meaningful occupations may be compromised (Burden, 1980; Crowe, Clark, & Qualls, 1996; Joosten, 1979). Mothers of children with disabilities may experience pressure to take on time-consuming activities such as advocating for their child with medical professionals (Lawlor & Mattingly, 1998), or they may be asked to assume responsibility for performing therapy and other interventions at home with their children (Allen & Hudd, 1987). Because of these competing demands, they may find themselves unable to continue discretionary roles such as friend, student, or hobbyist (Cant, 1993; Crowe, VanLeit, Berghmans, & Mann, 1997).

Nelson's (2002) metasynthesis of twelve qualitative studies examined the experiences of mothers of children with different challenges. She hypothesized that mothering children with disabilities involves a four-step process. The first step, "becoming the mother of a disabled child" (p. 520), is characterized by feelings of "injustice, fear, anxiety, grief, shock, disappointment, despair and guilt" (p. 522). During this time, mothers' ability to assume the maternal role as they may have previously envisioned is challenged by the intense involvement of medical professionals who may have great-

er influence on the decisions made for their child. In the second step, "negotiating a new kind of mothering" (p. 522), mothers redefine their maternal image to reflect their role as the mother of a child with special needs and learn how to become the expert caregivers of their child. In this stage, mothers of children with disabilities have an increased sense of responsibility for not only the child with a disability, but all members in their family. In the third stage, "dealing with daily life; it will never be the same" (p. 525), mothers "redefine their priorities, make personal sacrifices and alter their lifestyle to accommodate their new role" (p. 524). Their heightened sense of responsibility for their child's happiness results in patterns of behavior that often compromise their own well-being. In the fourth stage, "the process of acceptance/denial," Nelson (2002) suggested that mothers redefine normal to "affirm their maternal identity and their child's worth" (p. 527).

Accompanying occupational loss or change, mothers of children with disabilities may experience high levels of stress (Dyson, 1993; Traustadottir, 1993). Recent research has identified public perceptions and reactions toward people with disabilities, in addition to the daily responsibilities of caring for a child with a disability, as contributing factors in maternal stress (Green, 2003). In a qualitative study by Helitzer, Cunningham-Sabo, VanLeit, and Crowe (2002), women caring for children with disabilities reported that they some-

times felt overwhelmed, socially isolated, and without support.

A decade ago, Wallander (1993) found that mothers of children with disabilities have a higher risk of adjustment problems compared with mothers of children without disabilities. However, when researchers measured adjustment over time, they found that most mothers of children with disabilities either changed their classification toward good adjustment or maintained their previous status as having good adjustment (Thompson et al., 1994). In a more recent study, there was no association between the severity and type of a pediatric disability and the mother's reported adjustment (Wallander & Varni, 1998). Wallander and Varni found that the best predictors of resistance factors for maternal adjustment were the presence of family support, marital satisfaction, and access to a larger social support network.

Occupational therapists are just beginning to explore the occupational and time use strategies that mothers use to successfully care for their children and get through the day in a positive manner. For example, mothers of children with disabilities appear to "orchestrate" their daily occupations by using the processes of planning, organizing, balancing, interpreting, anticipating, forecasting, perspective shifting, and meaning making (Larson, 2000). These strategies allow the women to make sense of the past and plan for the future. Other strategies that mothers of children with disabilities may

Article Reprint Information: Reprinted with permission from McGuire, B. K., Crowe, T. K., Law, M., & VanLeit, B. (2004). Mothers of children with disabilities: Occupational concerns and solutions. *Occupational Therapy Journal of Research: Occupation, Participation and Health, 24*(2), 54-63.

Table 1
General Characteristics of Participants

Characteristic	Mean	SD	Min	Max
Mother's years of education	17.0	2.7	13.0	25.0
Mother's age, y	37.1	5.5	27.6	46.0
No. of children in household	2.3	1.0	1.0	5.0
No. of adults in household	1.8	0.4	1.0	2.0
Weekly hours of employment	16.4	20.0	0.0	80.0

SD = standard deviation.

use include enfolding occupations (to allow multi-tasking and efficient time use), and unfolding occupations by either changing the time sequence of a series of activities or finding another adult to take responsibility for some of the tasks (Segal, 2000).

To understand how these strategies do or do not work for any particular woman, it is necessary to attend to the alignment between individual mothers of children with disabilities, the specific occupations that they need or choose to do, and the environmental context in which their lives are occurring. These essential features of the Person–Environment–Occupation (PEO) model (Fearing, Law, & Clark, 1997; Law, Cooper, Strong, Stewart, Rigby, & Letts, 1996) interact in such a manner that they can enhance or hinder an individual's occupational performance and satisfaction (Strong, Rigby, Stewart, Law, Letts, & Cooper, 1999). For mothers of children with disabilities, one might ask: What are their interests, values, and expectations concerning mothering? Do they feel competent and capable to meet the occupational requirements of the special expectations of the mothering role when the child has a disability? Are adequate environmental resources available to meet their own and their children's needs? What type of social, financial, community, and institutional support do mothers have to succeed? How do they handle the time and organizational needs of an extremely complex maternal role with multiple occupational demands? These are just some of the questions that the PEO model poses in exploring the occupational performance of mothers of children with disabilities.

The PEO model was used to guide an occupational therapy program, called "Project Bien Estar" (well-being in Spanish), designed to increase the satisfaction, time use, and occupational performance of mothers of school-aged children with disabilities (Helitzer et al., 2002; VanLeit & Crowe, 2000, 2002). This psychosocial intervention involved both individual and group sessions. This article focuses on the rich content of the group discussions and individual reflections, providing a window into the world of women caring for children with disabilities.

Method

Participants

Twenty-three women who had children with disabilities participated in this study. The women had at least one preschool or school-aged child (ages 3 to 14 years) with significant functional disabilities. For women to qualify for this study, their children needed to require significant assistance in at least three functional domains (mobility, eating, toileting, communication, and play). Children had the following diagnoses as described by the mothers: autism or Asperger's syndrome (29%), cerebral palsy (21%), Down syndrome (13%), developmental delay (8%), and other (29%). Eighty-seven percent of the children with disabilities were boys. The mean age of the children was 7.4 years, with eight children from 3 to 6 years old, twelve children from 6 to 10 years old, and four children from 10 to 14 years old. Ages of other children (siblings of children with disabilities) ranged from 6 months to 14 years, with an average sibling age of 6.3 years.

Table 1 provides demographic data for the families. The ethnicity of the women included white (75%), Hispanic (17%), and other (8%). Five of the women had 1 child, twelve had 2 children, three had 3 children, two had 4 children, and one had 5 children. Seventy percent of the women were married, 13% were divorced, 13% were single parents, and 4% were separated from their partner. All of the women were fluent in English and all women resided in a greater metropolitan area of a city in a southwestern state in the United States. Three of the women worked 40 hours a week, one woman worked 80 hours a week, and most women worked 10 hours a week.

Procedures

Women were recruited from advocacy groups, public schools, private pediatric practices, a pediatric hospital, and programs that serve children with disabilities. Recruitment followed the University of New Mexico School of Medicine Human Research Review Committee guidelines and all participants signed a consent form.

Women were recruited in groups and participants were then randomly assigned to either an intervention group or a control group. Representatives from interested community organizations helped to identify mothers of children with disabilities, provided them with written materials about the project, and encouraged them to contact the researcher for more information. This article will focus on only the women who were in the intervention group.

There were five intervention groups with a total of 23 women participating. Groups of four or five women participated in a psychosocial occupational therapy intervention, which consisted of six weekly group sessions and an individual session at the beginning and end of the intervention. An experienced occupational therapist met with the participants individually and also facilitated the group sessions to help them enhance their ability to manage their complex and demanding occupational lives. The initial individual intervention sessions focused on exploring in detail their personal interests and goals, how the women felt they were handling daily activities and routines, and how they felt about their support systems and access to needed resources.

Following the individual sessions, which took place in the women's homes, the women were brought together for weekly meetings. Child care was provided. The weekly meetings focused on (1) self-awareness (both strengths and needs); (2) problem-solving individual situations; (3) examining strategies to communicate needs more effectively; (4) providing social support and exploring ways to increase support in everyday life; and (5) discussing ways to expand leisure role involvement. The occupational therapist facilitator did not choose the discussion topics, but encouraged the women to raise issues that they wished to discuss with the group and to share ideas about how to handle a range of concerns that arose (e.g., how to find good babysitters, how to make more personal time, and how to juggle paid work and child care). Each group session lasted from 75 to 90 minutes. Careful notes were taken by an occupational therapist or occupational therapy student during all of the intervention sessions summarizing the group discussions. After completing the group intervention sessions, each participant met individually with the occupational therapy facilitator for a 60-minute session. The women examined their participation and reflected on perceived accomplishments.

Outcome data were collected prior to the first individual session, following the second individual session, and 6 months after the intervention was completed. Outcomes of several measures (Time Perception Inventory, Time Use Analyzer, and the

Table 2
Emerging Themes From Group Discussion

Theme	Person	Environment	Occupation
Concerns/obstacles	Having the burden of responsibility	Inadequate support services and systems	Achieving occupational balance
	Feeling disorganized and physically drained	Lack of understanding from others	Developing new skills
	Confusion about self-identity	Hectic and unpredictable lifestyles	Assuming new roles
	Coping with feelings of isolation	Concern about child's safety outside of home	
Solutions	Actions, experiences, or attitudes that rebalanced lifestyle	Physical and emotional support from others	Performing activities directed toward looking after themselves
	Maintaining/accepting own identity	Knowing and using available resources	Participating in family activities with children
	Maintaining a positive outlook	Experiencing a change in physical surroundings	Doing things that were helpful to others
			Performing tasks that support child's functioning

Canadian Occupational Performance Measurement) have been previously reported (VanLeit & Crowe, 2002). Either an occupational therapist or an occupational therapy student collected the data. Data collectors were trained in the research protocol before the data collection phase and systematic procedural checks were made throughout the study. The women were paid an honorarium for their participation.

Coding Process

The data for this study came from two different sources. First, statements by the women were summarized during group sessions by an occupational therapist and divided into two categories: "concerns/obstacles" and "solutions." Second, at the end of the program, a questionnaire was administered to the mothers that focused on "things learned" and "changes made" as a result of the program. The original intent was to use the PEO model (Law et al., 1996) to further divide the mothers' statements into one of six categories: concerns/obstacles, potential solutions, factors that help, factors that hinder, things learned, and changes made. The data were reviewed to gain a preliminary idea of potential themes. In the second review, each statement was coded as containing person, environment, or occupation factors by two separate evaluators. Some statements contained elements of more than one of these factors, and were coded as such. For example, the statement "stress of trying to do it all" was coded as an obstacle under both person and occupation, because the personal consequence of increased stress was a result of the number of occupations in which the woman engaged.

As the data were coded, it became apparent that "concerns/obstacles" could not be separated from "factors that hinder", and "potential solutions" could not be separated from "factors that help." Therefore, statements were combined to give four final categories: "concerns/obstacles," "solutions," "things learned," and "changes made." Any

discrepancies in coding between the evaluators were resolved by a third evaluator.

Once person, environment, and occupation subthemes were identified within the four categories, similar statements within these subthemes were combined to provide overall themes for each category. For example, the two statements "car problems" and "other things that go wrong: furnace malfunctions, toilet breaks, illness of other family members, etc." were coded as environmental factors in the concerns/obstacles categories. They were grouped under the subtheme "unexpected problems," which then became a part of the overall theme "hectic/unpredictable lifestyle." The overall themes are listed in order of prevalence; therefore, themes that were identified most frequently in each category are presented first.

Results

Concerns/Obstacles

Person. The personal difficulties identified by the mothers in this study included having the burden of responsibility, feeling disorganized and physically drained, dealing with confusion about their self-identity, and coping with feelings of isolation (Table 2).

Many women in this study felt that they were the primary person responsible for the well-being of their child with a disability. This was true for both single mothers and women who lived with a spouse or partner. One mother felt that she had "to be the one to always have the good attitude or be okay in order for the day to go well for everyone." This sense of responsibility was often intrinsic in nature, rather than a result of attempting to meet the expectations of others. Mothers stated that they were uncomfortable leaving their child, expressed doubt about their own capability of meeting the needs of their child, often felt at a loss when dealing with their child's behavior, and experienced guilt that they were not doing everything possible for their child. Some

mothers acknowledged that they struggled with meeting their own expectations, but stated that these expectations were "hard to let. . .go."

The result of these expectations was often frustration at feeling disorganized. Many women felt their house was too messy, their lifestyle was too busy, and they could not schedule time just for themselves. Working mothers also felt disorganized in their job and indicated that their employment took away time that they would rather spend caring for their child. Although some felt that they had little control over their lives, others also attributed time management problems to their own difficulties with prioritizing. One mother stated that she felt "like everything needs to come first."

The mothers in this study often had health issues of their own, some of which might have stemmed from the physical demands of caring for a child with a disability. They spoke of feeling exhausted, burned out, and sometimes unmotivated, depressed, or sad. In one group discussion, a mother stated, "I don't know what stops me from taking care of myself," whereas another stated that she was "burning [herself] out meeting her children's needs."

For several mothers, parenting a child with a disability left them with feelings of confusion about their self-identity, making it difficult to adjust to new roles in adult environments such as school or work. One mother described herself as feeling "so empty." She felt as though she had "lost something," although she did "not know what." Other mothers felt shame over asking for financial and parental help. For instance, one mother stated, "The thought of telling my mom I can't pay the rent would be harder than jumping off a roof! I can't do it, even though I can't afford rent."

A lack of adult support contributed to feelings of isolation in the mothers. The mothers often equated a lack of support with a lack of understanding about what was important to them and their child, leading to a sense that they were fighting their battles alone.

Environment. The participants identified environmental factors more frequently than personal or occupational factors as obstacles to their well-being. These factors included inadequate support services and systems, lack of understanding from others, hectic and unpredictable lifestyles, and concern over their child's safety outside of the home (Table 2).

School systems were most often identified as failing to meet the needs of children and their parents. Issues within schools ranged from concerns about the curriculum to dealing with personnel to bus scheduling. Lack of healthcare services was also frequently singled out, followed by deficiencies in respite and social supports. The mothers were frustrated by a perceived lack of power, and felt that "everyone else was making the choices for the family." They were aware of the need for "constantly playing [the role of] advocate."

The women in this study indicated that one of the main factors contributing to inadequate supports and services was an underlying lack of understanding and sensitivity from others, including partners, extended family, friends, public officials, and the general public. "Even the kindest person" discriminated against children with disabilities, according to one mother. Another mother used the term "exclusion of society" to describe the "world's reaction" to disability.

An additional obstacle to the mothers' well-being was their hectic and unpredictable lifestyle. Unexpected family illness or problems with the house, car, or other belongings had a significant impact on the mothers' well-being because these problems often exacerbated preexisting concern over issues such as finances, attending appointments, and maintaining an organized home.

Mothers also faced challenges associated with their child's well-being in the environment. Depending on the nature of their child's disability, mothers routinely had to consider whether environments that may have been designed for most children, such as playgrounds, posed a safety hazard for their child. This was especially true for mothers of children with assistive devices such as wheelchairs or walkers.

Occupation. Factors related to occupation that hindered the mothers' well-being included achieving occupational balance, developing new skills, and assuming new roles (Table 2).

The mothers felt that they took on too many responsibilities and that they were not achieving their preferred occupational balance between self-care, productivity, and leisure activities. Primarily, they did not have enough time to devote to sleep, their personal leisure activities, or their partner. One mother stated that she was too "burnt out at the end of the day to do anything for [herself]." According to one mother, "even though women are in the workplace, they are still doing the majority of the housework." Working mothers debated lessening their responsibility at work to achieve more occupational balance in their life. Many stated that driving their child to therapy and other appointments was another significant demand on their time. They expressed the need for more quality family time and time to enjoy their children.

Some mothers had to develop new caregiving skills that were outside the realm of typical parenting, such as "mothering a medically fragile child who has a chronic health condition" or feeding their child with a feeding tube.

The women discussed the fact that they had assumed various new roles to ensure their child's needs were met. For many, the most frustrating role to fulfill was that of advocate for their child. The women found their experiences of challenging the school system, talking about their child to others, and applying for adequate financial support to be particularly challenging.

Solutions

Person. The women's own actions most frequently restored in them a sense of well-being. As a result, multiple statements were coded as both person and occupation factors. Person factors had a direct physical, cognitive, or affective benefit to the mothers. In this study, these factors included actions, experiences, or attitudes that helped the women rebalance their lifestyle, maintain and accept their own identity, and keep a positive outlook (Table 2).

The mothers examined how their circumstances were impacting them negatively, and took action to create positive feelings and experiences. One mother's goal was to "make a list of activities that are worthwhile and. . .resign from activities that are not rewarding." Another mother suggested it was important to "talk to [spouse] regarding problems in relating and negative patterns." They felt that changing their behavior was helpful, but that it had to be guilt-free to best contribute to their well-being. Typical behavior changes that the mothers discussed were "letting go," "giving [themselves] permission to have free time and do nothing,"

and "not to do everything." The participants developed their own system of prioritizing activities, which helped them feel more organized and allowed them to focus on immediate tasks. One mother stated, "you do what you need to do for yourself right now," whereas another recommended doing "the 'icky' things first, then you can say you accomplished it." The women in this study realized that, physically, it was important to "take mini-breaks," "pace [themselves]," and "learn to delegate chores to others."

Maintaining and accepting their own identity was another significant factor that contributed to the mothers' well-being. They recognized the importance of "asserting [their] own needs " and "doing activities. . .and things for [themselves]." One mother discussed the importance of "turning incredible caring on yourself along with sensitive caring towards your child." Forming an identity other than that of a mother of a child with a disability was a positive experience for the women in this study. One woman admitted that it was "nice sometimes to be away from [her] child and not be thought of as a family with a 'special needs' child." Several mothers felt they benefited from accepting their own identity and "not comparing [themselves] with others."

Frequently, mothers employed "self-talk" strategies to "counteract negative thought with positive thought." Several mothers relayed the importance of a positive attitude and "finding one thing to make [themselves] happy during the day." For one mother, this was the "blessing of the great love of a child, no matter who they are."

Environment. The mothers identified several environmental factors that contributed to their well-being. Physical and emotional support from others were most often cited as helpful, but the participants also benefited from knowing and using available resources and experiencing a change in their physical surroundings (Table 2).

The women in this study felt that "pulling strength from others" was a positive solution to their challenging lifestyle. The people they relied on included professionals, family, other parents, and their friends. For example, one mother appreciated "having a partner who really cares about my son," whereas others were grateful for "the therapist coming to my home versus taking my child to therapy." They discussed instances when they felt emotionally supported, such as when a teacher and other parents thanked a mother for integrating her child into the classroom and when parents came together "to create a proactive and positive voice." The mothers recognized positive experiences within schools, such as witnessing "children with special needs teaching other children; sharing respect, socialization and acceptance." Some mentioned that they felt Project Bien Estar was a positive addition to their lives, and they came "to the group to be heard."

The mothers identified numerous resources that they found helpful. Some enlisted the help of experienced disability advocates, who assisted their family in educating others about their unique circumstances. The women welcomed the opportunity to talk with professionals who were involved with their child, particularly teachers. One mother stated that "sharing personal situations with the [individual education plan] team to help them understand their family's situation helped to 'humanize' the situation."

The physical environment also played a role in the participants' well-being. Several mothers discussed strategies they used to help keep their house organized, such as "having a special place out of the way for junk to be dumped" and "hiring a housekeeper." Some mothers also changed their children's school environment to one that was more supportive of their child. In these instances, the mother's well-being was linked to their child's well-being.

Occupation. Occupations were most commonly associated by the mothers as positive influences on their well-being. Statements from the participants were coded as "occupational" factors if they expressed how the women spent their time. The women in this study felt they benefited from performing activities that were directed toward looking after themselves, participating in typical family activities with their children, doing things that were helpful to others, and performing tasks that supported their child's functioning (Table 2).

Most women felt that a major part of looking after themselves involved "setting aside time...for [themselves]." During this time, the mothers developed hobbies, spent "quality time" with friends or their partner, exercised, visited places they could not otherwise visit with their children, and relaxed. For one woman, "going to work" provided her time alone. The important thing was to "take care of [themselves] and stop taking care of everyone else." One mother stated that "time away from [her child] with special needs makes me a better parent. Even an hour makes a difference." Several mothers found it helpful to talk to other parents in similar situations, stating that "talking through [their] frustration helps the rest of the week go smoother."

Efficient multi-tasking was an important factor in the mothers' ability to take time for themselves. Several mothers shared their time management strategies, such as "prioritizing," "changing work hours," "cooking double amounts to have extra meals," "doing laundry every morning," "picking up as [they] go along," and "creating a 'to do' list." The women also recognized the importance of "defining [their] own boundaries, and what [they] can and cannot do." Delegating tasks to other family members and hiring personnel, such as a housekeeper and a personal organizer, were identified as alternate methods of dealing with their busy schedules. For the women in this study, looking after themselves also involved increasing or maintaining their independence. There were mothers who continued to develop their own identity by returning to school, working full- or part-time, and learning how to drive.

Several women found that doing fun activities with their children and going on family trips contributed positively to their well-being. One mother designated Sunday as "specifically for [her] kids." This provided further indication that the mothers' happiness was reflected by their children's happiness.

The mothers received great satisfaction from "taking action to help other people" in addition to their child(ren), which they felt "might facilitate [their] own well-being." This included incorporating activities to "improve their [partner's] outlook," altering their parental style, applying for and receiving financial assistance, and "being a firm advocate for [their] child."

Things Learned and Changes Made

In the questionnaire administered at the end of the program, the mothers indicated that participation in Project Bien Estar enabled them to gain insight into the lives of women in similar situations as themselves (Table 3). The opportunity to listen and speak with other parents of children with disabilities served to reassure the women that the struggles they faced were not uncommon. One mother stated that she discovered that she was "not alone—others have situations that are just as difficult," a feeling that was echoed by other participants. They realized that the expectations they set for themselves were often too high. One mother indicated that she learned "not to be so hard on myself," whereas another stated that she "started looking at things thinking I'm not supermom."

Interestingly, although "not comparing myself with others" was identified as a solu-

---

Table 3
Emerging Themes From Group Discussion
Things Learned/Changes Made

- Other families experience similar difficulties
- Mothers set high expectations for themselves
- Importance of taking care of self
- Devote more time to activities for self (e.g., exercise or reading)
- Decrease responsibilities or ask for help from others
- Improve time management

---

tion during group sessions, the perception that they were coping as well as others in similar situations appeared to be helpful for the mothers overall. This was particularly evident in the statement of one mother, "I realize how important it is to take care of myself and also I don't feel so bad when I have a day which is difficult to handle. I know it is normal."

Through participation in the intervention program, the women learned that taking care of themselves was an important coping strategy. "The experience has helped me to focus a little more on my own needs. Also, it has given me some coping strategies, for the most stressful times, and I feel better equipped to handle those times." One woman stated, "I. . .learned or was reminded of the importance of balance. I have to find time for those activities that nourish me in order for me to do this difficult, stressful job." The concept of learning how to achieve balance was reiterated in other statements from participants, as was the feeling of reevaluating their lives and developing a better sense of their own needs. One mother remarked, "I have a more clearly defined sense of how important taking care of the caregiver is. I have stronger ideas about what I need, to keep my balance." Some women increased their participation in exercise, reading, or continued education as a means of devoting more time to their own well-being.

In addition to participating in activities, the mothers identified changes such as giving "permission...[for] children to do things," and changing their attitudes to be "more accepting of things that cannot be done." A few mothers demonstrated this change in attitude by decreasing their responsibilities and making a concerted effort to ask for help from others. Time management was another common area in which the mothers identified a change in behavior. For example, one woman stated that the changes she made included "setting goals for the day and not doing things last minute, having more control."

Discussion

Obstacles

There was a perceived lack of occupational balance in the women's lives. Specifically, they did not have enough time to devote to occupations they considered important, such as sleep, their own leisure pursuits, and quality family time. As a result, the women struggled with burn out, questioned their self-identity, and experienced a loss of self-esteem. Similar to findings from Crowe et al. (1997), the mothers in this study would have liked to spend more time in roles that fulfilled their own needs. They found it challenging to establish priorities in the midst of such busy lives.

Lack of environmental supports were a significant obstacle to the mothers' well-being. In particular, the mothers felt that school and health systems, family, friends, and members of the general public did not understand what was important to them and their child. They were frustrated by the lack of opportunity to influence decisions made about their families within the school and health systems.

Research indicates that mothers of children with disabilities sometimes feel unsupported and socially isolated (Crowe, 1993). The women in this study felt they were the primary person responsible for the well-being of their child, regardless of whether they were raising their child(ren) with a partner. They expressed doubt and disappointment over their ability to meet the unique needs of their children and struggled to meet their own expectations for parenting. The women found it difficult to alter their expectations and accept that these might be consequences from ignoring their own needs.

Solutions

The women discovered that rebalancing their lifestyles was an important strategy to improve their sense of well-being. This process involved examining the negative influences in their lives, establishing priorities for their family, changing their expectations of themselves, and then actively attending to their own needs. By examining the negative influences in their lives, the women became more attuned to factors that made it difficult for them to maintain a positive attitude. Several women felt a positive outlook was a necessary component of personal well-being. Establishing priorities helped to provide the mothers with a systematic way of completing tasks throughout the day and, in turn, made the women feel more organized and effective at managing their time. Often, attending to their own needs was as simple as allowing time to relax and "do nothing" or admitting to a partner that they felt overwhelmed. Developing hobbies, exercising, and spending quality time with friends were positive experiences for the women in this study and helped to build identities that encompassed more than that of mother of a child with a disability.

Additional factors that contributed positively to the mothers' well-being included elements from social, institutional, and physical environments. They identified moments when they felt emotionally supported by partners, families, professionals, and friends who they felt understood what was important to them and subscribed to the same philosophies. Segal (2000) found that sharing responsibility with other adults was an adaptive coping strategy for mothers of children with disabilities. The women in this study appreciated interacting with people who took a special interest in their child or temporarily relieved them of some of their responsibilities. They also benefited from the use of community resources such as advocates and educators, and endorsed decision-making processes within institutional environments that incorporated their input. Physical environments such as organized homes and inclusive school grounds also gave the women less to worry about and more time to focus on their child's enjoyment within these environments.

The Effects of Participation in a Support Group

According to King, Stewart, King, and Law (2000), self-help groups provide "social support, practical information and a sense of shared purpose or advocacy" (p. 226). Feedback from the women in this study indicated that participation in Project Bien Estar was a positive experience that provided such benefits. The women were heartened to find that other people experienced similar problems, frustrations, and joys when parenting a child with a disability. The shared purpose of the women in the Project Bien Estar group was to improve their sense of well-being. Many of the changes they made before the end of the program appeared to reflect a commitment to reestablishing themselves as a priority in their lives. They realized that their own expectations often compromised their well-being by increasing their stress, and perhaps contributed to feelings of inadequacy as mothers. Overall, the changes the mothers made by the end of the program coincided with lessons learned from the program, and were directed toward improving their well-being.

Implications for Occupational Therapy

The results from this study provide detailed insight into the challenges and successes of a group of women raising children with disabilities. The use of the PEO model (Law et al., 1996) to extract themes and analyze discussion provided a framework for understanding the women's experiences from an occupational therapy perspective.

This study provides important information for occupational therapists working in multiple areas of practice. It is evident that occupational balance can be elusive to mothers of children with disabilities, because a great portion of their time is spent in the productive role of parent and less time is spent pursuing leisure activities as an individual. Ironically, the mothers in this study found that this imbalance negatively affected their satisfaction as a parent. Occupational therapists attending to the needs of a parent can play a valuable role in helping individuals increase their self-awareness, adopt efficient time-use strategies, and prioritize effectively so that they can achieve occupational balance.

Occupational therapists working with children should be aware that recommendations for additional activities or exercises to incorporate into a child's life may contribute to unrealistic expectations parents place on themselves. A parent's well-being is a necessary factor to consider when developing a plan to achieve goals for a child.

Another important consideration from this study is that school and health systems are often not meeting the needs of the families for which they are designed to serve. Professionals working within these systems who subscribe to principles of family-centered care are in a position to make important changes through advocacy and education.

Finally, the women in this study found it helpful to listen to and be heard by others in similar circumstances. The role of such a support group in contributing to a mother's well-being should not be underestimated. Occupational therapists can play a valuable role by facilitating the process of transforming shared experience into improved occupational performance.

Acknowledgments

This study could not have been conducted without the willingness of the women to honestly share their life stories. We greatly appreciate their time, knowledge, and support. We would also like to thank the numerous occupational therapy students at the

University of New Mexico who assisted us. Sarah Picchiarini was particularly helpful with several dimensions of this study. This study was partially funded by the American Occupational Therapy Foundation.

References

Allen, D., & Hudd, S. (1987). Are we professionalizing parents?: Weighing the benefits and the pitfalls. *Mental Retardation, 25,* 133-139.

Barnett, W. S., & Boyce, G. C. (1995). Effects of children with Down syndrome on parents' activities. *American Journal on Mental Retardation, 100,* 115-127.

Burden, R. L. (1980). Measuring the effects of stress on the mothers of handicapped infants: Must depression always follow? *Childcare, Health and Development, 6,* 111-125.

Cant, R. (1993). Constraints on social activities of care-givers: A sociological perspective. The *Australian Occupational Therapy Journal, 40,* 113-122.

Crowe, T. K. (1993). Time use of mothers with young children: The impact of a child's disability. *Developmental Medicine and Child Neurology, 35,* 621-630.

Crowe, T. K., Clark, L., & Qualls, C. (1996). The impact of child characteristics on mothers' sleep patterns. *Occupational Therapy Journal of Research, 16,* 3-22.

Crowe, T. K., VanLeit, B., Berghmans, K. K., & Mann, P. (1997). Role perceptions of mothers with young children: The impact of a child's disability. *American Journal of Occupational Therapy, 51,* 651-661.

Dyson, L. L. (1993). Response to the presence of a child with disabilities: Parental stress and family functioning over time. *American Journal of Mental Retardation, 98,* 207-218.

Eisner, C. (1993). *Growing up with a chronic disease: The impact on children and their families.* London: Jessica Kingsley Publishers.

Fearing, V. G., Law, M., & Clark, J. (1997). An occupational performance process model: Fostering client and therapist alliances. *Canadian Journal of Occupational Therapy, 64,* 7-15.

Green, S. E. (2003). "What do you mean 'what's wrong with her?'": Stigma and the lives of families of children with disabilities. *Social Science and Medicine, 57,* 1361-1374.

Helitzer, D. L., Cunningham-Sabo, L. D., VanLeit, B., & Crowe, T. K. (2002). Perceived changes in self-image and coping strategies of mothers of children with disabilities. *OTJR: Occupation, Participation and Health, 22,* 25-33.

Joosten, J. (1979). Accounting for changes in family life of families with spine bifida children. *Z Kinderchir, 28,* 412-417.

King, G., Stewart, D., King, S., & Law, M. (2000). Organizational characteristics and issues affecting the longevity of self-help groups for parents of children with special needs. *Qualitative Health Research, 10,* 225-241.

Larson, E. A. (2000). The orchestration of occupation: The dance of mothers. *American Journal of Occupational Therapy, 54,* 269-280.

Law, M., Cooper, B., Strong, S., Stewart, D., Rigby, P., & Letts, L. (1996). The Person–Environment–Occupation model: A transactive approach to occupational performance. *Canadian Journal of Occupational Therapy, 63,* 9-23.

Lawlor, M. C., & Mattingly, C. F. (1998). The complexities embedded in family-centered care. *American Journal of Occupational Therapy, 52,* 259-267.

Nelson, A. M. (2002). A metasynthesis: Mothering other-than-normal children. *Qualitative Health Research, 12,* 515-530.

Segal, R. (2000). Adaptive strategies of mothers with children with attention deficit hyperactivity disorder: Enfolding and unfolding occupations. *American Journal of Occupational Therapy, 54,* 300-306.

Strong, S., Rigby, P., Stewart, D., Law, M., Letts, L., & Cooper, B. (1999). Application of the Person–Environment–Occupation model: A practical tool. *Canadian Journal of Occupational Therapy, 66,* 122-133.

Thompson, R. J., Jr., Gil, K. M., Gustafson, K. E., George, L. K., Keith, B. R., Spock, A., et al. (1994). Stability and change in the psychological adjustment of mothers of children and adolescents with cystic fibrosis and sickle cell disease. *Journal of Pediatric Psychology, 19,* 171-188.

Traustadottir, R. (1993). Mothers who care: Gender, disability and family life. In M. Nagler (Ed.), *Perspectives on disability* (pp. 173-184). Palo Alto, CA: Health Markets Research.

VanLeit, B., & Crowe, T. (2000). Promoting well-being in mothers of children with disabilities. *OT Practice, 5*(13), 26-31.

VanLeit, B., & Crowe, T. (2002). Outcomes of an occupational therapy program for mothers of children with disabilities: Impact on satisfaction with time use and occupational performance. *American Journal of Occupational Therapy, 56,* 402-410.

Wallander, J. L. (1993). Current research on pediatric chronic illness. *Journal of Pediatric Psychology, 18,* 7-10.

Wallander, J. L., & Varni, J. W. (1998). Effects of chronic physical disorders on child and family adjustment. *Journal of Child Psychology and Psychiatry and Allied Disciplines, 39*(1), 29-46.

Caregivers' Self-Initiated Support Toward Their Partners With Dementia When Performing an Everyday Occupation Together at Home

Sofia Vikström, Lena Borell, Anna Stigsdotter-Neely, Staffan Josephsson

Key words: caregiving, dementia, home care

Abstract: The aim of this study was to identify the support caregivers provide by their own initiative when performing an everyday occupation together with their partner who has dementia. This is to identify what type of self-initiated caregiver support enhances or limits the performance of the person with dementia. Thirty cohabitating couples participated. One of the spouses in each couple was the primary caregiver for a partner with mild to moderate dementia. Observational data were collected in the participants' homes, where each couple was asked to prepare afternoon tea together. The performances were documented by video and supplementary field notes. Data were analyzed using a qualitative comparative approach. The results of the analyses identified two major themes related to support the caregivers provided: provision of a supportive working climate and provision of practical support. A third theme was related to negative aspects of caregiver support. The results of this study have implications for how occupational therapists and caregivers in dementia care can support and guide primary caregivers in their homes.

Sofia Vikström, OT (Reg.), Lena Borell, PhD, OT (Reg.), and Staffan Josephsson, PhD, OT (Reg.), are from The Department of Neurotec, Division of Occupational Therapy, Karolinska Institutet, Stockholm, Sweden. Anna Stigsdotter-Neely, PhD, is from the Department of Psychology, Umeå University, Umeå, Sweden. Address correspondence to Sofia Vikström at sofia.vikstrom@neurotec.ki.se.

Alzheimer's disease and other dementia diseases are known to have a limiting effect on the individual's ability to independently perform everyday occupations (American Psychiatric Association, 1994). The progressive deterioration in cognitive, social, and occupational skills gradually increases the dependency individuals with dementia develop toward others (Agüero Torres, Fratiglioni, Guo, Viitanen, von Strauss, & Winblad, 1998). The traditional definition of rehabilitation, to regain lost abilities, is not applicable for individuals with a dementia disease (Josephsson, Bäckman, Borell, Nygård, & Bernspång, 1994). Rather, finding solutions to solve and prevent problems in everyday life that are caused by the disease should be the focus of therapy (Borell, 1992; Fisher, 1998).

In line with such a suggestion, research in occupational therapy has stressed the importance of being actively engaged in daily occupations as long as possible to sustain present abilities and a sense of well-being in individuals with dementia (Bond & Corner, 2001; Bonner & O'Brien Cousins, 1996; Borell, 1992; Josephsson et al., 1994). It has been shown that individuals with dementia, who often tend to reduce their official and private occupational and social engagements, still strive to continue engaging in daily occupations (Öhman, Nygård & Borell, 2001).

In parts of the western world (i.e., the United States and Sweden), individuals with dementia continue to live in their homes for several years after their dementia has been diagnosed (Statistics Sweden, 1997). As a consequence, the emphasis of the care is often on home care (Agüero Torres, Fratiglioni, & Winblad, 1998; Schulz, 2000). Moreover, the most important provider of care at home is the spouse (Spencer, 2001). Despite the fact that most caregivers show a will and desire to care for their partners with dementia at home (Max, 1996), especially when the caregivers perceive themselves as being in good health, caregiving comes at a cost (Gold, Cohen, Shulman, Zucchero, Andres, & Etezadi, 1995). Research has shown that providing care for a relative with any kind of progressive dementia disease has profound implications for the caregivers' personal daily lives. Caregiving has been linked to increased levels of depression and anxiety, a prominent sense of burden, risk of social isolation, compromised immune function, and increased mortality (Almberg, Grafström, & Winblad, 1997; Grafström, Fratiglioni, Sandman, & Winblad, 1992; Ory, Hoffman, Yee, Tennstedt, & Schulz, 1999; Schulz & Beach, 1999).

As a consequence, research on caregivers' experiences of supporting their spouses in everyday life activities has called for the development of guidelines of practical support in caring for individuals with dementia in the home environment so that both partners can live together more satisfactorily and institutionalization can be avoided (Björkhem, Olsson, Hallberg, & Norberg, 1992; Melzer et al., 1996). In previous caregiving intervention studies, two major themes of supportive strategies can be identified. One approach has focused on alleviating the stressors for caring for an individual with dementia, usually by offering psychosocial support such as counseling and education for the caregiver. The second approach has focused on adjustments of the physical environment or the use of structured everyday occupational patterns (Gitlin et al., 2003; Schulz, 2000). Most of these studies have produced modest benefits for the caregiver and for the person with dementia in terms of well-being, mood, and caregiving burden (Schulz et al., 2002).

In light of such modest successes, questions have been raised concerning how healthcare professionals can best provide supportive strategies that can lead to increased well-being for both the caregiver and the person with dementia and offer advice on what support strategies work best for certain problems (Corcoran & Gitlin, 2001; Gitlin, Corcoran, Winter, Boyce, & Marcus, 1999; Schulz, 2000; Teri, 1999). There is thus a need to identify support behaviors that work for caregivers in everyday situations at home.

In line with Yerxa's (1998) suggestion that the task of the occupational therapist is

Article Reprint Information: Reprinted with permission from Vikström, S., Borell, L., Stigsdotter-Neely, A., & Josephsson, S. (2005). Caregivers' self-initiated support toward their partners with dementia when performing an everyday occupation together at home. *Occupational Therapy Journal of Research: Occupation, Participation and Health, 25*(34), 149-159.

Table 1
Participant Characteristics

Participants	Gender	Age (Y)	Education	MMSE Score[a]
Caregiver group	14 male, 16 female	58 to 84 (median = 74)	4 elementary, 8 high school, 10 college, 8 university	Range = 23 to 30, median = 28
Dementia group	16 male, 14 female	68 to 85 (median = 78)	5 elementary, 7 high school, 12 college, 6 university	Range = 16 to 24, median = 21

MMSE = Mini-Mental State Examination (Folstein et al., 1975).
[a]Maximum score = 30; higher score indicates better performance.

to learn how to assess individuals' current ability to provide support to clients based on the "just right challenge," the occupational therapist may need to help caregivers to identify and adjust the support needed so it applies to both the caregiver and the person with dementia. To accomplish this, we suggest that occupational therapists may benefit from knowledge about what support strategies caregivers naturally use, and thereafter guide and encourage caregivers to further develop these strategies.

There are several conceivable benefits to identifying support strategies already within the behavior repertoire of the couple. For example, these strategies may be more optimal to the cognitive functions of both the caregiver and the care-recipient, as well as more familiar to both partners as they relate to their common history. This may lead to a more optimal strategy utilization, foster compliance, and optimize transfer over time. In a recent study by Derwinger, Stigs-dotter-Neely, and Bäckman (in press) on self-generated strategy training in healthy older adults, it was shown that generating one's own strategies had benefits over strategies provided by the experimenter, especially for measures of long-term maintenance. These results lend support to our focus in this study.

Some empirical research on caregiver support does exist. There is research on general patterns of caregiving (Jansson, Nordberg, & Grafström, 2001) and on types of verbal support caregivers use when solving a cognitive task in collaboration with their spouse (Cavanaugh et al., 1989). There has also been research on healthy older adults on collaboration in everyday tasks, comparing performance between spouses and between strangers of opposite gender (Margrett & Marsiske, 2002), and on collaboration in story recall between married and unacquainted dyads (Gould, Osborn, Krein, & Martenson, 2002). These studies show that having insight into the spouse's thoughts and manners is beneficial when providing support in solving a task together. In addition, these studies again demonstrate

the potential benefits of focusing on self-initiated support strategies in caregivers and individuals with dementia.

As seen by the literature review above, the term support is used differently in different studies. In this study, we define support as verbal and physical helping acts that caregivers use in the interactions with their partner who has dementia that have an impact on the performance of the person with dementia in the fulfillment of the task.

A review of the literature has identified a need for research on self-initiated caregiver support strategies used in everyday occupations in the home environment. The aim of the current study was to identify self-initiated support strategies that caregivers provide when performing an everyday occupation together with their partner with dementia, and to identify negative aspects of caregiver support.

Methods

Selection of Participants

The sample consisted of 30 cohabitating couples, in which one of the spouses was the primary caregiver for a partner diagnosed as having mild to moderate dementia (Table 1). The Mini-Mental State Examination (MMSE) (Folstein, Folstein, & McHugh, 1975) was performed within 1 week prior to the data collection. The cut-off point for suspicion of a dementia diagnosis is 23 of 30 points. Subsequently, individuals with an MMSE score below 23 can be suspected of having cognitive impairment in one or several of the cognitive dimensions investigated.

The participating couples were recruited from two large outpatient memory investigation units in the Stockholm area. The individuals with dementia had been examined and diagnosed as having mild to moderate Alzheimer's disease or vascular dementia according to the criteria established by the *Diagnostic and Statistical Manual of Mental Disorders*, 4th ed. (American Psychiatric Association, 1994) within the 8 months prior to the study. All individuals had a cohabi-

tating significant other who was considered to be the primary caregiver. Additionally, individuals were required to have evidence in their records of problems in remembering and performing everyday occupations. Individuals with an MMSE score of less than 16 were excluded. Written or verbal medical approvals were received from the physicians responsible for the individuals with dementia regarding their ability to participate in the study.

All potential participants were then sent a letter with information about the study, including a request for their participation. The first 30 to accept the invitation to participate when contacted on the telephone were selected. Seventeen refused participation, citing reasons such as too little time or family-related reasons. All participating couples had a history of a long marriage or partnership. It should be noted that in this article we have chosen to call all participants "spouses" regardless of whether they were married.

During the first visit to each of the 30 participating couples' homes, verbal information on the aim and nature of the study was provided, and participants also gave their written consent to the planned video documentation of their performances in a common everyday activity. Their right to withdraw from the study at any time without any further notice and explanation was emphasized, as was the confidential use of documented data.

Data Collection

The data collection incorporated observational data from video recordings collected in the participants' homes. Each couple was informed about the desired details to be included in the everyday occupation that they were asked to perform together. The occupation agreed on was preparation of afternoon tea (including tea or coffee and cake), because such an occupation is highly prevalent in the culture of Swedish socializing. After a discussion concerning what should be included in the activity and how the couple usually prepared it, the ac-

Table 2
The Structure of Caregivers' Support Toward Their Partners in Everyday Occupations

Supportive working climate

Creates comfort

- Is attentive to the partner
- Offers time to think/remember
- Allows partner to take command
- Encourages the partner

Takes responsibility for the activity

- Reassures partner involvement
- Asks check-up questions
- Keeps track of the agreement

Supportive practical involvement

Adapts the physical space and objects

- Provides physical space
- Removes irrelevant objects
- Places objects relevant to the activity forward

Alters the activity to make it easier

- Prepares the activity
- Adjusts the activity

Supports the performance

- Provides guidance
- Provides reminders and clues
- Provides problem solutions

Negative aspects in the caregiver support

Provides insufficient support

- Lacks attentiveness
- Does not stay in the area
- Does not take responsibility for the task

Provides inappropriate support

- Provides unclear support
- Provides unproportional support

Failure to respond to support need

- Questions the partner's behavior
- Takes over

tivity was altered accordingly. For example, some couples made coffee by boiling it on the stove and some boiled water and added instant coffee powder or tea bags, but most used a coffee brewer. The agreement that had been made on what to include in the activity was thereafter verbalized, such as an instruction initiating the activity. The couples were then asked to begin the activity and to work naturally together as would please them best.

All verbal and practical performance of the couples in the activity was documented on videotapes using a camera fixed on a tripod in one corner of the kitchen. Field notes on aspects that might affect the performance of the activity were written by the first author, who conducted the data collection from all couples immediately following the home visits (Bogdan & Biklen, 1998). For example, field notes would include information on perceptions of the social or physical environment and background data on aspects of the couples' performances that could be important to accurately remember during analyses. The first author, who observed and filmed the couples' performances, did not take part in the activity and did not speak or interfere unless her actions or responses were sought. The time the participants used to perform the activity ranged from 10 to 25 minutes.

For each of the 30 couples, the entire dialogue and each spouse's acts were transcribed from the videotapes by the first author. To verify their accuracy, the detailed transcribed texts from the dialogues, along with the observations of the couples' interaction while performing the activity (e.g., pointing) and the recorded field notes were compared to the videotapes and adjusted when necessary by the first and fourth author. Such adjustments could concern explanations to certain remarks the spouses made to each other in the dialogues. For example, one person with dementia who wanted to set the table in the living room where they normally received guests had to be told to remain in the kitchen because the camera could not be moved from that setting.

Data Analysis

The analysis of the transcribed material was performed according to a constant comparative approach as described by Bogdan and Biklen (1998), starting with all texts being read through repeatedly to obtain a profound understanding of the contents. Then the first author searched for supports provided by caregivers that concerned the activity or were directed toward the person with dementia. Supports were coded line by line and read through repeatedly. In the coding process, each sign of verbal or nonverbal contact between the two spouses in the text was coded with a conceptual code. To stay close to the data, these codes were made in everyday language, as close as possible to the words or the acts used by the couple. The first and fourth authors then compared all transcript codes and systematically sorted them into emerging themes. The themes and the concept of the codes were again compared to the data on the

videotapes to see whether data supported the findings. In this way, all codes were compared in repeated processes. The aim of this procedure was to find overall themes and to discover how these themes could be related to one another.

To ensure credibility and truthfulness of the data, the codes and themes were compared yet again to the original data through a peer examination involving the first, second, and fourth authors and colleagues in the research group. Consensus was reached between the authors concerning codes and themes and the systematic relations between the found concepts.

Results

The results of the analyses showed that the caregivers seemed to put effort into two major aspects of their performance of the activity—creating a supportive working climate and using practical support when performing an everyday occupation together with their spouse. Analyses also revealed aspects of support that had a negative influence on the performance of the person with dementia (Table 2).

A Supportive Working Climate

The results show that the caregivers often contributed to a supportive working climate in two ways—by creating comfort and by taking responsibility for the task.

Creating Comfort in the Activity Situation. When creating comfort, the caregivers used four techniques: being attentive, offering time, being encouraging, and being permissive.

The analyses revealed signs of the caregivers' attentiveness toward the problems the person with dementia might come across. Most caregivers repeatedly turned toward and kept an eye on how the partner with dementia managed during the coffee- or tea-making activity. Sometimes the attentiveness was revealed in caregivers' comments on the performance of the partner and sometimes they provided the spouses with a chance to try to perform before offering their assistance. One common comment was, "I am over here if you need me." This laid-back attitude in combination with their readiness to offer assistance seemed to give the person with dementia time to think and act without pressure. For some caregivers, it was evident that offering time was a deliberate comforting act. This could be exemplified by the following quotes: "Take your time" or "Do not hesitate to grab me if you need me." Thus, the person with dementia had time to search in his or her mind for the steps in the activity that were included in the coffee- or tea-making agreement, and assistance could be provided if needed. This offering of time and assistance seemed to have a positive influence on how the person remembered what to do next.

Caregivers also used encouragement to contribute to the creation of a comfortable climate. One encouraging act was confirmation of the correctness in the partner's actions. Caregivers commonly would say, "That's the way to do it" or "Looks good that!" In the dialogues during the activity, caregivers often emphasized different skilful acts that the person with dementia used to possess or still possessed (e.g., "Julia is famous for her fantastic cakes!"). Furthermore, some caregivers chose to decrease their partners' shortcomings by demeaning themselves. One husband jokingly revealed that he had his own shortcomings: "I have never been a great brewer of coffee, but we will have to put up with whatever taste my attempt results in." A third comforting act commonly used was explanations from caregivers when the partner with dementia failed during the performance of the activity. One caregiver turned to the camera and stated, "We usually do this differently."

It also appeared to be comforting when most caregivers corrected their partners' mistakes tenderly. For example, one caregiver said to his wife, "Why don't we pour the milk into this porcelain jug now that we have guests visiting us? It's not a big deal, and our guests surely don't mind the tetra [carton] you brought out, but it is nice to use this porcelain jug once in a while, don't you agree?" Some caregivers would allow their partners to take command in the activity. One husband turned to his wife and asked, "Any ideas on how you want us to do this?" This permissive attitude also occurred when the performance of the activity did not live up to the agreement or to the standards the caregivers had in mind. A common caregiver comment was "We agreed on something else, but that doesn't matter." Sometimes the caregivers would make a discreet comment on the incorrectness of their partners' performance, but still accept the way their partners solved the problems even though it was apparent that the task, in their eyes, might have been better solved in another manner. There were also several occasions where the caregivers, discreetly and without remarks, corrected their partners' mistake to make the performance match what was agreed on earlier.

Taking Responsibility for the Activity. In this study, caregivers showed three different ways to take responsibility for performing the activity. These were reassuring partners'

involvement, asking check-up questions, and keeping track of the agreement.

Some caregivers' acts were characterized by their tendency to reassure their partners' involvement through verbalizing what they were about to do (e.g., "If I go and start with the coffee, will you take care of the cookies?"). Analyses also identified how caregivers would remind their partners of the activity agreed to by verbalizing it repeatedly. For example, if the person with dementia got stuck, the caregiver might say, "We agreed with the occupational therapist to do this and this. That is why I started with this and you can do that."

A common support when the person with dementia had problems performing was that caregivers asked check-up questions concerning the task to be solved. One type of check-up question was whether the partner with dementia could recall the agreement of the activity (e.g., "Do you remember what we just agreed on preparing?"). Another type of check-up question was used when the person with dementia stopped acting in the middle of performing an activity. The caregiver would then commonly ask what he or she was about to do when the memory failed. Still, the most common questions from caregivers to their spouses were check-up questions entailing offerings of assistance (e.g., "Do you want me to help you in any way?"). These questions almost always resulted in a dialogue where the person with dementia received the necessary assistance to proceed with the activity.

The analyses also showed that the caregivers took responsibility in completing the activity. For example, one caregiver shared his thoughts aloud: "Do we have the milk? Yes. And the sugar is set out. Good."

Supportive Practical Involvement

The analysis showed that, in addition to providing a supportive working climate, caregivers also supported their partners through the following practical involvements: adaptations of the physical space and objects, alterations of the activity to make it easier, and supports for the performance.

Adapting the Physical Space and Objects. The caregiver showed signs of adapting the physical space and objects in the performance area through providing space, removing irrelevant objects, and placing objects relevant to the activity forward.

Similar to the offering of time and assistance mentioned earlier, the analyses also showed how the caregivers often provided extra physical space for their partners by

stepping aside when they were about to perform a part of the activity. This was assumed to be out of consideration for the person with dementia, giving him or her space and room to think and act undisturbed. This assumption was also confirmed in their dialogues on those occasions. Common statements were, "Am I standing in your way now?" or "I'll leave you to start with your chores and go over here and start with mine." It seemed beneficial to the person with dementia when the caregivers placed themselves at a near distance, but still close at hand, to provide support when needed.

Another caregiver support related to the physical space was removing irrelevant objects from the activity arena. Sometimes the argument was that the objects stood in the way of the spouses' actions, but it was also common that objects were removed because they could appear to be irrelevant or perhaps disturbing to the activity performance. One example was a caregiver who removed medicine jars and a transistor radio from the kitchen table (to be set) and said, "We don't need these now" or " Let's put this away too for the moment."

One contrasting strategy was to alter the physical environment by placing forward objects relevant to the activity. Examples of these supports were fetching and placing forward the cutting board and knife so that the spouse could start cutting the bread if he or she would feel like it, or placing a porcelain milk jug from a cupboard and a milk carton from the refrigerator beside each other on the workbench. This presentation of objects entailed in the activity seemed helpful for the individuals with dementia, who almost always used the items placed forward, and seemed to be beneficial for the completion of the activity.

Altering the Activity to Make It Easier. Two kinds of alterations of the activity that caregivers provided seemed to have the purpose of making the tasks easier—preparing and adjusting the task. The first support used was altering the activity by preparing the first part of a task for the person with dementia. Examples of these acts were loading the coffee brewer with water or coffee or cutting the bread so that the spouse then could put the slices on a plate and place it on the table.

The other support used by caregivers was adjusting the tasks, such as fetching the heavy or not-easy-to-reach porcelain from the cupboards, tearing open the milk cartons, or cutting through tough plastic wrapping around the cookies that otherwise would be hard to open). The adjustments also concerned parts of the activity that could be difficult to understand or remember. For example, some individuals with dementia needed help to slide open the holder for the filter bag on the coffee brewer, and another person received support to understand the markings for the amount of water on the brewer. Most commonly, caregivers had to help switch on the electrical timer connected to the brewer. Most of these adjustments appeared to be necessary help for the person with dementia to complete the task properly.

Supporting the Performance. The caregivers showed signs of supporting their spouses in their performance by providing guidance, reminders and clues, and solutions to problems. The most common support by caregivers was provision of verbal guidance. The situations where the directives had a supporting impact on the partners' performance were when they were formulated as short instructions or reminders (e.g., "You need to fill the water up before you put the brewer on" or " Don't forget to bring teaspoons out").

However, caregivers sometimes dealt with the spouses' difficulties by providing them with clues, often as answers to an earlier question posed by the person with dementia. For example, if the person with dementia asked, "What do I do next?", the caregiver might say, "We have something to slice up, too. Something to chew on along with the coffee...."

Further analyses of the data showed that when the partners with dementia faced a situation where a choice had to be made (e.g., to use paper or woven napkins), most caregivers supported their partners by providing solutions on what to choose. Sometimes, the caregivers also prevented mistakes by suggesting an easier way of solving a problem. For example, one caregiver helped her husband to choose by saying, "Why don't you start with that one?" Another caregiver demonstrated how to fill up the coffee brewer and said, "I usually do it like this." Most partners with dementia did not seem offended by this form of support, but rather used the support provided and acted according to it.

Negative Aspects in the Caregiver Support

Some of the ways caregivers supported the performance of the person with dementia did not appear to be beneficial. This negative support created confusion in the individuals with dementia because it was provided either delayed, too late, or not at all.

Providing Insufficient Support. The analyses showed that failure in the performance of the person with dementia often was related to insufficient support from the caregiver. Sometimes caregivers lacked attentiveness toward their spouses, and other times they were not present and did not take responsibility for the task.

A common example of caregivers' lack of attentiveness toward their partners' needs was when the person with dementia showed signs of hesitation, insecurity, or frustration toward performing a task. These often apparent signs were sometimes insufficiently acknowledged by the caregiver.

In some couples, one spouse or both the spouse with dementia and the husband or wife left the room for some time. Examples of reasons for their absence were to collect a special piece of porcelain or to find paper napkins. One of the caregivers went away to smoke his pipe for a while, leaving his wife apparently bewildered and on her own. She kept searching in the different cupboards, presumably having difficulties finding what was needed and verbalized difficulties in deciding what porcelain to use. This seemed to be a case of the caregiver placing himself too much out of reach, so that the support need of the person with dementia was not met.

Similarly, some caregivers did not always take charge of steering the activity when the partner with dementia deviated from the prearranged "agreement" for performing other (supplementary) activities, which led them to make mistakes.

Providing Inappropriate Support. The data analyses also identified issues of existing caregiver support that led to failure in supporting the performance of the individuals with dementia. These included provision of unclear support and disproportional provision of support.

Unclear support could involve statements the individual with dementia found confusing or instructions that were given too quickly for the person with dementia to follow. The following example of unclear support concerned placing plastic placemats on the coffee table. The caregiver said, "Why do you do it like that? I told you to use the plastic things, whatever they are called...Those with the flowers on...The ones we always have, you know! Surely you know what I'm talking about!?"

Support that was delivered too quickly was also perceived to lead to failure. One of the caregivers watched her husband's every move without doing anything practical in the activity herself. As soon as her husband finished with one activity, she instructed him

to do something else. Such acts seemed to deprive him of the time to think for himself and have a fair chance to perform the specific task without instruction. This approach was also time-consuming because the specific caregiver's performance in the activity was limited to keeping her husband active.

Disproportional support involved caregivers' providing too little or too much support. One caregiver suggested, "OK, if I make the coffee you can start with the rest." This is an example of too little or incomplete support that seemed to create confusion in the individuals with dementia, who often had to ask the caregiver for additional support so they could complete the activity.

Too much support tended to result in the person with dementia forgetting the initial instruction and therefore failing to initiate the activity. An example of this was a caregiver who said to his wife, "So, if I brew the coffee, you could cut the bread and place it in this basket. Then we need to get 3 sets of the china with the flowers, the silver spoons, the plate with golden stripes for the cookies. After that we will see who places out the sugar, milk and napkins." His wife responded by asking, "What was that you said again?" The complexity of this kind of suggestion seemed to make the activity difficult to fulfill for most of the participants with dementia.

Failing to Respond to Support Need. During the performance of the activity, several of the caregivers repeatedly showed signs of confusion and sometimes resignation toward some of the questions asked by the person with dementia. This became evident in the responses the caregivers gave to the questions their partners posed, such as "You should not need to ask that" or "You know the answer to that question if you just think." Other caregivers reacted to questions from partners with dementia with reproach (e.g., "Why do you ask that? Do you not remember?"). Some caregivers showed puzzlement over the unpredictability of the partner with dementia's memory capacities (e.g., "You don't remember that? But we discussed it, and agreed on it just a moment ago.").

The analyses also showed several expressions of acts that seemed dominant. The caregiver could make decisions without consulting the person with dementia or interfere with and forestall the person with dementia's own planned doing. Finally, there were some occasions where the caregiver chose to take over and do tasks for the person with dementia, instead of supporting the partner with dementia in his or her own doing.

Discussion

The aim of the current study was to identify support that caregivers to individuals with dementia provided on their own initiative when performing an everyday occupation together. The result of this study contributes to the discussion on how support can be delivered to enhance occupational performance for individuals with a dementia disease.

The study showed that caregivers to individuals with dementia used a wide range of supports when working together with their partners. Most of these supports were shown to be beneficial to the occupational performance of the person with dementia. The findings are in line with studies on collaboration that point out the positive impact of having deep knowledge about the person you assist (Gould et al., 2002) and the consequences the dementia disease has on occupational performance (Cavanaugh et al., 1989; Jansson et al., 2001).

In this study, caregivers' knowledge about their spouses was shown through identification of comforting and supportive acts used to provide encouragement. Through emphasizing the skillful behaviors of the partner, and sometimes also through jokingly revealing his or her own shortcomings, the caregiver reduced the impact of the mistakes made by the partner in the coffee-making situation. This could be interpreted as natural skills in "empowering" the person with dementia, as described by Martin and Younger (2000). This finding may have implications on how future interventions are designed to support and enhance collaboration.

Further, it seemed beneficial for the person with dementia (and indirectly toward the fulfillment of the task) that the caregiver took on the responsibility for performing the activity. Apart from taking responsibility based on the obvious necessity to support due to the impact of the dementia disease, there could also be caregiver implications for such actions, as discussed by Weiss (1973). He argued that caregiving could be seen as a basic human need or an opportunity for nurturance (i.e., the impact of feeling responsibility toward another person's well-being) (Weiss, 1973). This important psychosocial aspect of caring corresponds well with findings by Max (1996) and Gold et al. (1995), who also state that caregiving might not necessarily be perceived by caregivers as an altogether burdensome experience.

Based on the findings in this study, there could be discussion about whether it is an advantage or a disadvantage for the partici-

pants to take on a collaborative approach when performing everyday activities. One disadvantage that has been identified in the analyses in this study is the time-consuming need for most caregivers to go back and check that the agreed tasks in the activity were fulfilled. This corresponds well with a study on collaboration effects on couples' mutual performances described by Andersson and Rönnberg (1995). The study showed that, even though the quality of the task performed benefited from collaboration, joint performance almost always had a negative effect on time consumption. Perhaps the extra effort the caregivers put into the activity so that the task was completed might partly explain findings of burden and stress that previous caregiver research has shown (Grafström et al., 1992; Ory et al., 1999). The extra time the performance of the activity takes when working together with a person with dementia might need to be emphasized to caregivers to motivate them to continue working together in everyday occupations.

Another implication of the findings that needs to be highlighted is that although the 30 participants with dementia had a mild to moderate stage of the disease, they seemed to need different amounts and types of support to be successful in their occupational performance. They also responded to the same kind of support differently. This might provide us with an understanding of why the difference in performance in cognitive assessments (e.g., MMSE) is not necessarily mirrored in occupational performance in a familiar environment (Kielhofner, 2002; Nygård, Amberla, Bernspång, Almkvist, & Winblad, 1998). For example, in this study, the person with the lowest MMSE score of the participants with dementia was not the one having the greatest need for support in performance of the activity. These variations between individuals might also underscore the importance of avoiding generally tailored interventions and treatment founded on the idea of increasing cognitive status when supporting occupational performance for individuals with dementia (Bond & Corner, 2001; Woods, 1999). As a consequence, interventions with the aim of having a supportive effect on the occupational performance of individuals with dementia would probably benefit from being individually tailored to each person and his or her specific environment.

The analysis further showed that it was difficult for the caregivers to provide an adequate amount of support to their partners. Our findings demonstrated that both provision of insufficient support and provision of

too much support at a time had a negative impact on the occupational performance of individuals with dementia. These findings underscore one of the great difficulties caregivers to individuals with dementia are facing, namely that the symptoms of the disease increase and change over time. Support given must therefore be flexible and adjusted to the partner's performance needs of the moment. Parallels could be drawn to the idea of providing "the just-right challenge" for the individuals who are in need of support (Yerxa, 1998). Thus, if the ambition is to provide support that corresponds with the just right challenge, the support must be easily revised to suit the person with dementia's current status.

This approach could possibly be achieved by introducing caregivers to a way of reasoning through the process of providing support in increasingly specified detail, starting with a small amount of support and increasingly providing more and more specific information until the person with dementia remembers what to do. Introducing such a process might be beneficial for both partners through reduced frustration.

Furthermore, findings showed that individuals with dementia reacted with signs of frustration when caregivers failed to provide sufficient or relevant support. In a study by Hepburn, Tornatore, Center, and Ostwald (2001), spouses of individuals with dementia were taught to view themselves as caregivers with an increased emotional distance toward their partners. Caregivers were taught that provision of help might not necessarily lower the self-esteem of the person with dementia. Rather, it might be beneficial to provide help to lower their frustrations. Shifts between the close role of being a spouse and the more emotionally distanced role as a caregiver might partly explain the ambiguous way the caregivers in this study supported their partners, providing both well adjusted support and support that resulted in failure. Results from that study, as well as results from this research, indicate a necessity for professionals to prepare caregivers for and guide them through the challenge of being a caregiver.

The identified types of support that led to occupational performance failure for the person with dementia underscore the need for professionals to also guide the individual caregivers in recognizing their own ways of supporting. When the different individual types of support have been identified, professionals could assist caregivers in choosing one or several of the "positive" supports found, rather than using the ones that lead to failure. Recognizing positive supports and supporting the caregiver in using them could, in conjunction with the implementation of the just-right challenge notion, be an important foundation for an individualized intervention strategy (Martin & Younger, 2000; Tannous, Lehmann-Monck, Magoffin, Jackson, & Llewellyn, 1999).

One methodological issue worth considering concerns the fact that the data were collected using a participant observation method including video-recordings. Although the participants were performing a familiar activity in their own home setting, an alteration of their performance due to the presence of the first author and the video camera cannot be excluded. However, actions were taken to make the participants relax and feel comfortable. For example, the first author spent time with the couples, drinking coffee, discussing everyday topics, and answering questions about the aim and implications of the data collection. The initial tensions might therefore only to a minor extent have had a negative impact on the couple's performance toward one another in the coffee-making activity. Still, validity concerning the genuineness of the individuals' performances (Patton, 1987) could be discussed.

However, pursuing an intervention, descriptive observational data would preferably be complemented with interview data from the participants on how they reason about and value their own different supportive acts, and what their preferences of focus in the intervention would be. Such data have been collected in conjunction to the observation and field note data reported in this study, but are reported elsewhere (Vikström, Josephsson, & Nygård, 2003).

Finally, findings from this study show that there are wide ranges of support that caregivers provide by their own initiative. Future studies might benefit from taking into account the findings from this study when planning and evaluating interventions aiming to support caregivers in their collaboration with individuals diagnosed as having dementia.

Acknowledgments

The research reported in this study was supported by grants from the Swedish Council for Social Research to Anna Stigsdotter-Neely and Staffan Josephsson, as well as grants from The Solstickan Foundation, the Gun and Bertil Stohnes Foundation, and The Swedish Association of Occupational Therapists to Sofia Vikström. We thank the families for their time and Marie Persson for competent assistance with the data.

References

Agüero Torres, H., Fratiglioni, L., Guo, Z., Viitanen, M., von Strauss, E., & Winblad, B. (1998). Dementia is the major cause of functional dependence in the elderly: 3-year follow-up data from a population-based study. *American Journal of Public Health, 88,* 1452-1456.

Agüero Torres, H., Fratiglioni, L., & Winblad, B. (1998). Natural history of Alzheimer's disease and other dementias: Review of the literature in light of the findings from the Kungsholmen Project. *International Journal of Geriatric Psychiatry, 13,* 755-766.

Almberg, B., Grafström, M., & Winblad, B. (1997). Major strain and coping strategies as reported by family members who care for aged demented relatives. *Journal of Advanced Nursing, 26,* 683-691.

American Psychiatric Association. (1994). *Diagnostic and statistical manual of mental disorders,* 4th ed. Washington, DC: Author.

Andersson, J., & Rönnberg, J. R. (1995). Recall suffers from collaboration: Joint recall effects of friendship and activity complexity. *Applied Cognitive Psychology, 9,* 199-211.

Björkhem, K., Olsson, A., Hallberg, I. R., & Norberg, A. (1992). Caregiver's experience of providing care for demented persons living at home. *Scandinavian Journal of Primary Health Care, 10,* 53-59.

Bogdan, R. C., & Biklen, S. K. (Eds). (1998). *Qualitative research for education: An introduction to theories and methods,* 3rd ed. Boston: Allyn & Bacon.

Bond, J., & Corner, L. (2001). Researching dementia: Are there unique methodological challenges for health services research? *Ageing and Society, 21,* 95-116.

Bonner, A. P., & O'Brien Cousins, S. (1996). Exercise and Alzheimer's disease: Benefits and barriers. *Activities, Adaption and Aging, 20*(4), 21-34.

Borell, L. (1992). *The activity life of persons with Alzheimer's disease.* Doctoral thesis, Karolinska Institutet, Stockholm, Sweden.

Cavanaugh, J. C., Dunn, N. J., Mowery, D., Feller, C., Niederehe, G., Fruge, E., et al. (1989). Problem-solving strategies in dementia patient-caregiver dyads. *The Gerontologist, 29,* 156-158.

Corcoran, M. A., & Gitlin, L. N. (2001). Family caregiver acceptance and use of environmental strategies provided in an occupational therapy intervention. *Physical & Occupational Therapy in Geriatrics, 19*(1), 1-20.

Derwinger, A., Stigsdotter-Neely, A., & Bäckman, L. (in press). Design your own memory strategies! Self-generated strategy training versus mnemonic training in old age: An eight months follow-up. *Neuropsychological Rehabilitation.*

Fisher, A. G. (1998). Uniting practice and theory in an occupational framework. *The American Journal of Occupational Therapy, 52,* 509-521.

Folstein, M. F., Folstein, S. E., & McHugh, P. R. (1975). "Mini-Mental State Examination": A practical method for grading the cognitive state of patients for the clinician. *Journal of Psychiatric Research, 12,* 189-198.

Gitlin, L. N., Belle, S. H., Burgio, L. D., Czaja, S. J., Mahoney, D., Gallagher, D., et al. (2003). Effect of multicomponent interventions on caregiver burden and depression: The REACH multisite initiative at 6-month follow-up. *Psychology and Aging, 18,* 361-374.

Gitlin, L. G., Corcoran, M., Winter, L., Boyce, A., & Marcus, S. (1999). Predicting participation and adherence to a home environmental intervention among family caregivers of persons with dementia. *Family Relations, 48,* 363-372.

Gold, D. P., Cohen, C., Shulman, K., Zucchero, C., Andres, D., & Etezadi, J. (1995). Caregiving and dementia: Predicting negative and positive outcomes for caregivers. *International Journal of Aging and Human Development, 41,* 183-201.

Gould, O. N., Osborn, C., Krein, H., & Martenson, M. (2002). Collaborative recall in married and unacquainted dyads. *International Journal of Behavioral Development, 26,* 36-44.

Grafström, M., Fratiglioni, L., Sandman, P.-O., & Winblad, B. (1992). Health and social consequences for relatives of demented and non-demented elderly: A population-based study. *Journal of Clinical Epidemiology, 45,* 861-870.

Hepburn, K. W., Tornatore, J., Center, B., & Ostwald, S. W. (2001). Dementia family caregiver training: Affecting beliefs about caregiving and caregiver outcomes. *Journal of the American Geriatrics Society, 49,* 450-457.

Jansson, W., Nordberg, G., & Grafström, M. (2001). Patterns of elderly spousal caregiving in dementia care: An observational study. *Journal of Advanced Nursing, 34,* 804-812.

Josephsson, S., Bäckman, L., Borell, L., Nygård, L., & Bernspång, B. (1994). Effectiveness of an intervention to improve occupational performance in dementia. *The Occupational Therapy Journal of Research, 15,* 36-51.

Kielhofner, G. (2002). *A model of human occupation: Theory and application,* 3rd ed. Philadelphia: Lippincott, Williams, & Wilkins.

Margrett, J. A., & Marsiske, M. (2002). Gender differences in older adults' everyday cognitive collaboration. *International Journal of Behavioral Development, 26,* 45-59.

Martin, G. W., & Younger, D. (2000). Anti oppressive practice: A route to the empowerment of people with dementia through communication and choice. *Journal of Psychiatry and Mental Health Nursing, 7,* 59-67.

Max, W. (1996). The cost of Alzheimer's disease: Will drug treatment ease the burden? *Pharmacoeconomics, 9,* 5-10.

Melzer, D., Bedford, S., Dening, T., Lawton, C., Todd, C., Badger, G., et al. (1996). Carers and the monitoring of psychogeriatric community teams. *International Journal of Geriatric Psychiatry, 11,* 1057-1061.

Nygård, L., Amberla, K., Bernspång, B., Almkvist, O., & Winblad, B. (1998). The relationship between cognition and daily activities in cases of mild Alzheimer's. *Scandinavian Journal of Occupational Therapy, 5,* 160-166.

Öhman, A., Nygård, L., & Borell, L. (2001). The

vocational situation in cases of memory deficits on younger-onset dementia. *Scandinavian Journal of Caring Sciences, 15,* 34-43.

Ory, M. G., Hoffman, R. R., III, Yee, J. L., Tennstedt, S., & Schulz, R. (1999). Prevalence and impact of caregiving: A detailed comparison between dementia and nondementia caregivers. *The Gerontologist, 39,* 177-185.

Patton, M. Q. (Ed.) (1987). *How to use qualitative methods in evaluation.* Thousand Oaks, CA: Sage Publications.

Schulz, R. (Ed.). (2000). *Handbook on dementia caregiving: Evidence-based interventions in family caregiving.* New York: Springer Publishing.

Schulz, R., & Beach, S. R. (1999). Caregiving as a risk factor for mortality: The Caregiver Health Effect Study. *JAMA, 282,* 2215-2219.

Schulz, R., O'Brien, A., Czaja, S., Ory, M., Norris, R., Martire, L. M., et al. (2002). Dementia caregiver intervention research: In search of clinical significance. *The Gerontologist, 42,* 589-602.

Spencer A. (2001) Ageing through occupation. *Asian Journal of Occupational Therapy, 1,* 15-21.

Statistics Sweden. (1997). *Statistisk årsbok* [in Swedish]. Stockholm, Sweden: Statistiska Centralbyrån.

Tannous, C., Lehmann-Monck, V., Magoffin, R., Jackson, O., & Llewellyn, G. (1999). Beyond good practice: Issues in working with people with intellectual disability and high support needs. *Australian Occupational Therapy Journal, 46,* 24-35.

Teri, L. (1999). Training families to provide care: Effects on people with dementia. *International Journal of Geriatric Psychiatry, 14,* 110-119.

Vikström, S., Josephsson, S., & Nygård, L. (2003, May). *Engagement in everyday activities in the home from the perspective of persons with dementia and their caregivers respectively.* Paper presented at the Nordic Congress of Rehabilitation, Copenhagen, Denmark.

Weiss, R. S. (1973). *Loneliness: The experience of emotional and social isolation.* Cambridge, MA: The MIT Press.

Woods, B. (1999). Promoting well-being and independence for people with dementia. *International Journal of Geriatric Psychiatry, 14,* 97-109.

Yerxa, E. J. (1998). Occupation: The keystone of a curriculum for a self-defined profession. *The American Journal of Occupational Therapy, 52,* 365-372.

The Effect of Constraint-Induced Movement Treatment on Occupational Performance and Satisfaction in Stroke Survivors

Nancy A. Flinn, Sue Schamburg, Jill Murray Fetrow, Jennifer Flanigan

Key words: stroke rehabilitation, occupational performance, constraint-induced movement treatment

Abstract: Stroke is a leading cause of disability and impaired arm function is a common consequence. Constraint-induced movement treatment is a technique used to increase weak arm use and to decrease motor deficits resulting from stroke. Eleven stroke survivors participated in a constraint-induced movement treatment protocol of 3½ hours of treatment per day for 8 days. Participants experienced significantly increased use of the weak arm in daily activities, which was measured by the Motor Activity Log, and a trend toward improved coordination in the weak arm, which was measured by the Wolf Motor Function Test. Participants did not report significant improvements in average performance or satisfaction in self-identified occupational performance problems. When these problems were analyzed individually, no significant differences were seen immediately post-treatment. However, significant improvements were seen for satisfaction at 4 to 6 months post-treatment. The occupational performance problems identified by the participants were equally divided between problems related to hand use and problems not related to hand use. Approximately half of the non-hand use problems involved endurance. Although participants in this study did make improvements in arm use and coordination, they did not identify improvements in average occupational performance or satisfaction as an outcome of constraint-induced movement treatment.

Nancy A. Flinn, PhD, OTR/L, is Associate Professor, Department of Occupational Science and Occupational Therapy, College of St. Catherine, St. Paul, Minnesota. At the time the article was written, Sue Schamburg, MA, OTR/L, Jill Murray Fetrow, MA, OTR/L, and Jennifer Flanigan, MA, OTR/L, were Masters Students in Occupational Therapy, College of St. Catherine, St. Paul, Minnesota. Sue Schamburg is currently Occupational Therapist, Missouri. Jill Murray Fetrow is currently Occupational Therapist, Sports Rehab and Professional Therapy Associates, Storm Lake, Iowa. Jennifer Flanigan is currently Occupational Therapist, Cumberland Memorial Hospital, Cumberland, Wisconsin. Address correspondence to Nancy A. Flinn, PhD, OTR/L, naflinn@stkate.edu.

Stroke is a leading cause of long-term disability in the United States (American Heart Association, 2000). It is estimated that 750,000 strokes occur in the United States each year. Impaired arm function is a common consequence for stroke survivors (Broeks, Lankhorst, Rumping, & Prevo, 1999) and stroke survivors with impaired arm function report decreased subjective well-being 1 year after experiencing a stroke, decreased independence in self-care, and decreased quality of life (Duncan et al., 1997; Nilsson, Aniansson, & Grimby, 2000; Sveen, Bautz-Holter, Sodring, Wyller, & Laake, 1999; Wyller, Sveen, Sodring, Pettersen, & Bautz-Holter, 1997).

Constraint-induced movement treatment (CIMT) is an intensive, short-term treatment consisting of movement drills and intensive use of the weak arm focused on increasing the amount of use and improving movement of the involved arm after stroke (Taub, 1980). CIMT has demonstrated improvements in the actual amount of arm use in daily activities with large effect sizes in the range of 1.5 to 3.3 (Liepert, Bauder, Miltner, Taub, & Weiller, 2000; Miltner, Bauder, Sommer, Dettmers, & Taub, 1999; Taub & Uswatte, 2000; Taub, Uswatte, & Pidikiti,

1999). In addition, CIMT has also been effective in improving upper extremity coordination with effect sizes in the range of 0.82 to 0.90 (Kunkel et al., 1999; Taub et al., 1999).

Treatment protocols for CIMT can vary, but they generally include 3 hours of direct therapy per day (Sterr et al., 2002) to 6 hours of therapy per day (Morris, Crago, DeLuca, Pidikiti, & Taub, 1997) for 8 to 10 days (Morris et al., 1997; Miltner et al., 1999). Although most CIMT protocols achieve significant improvement in both incorporation of the arm into daily activities and arm coordination, there appears to be a dose effect; protocols that provide more intervention achieve greater gains than those that provide less intervention. In a direct comparison, both 3 and 6 hours per day of therapy resulted in significant changes in both the amount of use of and coordination in the involved arm, but the 6 hour per day protocol resulted in greater improvement (Sterr et al., 2002). However, Sterr et al. concluded "significant and functionally relevant treatment effect can be obtained with 3 hours a day of training" (p. 1376).

The best candidates for CIMT are stroke survivors with active movement of their

involved limb, at least 45° of either active shoulder flexion or abduction, 10° of active elbow extension (D. Morris, personal communication, October 28, 2001), 20° of active wrist extension, and 10° of active finger extension in all joints of all five fingers (Taub et al., 1993). In addition, participants must score within normal limits on a cognitive screen, be able to participate in simple conversations, and be at least 6 months post-stroke (Liepert et al., 1998). Candidates must be limited in how much they use their involved arm in daily activities because there is a ceiling effect to treatment. They cannot have pain with movement of the arm (Kunkel et al., 1999). Some protocols also require a 24-hour caregiver (Morris et al., 1997), but other studies have not discussed the involvement of a caregiver in treatment (Miltner et al., 1999; Taub et al., 1993).

Although CIMT has been shown to be effective in increasing arm use in daily activities and improving arm coordination, only limited attention has been given to how these changes influence the daily lives of these participants. Specifically, occupational therapists are interested in the effect of CIMT in reducing problems with meaning-

Article Reprint Information: Reprinted with permission from Flinn, N. A., Schamburg, S., Fetrow, J. M., & Flanigan, J. (2005). The effect of constraint-induced movement treatment on occupational performance and satisfaction in stroke survivors. *Occupational Therapy Journal of Research: Occupation, Participation and Health, 25*(3), 119-127.

ful occupations of stroke survivors. Participation in meaningful occupation has been associated with both physical and mental health (Ostir, Markides, Black, & Goodwin, 2000), whereas decreases in participation in meaningful occupation are associated with decreases in self-perceived health and well-being (Law, Steinwender, & LeClair, 1998; Wilcock et al., 1998). This indicates that involvement in personally identified meaningful activities promotes health.

Gillot, Holder-Walls, Kurtz, and Varley (2003) used a mixed-methods single case design to evaluate changes in two stroke survivors receiving a modified program of CIMT. Through the use of the Canadian Occupational Performance Measure (COPM), these participants both reported improvements in performance, but one had increased satisfaction and the other had decreased satisfaction with performance (Gillot et al., 2003). These results raise questions about the relationship between occupational performance and CIMT.

The questions posed in this study are: Does this model of CIMT result in changes in arm use and coordination? Does CIMT change perceptions of participation in meaningful activities? To answer these questions, arm use in daily activity, coordination, and performance and satisfaction with personally identified problems in important activities were measured before and after CIMT treatment in a group of 11 stroke survivors.

Methods

This is a quasi-experimental cohort study examining effects of one model of CIMT on upper extremity use in daily activities, upper extremity coordination, and perceptions of performance and satisfaction with self-identified problems in occupational performance. These were measured by use of the Motor Activity Log (MAL), the Wolf Motor Function Test (WMFT), and the COPM, respectively. Participants completed the measures 1 to 3 weeks prior to the intervention, on the last day of the intervention, and at 4 to 6 months after the intervention. The exception to this schedule was that the MAL was completed by telephone 7 to 10 days after the study was performed. This was done because the measure refers to activities performed in the prior week, and participants were wearing their mitts for the week prior to the last day of treatment. This would have resulted in an artificially high score on the amount of arm use. The 4- to 6-month time frame was used for the second post-test because of problems with scheduling due to weather and transportation. Other evaluations were performed and

Table 1
Participant Demographics

Subject	Gender	Age (Y)[a]	Years Post-Stroke[b]	Mean Hours of Intervention Per Day[c]
1	F	64	11.4	2.76
2	M	64	2.0	3.34
3	M	79	.9	2.46
4	M	54	2.7	3.89
5	M	67	10.8	3.34
6	M	78	1.1	3.10
7	F	53	2.4	3.60
8	M	62	.8	3.00
9	F	80	.5	3.44
10	F	37	1.0	3.60
11	M	38	.8	3.14

[a]Mean (M) = 61.4 years; range (R) = 37–80 years; standard deviation (SD) = 14.98.
[b]M = 3.1; R = .5–11.4; SD = 4.
[c]M = 3.24; R = 2.76–3.89; SD = .41.

will be reported separately.

The study was publicized through presentations at stroke support groups and by posting flyers in community centers. In addition, professionals in the community were informed of both the study and the criteria for participation. Initial screening was performed by telephone, followed by an in-person screening. The inclusion criteria for the study included the most recent stroke occurring at least 6 months prior to the intervention date, but no outside limit was set because length of time since the stroke has not been shown to influence the outcome of this treatment technique (Miltner et al., 1999). Participants also needed to demonstrate independence in toileting and eating, pain free active range of motion in all joints of the arm (45° of shoulder abduction or flexion, 10° of elbow extension, 20° of wrist extension, and 10° of finger extension in all finger joints), muscle tone that allowed functional use of the arm (operationally defined as the ability to repeat each motion three times), cognitive function within normal limits as measured by scoring at least 24/30 on the Mini-Mental State Examination cognitive screen (Folstein, Folstein, & McHugh, 1975), language skills adequate for participation in simple discussions, and clearance from the individual's physician ensuring that the participant did not have any significant ongoing medical concerns. Participants scoring above 2.5 on the MAL were excluded because the ceiling effect of CIMT would limit the effect of treatment (Kunkel et al., 1999). In addition,

participants were asked to provide lunch and transportation to and from the treatment site each day. There was no charge for evaluation or treatment. The presence of a 24-hour caregiver was not required.

Participants

Forty-three individuals were screened, and 14 enrolled in the study. The primary reason individuals were excluded during the telephone screening was because they did not meet the diagnostic criteria, and the primary reason they were excluded at the in-person screening was inadequate active movement in the weak arm. Three participants who enrolled did not participate in the study, two because of medical problems that developed prior to the pre-test, and one who left treatment on the third day because treatment was too time-consuming. The 11 participants who completed the study had ages ranging from 37 to 80 years, and were from 0.5 to 11.4 years post-stroke (Table 1). After stroke survivors were accepted into the study, they were asked to make no changes in their arm use prior to treatment. Following a physician's clearance, each participant was evaluated by the treating therapists. Although the evaluations were not masked, precautions were taken to avoid bias. Shadish, Cook, and Campbell (2002) identify several methods to limit bias used in this study, including using several experimenters and observing experimenters to detect and reduce expectancy-inducing behavior.

Measurement Tools

The MAL used here was a modification of the original semi-structured interview used by Taub et al. (1993) with 30 questions focused on the use of the involved limb during activities of daily living (Constraint-Induced Movement Therapy Research Group, University of Alabama, Birmingham, personal communication, September 11, 2000). Using a 6-point scale, the participants were asked to identify how much they had used their arm in a particular task during the past week. Although there is also a "how well" scale for this measure only the "how much" scale was used in this study. The scores were averaged across all of the activities performed in the past week. The intraclass correlation coefficient ($ICC_{)(3,1)}$ ($r = 0.90$) between participant and caregiver scores obtained separately supports that both the participants and their caregivers have similar perceptions of the functional use of the limb (Uswatte & Taub, 1999). The MAL has also been shown to have "a perfect correlation to an observational measure of arm use" (Taub & Uswatte, 2000, p. 987).

The WMFT consists of 17 items: two strength items, six timed single joint movements, and nine timed functional movements involving more than one joint (Morris, Uswatte, Crago, Cook, & Taub, 2001; Wolf et al., 2001). The test is videotaped and timing is measured from the videotape. For the timed items at two points in time, the reliability was $ICC_{(3,1)}$ (inter-rater consistency) $r = 0.99$ to 0.97, and $ICC_{(2,1)}$ (inter-rater agreement) $r = 0.99$ to 0.97 (Morris et al., 2001).

The COPM is commonly used to evaluate participant perspectives of occupational performance (Law et al., 1998). Individuals identify activities in their daily lives that they want to do, need to do, or are expected to do that cause problems for them in the areas of self-care, productivity, or leisure. Individuals then rank their most important problems, and rate both how well they perform them and how satisfied they are with that performance (Law et al., 1998). Test–retest reliability of the COPM is satisfactory for stroke survivors, with $r = 0.89$ for performance and $r = 0.88$ for satisfaction (Cup, Scholte-op-Reimer, Thijssen, & van Kuyk-Minis, 2003). The COPM has been shown to be sensitive to change in the adult neurorehabilitation populations, but only when used for 4 weeks or longer (Cheng, Rodger, & Polatajko, 2002).

Intervention

The pre-test WMFT videotapes were viewed by the treating therapists and spe-cific movement difficulties were identified for each participant. For each movement difficulty, three or four activities were selected from the standard CIMT shaping and task practice activity list that was obtained from Dr. Edward Taub (E. Taub, personal communication, September 11, 2000). The selection of 59 tasks available for this study was a representative sample of the original tasks, based on equipment availability and cost. In addition, some tasks were modified and some new tasks were developed to match participants' interests and activities, and to use materials that were as ecologically valid as possible. For example, one of the CIMT shaping tasks had participants moving cones from one target to another while keeping their forearm in a neutral position. This task was modified in our project to require participants to pick up an empty or partially filled bottle and move it from a counter to a shelf.

The participants were treated in two consecutive groups of five and six participants, 2 weeks apart. The participants' arrivals were staggered by 30 minutes each day so that while one participant was working with the therapist, the other participant assigned to that therapist was working independently or resting. In that way, each participant's treatment was provided on a one-to-one basis. Three and one-half hours of individual therapy were scheduled during the 8 hours participants were scheduled to be at the facility. Several participants missed days because of illness or transportation problems, and these days were made up as possible, on a one-to-one basis with the same 30-minute practice, 30-minute rest schedule. Participants were encouraged to continue to practice activities independently during their rest periods.

Lunchtime was not included as treatment time in this project because supervision and feedback could not be provided at the same level of intensity as the individual therapy sessions, and it was decided not to treat these two levels of intensity of treatment as the same. Feeding adaptations such as built-up handled utensils or spill-proof mugs were provided as necessary and participants were strongly encouraged to feed themselves using their weak arms.

Participants were given daily logs to fill out for 2 weekdays and 1 weekend day prior to the start of treatment. At the beginning of the first day of treatment, participants were fitted with a padded safety mitt for their stronger arm. The mitts were adapted so that they could be put on and taken off independently (Morris et al., 1997; Taub et al., 1999). The daily logs completed by the participants were used to set up the behavioral contracts, which identified those daily tasks to be performed with the mitt and without the mitt (Morris et al., 1997). Participants were instructed that any tasks that involved water, transfers, or safety were to be performed without the mitt. Participants were asked to wear their mitt 90% of the time they were not in therapy.

As treatment began, the participants were allowed to select one of the tasks from the list identified for each specific movement difficulty. For each 30-minute treatment session, each practice trial was recorded and a graph of performance was shown to the participant (Morris et al., 1997). If participants fatigued during the session, they were allowed to rest briefly, the task was modified to make it easier, or a new task was introduced. If performance remained unchanged for more than 10 trials, the task was modified. Three occupational therapy graduate students provided this treatment and were directly supervised by a faculty member.

On each day of treatment, the participants filled out activity and mitt-wearing logs from the time they left in the afternoon until they returned the following morning (Morris et al., 1997). These were reviewed each morning to identify the activities they were doing at home, to provide assistance with problem solving for difficult activities, and to determine how much of the time they wore their mitts. At some point in the day, the home program was reviewed to identify daily activities and exercises they were to practice in their own home (Morris et al., 1997).

The protocol was 3½ hours of treatment for each participant for 8 days. This resulted in 28 hours of directly supervised treatment, which is slightly less than the total of 30 hours of treatment reported in the 3 hours a day protocol of Sterr et al. However, lunchtime was counted as treatment time in Sterr et al.'s protocol, but was not counted in this project, as explained earlier. The average number of hours of treatment actually provided per day was slightly below the goal of 3½ hours, at 3 hours and 14 minutes (range: 2 hours, 28 minutes to 3 hours, 53 minutes), primarily because of fatigue on the part of participants. No participants approached the mitt-wearing target, with reported mitt-wearing ranging from 1.2% to 79% of waking hours (average: 48.9%).

Data Analysis

The first question asked in this study was whether this particular protocol of CIMT resulted in changes in arm use and coordination. This was evaluated through a cohort analysis of the group comparing pre-test and immediate post-test data, and pre-test and 4- to 6-month follow-up data using the Wilcoxon signed ranks test. Cohen's measure of effect size (*d*) will be used to describe the treatment effect sizes (Portney & Watkins, 2000). The effect of changes in daily arm use and coordination produced by CIMT on self-identified problems in meaningful daily activities was explored in several ways. A cohort analysis of that data was performed, followed by an in-depth analysis of the types of problems identified by participants.

The inter-rater reliability for the tools and raters in this study were also established. For the MAL, the reliability for ten participants and four raters was $ICC_{(3,1)}$ (inter-rater reliability) $r = 0.96$. To avoid artificially inflating the scores at the immediate post-test by asking participants how they had used their arm while they had been wearing the mitt, the immediate post-test was performed by telephone 7 to 10 days after the study was completed. The inter-modal reliability established for one researcher performing both in-person and telephone MALs with nine participants familiar with the MAL was $ICC_{(2,1)}$ $r = 0.88$. For the WMFT, the inter-rater reliability was determined for 12 randomly selected evaluations of 33 videotaped measurements and scored by three researchers. The $(ICC)_{(2,1)}$ (inter-rater agreement) for timing from the videotape was $r = 0.99$. For the COPM, inter-rater reliability established between two raters and 10 subjects was $ICC_{(3,1)}$ $r = 0.90$ for performance, and $ICC_{(3,1)}$ $r = 0.89$ for satisfaction.

Results

The CIMT provided with this treatment protocol resulted in significant changes in actual use of the involved limb, as measured by the MAL. Because two comparisons were performed using the same data, a Bonferroni correction was used, with a resulting significance level of .025. The Wilcoxon signed ranks test comparing the pretest and immediate post-test data revealed significant differences (n = 11; *p* = .003). The Wilcoxon signed ranks test comparing the pre-test and the 4- to 6-month follow-up data also showed significant differences (n = 11; *p* = .003). The pre-test to immediate post-test effect size was *d* = 2.84, and the pre-test to 4- to 6-month follow-up effect size was *d* = 2.63. Both of these effect sizes are interpreted to be large (Table 2).

| | | *Table 2* | |
| | | *Motor Activity Log* | |
Subject	Pre-test[a]	Immediate Post-test[b]	4 to 6 Months Post-test[c]
1	1.50	2.24	2.18
2	.45	1.17	.81
3	1.07	2.69	2.46
4	1.12	3.76	3.84
5	.63	1.50	1.33
6	2.46	4.14	3.57
7	.87	3.76	3.73
8	.83	1.70	1.13
9	.98	2.13	2.83
10	1.14	3.89	3.03
11	1.04	2.67	3.55

[a]Mean (M) = 1.10; range (R) = .45–2.46.
[b]M = 2.70; R = 1.5–3.89.
[c]M = 2.59; R = .81–3.84.

| | | *Table 3* | |
| | | *Wolf Motor Function Median Scores* | |
Subject	Pre-test[a]	Immediate Post-test[b]	4 to 6 Months Post-test[c]
1	35.1	3.04	50.62
2	7.82	13.94	4.97
3	1.81	1.5	1.53
4	3.32	2.2	1.9
5	4.02	5.42	3.53
6	2.09	1.57	1.93
7	6.97	4.12	4.47
8	3.95	4.4	4.34
9	12.56	6.06	3.09
10	3.19	1.75	1.47
11	1.7	1.23	1.13

Note. All data in seconds.
[a]Median (M) = 3.95; Range (R) = 1.7–35.1; Standard Deviation (SD) = 9.71.
[b]M = 3.04; R = 1.23–13.94; SD = 3.66.
[c]M = 3.09; R = 1.13–50.62; SD = 14.47.

The WMFT evaluations revealed smaller effects (Table 3). Again, a Bonferroni correction was used with a resulting significance level of .025. The Wilcoxon signed ranks test showed no significant difference either from pre-test to immediate post-test (n = 11; *p* = .16), or from pre-test to 4- to 6-month follow-up data (n = 11; *p* = .09). Further analysis through comparisons of effect size, which reveals treatment effectiveness without regard to the number of subjects, was calculated to further explore the effect of this treatment program. Moderate treatment effects were revealed for the pre-test to immediate post-test measure with an effect size of *d* = 0.72, but a much smaller effect size for the pre-test to 4- to 6-month follow-up measure was found with an effect size of *d* = 0.04.

A closer analysis of the WMFT data revealed participant 1 as an outlier. Her WMFT times were 2.84 standard deviations slower than the median score for the group's pre-test, and 3.00 standard deviations slower than the median at the follow-up. When her data were removed from the data set, there was no significant change between pre-test and post-test data (n = 10, Wilcoxon signed ranks test, *p* = .285), but a significant change was present between pre-test and 4- to 6-month follow-up data (n = 10, Wilcoxon signed ranks test, *p* = .013). With her data removed from the pool, effect sizes are more in keeping with CIMT research as a whole, with a pre-test to immediate post-test effect size of *d* = 0.19 and

a pre-test to 4- to 6-month follow-up effect size of *d* = 1.11.

To begin analysis of the COPM data, a cohort analysis of the average performance and satisfaction scores for each participant was performed. Using the Wilcoxon signed ranks test and a Bonferroni correction, a level of significance of *p* = .025 was used for all comparisons. Analysis of the average performance scores (n = 11) revealed no significant findings; the pre-test to immediate post-test analysis was *p* = .506, (negative sum of ranks = 21, positive sum of ranks = 34), and the pre-test to 4- to 6-month follow-up analysis was *p* = .283 (negative sum of ranks = 17, positive sum of ranks = 38). Analysis of the average satisfaction scores (n = 11) also revealed nonsignificant findings; the pre-test to immediate post-test analysis was *p* = .262 (negative sum of ranks = 16.5, positive sum of ranks = 38.5), and the pre-test to 4- to 6-month follow-up analysis was *p* = .062 (negative sum of ranks = 12, positive sum of ranks = 54). Figure 1 provides the average performance and satisfaction scores.

A cohort analysis of the COPM data from pre-test to post-test and pre-test to 4- to 6-month follow-up data for the 55 individual problems was performed using a Wilcoxon signed ranks test and a Bonferroni correction with a level of significance of *p* = .025 for all comparisons. The Wilcoxon signed ranks test from pre-test to immediate post-

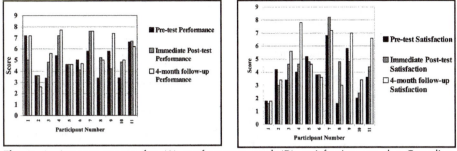

Figure 1. Average scores for (A) performance and (B) satisfaction on the Canadian Occupational Performance Measure.

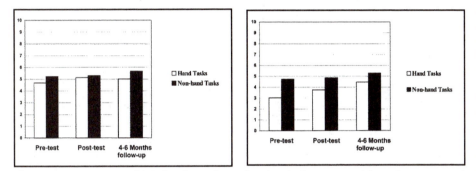

Figure 2. Comparison of hand tasks and non-hand tasks by average (A) performance and (B) satisfaction scores.

test (n = 55) revealed no significant differences, with a performance score of $p = .30$ (negative sum of ranks = 252, positive sum of ranks = 378) and a satisfaction score of $p = .11$ (negative sum of ranks = 232.5, positive sum of ranks = 433.5). The pre-test to 4- to 6-month follow-up findings for the 55 problems revealed a performance score difference of $p = .14$ (negative sum of ranks = 240.5, positive sum of ranks = 425.5) and a satisfaction score difference of $p = .007$ (negative sum of ranks = 172.5, positive sum of ranks = 530.5). Thus, significant differences were not seen in performance scores at either time-point, but significant differences were seen at the 4- to 6-month follow-up for satisfaction scores.

To explore the COPM problems further, a descriptive analysis was performed. One of the interesting characteristics of the problems identified by participants was that of the 55 activities identified by the 11 participants, only 29 were specifically related to arm and hand function (e.g., cooking faster, doing the dishes, knitting, weaving, typing, or writing). The other 26 problems were not related to hand function, but to other problems such as endurance for shopping, speech, reading, travel, socializing, getting outside more, or walking faster. To analyze this more fully, the performance and satisfaction averages of the tasks within the two categories, hand tasks and non-hand tasks, were calculated. Performance in hand tasks

improved an average of 7% during the course of the study, whereas performance in non-hand tasks improved an average of 8%, which would account for the nonsignificant findings in the performance score comparisons. Satisfaction with performance of hand tasks improved an average of 48% during the course of the study, whereas performance of non-hand tasks improved only an average of 12%. Not surprisingly, there were greater changes in satisfaction with the hand tasks than with the non-hand tasks. However, the fact that there were limited changes in performance scores and larger changes in satisfaction scores is somewhat surprising (Fig. 2).

The 26 non-hand task problems were related to other issues, and slightly more than half of them (14 of 26) had at least a component related to endurance (e.g., walking faster, tolerating standing when shopping, and being able to work part-time). These problems would not be expected to change as a result of a treatment focused on upper extremity use and function, but do represent an area that may benefit from occupational therapy treatment.

Discussion

This study asked whether this treatment protocol was representative of CIMT as a whole. This is an important question because this protocol did not require that participants have 24-hour caregivers, which is a departure from some standard protocols.

In addition, this treatment model provided only 3½ hours of treatment per day, which is at the lower range of previous protocols. In this study, it was found that this version of CIMT did result in improvements in the amount of arm use in functional activities; however, it was less effective in improving coordination.

One other notable finding was that the mitt-wearing rate reported by these participants was very low, whereas their gains in functional use of the weak arm remained similar to other reports. Some participants reported that they were afraid to wear the mitt when they were alone for fear they might fall. Because we did not require 24-hour caregivers, most of our participants were alone when they were at home. This suggests that stroke survivors who do not have 24-hour caregivers could benefit from the treatment and that extensive mitt wearing may not be necessary.

Another problem identified in this study was that many of the participants could not tolerate the 3½ hours of treatment that was scheduled, although they were allowed 30 minute breaks between the 30 minute treatment sessions. In fact, of the 11 participants in this study, only 4 were able to tolerate the scheduled amount of therapy. This raises questions about whether alternative formats for treatment might be more effective for individuals with fatigue. Fatigue has been identified as a significant issue for stroke survivors. In a sample of stroke survivors, 51% identified fatigue as their primary complaint (van der Werf, van den Broek, Anten, & Bleijenberg, 2001). Glader, Stegmayr, and Kjell (2002) found that 39% of respondents 2 years post-stroke stated that they always or almost always felt tired. Further investigation of the role of fatigue as a factor that may limit improvement from CIMT by limiting participation in the intervention needs to be considered.

Another purpose of this study was to explore the nature of the benefits of CIMT and changes in satisfaction and performance in self-identified occupational performance problems. Although the 11 participants in this project had increased arm use in daily activities and had small improvement in coordination, they reported no changes in average performance or satisfaction scores. When the problems were considered individually, there continued to be no changes from pre-test to immediate post-test, but there were changes in satisfaction at the 4- to 6-month follow-up. The lack of change in either performance or satisfaction scores at immediate post-test may be explained by the fact that the participants had not had time to integrate the changes in arm use and coordination into the identified activities because the COPM was performed on the last day of the study. They had attended the CIMT program for 8 of the previous 11 days, and this would have limited the opportunity to participate in the other activities.

The lack of change in performance scores in either the immediate or 4- to 6-month time frame for these participants indicated that the changes in arm use and coordination did not transfer to perceived improvements in performance in these important activities. It may be that although performance improved, it still was not what participants perceive as *normal* and so their assessment of performance did not change. It may also be because these identified problems are parts of complex activities and that changing motor performance does not translate into changes in overall performance. The cognitive, physical, psychosocial, cultural, and socioeconomic contexts within which these activities occur may lack the flexibility to allow changes in performance to be apparent.

This study was a cohort analysis of a small group of participants in one model of CIMT. There was no control for other events that may have occurred outside the treatment session, either during the intervention period or during the 4 to 6 months between the study and the post-test. Additionally, the small sample size resulted in decreased power in this study, which affected the ability of this study to reveal differences resulting from treatment. Further study of the occupational performance outcomes from CIMT should be done with a larger sample to verify these findings.

Other factors not analyzed in this study may also have influenced these results, including the use of a group setting for this project. Participants spent 8 hours per day with a group of stroke survivors and four therapists in a highly social environment and spent much of their time talking about shared experiences and frustrations. These group interactions may have influenced the way that they viewed themselves and their situations beyond the changes in arm use.

CIMT is an intervention that can improve incorporation of the weak arm into daily activities for stroke survivors and may increase satisfaction with performance of hand-related occupations. However, because of the complexity of the occupations in daily life, it does not appear to be successful in improving the perception of performance of these occupations.

Acknowledgments

This study was partially supported by a Faculty Development Grant from the College of St. Catherine, St. Paul, Minnesota.

References

American Heart Association. (2005). *Stroke statistics*. Retrieved May, 26, 2005, from http://www.americanheart.org/presenter.jhtml?identifier=4725.

Broeks, J. G., Lankhorst, G. J., Rumping, K., & Prevo, A. J. H. (1999). The long-term outcome of arm function after stroke: Results of a follow-up study. *Disability and Rehabilitation, 21*, 357-364.

Cheng, Y. H., Rodger, S., & Polatajko, H. (2002). Experiences with the COPM and client-centred practice in adult neurorehabilitation in Taiwan. *Occupational Therapy International, 9*, 167-184.

Cup, E. H. C., Scholte-op-Reimer, W. J. M., Thijssen, M. C. E., & van Kuyk-Minis, M. A. H. (2003). Reliability and validity of the Canadian Occupational Performance Measure in stroke patients. *Clinical Rehabilitation, 17*, 402-409.

Duncan, P. W., Samsa, G. P., Weinberger, M., Goldstein, L. B., Bonito, A., Witter, D. M., et al. (1997). Health status of individuals with mild stroke. *Stroke, 28*, 740-745.

Folstein, M. F., Folstein, S. E., & McHugh, P. R. (1975). "Mini-Mental State": A practical method for grading the cognitive state of patients for the clinician. *Journal of Psychiatric Research, 12*, 189-198.

Gillot, A. J., Holder-Walls, A., Kurtz, J. R., & Varley, N. C. (2003). Perceptions and experiences of two survivors of stroke who participated in constraint-induced movement therapy home programs. *American Journal of Occupational Therapy, 57*, 168-176.

Glader, E.-L., Stegmayr, B., & Kjell, A. (2002). Poststroke fatigue: A 2-year follow-up study of stroke patients in Sweden. *Stroke, 33*, 1327-1333.

Kunkel, A., Kopp, B., Muller, G., Villringer, K., Villringer, A., Taub, E., et al. (1999). Constraint-induced movement therapy for motor recovery in chronic stroke patients. *Archives of Physical Medicine and Rehabilitation, 80*, 624-628.

Law, M., Baptiste, S., Carswell, A., McColl, M. A., Polatajko, H., & Pollock, N. (1998). *The Canadian Occupational Performance Measure* (3rd ed.). Ottawa, Ontario, Canada: Canadian Association of Occupational Therapists Publications, Ace.

Law, M., Steinwender, S., & LeClair, L. (1998). Occupation, health and well-being. *Canadian Journal of Occupational Therapy, 65*, 81-91.

Liepert, J., Bauder, H., Miltner, W. H. R., Taub, E., & Weiller, C. (2000). Treatment-induced cortical reorganization after stroke in humans. *Stroke, 31*, 1210-1216.

Liepert, J., Miltner, W. H., Bauder, H., Sommer, M., Dettmers, C., Taub, E., et al. (1998). Motor cortex plasticity during constraint-induced movement therapy in stroke patients. *Neuroscience Letters, 250*, 5-8.

Miltner, W. H. R., Bauder, H., Sommer, M., Dettmers, C., & Taub, E. (1999). Effects of constraint-induced movement therapy on patients with chronic motor deficits after stroke: A replication. *Stroke, 30*, 586-592.

Morris, D. M., Crago, J. E., DeLuca, S. C., Pidikiti, R. D., & Taub, E. (1997). Constraint-induced movement therapy for motor recovery after stroke. *NeuroRehabilitation, 9*, 29-43.

Morris, D. M., Uswatte, G., Crago, J. E., Cook, E. W., III, Taub, E. (2001). The reliability of the Wolf Motor Function Test for assessing upper extremity function after stroke. *Archives of Physical Medicine and Rehabilitation, 82*, 750-755.

Nilsson, A. L., Aniansson, A., & Grimby, G. (2000). Rehabilitation needs and disability in community living stroke survivors two years after stroke. *Topics in Stroke Rehabilitation, 6*(4), 30-47.

Ostir, G. V., Markides, K. S., Black, S. A., & Goodwin, J. S. (2000). Emotional well-being predicts subsequent functional independence and survival. *Journal of the American Geriatrics Society, 48*, 473-478.

Portney, L., G., & Watkins, M. P. (2000). *Foundations of clinical research: Applications to practice* (2nd ed.). Upper Saddle River, NJ: Prentice-Hall, Inc.

Shadish, W. R., Cook, T. D., & Campbell, D. T. (2002). *Experimental and quasi-experimental designs for generalized causal inference.* Boston, MA: Houghton Mifflin.

Sterr, A., Elbert, T., Berthold, I., Kolbel, S., Rockstroh, B., & Taub, E. (2002). Longer versus shorter daily constraint-induced movement therapy of chronic hemiparesis: An exploratory study. *Archives of Physical Medicine and Rehabilitation, 83*, 1374-1377.

Sveen, U., Bautz-Holter, E., Sodring, K. M., Wyller, T. B., & Laake, K. (1999). Association between impairments, self-care ability and social activities 1 year after stroke. *Disability and Rehabilitation, 21*, 372-377.

Taub, E. (1980). Somatosensory deafferentation research with monkeys: Implications for rehabilitation medicine. In L. P. Ince (Ed.), *Behavioral psychology in rehabilitation medicine: Clinical applications* (pp. 371-401). Baltimore: Lippincott, Williams, & Wilkins.

Taub, E., Miller, N. E., Novack, T. A., Cook, E. W., III, Fleming, W. C., Nepomuceno, C. S., et al. (1993). Technique to improve chronic motor deficit after stroke. *Archives of Physical Medicine and Rehabilitation, 74*, 347-354.

Taub, E., & Uswatte, G. (2000). Constraint-induced movement therapy and massed practice [Letter to the Editor]. *Stroke, 31*, 983-991.

Taub, E., Uswatte, G., & Pidikiti, R. (1999). Constraint-induced movement therapy: A new family of techniques with broad application to physical rehabilitation: A clinical review. *Journal of Rehabilitation Research and Development, 36*, 237-251.

Uswatte, G., & Taub, E., (1999). Constraint-induced movement therapy: New approaches to outcome measurement in rehabilitation. In D. T. Stuss, G. Winocur, & I. H. Robertson (Eds.), *Cognitive neurorehabilitation* (pp. 215-

229). Cambridge, England: Cambridge University Press.

van der Werf, S. P., van den Broek, H. L. P., Anten, H. W. M., & Bleijenberg, G. (2001). Experience of severe fatigue long after stroke and its relation to depressive symptoms and disease characteristics. *European Neurology, 45*, 28-33.

Wilcock, A. A., van der Arend, H., Darling, K., Scholtz, J., Siddall, R., Snigg, C., et al. (1998). An exploratory study of people's perceptions and experiences of well-being. *British Journal of Occupational Therapy, 61*, 75-82.

Wolf, S. L., Catlin, P. A., Ellis, M., Archer, A. L., Morgan, B., & Piacentino, A. (2001). Assessing Wolf Motor Function Test as outcome measure for research in patients after stroke. *Stroke, 32*, 1635-1639.

Wyller, T. B., Sveen, U., Sodring, K. M., Pettersen, A. M., & Bautz-Holter, E. (1997). Subjective well-being one year after stroke. *Clinical Rehabilitation, 11*, 139-145.

Constraint-induced Movement Therapy for Hemiplegic Children With Acquired Brain Injuries

N. Karman, PT, MS, PCS, J. Maryles, MA, OTR/L, R. W. Baker, MA, E. Simpser, MD,
P. Berger-Gross, PhD

Key words: brain injury, children, hemiparesis, rehabilitation

Objective: To evaluate the feasibility and efficacy of constraint-induced movement therapy (CIMT) for impaired upper extremity (UE) function in children with acquired brain injury (ABI). **Design:** Multiple case studies. **Setting:** Inpatient pediatric rehabilitation. **Participants:** Seven consecutive ABI rehabilitation admissions with hemiparesis were recruited without regard to injury etiology, age, or cognitive capacities. **Main Outcome Measure:** The actual amount of use test (AAUT) was used to evaluate change in UE function. AAUT amount of use (AOU) and quality of movement (QOM) scales were obtained at baseline and follow-up. **Results:** AOU and QOM item improvements were significant, as were changes in activities of daily living. The effect sizes for these changes were large. **Conclusions:** Stringent CIMT training, previously only implemented with adults, can be used effectively with children when everyday elements of a child's life are integrated into adult protocols. The use of child-friendly UE shaping exercises, pushed into activities by professional therapists as well as trained teachers, paraprofessionals, and parents, was supported. Effects of impairment, injury, and behavior on outcomes are discussed. Larger controlled studies with additional outcome measures are indicated.

From the Traumatic Brain Injury Program, St. Mary's Hospital for Children, Bayside, NY, and the Department of Physical Therapy (Karman) at Hunter College of the City University of New York, NY. Corresponding author: P. Berger-Gross, PhD, TBI Program Director, St. Mary's Hospital for Children, 29-01 216th Street, Bayside, NY 11360. E-mail: pberger-gross@stmaryskids.org.

Constraint-induced Movement Therapy (CIMT) has received increasing scientific[1-4] and media attention[5] as the most promising rehabilitation technique for the affected upper extremity (UE) in stroke[6] and traumatic brain injuries[7] in adults. CIMT, characterized by short-term, high-intensity physical training accompanied by nearly constant restraint of the unaffected UE, has been demonstrated to provide superior immediate and long-term outcomes in comparison to standard therapies.[4]

CIMT was derived from a series of studies of "learned nonuse" in monkeys,[8] with a single deafferented forelimb. Animals with the naturally occurring chronic nonuse of the deafferented extremity rapidly reacquired functional forelimb use after restriction of the unaffected forelimb. Subsequent work showed that behavioral shaping of the neglected extremity was also effective in reinstating use of the limb in life situations.[9] Motor behavior shaping is the continuous reinforcement of each successive approximation of a skill. Typically, in CIMT, everyday tasks are used to train for accuracy, strength, and speed of movement in the affected UE. Initially, a checker might be placed in a child's hand to be inserted in columns of a "Connect Four" game board. Step by step the child would be given explicit feedback, in terms of the knowledge of results, for improved self-grasping, accuracy of release, and speed of repetitions.

Massed practice and positive feedback are combined to maximize the learning effects on the performance of motor tasks.

The improved motor performance and increased use of the affected extremity in the free situation of deafferented monkeys had profound implications for extending these techniques to humans with neurologically based UE dysfunction.[9] Although standard physical therapies often result in measured improvements in UE skills of hemiplegic individuals, those skills frequently fail to be employed after the individual leaves the therapeutic environment.[10,11] CIMT, with both restraint and motor skill shaping, produced long-term changes in both motor skills and everyday use of the affected limb.[1-7]

Experts in the field of brain injury recovery and rehabilitation have explained the recovery of function by invoking neural plasticity as a general concept. Other than functional gains there was little direct evidence of what specific parameters of intervention produced CNS changes. Following the research of Merzenich and others,[12-14] literature developed that described, in intact and lesioned animals and humans, the conditions under which cortical representation for perception and action could be changed in fully developed individuals. Those basic science papers suggested that such reorganization occurred only when an extraordinary number of trials occurred in a

short period. For example, as a result of intense practice, expert string musicians show greater cortical representation of fingering hand's digits.[13] Such changes frequently required some alteration in the "expected" way a stimulation or action took place, for example in the position the targeted item is placed or in the timing of presentation of items.[12,14] In CIMT, the altered expectation is accomplished by applying a constraint to the unaffected extremity, thereby forcing the subject to use the affected extremity to accomplish tasks. CIMT clearly includes these attributes of intensity and altered "expectation" (i.e., the constraint). The links in adult stroke patients among constraint training, functional improvement, and brain reorganization have recently been further supported by direct brain-mapping techniques. Training following ischemic infarct resulted in expansion of the cortical representation of the digits to areas adjacent to the infarct, as measured by intracortical microstimulation in adult squirrel monkeys.[15] This change correlated with improvements in hand function. Transcranial magnetic stimulation mapping demonstrated an increase in cortical representation of hand musculature in stroke patients following CIMT.[1]

Successful CIMT trials with adults inevitably evokes the question, will this work with children? Despite approximately 40,000 American children (5-14 years old) with hemiplegia, the CIMT literature is dominat-

Article Reprint Information: Reprinted with permission from Karman, N., Maryles, J., Baker, R. W., Simpser, E., & Berger-Gross, P. (2003). Constraint-induced movement therapy for hemiplegic children with acquired brain injuries. *Journal of Head Trauma Rehabilitation, 18*(3), 259-267.

ed by studies of adults. Children become hemiplegic as a result of stroke in sickle cell disease, perinatal vascular events, head traumas, or other acquired brain injuries (ABIs). Concerns about a minimal cognitive level suitable to training, the tolerance of youngsters for this restrictive and intensive therapy, and the ethics of using any experimental paradigm in youngsters, has resulted in only two published papers concerning children.[16,17] Those studies only employed "average"-IQ children with hemiplegic cerebral palsy. More importantly, they did not attempt to replicate the most effective CIMT protocols, because they lacked both shaping techniques and the intensity of training applied in adult populations. Crocker et al.[16] attempted to use constraint without explicit shaping. Only one of Crocker's two young subjects tolerated the 3-week treatment, showing a long-term increase in voluntary control and spontaneous use of the affected UE. Charles et al.[17] employed constraint for only 6 hours per day and provided 2 hours of therapeutic activities without shaping. Two of three study children demonstrated improved hand function, all had an improved two-point discrimination threshold, but "real world" adaptive skills were not assessed.

In contrast to earlier work in children, we have adhered closely to the CIMT protocol developed by Taub for the research program at the University of Alabama. The preliminary nature of this study of children made the use of experimental controls somewhat premature. Three of seven subjects had reached a plateau after long periods of standard therapies aimed at improving upper extremity function. These seven well-documented cases could demonstrate the likelihood that children have the capacity for persevering and progressing during CIMT. We will use individual case material to show the roles age, cognitive level, time since injury, type of injury, and psychosocial factors play in training adherence and functional improvement.

Beyond the lack of background concerning criteria for applying CIMT in children with TBI or other ABIs, young people present unique challenges to the goal of constant constraint and 6 hours per day of shaping activities. Children attend school, children should play and socialize, and (especially) younger children cannot be expected to perform tedious tasks for long periods. These unique challenges lead to our creation of a child-centered program that:

- "pushed-in" through all of the everyday activities of the child
- trained nontherapist staff (e.g., teachers,

recreation staff), friends, and families who were familiar to the children, from their school, nursing unit, and recreational activities to be "lay shapers"
- employed these individuals in their regular settings based upon the practical concerns raised in the CIMT and rehabilitation literature[18]
- minimized embarrassment caused by wearing a constraining device at all times; mitts were used and were often decorated with stickers, written messages, or self-selected designs
- provided a number of sessions involving parents and children in exposure to the constraining equipment and sample tasks to prepare them (especially cognitively compromised and younger children) for the training.

The main objectives of this investigation were to demonstrate that children could tolerate a standard CIMT protocol and to assess the effectiveness of CIMT in children with ABIs.

Methods

Research participants

This study was approved by the St. Mary's Healthcare System for Children Institutional Review Board. Seven successive children, admitted to the TBI unit for rehabilitation, who met criteria were enrolled. Six were admitted for subacute rehabilitation directly from acute care facilities. One "graduate" of the TBI rehabilitation program was readmitted for the purpose of undergoing CIMT after she reached inclusion criteria (21 months after injury and 1 year after her discharge from the rehabilitation unit). Participating children were screened by one of the investigators for possible inclusion by diagnosis of hemiplegia, examining active movement, asymmetry of hand function, and interest in participation. Prospective subjects were required to demonstrate some active movement in the impaired UE. Subjects were requested to lift their arm or to reach for the examiner's hand. Children who demonstrated initiation of movement, regardless of active range of motion or degree of synergy of movement, were included, as long as they could demonstrate volitional grasp and release. Asymmetry of hand function was measured by observation during motor tasks and by family/patient reports.

Ability to follow simple instructions and to attend to a task for at least 3 minutes was required for inclusion in this study. Although formal cognitive testing was performed as part of the admission assessment

for each patient, scores were not consulted before enrollment in this study.

After being identified as a possible subject, the child and his or her guardians were interviewed by the researchers to explain the methods and possible effects of the CIMT study and to determine interest. Then informed consent (and, if developmentally appropriate, assents) was obtained. Subjects were solicited without regard to their injury etiology, age, or cognitive capacities (though all could minimally understand and agree to the treatment). Three children were Hispanic, two were African-American, and two were Caucasian. Five lived in New York City and two lived in nearby suburbs of Long Island. Three children had sustained traumatic head injuries, two had had cerebrovascular events resulting from arteriovenous malformations, and two had had strokes. Four subjects were independently ambulatory; one with an assistive device. The three that were not independently ambulatory were maintained in their wheelchairs during the treatment day, but walked occasionally during nontreatment times. The child who used an assistive device, and the three children who were not independent ambulators, removed the mitt from their unimpaired hands while walking and replaced it when seated. Three had right (dominant)-sided and four had left (nondominant)-sided impairment. Table 1 provides individual subject characteristics.

Measures

Participants were assessed before treatment using the actual amount of use test (AAUT) as described by Taub et al.[19,20] The 18 AAUT items are scored for amount of use (AOU) with a 3-point scale and for quality of movement (QOM) with a 6-point scale (Tables 2 and 3, respectively). The 15 activities and the 3 other qualitative items were videotaped unobtrusively during the AAUT's upper extremity tasks (e.g., folding paper, opening a box, removing a videotape from its jacket, lifting a photo album, placing pictures in an album, writing). Upon completion of the 2-week CIMT training period, the AAUT was again administered to the children while they were unobtrusively videotaped. Pretraining and posttraining videotapes were scored separately by the two therapist authors. Both of these therapists had extensive pediatric TBI rehabilitation experience and underwent CIMT protocol training with members of the University of Alabama research staff. Intraclass reliability coefficients, measuring the degree of agreement between the two raters, for all of the items of each scale of

Table 1.
Characteristics of subjects

Subject	Age	Gender	Injury	Impaired upper extremity	Dominance before injury	Time after injury	Impairments	IQ	Shaping hours provided
S1	14 yr	F	Tr	R	R	2 yr	T, N, grasp	50	58
S2	9 yr, 9 mo	F	Tr	L	R	6 mo	T, N	60	45
S3	17 yr, 10 mo	M	Tr	R	R	4 wk	N	103	52
S4	15.5 yr	F	CVA	L	R	25 days	T, N	75	50
S5	12 yr	F	AVM	L	R	4 wk	T, N		45
S6	7 yr, 8 mo	M	AVM	L	R	4 wk	T (index finger), N	102	49
S7	13 yr	F	CVA	R	R	15 wk	F, N, grasp aphasic	70	41

Note: Tr, trauma; T, increased tone; N, neglect; CVA, cerebrovascular accident; AVM, arteriovenous malformation; F, flaccid.

the AAUT were obtained (two-way mixed model) to assure the reliability of outcome measure. Interrater reliability for items was high for both conditions of the two assessments (intraclass reliability coefficients: pretraining AOU = .96; posttraining AOU = .99; pretraining QOM = .91; posttraining QOM = .97; all $P < .001$). Because the interrater item reliability was quite high, mean ratings were generated for each item and used for data analysis.

Procedures

The 2-week treatment period began with the full-time use of a Posey mitt to prevent use of the less-impaired hand during all waking hours and the initiation of supervised shaping for 6 hours every weekday. All everyday activities were performed with the impaired hand; the more difficult tasks were modified to accommodate the patients' limitations (e.g., drinking from a straw to avoid spilling). Shaping exercises that targeted identified weaknesses of the particular patient and that progressively increased in difficulty were administered by the rehabilitation (occupational therapy, physical therapy, speech therapy, mental health), educational, recreation, and volunteer staff of St. Mary's Hospital for Children.

Recreational and educational material (e.g., computer keyboards, games, instruments, arts and crafts, sports) were selected by the staff administering the shaping sessions, taking into account the likes and dislikes of the individual child. Tasks included keyboarding, beading, writing, drawing, ball toss, manipulative games, card handling, bubble wrap popping, and sticker play. Tasks were selected to minimize cognitive demands and to place demands for controlled movements of the fingers, wrists, forearm, elbow, and shoulder. The person administering the shaping task modified activities to minimize frustration by allowing success on the part of the subject. Tasks included in the AAUT were excluded from

Table 2.
Amount of use scale ratings

0	Subject does not attempt to use affected arm to carry out task
1	Subject moves affected arm during task, but use of the affected arm is rudimentary and nonfunctional
2	Subject uses affected arm to carry out task, and the use of the affected arm is functional at some level. Subject uses affected UE at least 20% of the time that task is performed

Table 3.
Quality of Movement (QOM) Scale

0	Does not attempt with involved arm
1	Involved arm was moved during task, but not helpful (very poor)
2	The involved arm was of some use during the task, but needed some help from the stronger arm, moved very slowly or with difficulty, or required more than 2 attempts to complete (poor)
3	The involved arm was used for the purpose indicated, but the movements were influenced to some degree by syngery, or the movements were slow or were made only with some effort (fair)
4	The movements made by the involved arm were almost normal, but not quite as fast or accurate as normal
5	The involved arm was used for the task and the movement appeared to be normal (for the determination of normal, the uninvolved limb can be utilized as an available index for comparison, with premorbid limb dominance taken into consideration)

shaping. During shaping exercises, specific feedback including knowledge of results (i.e., speed, precision, magnitude) was provided continuously.

Staff and family members were instructed to remove the mitt for up to 5 minutes when a child complained of discomfort, or to offer small rewards (usually stickers or tokens) to avoid removal of the mitt. Over the weekend, unit and recreation staff members were instructed to maintain the mitt on the unimpaired hand for all waking hours. They were further instructed to encourage use of the impaired hand and were provided materials and activities for task practice.

Although at least 4 hours of CIMT were delivered per day by professional therapy staff, a significant portion of shaping practice was carried out by teachers, teaching assistants, nursing assistants, recreation staff, and parents. All rehabilitation professionals and all of the others administering CIMT training were instructed in appropriate task selection, use of feedback to enhance performance (i.e., shaping), and the importance of compliance in delivery

of all scheduled treatment hours. Training included individual instruction and videotaped examples. The authors observed training everyday for deviations from protocol and practice improvement. Shapers were required to submit record forms documenting the activities employed, time per activity, and numeric measures of shaping toward improved performance (e.g., greater number, speed, accuracy) for each hour of intervention (see Table 1).

Statistical analysis plan

Mean item ratings were used to obtain pretraining and posttraining overall scores for the AOU and QOM scale scores. This sample is too small to reliably test single score measures (i.e., AOU and QOM) with a repeated measure statistic. Consequently, no statistical test on scale means was planned. Means and standard deviations obtained for the seven children on the AOU and QOM before and after training would only be used to obtain a Cohen's d for estimating the "effect size" of the training.[21] With a small subject sample and no expec-

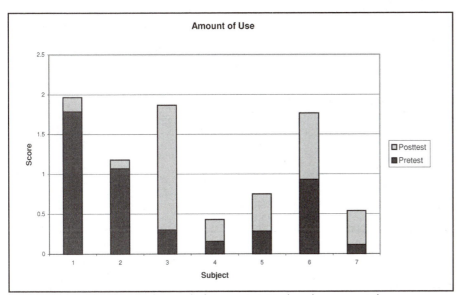

Fig 1. Amount of use at baseline and after constraint-induced movement therapy.

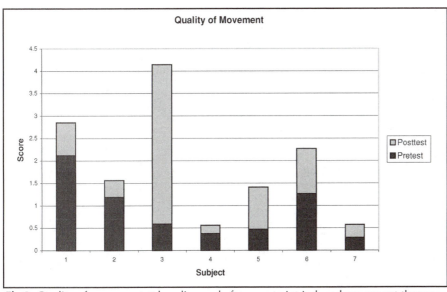

Fig 2. Quality of movement at baseline and after constraint-induced movement therapy.

tation of normal distributions, we planned to use the Wilcoxon sign-rank test for differences between (expectedly correlated) pretraining and posttraining item scores. Wilcoxon tests were planned to compare each child's before-training and after-training item scores for the AOU and the QOM. Analyses were two-tailed, with α set at .05.

Results

All seven children increased their AOU and QOM scores between the pretraining and posttraining period (Figs. 1 and 2, respectively). The mean item rating (used instead of the total score, because clinical factors led to different numbers of items being collected for certain subjects) on the AOU increased from 0.67 (standard deviation [SD] = 0.87) to 1.23 (SD = 0.92) indicating a large effect size (Cohen's d = .64). The mean item rating on the QOM increased from 0.96 (SD = 1.08) to 1.96 (SD = 1.63) with a large effect size (Cohen's d = .97). Three children showed significant differences and one showed a trend toward significance on AOU (Wilcoxon signed-ranks test: subject (S)3: P = .001; S4: P = .046, S5: P = .066; S6: P = .006; two-tailed). Four of the children showed a significant number of improved task performances and one showed a near significant trend on the QOM scale after training (S1: P = .013; S3: P = .001; S4: P = .083; S5: P = .024; S6: P = .009; two-tailed).

Discussion

These preliminary data suggest the promise of CIMT in the treatment of children with hemiparesis and some residual hand function. Despite regular fluctuations in motivation, very significant residual neuropsychologic deficits, and intellectual levels varying from average to mildly retarded, these children showed an effect of treatment that was clinically and psychometrically large. Several of the children were discomforted by the mitt restraint and all needed constant encouragement and concrete rewards. The oldest boy managed to misplace two mitts and then another accidentally fell into the ocean during a fishing trip! Nevertheless, he worked diligently during training and improved significantly. It was impossible to record every instance that the mitts were removed, but all nursing staff members were required to document observations of the mitt having been removed for more than 15 minutes. All of the children wore the mitt the vast majority of all waking hours, but S3 and S7 had about 10%-20% nonadherence during nontreatment times. The children appeared to maintain a high level of intrinsic motivation through the sets of shaping trials, driven by a competitive desire to best their previous scores.

In looking at the two children who failed to show significant improvement, we noted that neither had a parent that was able to provide shaping instruction. One of the parents actively attempted to interfere with training, to protect the child from the difficult work. Without parental support, these children were often observed during evening hours without their mitts; these parents also failed to support as much practice. Beyond the individual's characteristics, the AOU portion of the AAUT provides only one scale step between a no use score and a normal score (0 and 2, respectively). This restricted range made it very difficult to show improvement in children with some initial UE functional skills as well as to demonstrate the magnitude of change in some subjects who had actually made large functional gains. The subject that made the greatest amount of practical gains (S1) did not appear to have made as much improvement according to her AAUT scores. The subject who demonstrated the greatest amount of change was the most motivated subject in the group. Long-term follow-up of subjects was not possible in most cases, because of family moves with no forwarding address. One subject maintained close contact with the facility after discharge, and demonstrated continued improvement after the intervention. She now writes with her impaired hand, and her handwriting and artwork samples continue to show improving fine motor control. Despite instructional readings, training sessions with practice exercises and expert demonstrations, therapists, teachers, recreation staff, and parents all needed regular supervisory feedback to address their poor appreciation of the difference between practice and shaping.

Of the numerous scientific and pragmatic issues that must be addressed, the need for single-blinded controlled studies in children with ABIs that show reliable evidence of stability in UE function before intervention is foremost. The relationship between functional gains and CIMT will be supported by improving the documentation of UE function stability (before CIMT) through multiple baseline evaluations and standard therapy control subjects. We anticipate that larger samples and additional outcome measures will provide more precise information about the role of training parameters, age at injury, time since injury, and child and family characteristics in the improvement shown in distinct motor subdomains (e.g., ROM, targeting accuracy, pincer control). Because real-world use of rehabilitation trained skills is poor,[10] functional use tests (e.g., AAUT) should be supplemented by structured in vivo observational data concerning adaptive use of the affected limb. Future controlled efforts will avoid our limitation in being unable to provide scorers who were blinded to subjects' experimental status. Rather, we employed the only two trained AAUT scorers at the institution, who were involved in all phases of this study. Functional magnetic resonance imaging scanning in conjunction with CIMT may offer unique opportunities to understand cortical reorganization in children after brain injury.

Practical issues in increasing opportunities for CIMT research include the prohibitive expense of 6 hours per day of rehabilitation service and the lack of procedural control over how each therapist delivers a task. CIMT protocols have specified tasks for the participating therapists and intensity of training, but we intend to produce a complete manual that describes and provides means of documentation for task descriptions, task modifications for physical needs, and successive criteria points in all relevant training dimensions (e.g., speed, strength, accuracy, adaptive targeting). We believe that this will systematize the treatment for research purposes and provide clearer guidelines to clinicians who each use the tasks in their own idiosyncratic ways. A manualized protocol for a treatment that provides observable results in a short time frame would mobilize families, friends and community-based pediatric providers to pitch in to help provide treatment. Training nonprofessionals to provide shaping under professional supervision is a model that may address critical financial concerns.[22] These classes of individuals provide unique motivational influences for children, show high levels of interest in providing help, and render the treatment more contextually relevant to children's lives.

Though generalization of this study's findings is limited by the modest sample and lack of experimental controls, we have demonstrated the successful implementation of a rigorous CIMT protocol and its apparent effectiveness in children. We have shown that with the supervision of qualified professionals, people who are not rehabilitation experts, including parents, recreational workers, and teachers, can provide substantial hours of intervention. In fact, parental involvement and support of the CIMT program may be a key component of treatment effectiveness in children.

References

1. Liepert J, Bauder H, Wolfgang HR, et al. Treatment-induced cortical reorganization after stroke in humans. *Stroke.* 2000;31:1210-1216.
2. Kunkel A, Kopp B, Muller G, et al. Constraint-induced movement therapy for motor recovery in chronic stroke patients. *Arch Phys Med Rehabil.* 1999;80:624-628.
3. Wolf SL, Lecraw DE, Barton LA, et al. Forced use of hemiplegic upper extremities to reverse the effect of learned nonuse among chronic stroke and head-injured patients. *Exp Neurol.* 1989;104:125-132.
4. Morris DM, Crago JE, DeLuca SC, et al. Constraint-induced movement therapy for motor recovery after stroke. *NeuroRehabilitation.* 1997;9:29-43.
5. Blakeslee S. Therapies push injured brains and spinal cords into new paths. *New York Times.* August 28, 2001, Section F, p. 6.
6. Francisco GE, Shutter L, Wiggs L. *Constraint-induced movement therapy: Does it work in brain injury rehabilitation?* Symposium at the Annual Brain Injury Association Meeting: 2000, Chicago, IL.
7. Duncan PW. Synthesis of intervention trials to improve motor recovery following stroke. *Top Stroke Rehabil.* 1997;3:1-20.
8. Knapp HD, Taub E, Berman AJ. Movements in monkeys with deafferented forelimbs. *Exp Neurol.* 1963;7:305-315.
9. Taub E. Somatosensory deafferentiation research with monkeys: Implications for rehabilitation medicine. In: Ince LP, ed. *Behavioral psychology in rehabilitation medicine: Clinical applications.* New York: Williams & Wilkins; 1980.
10. Dunkin BH. Focused stroke rehabilitation programs do not improve outcome. *Arch Neurol.* 1989;46:801-703.
11. Andrews K, Stewart J. Stroke recovery: He can but does he? *Rheumatol Rehabil.* 1970;18:43-38.
12. Merzenich MM, Nelson RJ, Stryker MP, et al. Somatosensory cortical map changes following digit amputation in adult monkeys. *J Comparative Neurol.* 1984;224:591-605.
13. Elbert T, Pantev C, Wienbruch C, et al. Increased use of the left hand in string players associated with increased cortical representation of the fingers. *Science.* 1995;270:302-307.
14. Flor H, Elbert S, Knecht C, et al. Phantom limb pain as a perceptual correlate of massive cortical reorganization in upper limb amputees. *Nature.* 1995;375:482-484.
15. Nudo RJ, Wise BM, SiFuentes F, et al. Neural substrates for the effects of rehabilitation training on motor recovery following ischemic infarct. *Science.* 1996;272:1791-1794.
16. Crocker MD, MacKay-Lyons M, McDonnell E. Forced use of the upper extremity in cerebral palsy: A single case design. *Am J Occup Ther.* 1997;51:824-833.
17. Charles J, Lavinder G, Gordon A. Effects of constraint-induced therapy on hand function in children with hemiplegic cerebral palsy. *Pediatr Phys Ther.* 2001;13:68-76.
18. Blosser JL, DePompei R. A proactive model for treating communication disorders in children and adolescents with traumatic brain injury. *Clin Commun Disorders.* 1992;2:52-65.
19. McCullock K, Cook EW III, Fleming WC, et al. A reliable test of upper extremity ADL function [abstract]. *Arch Phys Med Rehabil.* 1988;69:755.
20. Taub E, DeLuca S, Crago JE. *Actual amount of use test (AAUT).* 1996. (Available from Edward Taub, Psychology Department, UAB, CH415, 11300 8th Ave. S., Birmingham, AL 35294).
21. Cohen J. *Statistical power analysis for the behavioral sciences.* 2d ed. Mahwah, NJ: Lawrence Erlbaum; 1980.
22. Holland D. The cost-effective delivery of rehabilitation psychology services: The responsible utilization of paraprofessionals. *Rehabil Psychol.* 1998;43:232-245.

From the General to the Specific: Using Meta-Analytic Reports in Clinical Decision Making

Linda Tickle-Degnen

The purpose of this article is to describe how health practitioners can interpret the results from published meta-analytic reports of intervention effectiveness and efficacy studies, and then communicate those results, in a manner that helps patients make critical clinical and life decisions. The problem of using research evidence in clinical decision making is one of moving from generalized findings about intervention effectiveness to a prediction for a specific patient. To move toward a reasonable prediction, practitioners need information from a meta-analytic report that enables them to identify and understand the distribution of outcome results that are most applicable to a specific patient. Relevancy, effectiveness, and interpretation forms of information are discussed in this article. The focus is on the interpretation of the effect size statistics d and r for understanding the variation in responses that the patient might experience with an intervention.

Author's note: Address correspondence to: Linda Tickle-Degnen, Ph.D., OTR, Department of Occupational Therapy, Sargent College of Health and Rehabilitation Sciences, Boston University, 635 Commonwealth Ave., Boston, MA 02138; e-mail: tickle@bu.edu.

In 1982, the evolutionary biologist Stephen J. Gould was diagnosed with abdominal mesothelioma, a form of cancer. On review of the medical literature, he found a "brutal message" (Gould, 1996, p. 47): The disease was incurable and had a median mortality of 8 months following diagnosis. He reported that the common interpretation of this message would be "I will most probably be dead in 8 months." His own interpretation, however, was informed by a recognition that the median is a measure of central tendency and does not describe the variation of mortality outcomes. He focused on the fact that some individuals lived for quite a long time after the diagnosis and interpreted the literature with a variation perspective:

Central tendency is an abstraction, variation the reality . . . I am not a measure of central tendency, either mean or median. I am one single human being with mesothelioma, and I want a best assessment of my own chances—for I have personal decisions to make, and my business cannot be dictated by abstract averages. I need to place myself in the most probable region of the variation based upon particulars of my own case; I must not simply assume that my personal fate will correspond to some measure of central tendency. (pp. 48-49)

If Gould had been less statistically sophisticated, he may have read the literature about mesothelioma and come away from that reading with the common interpretation of death in 8 months. Consequently, he may have resigned himself to his fate and then lived with the full expectation of impending death. The course he in fact followed was to attempt to position himself on the low mortality end of the distribution of results. Perhaps because he chose to try a new experimental treatment, or for other reasons, Gould is alive, almost two decades after his initial diagnosis, a prolific scholar, researcher, and teacher.

Gould's description of his personal experience and his reaction to the message of the research literature illustrate the central problem surrounding the use of a body of published research findings for making clinical decisions. This problem is to select and apply to a specific patient the generalized findings from studies of groups of patients that did not include the patient who is currently seeking clinical care (Glasziou et al., 1998; Mant, 1999; Rosser, 1999; Sackett, Richardson, Rosenberg, & Haynes, 1997). When patients seek the help of a health practitioner, they need information about their personal chances of increasing their survival time; of reducing physical, cognitive, or emotional impairments; of improving their performance in daily living activities; or of deriving more satisfaction from their lives. They need information to choose interventions that will maximize the potential for beneficial outcomes.

The purpose of this article is to describe how practitioners, who are the primary conduit of information from the research literature to the patient, can interpret the results from published meta-analytic reports with a variation perspective and communicate those results in a manner that helps patients make critical clinical and life decisions. Meta-analytic reports are particularly useful to practitioners for timely decision making because they provide efficient access to a large body of evidence that has been synthesized using systematic procedures. For the sake of focus, this article is about the use of meta-analytic reports of clinical intervention outcomes rather than about the use of reports concerned with the measurement properties of diagnostic tests or with risk factors associated with disease onset (although the variation perspective is relevant across all types of meta-analytic reports used in clinical decision making). Furthermore, because I work and teach practitioners in the area of medical, psychiatric, and pediatric rehabilitation, I have focused on meta-analytic reports related to intervention outcomes that are usually measured on a continuous scale, such as quality of life, rather than on a dichotomous scale, such as survival. Gould's life-or-death predicament is a riveting clinical example, yet the need for a variation interpretation of the research literature is just as critical in the seemingly mundane affairs of daily living.

Although in recent years there has been increasing attention in the literature to the problem of how to apply results from population-based studies to the individual client, most of this attention has been directed toward physician decision making, often with pharmacological or surgical treatments, biomedical outcomes, and statistics used in an epidemiological statistical paradigm (Glasziou et al., 1998; Mant, 1999; Rosser, 1999; Sackett et al., 1997). Although this literature is informative to practitioners in rehabilitation, many rehabilitation practitioners who are making decisions with clients are not physicians, but rather are therapists, nurses, and social workers. They apply physical, psychological, and social interventions that are often concerned primarily with quality-of-life outcomes and are trained in statistics used in a behavioral science paradigm. This article is meant to extend the discussion of the clinical use of research findings to the decision making made by a variety of health practitioners.

The Information Needs of Practitioners

Practitioners need at least three forms of information from a meta-analytic report to make a variation interpretation of the results and communicate it to patients. They can use this information to identify and understand the distribution of outcome results that are most applicable to the case of a specific patient. More important, from this information they can produce an evidence-based hypothesis about the patient's probable success with a given intervention and communicate this hypothesis during decision-making interactions. The content of this article consists of describing how practitioners can find and use the information in meta-analytic reports to make a variation interpretation. The three forms of information that they must find and use are the following:

1. *Relevancy information.* This type of information describes the circumstances and attributes of the research participants involved in the studies included in the meta-analytic report. The practitioner can use this type of information to determine the degree to which the circumstances and attributes of a specific patient were represented in the primary (single) studies compiled in the meta-analysis.

2. *Effectiveness information.* This type of information describes how research participants responded to intervention, particularly participants whose situation was most relevant to the specific patient. The practitioner can use this type of information to hypothesize about the specific patient's probability of responding favorably to an intervention.

3. *Interpretation information.* This type of information explains the statistical results of the meta-analysis. The practitioner can use this type of information to make a variation interpretation of the findings.

Although a meta-analytic report may not include all three forms of information in the detail that I describe below, recent advances in the methodological conduct and reporting of meta-analyses promise to make this level of reporting detail common practice (Cooper & Hedges, 1994; Moher et al., 1999; Pogue & Yusuf, 1998; Stock, Benito, & Lasa, 1996; Stroup et al., 2000). Meta-analytic reports have become more usable for clinical decision making, particularly within the past 5 years.

Need No. 1: Are the Conditions and Attributes of This Specific Patient Represented in the General Sample?

One of the strengths of a meta-analytic report is that it represents the outcomes of a large number of research participants whose circumstances differed from one another (Hall, Rosenthal, Tickle-Degnen, & Mosteller, 1994). Besides having participated in different research studies, these participants may have varied in their personal attributes, in the type of intervention they experienced, or in the type of outcome that was monitored. The practitioner seeking information about the value of a particular intervention for a specific patient from a meta-analytic report must first know the degree of fit between the specific patient's situation and those of the research participants compiled in the meta-analytic report. They should review the report with the following questions in mind (see also Sackett et al., 1997):

1. Were there research participants that were of the same clinical population, gender, age, ethnicity, and socioeconomic status, as my specific patient? The types of attributes in this list would be the ones that theoretically would be most related to intervention outcomes. For example, patients who have experienced strokes may have a very different response to a hand therapy intervention compared with patients with work-related hand injuries. Males may have very different outcomes than females in an intervention designed to improve interpersonal relations. Older adults may have different responses to an assertiveness training program than younger adults.

2. Were there interventions that would be practical and suitable for my specific patient's life circumstances, values, skills, and interests and that would be feasible for me to implement in my clinical setting? This list would be highly personalized in relation to the patient, the diagnosis, and the clinical context. For example, a practitioner may be looking for information about the efficacy of interventions for improving independent participation in daily living activities among working-age adults with disabilities. The practitioner may want to know the location of the intervention (e.g., home, community, or clinic), the content of the intervention (e.g., training during actual performance of daily activities or lectures on how to do the activities), or the nature of the time commitment for patient and practitioner.

3. Were there outcome measures pertinent to my specific patient's needs? For example, if the outcome of interest was to improve a child's ability to socialize with children other than siblings, were there measures of change in peer social skills, or were the measures primarily associated with social behavior in the family?

Meta-analytic reports typically address these relevancy information needs by describing the characteristics of the primary studies compiled in the meta-analysis. One location of this information is in the methods section, where there is usually a list of inclusion and exclusion criteria. These criteria describe what types of research participants, interventions, and outcome measures were acceptable for inclusion within the meta-analysis. From this information, the practitioner can learn whether the meta-analytic report is at all relevant to the specific case.

Relevancy information is also included in the results section of a report, where there is usually a summary of the primary studies' characteristics. In the text of this section, total numbers, percentages, ranges, and averages describe the participants, interventions, and measures across the spectrum of studies. From a clinical-use perspective, the most valuable presentation of relevancy information is a table that lists information separately for each study. In this table, there are columns that identify primary study authors, year of publication, and information about the most relevant categories associated with intervention outcomes. The practitioner can scan this table to rank the studies from most to least relevant for a specific case, and if interested, use the author and year citations to retrieve and directly read the most relevant primary studies. One advantage of using meta-analytic evidence, however, is that it allows the practitioner to see the evidence from many studies all at once, without having to retrieve each primary study. Using the table, the practitioner can compare the single study with the entire set of other studies. This comparison helps the practitioner to identify whether the findings of the studies most relevant to the client are different or similar to the findings of less relevant studies. If the findings are similar, the practitioner may feel comfortable with generalizing the overall results of the meta-analysis to many different clients, including the specific client of interest.

Unfortunately, the table form of presentation is not feasible when the meta-analysis involves a large number of primary studies (perhaps more than 30), particularly if the journal in which the report has appeared operates under a strict manuscript length requirement. In that case, the practitioner must rely on summarized information in the text and on title names of primary studies that are listed in the reference section or appendices of the report. The content of the titles of primary studies may give a lead as to which studies are most relevant to the specific patient, but the attributes and findings of the studies cannot be easily and quickly compared.

Need No. 2: How Did Research Participants Who Were Similar to the Specific Patient Respond to Intervention?

The second information need of the practitioner is to determine the effectiveness of the intervention, especially for people like the specific patient. One important quality of meta-analysis is that its compilation of different primary studies enables the meta-analytic researcher to systematically examine several sources of variation in the effectiveness of an intervention, sources that individual primary studies had not necessarily examined. The findings of studies A and B may vary from one another simply because of sampling error (chance), differences in the quality of their research designs and internal validity, or differences in the attributes of their participants, interventions, or outcome measures. The meta-analyst conducts a statistical test of homogeneity (e.g., Shadish & Haddock, 1994) to decide whether the differences between effectiveness in studies is likely to be due to sampling error or not. If the results of this test, usually reported in the text or tables of the results section, suggest that the variation is likely to be due to sampling error, then the effects from all of the primary studies can be averaged and it is assumed that the best estimate of the effectiveness of the intervention is the overall average. Consequently, the effectiveness can be generalized with some confidence directly to a large number of intervention studies similar to those compiled

in the meta-analysis and, subsequently, indirectly to a large group of patients under diverse conditions. The practitioner can use the overall effectiveness estimate (i.e., the mean effect size) to develop a hypothesis about effectiveness for all types of patients included in the meta-analysis, including people like the specific patient. In other words, the findings for all studies are potentially useful for making an evidence-based hypothesis for the specific patient.

An alternative finding of the statistical test of homogeneity is that variation among studies is unlikely to be due to chance and is more likely to be due to some systematic source of variation. In this case, studies A and B have different findings that are probably due to some difference in the studies' designs, participants, interventions, or outcome measures. Often, meta-analysts examine this systematic variation through sensitivity or moderator analyses (Greenhouse & Iyengar, 1994). These analyses consist of breaking the studies down into subgroups on the basis of methodological features of the studies (such as type of research design and whether participants and practitioners in the study were blind to hypotheses) or features of the study that theoretically may be associated with differences in intervention effectiveness (such as attributes of the research participants, intervention, or outcome measures). The results of sensitivity or moderator analyses may enable the practitioner to determine which subgroups of study effects are most relevant for the specific patient (although see Oxman & Guyatt, 1992, for statistical concerns related to using subgroup analyses exclusively in decision making).

If the number of primary studies is not too large (perhaps less than 30), then effectiveness information is often presented in table form. If there is a column in the table that displays a statistical coefficient that describes the intervention effect (i.e., an effect size) for each primary study, in addition to the columns containing relevancy information, the practitioner can examine the range and average of the effects of the most relevant studies for the specific case. The practitioner who does this is performing a meta-analysis that is individualized for the specific patient on a subset of studies included in the report.

If the homogeneity test of the effect sizes within the meta-analysis suggests that subgroups of effects need not be examined (i.e., the effect sizes are relatively homogeneous), the practitioner derives a hypothesis for the specific patient's probability of benefiting from the intervention from the mean

effect size for the entire group of primary studies. If, on the other hand, the homogeneity test suggests that subgroups of effects should be examined (i.e., the effect sizes are somewhat heterogeneous), the practitioner derives a hypothesis from the mean effect size for the subgroup or subgroups of studies that are most relevant to the specific patient's case.

Need No. 3: What Are the Meanings of the Statistical Results for a Variation Interpretation?

The third type of information that a practitioner needs is information about how to interpret the statistics. Practitioners may not have specialized statistical training to translate meta-analytic statistics into usable interpretations. More and more frequently, as meta-analysts are producing their reports for clinical use and policy development, not only for research and theory development purposes, they include these translations in either the results or discussion section (McCartney & Rosenthal, 2000; Ottenbacher & Jannell, 1993).

From a clinical perspective, the major result of meta-analyses of intervention outcomes is the mean of the effect size estimates calculated for primary studies.[1] There are different types of effect size estimates, but the most common ones for outcomes that are measured on a continuous scale (such as physical strength, cognitive performance, independence in activities of daily living, or life satisfaction) are the effect size *d* and the effect size *r*. The mean effect size, whether it is an average *d* or *r*, contains two pieces of information: one piece that translates easily into a central tendency interpretation and a second piece that translates more readily into a variation interpretation.

The mean effect size indicates whether, on the average, participants who received the intervention condition had better outcomes than participants who received a control condition. Better average outcomes for the intervention versus control conditions are indicated by a positive mean effect size, equal average outcomes by a zero mean effect size, and worse average outcomes by a negative mean effect size, regardless of whether the effect size is measured as a *d* or an *r*. A central tendency interpretation of the effect size, akin to the kind that Gould (1996) discussed, is one that relies solely on the sign and zero versus nonzero status of the effect size for drawing a conclusion about effectiveness. This interpretation would be something like

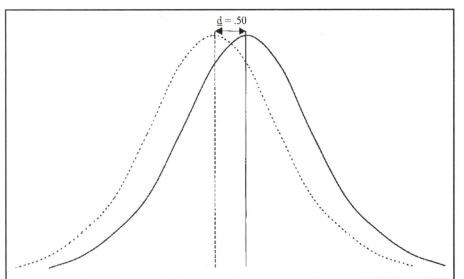

Figure 1: The Effect Size d. NOTE: The dashed normal curve represents the control group outcomes and the solid line curve represents the intervention group outcomes. The vertical straight lines through the peaks of the distributions are the average outcome score for each group, respectively. The effect size *d* is a measure of the difference, in standard deviation units, between the average response of the control versus intervention participants. In this example, the averages of the two distributions differ by one half of a standard deviation (.50).

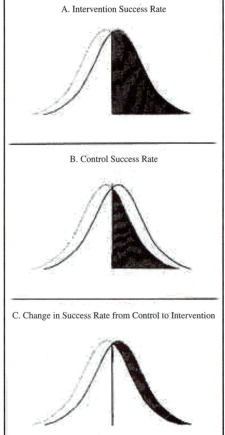

Figure 2: Success Rates of the Control and Intervention Conditions. NOTE: Dashed curve shows control group distribution of outcomes. Solid curve shows intervention group distribution of outcomes. Panel A shows the portion of the response distribution for the intervention condition that is above the average response of the entire sample (control plus intervention). For *d* = .50, approximately 60% of the scores fall above this average. Panel B shows the portion of the distribution for the control condition that is above average: here, approximately 40% of the responses. Panel C shows the difference between the portions shown in Panels A and B. This portion is roughly equivalent to the effect size *r*.

this: "The intervention works," for a positively signed effect size; "The intervention does not work," for a zero effect size; or "The intervention is harmful," for a negatively signed effect size. The problem with this interpretation is that it is drawn simply from the average outcomes of groups of participants in the intervention conditions compared with the average outcomes of groups of participants in the control conditions. It does not account for the fact that there were variations among individuals in these conditions, with many participants in the studies performing below and above the average within each condition.

It is the magnitude of the mean effect size (i.e., how big it is) that indicates variation of research participants' responses. Specifically, it is a measure of the variation of responses between intervention and control conditions compared with the variation of individuals within each condition. More simply speaking, the effect size (*d* or *r*) is an estimate of the degree to which two conditions (such as intervention vs. control) differ in terms of their therapeutic effectiveness, or, alternatively, the degree to which involvement in intervention had a relatively more successful or beneficial outcome for research participants than involvement in a control condition. The terms *degree* and *relatively* are important in this case because they indicate that outcomes are variable rather than fixed or absolute. The variation

interpretations of these two effect sizes are given below.

The effect size d

The effect size *d* is the difference between the mean outcomes for two conditions in standard deviation units. Figure 1 depicts *d* as the difference or distance between the two peaks of normally distributed outcomes. In Figure 1, the *d* is equal to .50, a medium-sized effect (Cohen, 1988). For this *d*, the average intervention outcome was one half of a standard deviation higher than the average control outcome. Because *d* is a standard normal deviate, it can be used with the information known about normal distributions to describe different characteristics of the variation of individuals' responses around the average outcomes. Cohen (1988, p. 23) provides three variation interpretations of *d* called *U* measures. These measures are percentages of participants under different areas of the curves of the distributions.[2]

I focus on one of the *U* measures here, *U*2, because, as will be shown, its interpretation can be very similar to the interpretation of the effect size *r*. When *d* is positive, the *U*2 measure describes the percentage of participants in the intervention condition whose scores were successful. Success is defined here as receiving a score that is higher than the combined average of both the intervention and control condition.[3] For

a *d* of .50, the *U*2 is approximately 60%. In other words, 60% of the participants who received intervention had a successful outcome. *U*2 can also be used to calculate the percentage of participants in the control condition who had a successful outcome. The successful outcome for the control condition is 100% minus *U*2. Therefore, when *d* is .50, the success rate of participants in the control condition is 40% (100% – 60%). Figure 2 shows where these percentages are coming from in the two distributions. Be-

Table 1
Effect Sizes and Success Rates

Magnitude of Effect[a]	d[b]	Success Rates			r[f]	r Success Rates		
		Control[c] (%)	Intervention[d] (%)	Change[e] (%)		Control[g] (%)	Intervention[h] (%)	Change[e] (%)
Zero	0	50	50	0	0	50	50	0
Small	0.20	46	54	8	.10	45	55	10
Medium	0.50	40	60	20	.24	38	62	24
Large	0.80	34	66	32	.37	32	69	37
Very large	2.00	16	84	68	.71	15	86	71

NOTE: All calculations and estimations are based on the assumption of a binomial distribution of the outcome measure, with approximately equal number of cases and approximately equal variances within each condition. All rates here are success rates. To calculate failure rates, subtract any success rate from 100%.

[a] Interpretations of Cohen (1988) and Rosenthal and Rosnow (1991).

[b] $d = (M\text{intervention} - M\text{control})/\sigma$ pooled.

[c] d control success rate = 100% − U2.

[d] Intervention success rate = U2 (Cohen, 1988). U2 is the percentage of the population (one-tailed p) of cases falling above or below $z = d/2$ on a table of standard normal deviates (cumulative normal probabilities).

[e] Change in success rate = intervention rate − control rate. This change, divided by 100, is equal to the phi coefficient (a product-moment correlation) calculated from the dichotomous independent variable (intervention vs. control) and a dichotomized (median split) outcome variable. For d, the change rate is exact, given that the assumptions described in the Note are met. For r, the change rate is approximate (see Rosenthal & Rubin, 1982) because the r is actually based on a continuous outcome variable.

[f] r is the point-biserial correlation between the dichotomous independent variable and the continuous outcome variable (see Rosenthal, 1994, for various means of calculating r).

[g] r control success rate = 50% − ½(r*100), calculated from the Binomial Effect Size Display (Rosenthal & Rubin, 1982).

[h] r intervention success rate = 50% + ½(r*100), calculated from the Binomial Effect Size Display.

cause 60% minus 40% is equal to 20%, the success rate increases by 20% from the control to the intervention conditions.

The effect size r

The effect sizes d and r are two different ways of describing the same variation in outcomes. Whereas the d is a measure of difference, the r is a measure of association. The effect size r is a point-biserial correlation or partial correlation coefficient that indicates the degree to which the independent variable (intervention vs. control) is associated with the outcome scores (see Cohen, 1988, p. 23). An r of a small magnitude indicates a small association between intervention and outcome, whereas an r of a larger magnitude indicates a larger association.

Rosenthal and Rubin (1982) have shown that the magnitude of the r (multiplied by 100) can most easily be understood as an estimate of the change in success rates across two conditions. They created a simple, practical tool, called the Binomial Effect Size Display, for translating the effect size r into intervention success rates. Table 1 shows that for the same magnitude of intervention effect, the r-related rates are slightly different from the d-related rates, but either rate gives a useful approximation of the difference in success rates (see the Note of Table 1 for more explanation). For example, the medium effect of d at .50 is equal to an r of .24. The success rates for the

control group are 40% for d and 38% for r, the success rates for the intervention group are 60% for d and 62% for r, and, therefore, the change in success rates is 20% for d (60% − 40%) and 24% for r (62% − 38%). These rates are fairly close to one another.

In this example of $d = .50$ or $r = .24$, both effect size estimates indicate that the intervention was successful for more people than was the control condition and the failure rate was lower for the intervention than control condition, suggesting that for a large number of people the intervention was generally effective. Of crucial importance for a variation interpretation is that there were still a number of people (approximately 40%) for whom the intervention was not successful and a number of people (approximately 40%) whose outcome was successful even though they were in the control condition.

Variation around the mean effect size.

The effect sizes for separate studies tend to be different from one another, as discussed in the section on effectiveness information above. The true intervention effect size, the one that is likely to generalize to other instances of the intervention, is likely to fall within a range around the mean effect size. If a meta-analyst reports the confidence interval or a standard error, the practitioner can use the lower and upper range effect sizes of the interval to estimate the likely range of success rates for the

intervention compared with control conditions.[4] For example, if a group of studies had a mean effect size d of .50 and a 95% confidence interval of .20 to .80, then the practitioner could with some confidence infer that the true intervention success rate in the population would range between 54% and 66% (see Table 1). If a confidence interval or standard error is not included in the report, the practitioner could use the lowest and highest effect sizes (i.e., the range) in the most relevant group of studies to discuss variation in success rates.

Using a Variation Interpretation of the Meta-Analytic Evidence in Decision Making

The practitioner uses the relevancy, effectiveness, and interpretation information found in the meta-analytic report to develop a preliminary hypothesis about the specific patient's probable response to the intervention. After intervention, the specific patient may be more similar to the group of individuals who have a successful outcome or to the group of individuals who have an unsuccessful outcome. The likelihood of having a successful response to intervention is hypothesized to be the success rate or range of success rates found in the group of studies most relevant to the specific patient's circumstances. In addition, the practitioner can hypothesize about the specific patient's success rates for participating in alternative interventions or no intervention (the control success rate).

To help illustrate how hypothesis formulation could occur, consider the following potential scenario. A 65-year-old woman, Mrs. Jones, had a stroke (middle cerebral artery) 3 years ago. Due to declining ability to perform her activities of daily living, such as bathing, independently, she and her family are seeking rehabilitation therapy services. They are wondering whether it is worth the woman's effort to engage in a more intensive or less intensive program of physical and occupational therapy. She is willing to engage in a more intensive form of therapy if the outcomes are more likely to improve her independence in daily living activities. On searching the recent stroke literature, the practitioner finds a meta-analytic study by Kwakkel, Wagenaar, Koelman, Lankhorst, and Koetsier (1997) that investigated the effects of intensity of rehabilitation after stroke. Before formulating the hypothesis, the practitioner determines the relevancy of meta-analytic findings for Mrs. Jones's case. A table of study characteristics indicates that the age of the participants in the nine primary studies included in the meta-analysis averaged 66 years, close to Mrs. Jones's age. In addition, there were two studies (Wade, Collen, Robb, & Warlow, 1992; Werner & Kessler, 1996) that investigated rehabilitation approximately 3 to 4 years post stroke, with one of those studies (Werner & Kessler, 1996) entirely composed of participants with middle cerebral artery strokes. Among the outcome variables studied in the meta-analysis is the one of relevance to Mrs. Jones: activities of daily living.

After determining that the meta-analytic report is relevant for the case of Mrs. Jones, the practitioner determines the effectiveness of engaging in more versus less intensive rehabilitation. The overall finding for activity of daily living outcomes was a mean effect size d of .34 with a 95% confidence interval of .21 to .48.[5] From the positive sign of this range of effect sizes, with the confidence interval not inclusive of a zero effect size, it is appropriate to hypothesize that individuals with strokes are more likely to benefit from more intensive than from less intensive therapy. Kwakkel et al. (1997) reported that the test of homogeneity of the effect sizes is nonsignificant, indicating that the magnitude of the effect sizes varied by chance and not because of systematic variation. Therefore, the practitioner can feel somewhat confident that the mean effect size for the entire set of nine primary studies gives a reasonable estimate of the

effect of intensity for a wide variety of types of strokes, participants, and settings.

Once the potential effectiveness of intense rehabilitation is established, the practitioner can interpret the effect sizes with a variation perspective. For ease, the reported confidence interval for the mean effect size of .21 to .48 can be approximated to be from .20 to .50, for comparability to the success rates shown in Table 1 of the current article. From Table 1, we can see that approximately 54% to 60% of the participants in the more intensive program were likely to have successful activities of daily living outcomes, whereas approximately 40% to 46% in the less intensive program were likely to achieve successful outcomes. The range of these success rates indicates that although the majority of participants were likely to benefit from more versus less intensive therapy, it is a small to moderate majority, not a large majority.

Even though the effect sizes are relatively homogeneous across the primary studies, it is useful to look at the primary study results specifically for the Werner and Kessler (1996) study, which was most relevant to Mrs. Jones's case. Kwakkel et al. (1997) used a line graph to show the effect size and confidence interval for that study. From this line drawing, the mean effect size appears to be approximately .60, with a 95% confidence interval from .20 to 1.00, suggesting that people like Mrs. Jones may derive even more benefit from intensive therapy than people who have experienced other types of strokes and post stroke periods.

This body of meta-analytic evidence will not tell the practitioner whether intensive therapy will work for Mrs. Jones. Rather, it indicates the probability of the therapy working for a client like Mrs. Jones.[6] This probability forms the basis for a hypothesis to communicate to the patient. Communicating the hypothesis starts the dialogue for mutual decision making, taking into consideration the patient's concerns (also, see Tickle-Degnen, 1998, for other communication examples). In the case of Mrs. Jones, the practitioner might communicate the hypothesis in the following manner:

You asked me whether it is worth it to become involved in an intensive rehabilitation program. Your concern is understandable given the effort required to do the treatment. A recent review of the research on the effectiveness of intensive rehabilitation programs found that a minority of patients had positive results in their ability to do daily living activities with no treatment or less intensive treatment, whereas a small to moderate

majority of patients had positive results with intensive treatment. A study involving people like you, who had middle cerebral artery strokes, found a slightly larger majority of patients who received benefit from an intensive form of therapy. These results suggest that you may benefit from intensive therapy. However, you are unique. You may or may not benefit from a more intensive program of therapy. Let's talk more about the benefits and costs of you participating in this intensive program.

Conclusion

Gould (1996) stated, "Old distributions offer no predictions for new situations" (p. 50). It may be true that they offer no predictions in a deterministic sense; however, with caution, they offer material for the development of hypotheses about what may happen in a new situation. Certainly, old distributions offer one of many sources of information that generate possible solutions to patients' problems. From this perspective, the practitioner does not replace clinical expertise and wisdom with research results. Rather, the practitioner uses the research evidence gleaned from meta-analyses and primary studies with a variation perspective, and in an individualized manner, to supplement other individualized evidence (self and family report, clinical observation and testing, expert opinion, past experience) that exists about the patient.

Notes

1. This article is about the interpretation of effect sizes rather than significance tests of intervention effects. Effect sizes lend themselves to variation interpretations. On the other hand, significance tests (and their p values) lend themselves to a dichotomous decision about whether to trust the results. If trust is high (i.e., the p value is low), there is a general inclination to conclude that the intervention works. If the trust is low (i.e., a high p value), the inclination is to conclude that the intervention does not work. Such conclusions are inconsistent with a variation interpretation.

2. The calculation, description, and interpretation of the effect size measures are based on the assumption that responses follow a normal distribution within each condition. The U measures get larger in magnitude as the distribution of the scores in the intervention and control conditions become less overlapping (i.e., the distance or d between them gets larger).

3. The *U*3 measure can be used as a stricter criterion for success. In that case, success is defined as receiving a score that is higher than the intervention condition's average score.

4. No distinction is made here between fixed-effect versus random-effect confidence intervals. Fixed-effect intervals will be smaller than random-effect intervals. The random-effect intervals are more easily generalized to different forms of an intervention. For a technical discussion, see Cooper and Hedges (1994). If the meta-analyst uses a fixed-effect model, then the practitioner may want to think of the actual confidence interval as being larger than the reported confidence interval.

5. Kwakkel et al. (1997) calculated the effect size *g*, which is a *d* = index that is calculated with the sample rather than population standard deviation. The effect size discussed in the current paper was the one weighted by intensity of treatment.

6. This phrasing was suggested by an anonymous reviewer. It clarifies the importance of using the meta-analytic evidence for forming possible rather than absolute answers to difficult clinical questions, such as, "Will this intervention work with Mrs. Jones?"

References

Cohen, J. (1988). *Statistical power analysis for the behavioral sciences* (2nd ed.). Hillsdale, NJ: Erlbaum.

Cooper, H. M., & Hedges, L. V. (Eds.). (1994). *The handbook of research synthesis*. New York: Russell Sage.

Glasziou, P., Guyatt, G. H., Dans, A. L., Dans, L. F., Straus, S., & Sackett, D. L. (1998). Editorial: Applying the results of trials and systematic reviews to individual patients. *ACP Journal Club, 129*(3), A15-16.

Gould, S. J. (1996). *Full house: The spread of excellence from Plato to Darwin*. New York: Three Rivers.

Greenhouse, J. B., & Iyengar, S. (1994). Sensitivity analysis and diagnostics. In H. M. Cooper & L. V. Hedges (Eds.), *The handbook of research synthesis* (pp. 383-398). New York: Russell Sage.

Hall, J.A., Rosenthal, R., Tickle-Degnen, L., & Mosteller, F. (1994). Hypotheses and problems in research synthesis. In H. M. Cooper & L. V. Hedges (Eds.), *The handbook of research synthesis* (pp. 17-28). New York: Russell Sage.

Kwakkel, G., Wagenaar, R., Koelman, T. W., Lankhorst, G. J., & Koetsier, J. C. (1997). Effects of intensity of rehabilitation after stroke: A research synthesis. *Stroke, 28*, 1550-1556.

Mant, D. (1999). Can randomised trials inform clinical decisions about individual patients? *Lancet, 353*, 743-746.

McCartney, K., & Rosenthal, R. (2000). Effect size, practical importance, and social policy for children. *Child Development, 71*, 173-180.

Moher, D., Cook, D. J., Eastwood, S., Olkin, I., Rennie, D., & Stroup, D. F. for the QUOROM Group. (1999). Improving the quality of reports of meta-analyses of randomised controlled trials: The QUOROM statement. *Lancet, 354*, 1896-1900.

Ottenbacher, K. J., & Jannell, S. (1993). The results of clinical trials in stroke rehabilitation research. *Archives of Neurology, 50*, 37-44.

Oxman, A. D., & Guyatt, G. H. (1992). A consumer's guide to subgroup analyses. *Annals of Internal Medicine, 116*, 78-84.

Pogue, J., & Yusuf, S. (1998). Overcoming the limitations of current meta-analysis of randomised controlled trials. *Lancet, 351*, 47-52.

Rosenthal, R. (1994). Parametric measures of effect size. In H. M. Cooper & L. V. Hedges (Eds.), *The handbook of research synthesis* (pp. 231-244). New York: Russell Sage.

Rosenthal, R., & Rosnow, R. (1991). *Essentials of behavioral research: Methods and data analysis* (2nd ed.). New York: McGraw-Hill.

Rosenthal, R., & Rubin, D. B. (1982). A simple general purpose display of magnitude of experimental effect. *Journal of Educational Psychology, 74*, 166-169.

Rosser, W. W. (1999). Application of evidence from randomised controlled trials to general practice. *Lancet, 353*, 661-664.

Sackett, D. L., Richardson, W. S., Rosenberg, W., & Haynes, R. B. (1997). *Evidence-based medicine: How to practice and teach EBM*. New York: Churchill Livingstone.

Shadish, W. R., & Haddock, C. K. (1994). Combining estimates of effect size. In H. M. Cooper & L. V. Hedges (Eds.), *The handbook of research synthesis* (pp. 261-281). New York: Russell Sage.

Stock, W. A., Benito, J. G., & Lasa, N. B. (1996). Research synthesis: Coding and conjectures. *Evaluation & the Health Professions, 19*, 104-117.

Stroup, D. F., Berlin, J. A., Morton, S. C., Olkin, I., Williamson, G. D., Rennie, D., Moher, D., Becker, B. J., Sipe, T. A., & Thacker, S. B. for the MOOSE Group. (2000). Meta-analysis of observational studies in epidemiology: A proposal for reporting. *Journal of the American Medical Association, 283*, 2008-2012.

Tickle-Degnen, L. (1998). Communicating with patients about treatment outcomes: The use of meta-analytic evidence in collaborative treatment planning. *American Journal of Occupational Therapy, 52*, 526-530.

Wade, D. T., Collen, F. M., Robb, G. F., & Warlow, C. P. (1992). Physiotherapy intervention late after stroke and mobility. *British Medical Journal, 304*, 609-613.

Werner, R. A., & Kessler, S. (1996). Effectiveness of an intensive outpatient rehabilitation program for postacute stroke patients. *American Journal of Physical Medicine and Rehabilitation, 75*, 114-120.

Controversial Practices: The Need for a Reacculturation of Early Intervention Fields

R. A. McWilliam

Address: R. A. McWilliam, Frank Porter Graham Child Development Center, CB# 8180 University of North Carolina, Chapel Hill, NC 27599-8180; e-mail: Robin_McWilliam@unc.edu.

As if families didn't have enough to contend with, the fields designed to help them now include more and more practices that have little research basis, provoke intense debate among professionals, and usually require a disruption of the family's life. This article explores what makes controversial practices controversial, what some of them are, what makes people adopt them, and what the early intervention field should do now. The purposes of this article are to raise awareness about controversies in the field, to give a few examples, and to present some issues for further debate. I do not claim to provide a comprehensive evaluation of specific treatments or even a comprehensive review of their advantages and disadvantages. The very act of labeling practices as controversial is controversial, because supporters of those practices do not like to have aspersions cast on them. Even the criteria for what makes a practice controversial could spur debate.

What Makes Practice Controversial?

What makes a practice controversial in any field is worthy of an article itself. In discussing treatment approaches for children with learning disabilities, Silver (1995) considered them controversial if (a) the approach was presented before any studies were available or when pilot studies had not been replicated, (b) the presented treatment went further than the data, or (c) the treatment was used in an isolated way when a multimodal assessment and treatment approach was needed. In this article, I propose five similar criteria for what constitutes a controversy: claims that the practice produces a cure, requirement of practitioner specialization, questionable research, high intensity requirement, and legal action.

Cure Claims

If a practice is claimed to cure a disability that theoretically cannot be cured, it is controversial. Thus, claims that the Lovaas (1987) treatment results in children with autism no longer needing special education and claims that Upledger's (1978) craniosacral therapy cures cerebral palsy render these practices dubious.

Practitioner Specialization

If a practice requires people who are already specialists to undergo even more specialized training, it is probably controversial. The stipulation that only certain disciples can practice the treatment ensures that the market will be stable and increases the mystique of the practice. Thus, special training for neurodevelopmental therapy, sensory integration, and Lovaas therapy make those treatments abstruse (and their practitioners valuable). Some practices appear to belong to certain disciplines, which hinders the adoption of transdisciplinary approaches to service delivery (see McWilliam & Bailey, 1994). If occupational therapists are the people to call for sensory integration techniques, physical therapists for craniosacral therapy, and speech-language pathologists for Fast ForWord, it is in those practitioners' interest to vaunt the practices.

Questionable Research

An important link between research and practice is the development of clinical treatment approaches based on theoretical frameworks and scientifically validated findings. This link has historically been tenuous in physical therapy and occupational therapy, according to Darrah and Bartlett (1995). No longer can these fields continue to rely on personal sources of authority rather than scientific knowledge.

When there are no published true experimental studies demonstrating the effectiveness of one treatment (e.g., craniosacral therapy) over other treatments, nothing adequately separates the treatment in question from a placebo effect. Upledger's (1978) study, showing how craniosacral motion examinations could be used to help diagnose a variety of disorders, was criticized, in a letter to the journal in which his study was published, on the basis of unreliable disorder definitions and unreliable cranial rhythmic measures (Steiner, 1979). One of the arguments for labeling practices as controversial, therefore, concerns the validity of the research to prove effectiveness (Rogers & Witt, 1997).

It should be noted, however, that most studies could be criticized on methodological grounds. If readers or reviewers really do not like the finding, they can always question the quality of a study. Similarly, if they like the finding (i.e., they agree with the theory, or they have been acculturated to accept the practice), they may overlook methodological flaws.

Matthews (1988) noted that many of the treatments for the management of cerebral palsy were developed first from clinical observation; later, a theoretical framework was forged to account for the feasible neurological and physiological principles. Rogers and Witt (1997) suggested that qualitative research could provide an understanding of how and why craniosacral therapy might help a child, but we still need controlled single-subject studies and randomized clinical trials to provide outcome support for the practice. It is imperative that readers, researchers, and reviewers become well versed in yardsticks of good qualitative research so as not to confuse unanalyzed opinions and anecdotes with qualitative investigation.

Intensity

Intense treatment appeals to parents and professionals, if not to administrators. The more-is-better phenomenon has been identified as a theme in studies about service utilization (McWilliam, Tocci, & Harbin, 1995) and service integration (McWilliam, Young, & Harville, 1996). This apparently explains the appeal of therapy services as a whole,

---

with early intervention teams planning for therapy on the basis of the child's diagnosis rather than as a support to meeting functional goals (McWilliam et al., 1996). Thus, any therapeutic practices can become controversial when they are described as needing to occur for a certain amount of time per week. Families are likely to think that doubling that amount of time, whatever its duration, would increase the likelihood of the therapy being effective with their child. This is particularly likely if the therapy has also promised a cure.

The Lovaas (1987) program, although very popular with parents, has not been embraced as enthusiastically by all professionals in the field. The Lovaas treatment features the systematic application of contingencies to reinforce desired behaviors; this is known as applied behavioral analysis. The analysis refers to the careful collection and graphing of data, which is an important aspect of the intervention. The reason for professional skepticism might be twofold. First, it is an educational rather than a therapeutic practice (therefore having less mystique). Professionals, especially special educators, can examine the treatment and determine for themselves whether 40 hours a week is unnecessary. This is the second reason for skepticism: The time required is excessive. Professionals might advocate greater intensity for other treatments in early intervention—but that would be for fewer than 5 hours a week. Thus, familiarity and excess might explain why professionals are not as enthusiastic about the intensity of the Lovaas program. Lest this seem like professionals are entirely justified in their disaffection, it is remarkable how seldom behavior analysis—at any intensity—appears to be implemented. Professionals' skepticism would be more credible if they used more systematic instruction, at whatever rate (see Strain et al., 1992).

The problem with intensive treatments for many early intervention programs (and for states) is the associated costs. As soon as parents, sometimes in collusion with professionals, want a costly service, a dispute (i.e., a controversy) is likely to arise about its necessity and effectiveness. When parents sense that administrators or state officials are balking at providing a service because of its cost, they don't know whether to trust what they hear about the treatment. This has been at the root of many lawsuits in early childhood special education. Groups that deliberating encourage families to sue school systems and states are capitalizing on this distrust.

Legal Action

The Lovaas controversy continues to be instructive about what makes a practice controversial with regard to legal action. Almost by definition, as soon as the merits of a practice are debated in court, it is controversial.

If a practice meets one of these five criteria—cure claims, practitioner specialization, questionable research, intensity, or legal action—it is likely to be controversial in early intervention. If it meets more than one criterion, which often happens (each criterion tends to lead to others), it almost certainly qualifies as a controversy. Ultimately, however, controversy begins when someone casts aspersions on a practice that others are promoting. It is not simply a question of whether the practice is good or bad. Controversy arises when people react to practices. Hence, I have considered evaluative reviews of research as well as the primary sources themselves.

Some Controversial Treatments

The decision about what to include in the list of controversial treatments might itself be controversial. Advocates for treatments mentioned in this article may argue that their treatments are effective and, therefore, should not be controversial. Others might argue that treatments they dislike should have been included. The treatments I include here do not constitute an exhaustive list; they merely represent some that generate arguments in state-level corridors, Individualized Family Service Plan (IFSP) or Individualized Education Program (IEP) meetings, or professional conferences.

Controversial treatments in early intervention can be grouped into the following three broad areas: medical, educational, and therapeutic. I hesitate to separate the last two, because I don't want to exacerbate the already insidious problem of discipline overspecialization (McWilliam, 1996; McWilliam et al., 1996; McWilliam & Sekerak, 1995). Nevertheless, the roots of the treatments I discuss are in the specific disciplines, and therefore, anything we do about the controversies needs to be addressed accordingly. Medical controversies are addressed relatively superficially, because most readers of this journal will have more to do with educational and therapeutic treatments.

Medical

Alternative therapies are becoming a great interest in the medical field. National surveys confirm that there has been a statistically significant increase in the percentage of the population using alternative medicine between 1990 and 1997 (Eisenberg et al., 1998). The therapies with the most increased usage were herbal medicine, massage, megavitamins, self-help groups, folk remedies, energy healing, and homeopathy. Using my proposed criteria for controversial treatments, these approaches are controversial primarily because of cure claims and questionable research. The medical profession's penchant for seeking a cure is reflected in medical early intervention practices. Although medical research is often guided by methodological rigor (e.g., double-blind clinical trials), the theoretical rationale or causal implications are not always convincing. For example, we sometimes learn that group differences are found but cannot infer that the treatment accounted for these differences. Medical practices that have been considered controversial in early intervention include diets, surgical procedures, and drug treatments.

Diet. Vitamin supplementation has been proposed for numerous behavioral and cognitive disorders in children with mental retardation. A review of the literature has shown that vitamin B_6 was ineffective in treating children with Down syndrome, folic acid treatment had very limited effects on some children with fragile X syndrome, megadose multivitamin supplements have not been effective with cognitive disorders or attention-deficit disorders, and multivitamins and minerals have not been effective with Down syndrome or other forms of mental retardation (Kozlowski, 1992). To judge the efficacy of diets requires an examination of the primary sources (i.e., the original studies), but the controversy has arisen because of people's *interpretations* of the pros and cons of a practice. Therefore, this article relies on both primary and secondary sources.

Much of the controversy with early intervention treatments is based on the belief that, if a little is good, more must be better (Haslam, 1992; McWilliam et al., 1996). Megavitamin therapy has been defined as "treatment with quantities of one or more times the recommended dietary allowance" (Haslam, p. 303). Haslam conducted a clinical trial comparing 41 children diagnosed with attention-deficit/hyperactivity disorder with a control group of 75 children. The two groups did not differ in teacher, mother, and father behavioral ratings of the child. Other dietary treatments generating controversy have included sugar reduction to control behavior and macrobiotics for overall (including developmental) well-being. The dietary practices mentioned here are only a sampling of the treatments suggested in early intervention. They are controversial, according to the criteria proposed in this article, because the research is questionable. The link between the diet and the conditions that the diet is designed to cure or ameliorate is often tenuous. It could also be argued that dietary approaches are controversial because practitioners have to be specialized (i.e., nutritionists).

Surgery. Because of their invasiveness, surgical procedures tend to generate controversy. One neurosurgical treatment is dorsal rhizotomy for spasticity. Peacock, Arens, and Berman (1987) developed a method of stimulating rootlets to produce sustained muscle contraction or spread, resulting in reduced spasticity and significant gains in some children. The major concern is that more effectiveness evidence, acceptable protections, and selection parameters are needed before the technique is widely used (Matthews, 1988). Another fairly common surgical procedure that is not totally accepted is cutting the tight heel cords.

Perhaps the most controversial surgical procedure is plastic surgery for children with Down syndrome. This is controversial because elimination of one of the defining characteristics of the syndrome, facial features, can be construed as denial and lack of acceptance. Cochlear implants have generated a similar controversy: some members of the Deaf culture have declared the surgical implant to be a repudiation of the person's innate culture. They maintain that professionals with hearing are convincing parents of deaf children to agree to the implants. The examples of cosmetic surgery and cochlear implants introduce the element of cultural values to the controversy of a practice. Surgery is therefore controversial because procedures involve cure claims and, in some cases (e.g., rootlet stimulation), because the research is questionable (see Note).

Drugs. Few medications elicit such strong reactions as Ritalin, because many people feel that it is overprescribed and overdemanded. Ritalin is a stimulant that helps children with attention-deficit disorder with or without hyperactivity to focus, thus causing hyperactive children to calm down. Some suggested alternatives, such as craniosacral therapy, biofeedback, traditional Chinese medicine, homeopathy, the Feingold diet, and minerals (see "Alternatives," 1998), are no less controversial. The main controversy about Ritalin is that it might be prescribed too quickly, before less invasive (i.e., nonmedical) practices, such as be-

havior modification, have been adequately tried. Parents and teachers have been criticized for jumping on the Ritalin bandwagon. The effectiveness of Ritalin with many children is well documented, which is one reason for its popularity. Documentation alone does not, however, make a practice popular. Adding to the controversy about Ritalin is the fact that the manufacturer has subsidized the largest parent support group for children with attention-deficit disorder.

Another drug practice that is becoming increasingly controversial is the prescription of Prozac for children with autism. One controversial aspect of these drug treatments is that they are largely prescribed for disabilities for which many cures are sought and submitted: attention-deficit disorder, hyperactivity, learning disabilities, and autism. Wherever these disabilities are found, so are all kinds of practices. Drugs are controversial, according to the criteria used in this article, because of cure claims and questionable research.

Educational

Educational practices tend to be controversial because of all the criteria listed earlier: cure claims, practitioner specialization, questionable research, intensity, or legal action. In special education, two practices have generated enormous controversy in the United States: intensive applied behavior analysis and facilitated communication. In early intervention and early childhood special education in the United States, there has been some debate about developmentally appropriate practice. We also need to be aware, however, of conductive education, a Hungarian program sure to generate argument once it becomes better known in this country.

Lovaas Approach to Autism Treatment. Nothing approaches the controversy of intensive behavioral therapy for the treatment of autism, and Lovaas therapy is the most controversial of all. The program calls for 40 hours a week of one-on-one therapy provided by specially trained personnel and by the parents. It is, therefore, very costly, which partly explains the enormous debate it has generated. Estimates of the cost have ranged from $12,000 to $22,000 a year ("Requests," 1995). Because of the costs, litigation has ensued, with some case (e.g., *Delaware County Intermediate Unit v. Martin and Melinda K.*, 1995) ruling in favor of parents demanding Lovaas therapy and others (e.g., *Fairfax County Public Schools*, 1995) ruling in favor of schools' alternatives to Lovaas therapy. This program has been substantiated by studies examining

the short- and long-term outcomes for children with autism (Lovaas, 1987; McEachin, Smith, & Lovaas, 1993). By 7 years of age, 19 children who had received a very intensive behavioral intervention as preschoolers achieved less restrictive school placements and higher IQs than did a control group of 19 similar children who had received less intensive intervention (McEachin et al., 1993). At age 13 for the experimental group and age 10 for the control group, the gains of the experimental group had been maintained. The 9 children in the experimental group who had achieved the best outcomes received intensive evaluations that showed them to be indistinguishable in intelligence and adaptive behavior from typically developing children. Schopler and his colleagues (Campbell, Schopler, Cueva, & Hallin, 1996) have criticized Lovaas's research methods for using placement in a mainstream program as an outcome, which says more about the school's philosophy than about the treatment's efficacy. An important consideration, however, is that the autism controversy often pits Lovaas therapy against the Treatment and Education of Autistic and Communication Handicapped Children (TEACCH) program, which is Schopler's creation. Ironically, the TEACCH program is also extremely structured.

Wolery (1997) has thrown common sense into the autism debate with four notions about children with autism. First, children with autism are children, and there are few, if any, autism-specific educational practices. Second, children with autism grow up, and we ought to maintain a longitudinal perspective, because the reversibility of human behavior is a well-established fact. Third, children with autism have families who must be intimately involved in making decisions about what to teach their children and about their involvement in instructional activities. Fourth, children with autism live in communities, and the curriculum—even at the preschool level—should be community referenced. Wolery's points are related to education placement and services; these four points demonstrate that children need vital learning environments with many supporters. They also demonstrate the tragedy of the current autism controversy, which assumes that there are autism-specific practices, that certain practices absolutely must be employed in the preschool years, that parents need to become teachers as well as parents, and that special settings are necessary. The Lovaas approach is, therefore, controversial because claims of recovering from autism have been made (e.g., Maurice, 1993), specially trained practitioners are needed, an extremely intensive regimen is required, and parents and states have gone to court to demand or repudiate—respectively—this particular treatment. It should be noted that, although practitioners of the Lovaas approach need specialized training, the requirements are not as demanding as the requirements for some other controversial practices. Most special education teachers, for example, can be trained to administer the Lovaas approach.

Conductive Education. Conductive education has not yet caught on in the United States, but it has become very popular in parts of Europe. It is an approach for people with motor disabilities caused by damage to the central nervous system, and it involves active learning. It was developed by András Petö in Hungary in the 1940s (see Kozma & Balogh, 1995), who believed that a child could learn even if challenged by his or her disability (usually what we would call cerebral palsy). The key to conductive education is the *conductor*—that is, the interventionist. Kozma and Balogh—who are the director general and associate director general of the Petö András Institute for Conductive Education of the Motor Disabled and Conductors' College—described conductive education as the development of personality, not a therapy. Supposedly, the treatment is integrated into family routines, and prevents disruptions in families' lives. Children are taught to perform the following age-appropriate skills, regardless of their "motor dysfunctions": changing position, task series, speech, self-help skills, successful actions, and preparation for kindergarten.

The treatment itself revolves around the two basic meanings of conductive education: (a) orchestration by the conductor who has had special education training and combines the skills of occupational, physical, and speech-language therapists; and (b) an emphasis on the child's completing an action once it has been initiated (see Spivack, 1995). Conductive education has been described as a classroom-based approach, in which *rhythmic intention* (children being taught sing-song rhymes to accompany their intended actions—the actions the conductor wants them to intend) is a primary teaching principle. Other characteristics of the approach are that the conductor deliberately plans to motivate the children and that the children learn in groups. Research on conductive education has been scant, with very few children but with data subjected to statistical analyses (Bairstow, Cochrane, & Hur, 1993; Russell, 1994; Weber & Rochel, 1992). An evaluation of German and Brit-

ish studies concluded that neither the most hopeful expectations nor the worst apprehensions about conductive education were confirmed. Notably, Spivack reported that efficacy studies have been tried in his own conductive education center in the United States (in Brooklyn, NY), "but the most dramatic are the personal reports from parents and children after leaving the program" (p. 84). One of the claimed advantages of the model is that the conductor takes the majority of the work away from highly paid physical and occupational therapists, who are used mostly as evaluators. One problem for the New York center is that state agencies do not endorse conductors as a separate professional program; conductors must have masters' degrees in special education.

Conductive education has been embraced by some factions in the United Kingdom, as a result of British families who had been to Hungary and returned with success stories. It is well known in Britain that parents have played an important role in pushing for the method's use (Taylor & Emery, 1995). Using the proposed criteria, conductive education qualifies for controversy because specially trained practitioners (not to mention special schools) are required, the research is questionable, and the treatment is very intensive. It is also controversial because it breaches American values about remediation of children with cerebral palsy (it doesn't even acknowledge that diagnostic label because of its finality), it pits conductors against allied health practitioners, and it violates American values about child initiation in interactions.

Facilitated Communication. One of the most controversial treatments for children with disabilities has been facilitated communication. It has been tried with children with autism and other significant communication and behavior disorders. The approach consists of a child's typing answers to questions while receiving hand-over-hand assistance from an adult. Witnesses have been amazed to see users pressing keys without even looking at the keyboard or having their hands anchored on the keyboard (e.g., beginning with index fingers on the F and J keys). Meanwhile, however, the facilitator is watching the keyboard. The evidence in support of facilitated communication has been equivocal. As with many controversial practices, much of the research has been conducted by the developer of the practice. In the case of facilitated communication, that person has been Biklen (1990, 1992, 1993; Biklen & Schubert, 1991). In a study by others, several participants were able to complete simple set work and related re-

sponses to requests and questions when the facilitators knew the answers (Simpson & Myles, 1995). On the other hand, when the facilitators did not know the answers, the students were unable to respond correctly. The controversy of facilitated communication first arose because of wild statements that the users supposedly made, including accusations of abuse by their parents. Using the proposed criteria for controversy, however, this practice is controversial because of questionable research.

Developmentally Appropriate Practice. The effectiveness of developmentally appropriate practice (DAP; Bredekamp, 1987) has been deliberated in numerous articles in *Topics in Early Childhood Special Education* (e.g., Carta, Schwartz, Atwater, & McConnell, 1991; Johnson & Johnson, 1992; Mahoney, Robinson, & Powell, 1992; Mallory, 1992), including the last time controversies were deliberately addressed in this journal. Because these articles are easily available, I will not dwell on the arguments here. Suffice it to say that the original concept of the practice as defined by the National Association for the Education of Young Children (see Bredekamp) appeared to offer too little structure for actual instruction to occur. Some early childhood special educators thought that specific instruction was necessary especially for children with disabilities. Over time, and in collaboration with early interventionists (Wolery, Strain, & Bailey, 1996), the National Association for the Education of Young Children has clarified or actually modified its position on instruction to allow for the possibility of systematic instruction within the framework of developmentally appropriate practice. The controversy of DAP arose first because it was presented as an alternative to the status quo—as the approach that would be most consistent with the values of normalization and inclusion. It was presented as a replacement for behavioral practices, which were deemed too unnatural. Unfortunately for the proponents of DAP, however, they were trying to replace a well-researched approach with a poorly researched one. DAP is controversial because of the questionable research criterion.

Therapeutic

The allied health fields are particularly prone to controversial practices. What they do is less familiar to everyday parents and professionals, so some practices become widely adopted with little questioning. I describe a number of treatments, ranging from prevalent ones such as sensory integration therapy to little known ones such as Fast

ForWord. The list at the end of this section indicates the huge number of practices potentially bewildering to early intervention teams.

Sensory Integration. Perhaps the most pervasive controversial practice in early intervention is sensory integration. The fact that many professionals and parents will wonder what is controversial about it indicates how well accepted it has become in the field, particularly among occupational therapists. Yet, the claim that sensory integration is effective has not been substantiated by empirical studies (e.g., Matthews, 1988).

Sensory integration (SI) is both a theory and a practice. It is based on the work of Ayres (1972a), who theorized that sensory input from motor movement and touch provides feedback to the integration process occurring at different levels of the nervous system. The treatment emphasizes tactile and vestibular stimulation of motor and sensory input. Ayres claimed that improvement in sensorimotor integration would result in improvement in motor skills, academic achievements, language abilities, and emotional tone. Most studies with reasonable guards against threats to internal validity have borne out the first claim—to a degree (e.g., Montgomery & Richter, 1977; Ottenbacher, 1982). Some research has supported the claim of improved motor and academic functioning of children with learning disabilities (e.g., Ottenbacher's meta-analysis). Serious methodological problems exist with most SI studies, however. None of them included an examination of the effectiveness of SI in relation to other therapies; they did not control for the heterogeneity of the participant groups; the studies conducted by Ayres (e.g., 1972b, 1978) and many of the studies reviewed by Ottenbacher employed inadequate sampling and matching procedures and failed to control for a placebo effect.

In a review of seven studies involving children with both a learning disability and a diagnosed "sensory integration dysfunction" and at least one comparison group with random assignment to groups, each study was reported to show improvement on both academic and motor variables over time *regardless of the treatment*. One study showed that academic tutoring seemed to influence the motor skills of children with learning disabilities (Wilson, Kaplan, Fellowes, Gruchy, & Faris, 1992). Other authors (e.g., Kavale & Mattson, 1983) have speculated that much of the improvement seen in SI treatment research and in research involving other forms of therapy

might be the result of the extra attention that these children received. Unfortunately, this potential variable has not been isolated and studied. In general, the many studies purporting to show the effectiveness of SI are highly unconvincing when held under reasonable scrutiny (see Arendt, MacLean, & Baumeister, 1988). This is especially worrisome given the popularity of SI with families who have a child with Fragile X syndrome. Although the effectiveness of the practice with these particular children has not yet been documented, research showing positive outcomes in people with mental retardation (some of whom we can assume had Fragile X syndrome) could easily be explained by alternative theories. The conceptual foundation of sensory integration therapy has been seriously discredited (see Arendt et al.). For example, one popular aspect of sensory integration is the diagnosis of tactile or sensory defensiveness, which is typically treated with brushing programs, oral-motor stimulation, and a "sensory diet" (Wilbarger & Wilbarger, 1991). In a randomized study, no group differences could be detected on any measure between children with learning disabilities who received sensory integration therapy and those who received perceptual-motor therapy (Polatajko, Law, Miller, Schaffer, & Macnab, 1991). A subsequent study did find that children receiving perceptual-motor therapy showed more gains, especially in gross motor performance, than groups receiving either sensory integration therapy or no therapy (Humphries, Wright, Snider, & McDougall, 1992). The SI group did show more gains in motor planning. Despite the widespread adoption of sensory integration practices, the theory supporting SI is poorly defined, and efficacy research is practically nonexistent. Sensory integration and its associated techniques are controversial because the claims exceed what they logically or empirically can treat, because specialized practitioners are needed, and because the research in support of SI is highly questionable.

Patterning. Perhaps the most controversial treatment in early intervention has been the Doman-Delacato pattering approach for children with cerebral palsy (American Academy of Pediatrics, 1982), in which a set of exercise mimicking locomotion states of animals was repeated throughout the day. The idea was to establish cerebral dominance and normalization of function by unlocking reflexes and by positioning. The research base for this approach was sketchy at best, but the controversy was primarily provoked by the intensity of the treatment.

The developers of patterning claimed that it only worked with many hours of application every day. Families therefore had to recruit a small army of volunteers to help them with this intensive treatment. The cost to families, and their feelings of guilt about what their child had to endure, eventually caught up with many of them. The approach also stressed the resources of agencies serving children with cerebral palsy. At the same time, many parents developed a strong belief that this was the right and the only treatment for their child. These characteristics are disturbingly similar to the situation today with the Lovaas approach to treating children with autism. Yet we appear to have learned little from history. Patterning, according to the criteria used in this article, is controversial because of cure claims, questionable research, and intensity.

Craniosacral Therapy. Whereas sensory integration is the controversial therapy most closely associated with occupational therapy, craniosacral therapy and myofascial release represent the emerging controversies in physical therapy. There are others, but these are likely to generate the most heated debate. Because the two practices overlap, I will discuss only craniosacral therapy.

Craniosacral therapy shares with cranial osteopathy the theoretical belief in cranial bone motion. Craniosacral therapists propose that repeated oscillations in cerebrospinal fluid pressure cause rhythmic motion of the cranial bones and sacrum—the craniosacral rhythm. By putting careful pressure on the cranial bones, they manipulate this craniosacral rhythm to effect a therapeutic outcome in their patients. Although cranial bone motion has been embraced by a number of physical therapists, some are skeptical and consider the approach controversial (see Rogers & Witt, 1997). Conventional physiologists do not conceive of the cranial sutures as playing any significant role in this intervention, which is focused on a belief that unfused sutures can move throughout life. Efficacy studies have been reported to contain inadequate information and have often been conducted by colleagues of John Upledger, the founder of this approach (e.g., Retzlaff, Jones, Mitchell, Upledger, & Walsh, 1982; Retzlaff, Micheal, Roppel, & Mitchell, 1976; Retzlaff, Walsh, Mitchell, & Vredevoogd, 1984). Claims that palpation of the craniosacral rhythm can be reliably measured have been shown to be exaggerated when subjected to statistical analysis (Wirth-Pattullo & Hayes, 1994). Upledger's (1978) study on the relationship of craniosacral examination findings in grade school children with developmental problems was criticized by a fellow osteopath (Steiner, 1979) as "combining figures derived from personal impressions of motion with un-coordinated personal opinions concerning behavior....No justifiable conclusions can be drawn from the paper" (p. 386). Upledg-er (1979) replied, basing much of his de-fense on low *p* values associated with low correlations, which could be explained by his high (203) sample size. Questionable research, the fact that only specially trained practitioners can use the method, and cure claims all qualify craniosacral therapy as controversial.

Auditory Integration Training. Guy Be-rard, a French doctor, developed this ap-proach to speech therapy. It is based on the theory that some people are extremely sensitive to certain sounds, hear distortions of sounds, or hear certain sounds in the nor-mal range that make them uncomfortable. Treatment consists of playing compact disks through a device (which has been banned by the Food and Drug Administration) that amplifies certain sounds and filters others, according to individual needs. Silver (1995) reported that the literature sent by provid-ers of the service was "full of claims of suc-cess. Parents are almost made to feel guilty if they do not avail their child (sic) of this treatment. No research supports the theo-ry or claims" (p. S98). In fact, two studies have found reductions in hearing problems as well as improvements in behavior (Rim-land & Edelson, 1992), 1994). Neverthe-less, controversy about the approach is still widespread (see Berkell, Malgeri, & Streit, 1996). One area of concern is that many unlicensed practitioners are offering audito-ry integration training (AIT). Other concerns are that AIT's efficacy for treating people with autism is unclear and that the devices might be unsafe. According to Berkell et al., "there are no published research reports which meet scientific standards to support or refute the validity of AIT as an effective treatment" (p. 70).

Gravel (1994) has expressed grave reser-vations about AIT, noting that within 4 years of its introduction to the United States it had been used with more than 10,000 children (citing Georgiana Organization, Inc., per-sonal communication). Gravel takes issue with three premises on which AIT is found-ed. First, auditory distortions are claimed to underlie autism, but there is no scientific support for the idea that auditory distortions as described by Berard exist. Furthermore, no research supports the notion that periph-eral distortions exist in people with autism. Second, the claim that AIT "straightens out" the peaks and valleys of the conven-tional audiogram cannot be substantiated, because variations of ± 5 db are normal in conventional audiograms and need not be eliminated. Third, the claim that AIT is a safe procedure does not convince many speech-language pathologists and audiolo-gists, because there are no data to verify that threshold shifts could not occur, especially in young listeners. Using the criteria for controversy presented earlier, AIT qualifies as controversial because of questionable research.

Fast ForWord. Another treatment touted as helping children's language skills is the Fast ForWord system, a program rooted in how infants hear and how they learn lan-guage. Paula Tallal hypothesized that some children might not be able to process fast elements of speech because of a deficit in the rate at which they process information (Tallal & Merzenich, 1997). Preliminary re-search indicated that these children could discriminate speech syllables that had been modified to emphasize the rapid acoustic elements. The Fast ForWord exercises thus consist of identifying and repeating comput-er-made speech sounds that are stretched and in which the important acoustic dif-ferences are emphasized. According to Tal-lal, the program can only be provided by a licensed and trained clinician or educator, and it only works when a child performs the exercises daily for 100 to 140 minutes, 5 days a week (information from Scientific Learning Corporation Web site, http://www.fastforword.com). According to the Web site, children make on average 1.5 years of language gains after 4 to 8 weeks of train-ing. Fast ForWord is backed by a corpora-tion with impressive marketing that includes a comprehensive Web site, many publica-tions, and an elaborate conference display booth. This company, recognizing the need for validating a practice that was only intro-duced in 1997, emphasizes peer-reviewed articles demonstrating the effectiveness of Fast ForWord (e.g., Merzenich et al., 1996; Tallal et al., 1997), and the national field trial preceding its introduction (http://www.scientificlearing.com). This practice qualifies as controversial because specially trained practitioners are needed and because the practice requires intensive application. These two criteria alone may not make a practice controversial, so it is perhaps the newness of Fast ForWord, the remarkable efficacy claims, the polished marketing, and the strangeness of the intervention that qualify it for inclusion in this list.

Neurodevelopmental Therapy. Neuro-developmental therapy (NDT) has been described as the most widely used method for treating children with cerebral palsy (see Matthews, 1988). This method is based on the premise that cerebral palsy is a disorder of the postural mechanism and that treat-ment should emphasize normal movement, decrease or increase in muscle tone, and the reduction of abnormal postures. The approach has gone out of fashion as motor learning and dynamic systems theory have replaced it (see Darrah & Bartlett, 1995). At one time, it was de rigueur for early inter-vention physical therapists and others to be specially trained in NDT. This practice is de-rived from a neuromaturational perspective of motor development—along with sensory integration (Adams & Snyder, 1998). This perspective holds that, as the nervous sys-tem matures, adaptive behavior emerges; therefore, more elaborate behaviors repre-sent higher levels of organization within the central nervous system. Whereas sensory integration is well entrenched in the field, however, NDT is now controversial be-cause many physical therapists have moved away from it. The motor field, especially occupational therapy, presents a confusing message: Although neuromaturational ap-proaches are being criticized, occupational therapists continue to be trained in sensory integration. Practitioners' gradual rejection of NDT is related to the controversy crite-rion of practitioner specialization: The very people who were trained in the approach are now eschewing it. Furthermore, the well-conducted research examining NDT has not supported it strongly.

This concludes the discussion of certain, somewhat arbitrarily selected, controversial practices. Even though many practices were discussed, these are not the only ones. Par-ents and practitioners are faced with even more options rife with controversy. To illus-trate the extent of these controversial treat-ments, I am listing some others, although it is beyond the scope of this article to discuss them. It might be useful for readers to be aware that, if someone suggests applying one of these treatments, it is worth investi-gating whether cures are claimed, whether practitioners have to be specially trained, whether the research is solid, whether the treatment is very intense, or whether legal action has ensued (the five controversy criteria). In no particular order, other con-troversial practices are relaxation and bio-feedback for children with cerebral palsy, functional electrical stimulation and epi-dural electrical stimulation over the dorsal column (Matthews, 1988), optometric visu-al training (eye exercises) for children with learning disabilities, cerebellar-vestibular dysfunction (antimotion sickness medication to treat dyslexia), applied kinesiology (manipulation of the sphenoid and temporal bones in the cranium), tinted lenses (also known as Irlen lenses, claiming to help people with reading problems who have scotopic sensitivity syndrome; Silver, 1995), the Snoezelen experience (using intensive sensory experiences to diagnose and treat children with severe learning disabilities; Whitaker, 1994), myofascial release (similar to craniosacral therapy but involving release of cerebrospinal fluid), articulation therapy (controversial because it is exceedingly common and unquestioned in application with children who are not yet developmentally able to articulate well), auditory enhancement (increasing volume through amplification to improve concentration), acupressure (for motor improvement, based on Chinese acupuncture theory), oral-motor strategies (noncontingent stimulation similar in theory to sensory integration techniques—and almost equally unquestioned by practitioners), and chiropractic treatment (historically controversial as an alternative to orthopedic medicine or physical therapy), Adams and Snyder (1998) provided a thoughtful discussion of options for the treatment of cerebral palsy. When considering how to help a child, why do professionals and parents sometimes choose these controversial practices over more parsimonious and usually better proven ones?

Reasons for Adopting Unproven Practices

An area ripe for and desperately warranting research is the cause of professionals' and parents' adopting unproven practices. From research on service utilization and integrated therapy (McWilliam & Bailey, 1994; McWilliam et al., 1995, 1996), I speculate as follows:

Proven Practices Are Not Necessarily the Easiest to Implement. For example, techniques for integrating therapeutic elements into a generalist model of service delivery exist, but home visitors and classroom teachers might not be using them because it is easier to stick to educational activities and leave therapy to the specialists.

Some Unproven Practices Reinforce the Specialization of the Professional. To preserve their identity as a valuable service provider, professionals often have a vested interest in letting everyone know that the child needs the particular treatment that only they can provide. For example, if a therapist trained in sensory integration can make the case that the child has "sensory problems," then that therapist will become

invaluable. It is hardly surprising that such therapists might find sensory problems in most children they see.

Professionals Do Not Read the Literature. The bridge from research to practice is weak (Shavelson, 1988), and many proponents of controversial therapies spout sound bite findings that cannot be substantiated by either the actual findings or the quality of the research quoted. For example, sensory integration advocates appear to be unaware of the methodological and conceptual problems with Ayres's research.

People Only Believe the Research That Supports Their Values. As mentioned earlier, acceptance of research findings depends to a considerable extent on the consumer's willingness to be influenced.

Professionals Believe What Other Professionals Tell Them. The mystique of controversial practices is related to arcane language, which only certain professionals—those who have received the relevant special training—have mastered. When a specialist, therefore, tells the team that a certain problem exists and that a certain treatment is warranted, the other professionals and parents have little reason to question the suggestion. This is an instance of specialist-to-generalist influence. An instance of specialist-to-specialist influence is the acculturation that exists within disciplines. For example, sensory integration is well established in occupational therapy, even among experts who promote an integrated approach (see Dunn, 1996).

A Parent's Job Is to Have Hope, and These Practices Offer Hope. Families understandably think that they should accept and fight for any practice that claims to be beneficial for their children. By definition, controversial treatments have pros and cons, and families feel that they cannot afford to ignore the potential advantages. Often the battle is between values and data, and we cannot count on data to win. This point has been made in the context of inclusion (Bailey, McWilliam, Buysse, & Wesley, 1998), which could well have been listed among the educational controversies, particularly for children with sensory impairments and those with autism.

These speculative reasons for the adoption of controversial practices are clearly not exhaustive. To improve early childhood special education and its accompanying disciplines, we should study the factors that lead to the adoption of controversial practices.

What Should the Field Do Now?

This article has described numerous

controversial practices that are currently popular and has alerted readers to others that might gain in popularity. Criteria that make certain treatments controversial have been proposed so that we can more clearly understand the nature of controversy in early intervention. Inherent in the problem is the eagerness of professionals and parents to adopt unproven practices. I have tried to make the case that we are at a point in the evolution of early intervention where we need do something about these practices. Five recommendations are provided.

Evaluate and Summarize the Research

The problems of studying controversial practices are multifaceted. Simply grasping and analyzing the existing research is a big enough endeavor considering the many disciplines involved. This should probably be accompanied by reviews of research into the development of cultural models related to early intervention practices, to understand better the phenomenon of belief in unproven treatments, especially by professionals.

As mentioned earlier, evaluators of the existing research will need to make careful assessments of the anecdotal evidence that permeates these practices. My own fairly cursory reviews have convinced me that the evidence is typically no more than that—anecdotes. But the proliferation of qualitative research in early intervention necessitates clear demarcations between mere vignettes or simple quotations and true narrative data with sophisticated qualitative analysis. The best vehicle for handling the large task of summarizing and evaluating all this research would be an early childhood research institute funded by the Office of Special Education Programs. This competition has a rich history of funding research on important topics in early intervention.

Conduct Comparative Research

Although an institute to analyze the existing research is necessary to understand the state of the art, the future requires comparative research. On the principle that—despite proponents' protestations to the contrary—there is no one right way to address a problem, two or more practices should be compared. Methods for conducting such research exist within the statistical, group-design paradigm (see Burchinal, Bailey, & Snyder, 1994) and within the single-subject, applied behavior analysis paradigm (see Wolery, Bailey, & Sugai, 1988).

Legislate Practice Guidelines

Practice guidelines exist to direct teams to appropriate types and levels of service delivery. For example, the State of New York is currently reviewing the appropriate intensity, locations, and personnel for working with children with autism. Although such guidelines have the appearance of removing the autonomy of the individual child's team, they are designed to provide parameters. The development of such guidelines gives states the opportunity to stop and evaluate many of the practices listed here. Without such a step, teams have blundered ahead with little direction. Although the legal system has been used effectively for ensuring needed services, it has also been used as a tool to force states and communities to provide the practice du jour. Thus, practice guidelines would help decrease the inappropriate use of the courts in determining appropriate practices.

Prepare Expert Witnesses

Because litigation will continue at some level, we need to have experts prepared to speak clearly, concisely, and knowledgeably about the evidence and the costs of these different practices. Court testimony is an unfamiliar art to most researchers, so they will need to be prepared.

Reacculturate the Field About the Role of Specialists

The introduction of more and more controversial practices goes hand in hand with a pernicious slide toward the overspecialization of early intervention (see McWilliam et al., 1996). Currently, early intervention professionals from different disciplines are usually trained separately, both at the preservice and inservice levels, although efforts have been made to bring them together for some courses and activities. As long as specialists continue to think that their role is to provide direct, hands-on therapy, we can expect the advocacy of dubious treatments to continue. When specialists realize that nearly all the intervention occurs *between* specialists' visits (i.e., primary caregivers are providing the real intervention in daily routines), we might see common sense prevail.

The two outcomes needed from this reacculturation are a demystification of the field and honesty by practitioners. The more controversial treatments we have, the more esoteric the field appears. This promotes the notion that only highly trained individuals can have positive effects on children. In fact, we need the highly trained individuals to fashion their knowledge to match the daily demands of primary caregivers. When those caregivers are empowered, services will be less expensive, and specialists will

be able to have a wider influence. Practitioners need the assurance that their new role as consultants to primary caregivers will be just as valued as their old role as direct healers of children. Research, policy, management, and personnel preparation will need to play a part in this reacculturation.

Note

For a good example of discussion of this controversy, see www.deafworldweb.org/chat

References

Adams, R. C. & Snyder, P. (1998). Treatments for cerebral palsy. Making choices of intervention from an expanding menu of options. *Infants and Young Children, 10*(4), 1-22.

Alternatives to Ritalin. (1998, January). *Learning: Information to Help Children with Learning Differences*, 1-2.

American Academy of Pediatrics. (1982). The Doman-Delacato treatment of neurologically handicapped children. *Pediatrics, 70,* 810-812.

Arendt, R. E., MacLean, W. E., & Baumeister, A. A. (1988). Critique of sensory integration therapy and its application in mental retardation. *American Journal on Mental Retardations, 92*, 401-411

Ayres, A. J. (1972a). *Sensory integration and learning disorders*. Los Angeles: Western Psychological Services.

Ayres, A. J. (1972b). Improving academic scores through sensory integration. *Journal of Learning Disabilities, 5*, 24-28.

Ayres, A. J. (1978). Learning disabilities and the verstibular system. *Journal of Learning Disabilities, 11*, 30-41.

Bailey, D. B., Jr., McWilliam, R. A., Buysse, V., & Wesley, P. W. (1998). Inclusion in the context of competing values in early childhood education. *Early Childhood Research Quarterly, 13*, 27-41.

Bairstow, P., Cochrane, R., & Hur, J. (1993). *Evaluation of conductive education for children with cerebral palsy* (Parts I and II). London, England: HMSO.

Berkell, D. E., Malgeri, S. E., & Streit, M. K. (1996). Auditory integration training for individuals with autism. *Education and Training in Mental Retardation and Developmental Disabilities, 31*(1), 66-70.

Biklen, D. (1990). Communication unbound: Autism and praxis. *Harvard Educational Review, 60*, 291-314.

Biklen, D. (1992). Typing to talk: Facilitated communication. *American Journal of Speech and Language Pathology, 1*(2), 15-17.

Biklen, D. (1993). *Communication unbound: How facilitated communication is challenging traditional views of autism and ability/disability*. New York, Teachers College Press.

Biklen, D., & Schubert, A. (1991). New words: The communication of students with autism. *Remedial and Special Education, 12*(6), 46-57.

Bredekamp, S. (1987). *Developmentally appro-*

priate practice in early childhood programs serving children from birth through age 8: Expanded edition. Washington, DC: National Association for the Education of Young Children.

Burchinal, M. R., Bailey, D. B., Jr., & Snyder, P. (1994). Using growth curve analysis to evaluate child change in longitudinal investigations. *Journal of Early Intervention, 18*, 403-423.

Campbell, M., Schopler, E., Cueva, J., & Hallin, A. (1996). Treatment of autistic disorder. *Journal of the American Academy of Child and Adolescent Psychiatry, 35*, 134-143.

Carta, J. J., Schwartz, I. S., Atwater, J. B., & McConnell, S. R. (1991). Developmentally appropriate practice: Appraising its usefulness for young children with disabilities. *Topics in Early Childhood Special Education, 11*(1), 1-20.

Darrah, J., & Bartlett, D. (1995). Dynamic systems theory and management of children with cerebral palsy: Unresolved issues. *Infants and Young Children, 8*(1), 52-59.

Delaware County Intermediate Unit v. Martin and Melinda K., 20 IDELR 363.

Dunn, W. (1996). Occupational therapy. In R. A. McWilliam (Ed.), *Rethinking pull-out services in early intervention: A professional resource* (pp. 267-314). Baltimore: Brookes.

Eisenberg, D. M., Davis, R. M., Ettner, S. Il, Appel, A., Wilkey, S., Van Rompay, M., & Kessler, R. C. (1998). Trends in alternative medicine use in the United States, 1990-1997. *Journal of the American Medical Association, 280*, 1569-1575.

Fairfax County Public Schools, 22 IDEIR 80 (SEA VA 1995).

Gravel, J. Sl. (1994). Auditory integration training: Placing the burden of proof. *American Journal of Speech-Language Pathology, 3*(4), 25-29.

Haslam, R. H. A. (1992). Is there a role for megavitamin therapy in the treatment of attention-deficit/hyperactivity disorder? *Advances in Neurology, 58*, 303-310.

Humphries, T., Wright, M., Snider, L., & McDougal, B. (1992). A comparison of the effectiveness of sensory integrative therapy and perceptual-motor training in treating children with learning disabilities. *Journal of Developmental and Behavioral Pediatrics, 13*, 31-40.

Johnson, J. E., & Johnson, K. M. (1992). Clarifying the developmental perspective in response to Carts, Schwartz, Atwater, and McConnell. *Topics in Early Childhood Special Education, 12*, 439-457.

Kaval, K., & Mattson, P. D. (1983). "One jumped off the balance beam": Meta-analysis of perceptual-motor training. *Journal of Learning Disabilities. 16*, 165-173.

Kozlowski, B., W. (1992). Megavitamin treatment of mental retardation in children: A review of effects on behavior and cognition. *Journal of Child and Adolescent Psychopharmacology, 2*, 307-318.

Kozma, I., & Balogh, E. (1995). A brief introduction to conductive education and its application at an early age. *Infants and Young Children, 8*(1), 68-74.

Lovaas, O. I. (1987). Behavioral treatment and normal educational and intellectual functioning in young autistic children. *Journal of Consulting and Clinical Psychology, 55*(1), 3-9.

Mahoney, G., Robinson, C., & Powell, A. (1992). Focusing on parent-child interactions: The bridge to developmentally appropriate practices. *Topics in Early Childhood Special Education, 12*, 105-120.

Mallory, B. L. (1992). Is it always appropriate to be developmental? Convergent models for early intervention practice. *Topics in Early Childhood Special Education, 11*(4), 1-12.

Matthews, D. J. (1988). Controversial therapies in the management of cerebral palsy. *Pediatric Annals, 17*, 762-764.

Maurice, C. (1993). *Let me hear your voice: A family's triumph over autism.* New York: Different Roads to Learning.

McEachin, J. J., Smith, T., & Lovaas, O. I. (1993). Long-term outcome for children with autism who received early intensive behavioral treatment. *American Journal on Mental Retardation, 97*, 359-372.

McWilliam, R. A. (Ed.). (1996). *Rethinking pullout services in early intervention: A professional resource.* Baltimore: Brookes.

McWilliam, R. A. & Bailey, D. B. (1994). Predictors of service delivery models in center-based early intervention. *Exceptional Children, 61*, 56-71.

McWilliam, R.A., & Sekerak, D. (1995). Integrated practices in center based early intervention: Perceptions of physical therapists. *Pediatric Physical Therapy, 7*, 51-58.

McWilliam, R. A., Tocci, L., & Harbin, G. (1995, August). Services are child-oriented and families like it that way—but why? *Early Childhood Research Institute: Service Utilization Findings*, 1-5.

McWilliam, R. A., Young, H. J., & Harville, K. (1996). Therapy services in early intervention: Current status, barriers, and recommendations. *Topics in Early Childhood Special Education, 16*, 348-374.

Merzenich, M. M., Jenkins, W. M., Johnson, P., Schreiner, C., Miller, S. L., & Tallal, P. (1996). Temporal processing deficits of language-learning impaired children ameliorated. *Science, 271*, 77-81.

Montgomery, P., & Richter, F. (1977). Effect of sensory integrative therapy on the neuromotor development of retarded children. *Physical Therapy, 57*, 799-806.

Ottenbacher, K. (1982). Sensory integration therapy: Affect or effect? *American Journal of Occupational Therapy, 36*, 571-577.

Peacock, W. J., Arens, L. J. & Berman, B. (1987). Cerebral palsy spasticity: Selected posterior rhizotomy. *Pediatric Neurosurgery, 13*, 61.

Polatajko, H. J., Law, M., Miller, J., Schaffer, R., & Macnab, J. (1991). The effect of a sensory integration program on academic achievement, motor performance and self esteem in children identified as learning disabled: Results of a clinical trial. *The Occupational Therapy Journal of Research, 11*, 155-176.

Requests for Lovaas therapy raise questions for early intervention programs. (1995, October). *Early Childhood Report*, pp. 1, 6-8.

Retzlaff, E. W., Jones I., Mitchell, F., Upledger, J., & Walsh, J. (1982), Possible autonomic innervations of cranial sutures of primates and other mammals. *Anatomy Record, 202*, 156A.

Retzlaff, E. W., Micheal, D., Roppel, R., & Mitchell, F. (1976). The structure of cranial bone sutures. *Journal of the American Osteopath Association, 75*, 106-107.

Retzlaff, E. W., Walsh, J., Mitchell, F., & Vredevoogd, J. (1984). Histological detail of cranial sutures as seen in plastic embedded specimens. *Anatomy Record, 208*, 145A.

Rimland, B., & Edelson, S. (1992). *Improving the auditory functioning of autistic persons: A comparison of the Berard auditory training approach with the Iomatis audio-psycho-phonology approach.* (Technical Report 111). San Diego, CA: Autism Research Institute.

Rimland, B., & Edelson, S. (1994). The effects of auditory integration training on autism. *American Journal of Speech-Language Pathology, 3*(2), 16-24.

Rogers, J. S., & Witt, P. L. (1997). The controversy of cranial bone motion. *Journal of Orthopedic and Sports Physical Therapy, 26*, 95-103.

Russell, A. (1994). *Evaluation of conductive education: A statistical overkill challenging the scientific validity and harsh conclusion of a University of Birmingham trial.* London: England Acorn Foundation.

Shavelson, R. J. (1988) Contributions of educational research to policy and practice: Constructing, challenging, changing cognition. *Educational Researcher, 17*, 4-12, 22.

Silver, L. B. (1995). Controversial therapies. *Journal of Child Neurology, 10*(1), 596-5100.

Simpson, R. L., & Myles, B.S. (1995). Effectiveness of facilitated communication with children and youth with autism. *The Journal of Special Education, 28*, 424-439.

Spivack, P. (1995). Conductive education perspectives. *Infants and Young Children, 8*(1), 75-85.

Steiner, C. (1979). Subjectivity-unsound basis for craniosacral research (Letter to the Editor). *Journal of the American Osteopathic Association, 78*, 386.

Strain, P. S., McConnell, S. R., Carta, J. J., Fowler, S. A., Neisworth, J. T., & Wolery, M. (1992). Behaviorism in early intervention. *Topics in Early Childhood Special Education, 12*, 121-142.

Tallal, P., & Merzenich, M. (1997, November 21). *Temporal training for Language impaired children: National clinical trial results.* Paper presented at the American Speech-Hearing Language Association Conference, Boston.

Tallal, P., Miller, S. L., Bedi, G., Byma, G., Wang, X., Nagarajan, S. S., Schreiner, C.., Jenkins, W. M., & Merzenich, M. M. (1997). Language comprehension in language-learning impaired children improved with acoustically modified speech. In M. E. Hertzig & E. A. Farber (Eds.), *Annual progress in child psychiatry and child development: 1997* (pp. 193-200). Bristol, PA: Brunner/Mazel.

Taylor, M., & Emery, R. (1995). Knowledge of conductive education among health service professionals. *European Journal of Special Needs Education, 10*, 169-179.

Upledger, J. E. (1978). The relationship of craniosacral examination findings in grade school children with developmental problems. *Journal of the American Osteopathic Association, 77*, 760-775.

Upledger, J. E. (1979). Author's reply. *Journal of the American Osteopathic Association, 78*, 386-388.

Weber, K. S., & Rochel, M. (1992). *Konduktive Forderung for cerebral geschadigte Kinder* [Conductive education for children with cerebral palsy]. Bon, Germany: Bunderministerium Fur Arbeit and Sozialordnung.

Whitaker, J. (1994). Can anyone help me to understand the logic of "Snoezelen." *Inclusion News, 1993-1994, 5* (Centre for Integrated Education and Community, Toronto Canada).

Wilbarger, P., & Wilbarger, J. L. (1991). *Sensory defensiveness in children aged 2-12: An intervention guide for parents and other care takers.* Santa Barbara, CA: Avanti Educational Programs.

Wilson, B. N., Kaplan, B. J., Fellowes, S., Gruchy, C., & Faris, P. (1992). The efficacy of sensory integration treatment compared to tutoring. *Physical and Occupational Therapy in Pediatrics, 12*, 1-36.

Wirth-Pattullo, V., & Hayes, K. W. (1994). Inter-rater reliability of craniosacral rate measurements and their relationship with subjects and examiner's heart and respiratory rate measurements. *Physical Therapy, 74*, 908-916.

Wolery, M. (1997, July 13). *Children with autism.* Paper presented at the NECTAS Meeting on Developing State and Local Services for Young Children with Autism and Their Families. Denver, CO.

Wolery, M., Bailey, D. B., & Sugai, G. M. (1988). *Effective teaching: Principles and procedures of applied behavior analysis with exceptional students.* Boston: Allyn & Bacon.

Wolery, M., Strain, P. S., & Bailey, D. B. (1996). Applying the framework of developmentally appropriate practice to children with special needs. In S. Bredekamp & T. Rosegrant (Eds.), *Reaching potentials: Curriculum and assessment for 3 to 8 year olds* (pp. 92-113). Washington, DC: NAEYC.

Controversial Therapies for Young Children with Developmental Disabilities

Robert E. Nickel, MD

Key words: autism, controversial therapy, developmental disability, Down syndrome

The search for a magical cure may be one stage in a parent's adjustment to the diagnosis of a developmental disability in his or her child. The parent may try controversial treatments as part of this search. In this article, the author discusses the reasons parents chose alternative treatments, reviews a few specific treatments, and provides recommendations to professionals on how to talk to families about controversial therapies.

Robert E. Nickel, MD, Associate Professor, Department of Pediatrics, Oregon Health Sciences University, Portland, Oregon, Clinical Director, Regional Service Center, Child Development and Rehabilitation Center, Eugene, Oregon.

I am an optimist and a realist. I know there are no miracle cures for autism. Yet, I am not afraid to dream of the day when there might be. I still hold on to that dream, even if it is with the nail on my little finger.

—Parent of a child with autism[1(pvii)]

Parents may react to the diagnosis of a developmental disability in their child with anger, shock, confusion, guilt, or extreme sadness. The search for a magical cure often is one stage in their adjustment to that diagnosis.[2] They may try one or more controversial therapies as part of their search for a magical solution. Proponents of such therapies often offer a cure or dramatic improvement, especially if therapy is started early. In addition, popular media may encourage parents to try such therapies by uncritical and, at times, sensationalistic coverage, such as a recent episode of the TV program, Day One: "Down Syndrome: A Breakthrough Treatment." The reporter concluded, "And there is another bit of good news: The formula (vitamins, minerals, amino acids, and piracetam) is also being used with older children and teenagers with Down syndrome and it appears to be working for them as well."[3(p6)]

In a recent survey of parents with children who were receiving services from the Regional Program for Autism, Oregon Department of Education, 50% (228 of 455) indicated that they had tried at least one nonstandard therapy.[4] Thirty-two percent of those surveyed had tried two or more nonstandard therapies. A variety of terms has been used to refer to controversial therapies, including nonstandard, alternative, irrational, unproven, and nontraditional. Many previous articles offer comprehensive reviews of specific alternative treatments

for various developmental disabilities.[5-10] In this article, the characteristics of controversial therapies and the reasons parents may choose to try such therapies will be discussed, a few specific nonstandard therapies will be reviewed in detail, and finally, recommendations will be provided for professionals on how to support parents in making decisions about these therapies.

What Is a Controversial Treatment?

In general, a standard treatment is widely accepted by the professionals serving children with developmental disabilities and their families. It has a sound scientific basis and is supported by research studies. However, a number of standard therapies in current practice have not undergone rigorous scientific review, and some alternative therapies have been used extensively. Thus, the definition of alternative or controversial therapy cannot be primarily based on whether it is supported by research or how many professionals recommend its use. In this article, the following list of characteristics of these therapies and the claims of their proponents will be used as an operational definition[8]:

- Treatments that are based on overly simplified scientific theories—for example, the importance of crawling as a stage of motor development in Doman-Delacato treatment programs.
- Therapies purported to be effective for a variety of conditions (Table 1)—for example, patterning therapy (Doman-Delacato treatment principles) has been used to treat children with developmental delay/mental retardation, Down syndrome, cerebral palsy, autism, and learning disabilities.

- Treatment claims that most children will respond dramatically and that some may be cured, particularly if treatment is started early—for example, this statement from the Trisomy-21 Research, Inc. regarding treatment with piracetam and vitamin and mineral supplements: "It is now possible to treat Down syndrome to the degree that the child should not be severely mentally or physically disabled...those who have benefit of therapy usually escape the range of mental retardation altogether and are only somewhat learning disabled."[11(p1)]
- Treatments supported by a series of case reports or anecdotal data and not by carefully designed research studies. If careful research studies have failed to support their claims, proponents of these therapies often respond emotionally and defensively.
- Treatments initiated with little or no attention to identifying specific treatment objectives or target behaviors. A positive response that is noted from 1 day to several months after the initiation of treatment may be claimed as proof that the therapy is working.
- Therapies that are said to have no or unremarkable side effects; thus, there is no reason to do controlled studies.[12] However, a review of side effects also should include the cost to the family in time and money, and the possible delay in instituting effective treatments. Some controversial treatments do have the potential for serious side effects, such as cell therapy and growth hormone therapy for children with Down syndrome. Cell therapy uses the cells from different organs (including the brain) of fetal sheep.[13] There is a risk of transmission of slow virus infection with resultant progressive brain infection

Article Reprint Information: Reprinted with permission from Nickel, R. E. (1996). Controversial therapies for young children with developmental disabilities. *Infants and Young Children, 8*(4), 29–40.

and further loss of function. The use of growth hormone for children with Down syndrome may increase the risk of developing leukemia.[14]

In addition, proponents of controversial therapies often use scientific or traditional medical names for their treatment centers. For example, the Hope Center (patterning treatment) in Newburg, Oregon has recently changed its name to the Northwest Neurodevelopmental Training Center. Health and educational professionals must keep in mind that practitioners of alternative therapies strongly believe in their treatment programs, provide parents a great deal of anecdotal information about the treatment's positive effects, and in general establish supportive relationships with children and families.

Why Do Parents Try Controversial Treatments?

A variety of factors determines a family's choice to pursue alternative treatments. As stated above, the search for a magical cure may be one stage in a parent's adjustment to the diagnosis of a developmental disability in his or her child.[2] Certain characteristics in the child make the search for a magical solution more likely (for example, a child with severe disabilities, or with marked problem behaviors without a specific etiologic diagnosis). In addition, the treatment of developmental disabilities is primarily behavioral and educational, not medical. Rarely is there a specific medical treatment for the cause of the disability. If available, such treatments are largely preventive in nature and of limited benefit if started after the diagnosis of the developmental disability (eg, thyroid supplementation for congenital hypothyroidism and dietary treatment of phenylketonuria).

The care needs of children with disabilities and their families are often complex. Standard or traditional treatments can be time consuming, costly, and difficult to access. Parents may become confused and overwhelmed by multiple, and at times, conflicting treatment recommendations. They may feel out of control and excluded from important treatment decisions. The support, information, and hope of improvement offered by proponents of controversial therapies may be particularly attractive to these families. Parents readily can obtain referral information about practitioners of a variety of controversial therapies through many local parent support groups for families of children with disabilities.

Furthermore, a current focus of a large segment of American society is on personal

---

Table 1
Claims for controversial therapies—what are they good for?

Therapy	Condition
Megavitamins and minerals	ADHD/LD,* autism, DD/MR†
Vitamin B_6 and magnesium	ADHD/LD, autism, DD/MR
Facilitated communication	Autism, DD/MR, CP‡
Sensory integration therapy	ADHD/LD, autism, DD/MR, dyspraxia
Antifungal treatment (diet and medication)	ADHD/LD, autism
Patterning (Doman-Delacato)	ADHD/LD, autism, DD/MR, CP

*Attention-deficit/hyperactivity disorder/learning disability.
†Developmental delay/mental retardation.
‡Cerebral palsy.

Table 2
Controversial therapies for children with autism and pervasive developmental disorders

Medications, vitamins, and diet	Behavioral therapies
Feingold diet	Facilitated communication[18-23]
Hypoallergenic diet for cerebral allergies	Auditory integration training
Megavitamins and minerals	Craniosacral therapy[24,25]
Vitamin B_6 and magnesium	Patterning (Doman-Delacato)[26-28]
Dimethylglycine (DMG)[12]	Music therapy
Antifungal therapy (diet and medication)[17]	Hold therapy (squeeze machine)
Intravenous immunoglobulin treatment	Rhythmic entrainment
	Brushing/massage

Table 3
Controversial therapies for children with developmental delay or Down syndrome

Medications, vitamins, and diet	Behavioral therapies	Surgeries
Megavitamins and minerals	Facilitated communication	
Useries (Turkel)	Craniosacral therapy	Facial surgery (for Down syndrome)[30,31]
Thyroid supplementation	Patterning (Doman-Delacato)	
Cell therapy[13]		
Dimethylglycine (DMG)		
Piracetam (nootropics)		
Growth hormone[14]		

---

fitness, preventive health care, the effects of nutrition and diet on health, and the use of alternative treatments. Pauling helped foster this interest by his theory regarding the use of megavitamin therapy or orthomolecular medicine for "the treatment of mental disorders by the provision of the optimal molecular environment for the mind."[15(p265)] In 1990, one of every three Americans was using unconventional therapies for the treatment of illness, with a total expenditure of nearly $14 billion.[16] In that year, Americans made more visits to practitioners of alternative therapies than to all types of primary care physicians.[16]

Controversial Therapies for Autism, Developmental Delay, and Down Syndrome

Controversial therapies can be categorized as: (1) medicines, vitamin and mineral supplements, and dietary treatments; (2) behavioral therapies; and (3) surgeries. Tables 2 and 3 list examples of controversial or nonstandard therapies for autism, developmental delay, and Down syndrome. These lists include the most commonly practiced treatments. Many of these therapies are being used in infants and young children. In addition, any new or standard therapy can become a controversial treatment based on how it is used or on claims made by proponents. Growth hormone treatment of children with Down syndrome is an example of a standard therapy being used for indications unrelated to its proven effectiveness. Piracetam is a treatment that is supported by encouraging animal research data but has had equivocal or disappointing results in clinical trials. Nevertheless, proponents often claim the possibility of a cure or dramatic improvement based on single case studies.

In this article, only a few of the controversial therapies listed in Tables 2 and 3 will be reviewed in detail. However, references are provided for many of the therapies listed. First, the uses of vitamin B_6 and magnesium, and auditory integration training to treat young children with autism will be discussed. Next, the use of megavitamins and piracetam for young children with Down syndrome will be examined. Finally, two new treatments, intravenous immunoglobulin and melatonin, will be discussed.

Vitamin B₆ and Magnesium

In a recent survey, vitamin B_6 (pyridoxine) with magnesium was the most frequently used controversial therapy (23%) by parents of children with autism.[4] Practical information on the use of vitamin B_6 and magnesium (dose, cost, where to order) is available at parent support groups in Oregon and through the Autism Research Institute, San Diego, California. Pyridoxine is an essential co-factor in amino acid metabolism and in normal brain metabolism, including the formation of serotonin, a neurotransmitter.[32] Deficiency of pyridoxine or magnesium can lead to significant health problems, including seizures. Thus, documented B_6 or magnesium deficiency is an established indication for administering vitamin B_6 or magnesium. However, pyridoxine also has been used to treat individuals who do not have documented deficiency states, but have a number of neurologic disorders, including seizure disorders, headaches, peripheral neuropathies, movement disorders, and depression. Clinical results have been variable.[32,33] Of note, chronic use of pyridoxine in high doses (2 to 6 g per day) can cause peripheral neuropathy.[32,34] This side effect has not been reported in children; however, no studies are available on children who start high doses of pyridoxine treatment at preschool age. Cohen and Bendich suggest that the relationship between daily dose and duration of use (the total dose) is the critical issue.[34] Thus, children treated with modest doses over long periods may be at risk for side effects.

A review of available research studies does not demonstrate a consistent, positive effect from supplemental vitamin B_6 and magnesium therapy for children with autism. Rimland has reviewed 16 studies of the use of vitamin B_6 and magnesium in autism.[35] Six studies were noted to be double-blind with placebo controls; however, several were open-label studies or a series of single-case reports. He concluded that published studies prove beyond a doubt that a substantial portion of autistic children and adults show benefits from a large daily dose of vitamin B_6 or magnesium given alone.[35] However, Kleijnen and Knipschild[36] reviewed 55 controlled trials of vitamin B_6 with or without magnesium given to children with autism. They con-

cluded that virtually all trials showed serious methodologic shortcomings: "Only in autistic children are some positive results found with very high doses of vitamin B_6 combined with magnesium; but further evidence is needed before more definitive conclusions can be drawn."[36(p931)] Three of the five studies did report positive results. All of these studies were small (fewer than 50 subjects per treatment group). None of the studies demonstrated adequate matching of the treatment group and controls, and none of the studies provided an adequate description of baseline data. Finally, a recent study by Tolbert and coworkers demonstrated no effect of low dose vitamin B_6 and magnesium administered to a group of children with autism.[37]

Auditory integration training

Auditory integration training (AIT) is based on the work of the French physician Guy Berard. In 1982, he reported the results of his treatment program with over 8,000 individuals who had unusual auditory sensitivity, including 48 individuals with autism.[38] He theorized that extreme auditory sensitivity interfered with cognitive processing and that treatment with broad band sound that had been filtered to eliminate the peaks of auditory sensitivity would result in decreased hearing sensitivity and improvement in cognitive and behavioral functioning. The therapy consisted of listening to 10 hours of electronically modulated music through earphones over a 10-day period. This therapy has been popularized by the book, *The Sound of a Miracle*,[39] a case report of a child with autism who was "cured" by AIT, a related article in the *Reader's Digest*, and the television show 20/20. AIT is now available from over 120 practitioners, and the cost is approximately $1,000 for the 10-day treatment. It has been used to treat preschool-age and older children with autism. It also has been used to treat attention-deficit/hyperactivity disorder, tinnitus, dyslexia, and other learning and behavior problems.[40]

Rimland and Edelson have reported the results of a pilot study of AIT treatment of autism.[41] This study involved nine matched pairs of children; however, one experimental subject subsequently dropped out. Significant positive effects were noted in favor of the experimental group for certain behaviors on parent-completed checklists, but no differences were noted for hearing acuity or sound sensitivity. Unfortunately, subjects were not matched on the severity of autism or behavior problems, and the experimental group did have significantly more auditory

and behavior problems. In fact, the statistical analyses of the data were conducted using group differences rather than matched pair differences. Thus, the positive effects of AIT that were noted may have been due solely to the initial differences between the experimental and control groups.

Rimland and Edelson also have recently reported a follow-up study of AIT of 445 children with autism.[42] This study was accompanied by several commentaries regarding the use of AIT.[40,43-45] It appears to have been an open-label study of consecutively treated children. No control group was identified. Data from the nine control children in the pilot study were used for comparison. Three different AIT devices and five different filtering conditions were used. A significant reduction in sound sensitivity and a reduction of problem behaviors were noted. No differences were demonstrated when AIT was performed with or without filters for the auditory peaks or with the three different AIT devices. Interestingly, lower functioning individuals showed greater improvement. Is AIT effective? This study shed no light on this question because there was no randomly assigned control group; complete audiologic data were not obtained; 55% of subjects did not have full audiometric data, and 34% (164 of the 445) had no audiologic data[42]; and other methodologic flaws existed.

There are a number of problematic issues with AIT. The rationale and time course of the treatment do not correspond with current knowledge or experience with conventional interventions for audiologic and communicative disorders.[43] No published statements are available on who is a good candidate.[44] Hearing testing and the use of filters are now said to be unnecessary for the treatment.[42] This statement appears to invalidate the basic premise for AIT that auditory peaks and distortions lead to cognitive and behavior problems. Practitioners of AIT vary widely in their educational background and experience.[40] The AIT practitioner training program in the United States has no consistent standards for trainees, and a certificate of course completion can be obtained in 4 or 5 days.[40]

Megavitamins and minerals

In 1981, Harrell and coworkers reported dramatic improvement in cognition and behavior in children with mental retardation who received supplementation of 11 vitamins and 8 minerals.[46] Children with Down syndrome also were noted to experience a significant change in physical appearance. Five children with mental retardation (two with Down syndrome) participated in a 4-month, placebo-controlled trial, and 16 children (five with Down syndrome) participated in an additional 4-month, open-label trial. However, the study had a number of methodologic problems. Kleijnen and Knipschild reviewed this study and nine additional studies that have attempted to replicate the results in children with Down syndrome.[36] Six of the subsequent nine studies were rated higher in research design than the study by Harrell et al.[46] None of the nine studies found any significant effect of multivitamin and mineral supplementation on developmental progress or behavior. Pruess et al[47] also have reviewed the published research studies concerning vitamin therapy in children with Down syndrome. Three studies replicated and expanded the Harrell et al research design by eliminating the methodologic problems and focusing on home-reared children with Down syndrome. Again, no significant differences were found on any measure of development or behavior.

Piracetam (nootropics)

Piracetam belongs to a group of chemicals referred to as nootropics or cognitive-enhancing drugs. It was first used to treat motion sickness in 1966, and its apparent effect on memory was first noticed in 1968.[48] A variety of animal experiments has documented apparent memory-enhancing properties, including protective effects on memory deficits induced by scopolamine, hypoxia, electric shock, and prenatal alcohol exposure.[48] In clinical trials, piracetam has been studied in adults with dementia, Parkinson's disease, and traumatic brain injury, as well as in children with learning disabilities.[49-59] No consistent positive effects have been demonstrated in clinical trials in contrast to the encouraging results from animal studies. In fact, one investigator has speculated that the animal models currently in use to screen potential antidementia drugs may not be valid predictors of therapeutic efficacy.[55] Few side effects have been reported with the use of piracetam; however, no long-term studies of the use of piracetam in young children are available. Its mechanism of action is unknown.

Piracetam has not been studied in children with developmental delay or Down syndrome. As stated in the introduction, its use for infants and children with Down syndrome was recently popularized by the television program, Day One. Following this program, the National Down Syndrome Society (NDSS) was flooded with calls requesting further information regarding

this treatment. The NDSS does not recommend the use of piracetam because of the absence of research data that would support its effectiveness.[60] Piracetam should be evaluated by the same process as any new medical treatment. Single-case studies that demonstrate dramatic improvement are perhaps useful for indicating potential new treatment directions; however they are inherently biased and subjective, and do not establish the validity of a therapy.[9] They must be followed by carefully constructed placebo-controlled, blinded, research trials with sufficient numbers of children.

Intravenous immunoglobulin

Two new therapies are intravenous immunoglobulin (IVIG) for the treatment of children with autism, and melatonin for the treatment of sleep disorders in children with autism or other disabilities. A great deal of research has explored possible immunologic causes of autism and other neurologic disorders,[61-66] and IVIG has been used to treat other neurologic disorders that have an autoimmune basis.[67-69] Recent individual case studies of the use of IVIG in children with autism have resulted in claims of a possible cure with this treatment. However, there are no published research data that support this theory or that autism is caused by autoantibodies or immune complexes.

Gupta and coworkers have submitted a study for publication involving 10 children with autism 3 to 8 years of age who were treated with monthly IVIG therapy for 6 months or more.[70] No criteria for patient selection were used other that the diagnosis of autism. Initially, patients who had mothers with high titers of rubella antibody were offered treatment. Gupta et al speculate that the children of mothers with high antibody titers would have preexisting antibody in infancy and would develop immune complexes after immunization (exposure to antigen), which could cause brain dysfunction and, thus, antibody titers in mothers did not predict which children would respond to IVIG in their series.[70]

At least five other children have been treated at four other centers.[70] The cost of the treatment program is approximately $5,000. One infusion of IVIG takes 1½ to 2 hours. Many physicians who use IVIG will require that the first infusion be done in the hospital because of the associated low risk of serious allergic reactions (anaphylaxis) and other minor side effects during the infusion. Use of this treatment should be restricted to carefully selected children as part of a rigorous research trial. Gupta does plan to do a research trial with 3 to 5 year

old children; however, he comments that identifying an appropriate control group will be difficult because parents likely will choose not to participate in a placebo-controlled study.[70]

Melatonin

Melatonin is a naturally occurring peptide secreted by the pineal glad, which helps to determine sleep/wake cycles.[71] Recent studies have demonstrated its effectiveness in adults with delayed sleep onset and visually impaired, multihandicapped children with sleep disorders.[71-74] Its use to treat sleep disorders is supported by sound scientific rationale and careful animal studies, as well as the few clinical trials with adults and young children. Other benefits have been suggested, including treatment of jet lag and insomnia, cancer prevention, and even prolonging life.[75] Melatonin is sold as a food supplement at health food stores. A 1 month supply costs approximately $10. No or minimal side effects have been reported. However, no information is available on the interaction of melatonin with other medications (eg, methylphenidate hydrochloride or fluoxetine hydrochloride). In addition, because it is sold as a food supplement, the purity of the preparation is unknown. Serious medical illness has resulted from impurity in L-tryptophan supplements were identified as the cause of a serious medical illness, eosinophilic myalgia syndrome.[76,77]

Continued use of melatonin in well-designed research trials is appropriate; however, melatonin may become a popular alternative treatment because of its availability, low cost, and the claims of a possible cure. In their study, Jan and coworkers noted that 13 of 15 children responded partially to treatment with melatonin.[74] However, an article on melatonin in *Newsweek* highlighted Jan's comments about one child: "We [physicians] had tried everything … but nothing worked …" (after one dose of the hormone) "the parents called me and said, 'It's a miracle! A miracle!' The child slept through the night."[75(p46)]

How to Talk to Families About Controversial Treatments

This is a subject that must be dealt with openly, honestly, and compassionately. Recommendations on how professionals can support families in decision making about controversial therapies are presented in the Box. The first step is ensuring that families collaborate with service providers and contribute to all treatment decisions. Families must be provided with sufficient informa-

Parents are likely to access some information about controversial treatments before professionals through parent support groups, national advocacy groups, newsletters, practitioners of alternative therapies, and the Internet. Health and education professionals can obtain information from these sources as well as professional journals and organizations. In addition, families can be referred to a developmental pediatrician or similar specialist for further information about controversial treatments.

Schedule ample time to discuss controversial treatments and make sure that it is clear that the discussion is not an endorsement of the treatment. Parents need all available information to enable them to make their best decision. Carefully describe the placebo effect and the importance of a controlled, blinded, research trial to establish a treatment's effectiveness. A tongue-in-cheek editorial by Strayhorn provides information regarding rival explanations for treatment effects to use in discussion with some families.[78] A review article on facial surgery for children with Down syndrome provides another useful example of the importance of controlled research trials.[30] In this review, the studies that had qualitative design with no control group reported positive results in facial appearance and physical (speech or motor) function after surgery. However, the studies that utilized qualitative and quantitative outcome measures with a control group demonstrated no significant differences on any outcome measure. If parents chose to pursue an alternative treatment, recommend that they consider an ABAB single subject design. For example, provide the treatment for 1 month, then stop for 1 month, put the patient back on the treatment for 1 month, and then, finally discontinue the treatment.

Also provide parents with information about the decision-making process. The author uses the handout, "Parents: Questions To Ask Yourself Regarding Specific Treatments," (see Box).[79] It was developed as part of a master's thesis on parents of children with autism by Valda Fields, the mother of a boy with autism. It is a useful outline to guide discussion with families who have children with any disability. In addition, identify any confounding factor, such as finances or the opinions of relatives, friends or clergy regarding a particular therapy. Be willing to support a trial of therapy in selected situations (eg, sensory integration treatment for young children with dyspraxia). However, require defined treatment goals and objectives and a specific treatment plan with pre- and posttesting

tion about the diagnosis and its treatment and community resources, and they must have access to appropriate services. Medical professionals also should perform all appropriate tests in an attempt to determine the etiology of the child's developmental problems. A specific etiologic diagnosis will help clarify the natural history, associated problems and appropriate treatments. Health and early intervention/early child special education staff must establish and maintain effective communication with each other and other service providers, particularly if there is disagreement over a specific treatment or intensity of a treatment.

When should professionals discuss controversial therapies with families? Controversial treatments should be discussed as part of the initial management plan and whenever parents ask questions about such therapies. If parents do not receive information directly from health and educational staff, they will obtain that information from the proponents of those therapies and/or other parents. The information they receive likely will be limited and biased. In addition, any subsequent information that health or education professionals provide may be discredited in the parents' eyes by the initial failure to have discussed the treatment.

to document any response to the therapy.

Finally, medical and education professionals should remain actively involved and available to parents to discuss the effects of any treatment that parents may choose. Support is essential to assist them in monitoring the effects of the therapy.

...Regarding treatment for autism, what works wonders for one individual may have absolutely no effect on another.... What makes a successful treatment? To me, a successful treatment improves the quality of my son's life or my family's life, often in small but significant ways.
—Parent of a child with autism[1](ppvii-viii)

An open discussion of controversial therapies should lead to reexamination of what is meant by success or failure in treatment.[44] This quote emphasizes the importance of incorporating family values and meaningful treatment objectives into clinical trials and treatment programs. The interest of parents of children with disabilities in controversial treatments will not diminish because of the nature of developmental disabilities and the nature of hope. The role of medical and education professionals is to support parents by providing a realistic framework for hope. "It is our responsibility to present facts and carefully considered opinions and let families make their own choices,"[44(p32)] and to continue to support families when they persist in holding onto a "dream, even if it is with the nail on my little finger."[1(pvii)]

References

1. Gerlach EK. *Autism Treatment Guide*. Eugene, Ore: Four Leaf Press; 1993.
2. Freeman BJ. The syndrome of autism: update and guidelines for diagnosis. *Inf Young Children*. 1993;6(2):1-11.
3. Sawyer F. *Down Syndrome: a breakthrough treatment* (transcript). Day One. 1995:4-6.
4. Nickel R, Stratton J. Unpublished data. 1995.
5. Starrett A. Nonstandard therapies. In: Capute AJ, Accardo PJ, eds. *Developmental Disability in Infancy and Childhood*. Baltimore, Md: Brookes Publishing Company; 1991.
6. Landman GB. Alternative therapies. In: Levin JD, Carey WB, Crocker AC, eds. *Developmental-Behavioral Pediatrics*. Philadelphia, Pa: W.B. Saunders; 1992.
7. Golden GS. Controversies in therapies for children with Down syndrome. *Pediatr Rev*. 1984;6(4):116-120.
8. Golden GS. Nonstandard therapies in developmental disabilities. *Am J Dis Child*. 1980;134:487-491.
9. Sieben RL. Controversial medical treatments of learning disabilities. *Acad Ther*. 1977;13(2):133-147.
10. Silver LB. Acceptable and controversial approaches to treating the child with learning disabilities. *Pediatrics*. 1975;55(3):406-415.
11. Lawrence D. Letter; information on piracetam. Trisomy 21 Research, Inc. August 1, 1994
12. Rimland B. Dimethylglycine (DMG), a nontoxic metabolite, and autism. *Autism Res Rev Int*. 1990;4(2):3.
13. Van Dyke DC, et al. Cell Therapy in children with Down syndrome: a retrospective study. *Pediatrics*. 1990;85(1):79-84.
14. Lawson Wilkins Pediatric Endocrine Society Commentary. Growth hormone for children with Down syndrome. *J Pediatr*. 1993;123(5):742-743.
15. Pauling I. Orthomolecular-psychiatry. *Science*. 1968;160:265.
16. Eisenberg DM, Kessler RC, Foster C, Norlock FE, Calkins DR, Delbanco TL. Unconventional medicine in the United States. *N Engl J Med*. 1993;328(4):246-283.
17. Rimland B. San Diego, Calif: Institute for Child Behavior Research; 1994. Pub. No. 65.
18. Biklen D. Communication unbound: autism and praxis. *Harvard Educ Rev*. 1990;60:291-314
19. Crossley R, McDonald A. *Annie's Coming Out*. New York, NY: Penguin; 1980.
20. Cummins R. Questions about facilitated communication and autism. *J Autism Dev Disord*. 1992;23:331-338.
21. Regal R. Rooney J, Wandas T. Facilitated communication: an experimental evaluation. J Autism Dev Discord. 1994;24:345-355.
22. Simon E, Toll D, Whitehair P. A Naturalistic approach to the validation of facilitated communications. *J Autism Dev Disord*. 1995;24:647-657.
23. Wheeler D, Jacobson J, Paglieri, Schwartz A. An experimental assessment of facilitated communication. *Ment Retard*. 1993;31:49-60.
24. Greenman P, McPartland J. Cranial findings and iatrogenesis from craniosacral manipulation in patients with traumatic brain syndrome. *J Am Osteopath Assoc*. 1995;95:182-191.
25. Upledger J, Vredevoogd J. *Craniosacral Therapy*. Seattle, Wash: Eastland Press; 1983.
26. Sparrow S, Ziegler E. Evaluation of patterning treatment for retarded children. *Pediatrics*. 1978;62(2):137-150.
27. American Academy of Pediatrics Policy Statement. The Doman-Delacrato treatment of neurologically handicapped children. *Pediatrics*. 1982;70(5):810-812.
28. Official Statement. The Doman-Delacato treatment of neurologically handicapped children. *Arch Phys Med Rehabil*. April 1968:183-186.
29. Van Dyke DC, et al. Cell therapy in children with Down syndrome: a retrospective study. *Pediatrics*. 1990;85(1):79-84.
30. Katz S, Kraveta S. Facial plastic surgery for persons with Down syndrome: research findings and their professional and social implications. *Am J Ment Retard*. 1989;94(2):101-110.
31. May DC, Turnbull N. Plastic surgeons' opinions of facial surgery for individuals with Down syndrome. *Ment Retard*. 1992;30(1):29-33.
32. Berstein AL. Vitamin B6 in clinical neurology. *Ann NY Acad Sci*. 1990;585:250-260.
33. Kasdan ML, Janes C. Carpal tunnel syndrome and vitamin B6. *Plast Reconstr Surg*. 1987;79:456-466.
34. Cohen M, Bendich A. Safety of pyridoxine-A review of human and animal studies. *Toxicol Let*. 1986;34:129-146.
35. Rimland B. the use of megavitamin B and magnesium in the treatment of autistic children and adults. *Neurobiol Issues Autism*. 1987;81:389-405.
36. Kleijnen J, Knipschild P. Niacin and Vitamin B in mental functioning: a review of controlled trials in humans. *Biol Psychiatry*. 1991;29:931-941.
37. Tolbert L, Haigler T, Waits MM, ennis T. Brief report; lack of response in an autistic population to a low dose clinical trial of pyridoxine plus magnesium. *J Autism Dev Disord*. 1993;23(1):193-199.
38. Berard G. *Hearing Equals Behavior*. New Canaan, Conn: Keats Publishing Co; 1993.
39. Stehi A. *The Sound of a Miracle*. New York, NY: Doubleday; 1991.
40. Veale TK. Auditory integration therapy: the use of a new listening treatment within our profession. *Am J Speech Lang Path*. 1994;3(2):12-15.
41. Rimland G, Edelson S. *Auditory Integration Training in Autism: A Pilot Study*. San Diego, Calif: Autism Research Institute; 1992.
42. Rimland R, Edelson SM. The effects of auditory integration training on autism. *Am J Speech Lang Path*. 1994;3(2):16-24.
43. Gravel JS. Auditory integration training; placing the burden of proof. *Am J Speech Lang Path*. 1994;3(2):25-29.
44. Friel-Patti S. Commitment to theory. *Am J Speech Lang Path*. 1991;3(2):30-34.
45. Veale TK. Weighing the promises and the problems: AI maybe a risk worth taking. *Am J Speech Lang Path*. 1994;3(2):35-37.
46. Harrell RF, Capp RH, David DR, Peerless J, Ravitz LR. Can nutritional supplements help mentally retarded children? An exploratory study. *Proc Natl Acad Sci USA*. 1981;78(1):574-578.
47. Pruess JB, Fewell RR, Bennett FC. Vitamin therapy and children with Down Syndrome: a review of research. *Except Child*. 1989;55(4):336-341.
48. Gouliaev AH, Senning A. Piracetam and other structurally related nootropics. *Brain Res Rev*. 1194;19:18-222.
49. Gottfries CG. Pharmacological treatment strategies in Alzheimer type dementia. *Eur Neuropsychopharmacol*. 1990;1(1):1-5.
50. Herrmann WM, Stephan K. Efficacy and clinical relevance of cognitive enhancers. *Alzheimer Dis Assoc Disord*. 1991;5(1):S7-S12.
51. Hermann WM, Stephan K. Moving from the question of efficacy to the question of therapeutic relevance: an exploratory reanalysis of a controlled clinical study of 130 in patients with dementia syndrome taking piracetam. *Int Psychogeriatrics*. 1992;4(1):25-44.
52. Israel L, Melac M, Milinkevitch D, Dubos G. Drug therapy and memory training programs: a double blind randomized trial of general practice patients with age-associated memory impairment. *Int Psychogeriatrics*. 1994;6(2):155-170.
53. Sano M, Stem Y, Marder K, Mayeux R.A. controlled trial of piracetam in intellectually impaired patients with Parkinson's disease. *Mov Disord*. 1990;5(3):230-234.
54. Vernon MW, Sorkin EM. Piracetam. An overview of its pharmacological properties and a review of its therapeutic use in senile cognitive disorders. *Drugs Aging*. 1991;1(1):17-35.
55. Claus JJ, Ludwig C, Mohr E, Giuffra M, Blin J, Chase TN. Nootropic drugs in Alzheimer's disease: symptomatic treatment with pramiracetam. *Neurology*. 1991;41:570-574.
56. Deberdt W. Interaction between psychological and pharmacological treatment in cognitive impairment. *Life Sci*. 1994;55(25-26):2057-2066.
57. Ackerman PT, Dykman RA, Holloway C, Paal NP, Gocio My. A trial of piracetam in two

subgroups of students with dyslexia enrolled in summer tutoring. *J Learning Disabilities.* 1991;24(9):542-549.

58. Wisher CR. A brief review of studies of piracetam in dyslexia. *J Psychopharmacol.* 1987;1:95-100.

59. Nicholson CD. Pharmacology of nootropics and metabolically active compounds in relation to their use in dementia. *Psychopharmacol.* 1990;101(2):147-159.

60. *Drug Alert on Piracetam.* New York, NY: National Down Syndrome Society. 1995.

61. Singh VK, Warren RP, Odell JD, Cole P. Changes of soluble interleukin-2, interleuking-2 receptor, T8 antigen, and interleukin-1 in the serum of autistic children. *Clin Immunol Immunopathol.* 1991;61:448-455.

62. Stubbs EF, Rito ER, Mason-Brother A. Autism and shared paternal HLA antigens. *J Am Acad child Adolesc Psychiatry.* 1985;24:182-185.

63. Stubbs EG, Crawford ML, Burger DR, Vanderbark AA. Depressed lymphocyte responsiveness in autistic children. *J Autism Child Schizophrenia.* 1977;7:49-55.

64. Warren RP, Yonk LJ, Burger RA, et al. Deficiency of suppressor-inducer (CD4+CD45RA+) T cell in in autism. *Immunol Invest.* 1990;19:245-251.

65. Warren RP, Cole P, Odell D, et al. Detection of maternal antibodies in infantile autism. *J Am Acad Child Adolesc Psychiatry.* 1990;29(6):873-877.

66. Weizman A. Weizman R, Szekely GA, Wijsenbeek H, Livni E. Abnormal immune response to brain tissue antigen in the syndrome of autism. *Am J Psychiatry.* 1982;7:1462-1465.

67. Leger JM, Younes-Chennoufi AB, Chassande B, et al. Human immunoglobulin treatment of multi-focal motor neuropathy and polyneuropathy associated with monoclonal gammopahy. *J Neurol Neurosurg Psychiatry.* 1994;57(suppl):46:49.

68. Van Dorn PA. Intravenous immunoglobulin treatment in patients with chronic inflammatory demyelinating polyneuropathy. *J Neurol Neurosurg Psychiatry.* 1994;57(suppl):38-42.

69. Allen AJ, Leonard HL, Swedo SE. Case study: a new infection-triggered, autoimmune subtype of pediatric OCD and Tourette's syndrome. *J Am Acad Child Adolesc Psychiatry.* 1995;34(3):307-311.

70. Gupta S. Personal Communication. August 1995.

71. Brown GM. Light, melatonin and the sleep-wake cycle. *J Psychiatry Neurosci.* 1994;19(5):345-353.

72. Alvarez B, Dahlitz MJ, Vignau J, Parkes JD. The delayed sleep phase syndrome: clinical and investigative findings in 14 subjects (see comments). *J Neurol Nueurosurg Psychiatry.* 1995;58(3):379.

73. Oldani A, Fewrini-Strambi L, Zucconi M, Stankov B, Fraschini F, Smime S. Melatonin and delayed sleep phase syndrome: ambulatory polygraphic evaluation. *Neuroreport.* 1994;6(1);132-134.

74. Jan JE, Espezel H, Appleton RE. The treatment of sleep disorders with melatonin. *Dev Med Child Neurol.* 1994;36:97-107.

75. Cowley G. Melatonin. *Newsweek.* 1995;125(32):46-49.

76. Mayeno AN, Gleich GJ. Eosinophilia-myalgia syndrome and tryptophan production: a cautionary tale. *Trends Biotechnol.* 1994;12(9):346-352.

77. Tazelaar HD, Myers JL, Drage CW, King TEJr, Aguayo S, Colby TV. Pulmonary disease associated with L-tryptophan-inuced eosinophilic myalgia syndrome. Clinical and pathologic features. *Chest.* 1990;97(5):1032-1036.

78. Strayhorn JM. The vitamin and mineral mystery. *J Am Acad Child Adolesc Psychiatry.* 1994;33(9):1346-1347.

79. Field V. *Autism. Advocacy in Lane County, Oregon: A Handbook for Parents and Professionals.* Eugene, Ore: University of Oregon; 1993. Thesis.

Index

WAIT

...There's More!

SLACK Incorporated's Health Care Books and Journals offers a wide selection of products in the field of Occupational Therapy. We are dedicated to providing important works that educate, inform and improve the knowledge of our customers. Don't miss out on our other informative titles that will enhance your collection.

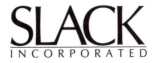